Handbook of
Behavioral Neurobiology

Volume 2
Neuropsychology

HANDBOOK OF BEHAVIORAL NEUROBIOLOGY

General Editor:
Frederick A. King
Yerkes Regional Primate Research Center, Emory University, Atlanta, Georgia

Editorial Board:
Vincent G. Dethier
Robert W. Goy
David A. Hamburg
Peter Marler
James L. McGaugh
William D. Neff
Eliot Stellar

Volume 1   Sensory Integration
Edited by R. Bruce Masterton

Volume 2   Neuropsychology
Edited by Michael S. Gazzaniga

A Continuation Order Plan is available for this series. A continuation order will bring delivery of each new volume immediately upon publication. Volumes are billed only upon actual shipment. For further information please contact the publisher.

Handbook of
Behavioral Neurobiology

Volume 2
Neuropsychology

Edited by

Michael S. Gazzaniga

Division of Cognitive Neuroscience
Cornell University Medical College
New York, New York

PLENUM PRESS · NEW YORK AND LONDON

Library of Congress Cataloging in Publication Data

Main entry under title:

Neuropsychology.

(Handbook of behavioral neurobiology; v. 2)
Includes bibliographies and index.
1. Brain — Diseases — Diagnosis. 2. Neuropsychology. I. Gazzaniga, Michael. S II. Series.
[DNLM: 1. Psychophysiology. 2. Language. 3. Language disorders.
RC386.5.N473   616.8   78-21459
ISBN 0-306-35192-7

© 1979 Plenum Press, New York
A Division of Plenum Publishing Corporation
227 West 17th Street, New York, N.Y. 10011

Printed in the United States of America

To
Charlotte

Contributors

DAVID M. BEAR, *Research Fellow, Massachusetts General Hospital, Boston, Massachusetts*

JASON W. BROWN, *Department of Neurology, New York University Medical Center, Goldwater Memorial Hospital, Roosevelt Island, New York*

ELISABETH O. CLARK, *Department of Psychology, New York University, New York, New York*

MICHAEL S. GAZZANIGA, *Department of Neurology, Cornell University Medical College, New York, New York*

MURRAY GLANZER, *Department of Psychology, New York University, New York, New York*

HAROLD GOODGLASS, *Boston Veterans Administration Medical Center and Department of Neurology, Boston University, Boston, Massachusetts*

HENRY HÉCAEN, *Unité de Récherches Neuropsychologiques et Neurolinguistiques, Ecole des Hautes Etudes en Sciences Sociales, Paris, France*

KENNETH M. HEILMAN, *Department of Neurology, College of Medicine, University of Florida, and Veterans Administration Hospital, Gainesville, Florida*

STEVEN A. HILLYARD, *Department of Neurosciences, University of California, San Diego, La Jolla, California*

MARC JOUANDET, *Department of Neurology, Cornell University Medical College, New York, New York*

EDITH KAPLAN, *Boston Veterans Administration Medical Center and Department of Neurology, Boston University, Boston, Massachusetts*

SHARON V. KREDER, *Department of Psychology, State University of New York, Stony Brook, New York*

JOSEPH E. LEDOUX, *Department of Neurology, Cornell University Medical College, New York, New York*

OSCAR S. M. MARIN, *Department of Neurology, Baltimore City Hospitals, and The Johns Hopkins University School of Medicine, Baltimore, Maryland*

MORRIS MOSCOVITCH, *Erindale College, University of Toronto, Mississauga, Ontario, Canada*

FREDA NEWCOMBE, *Neuropsychology Unit, Department of Clinical Neurology, The Churchill Hospital, Oxford, England*

FERNANDO NOTTEBOHM, *The Rockefeller University, New York, New York*

GRAHAM RATCLIFF, *Neuropsychology Unit, Department of Clinical Neurology, The Churchill Hospital, Oxford, England*

ELEANOR M. SAFFRAN, *Department of Neurology, Baltimore City Hospitals, and The Johns Hopkins University School of Medicine, Baltimore, Maryland*

MYRNA F. SCHWARTZ, *Department of Neurology, Baltimore City Hospitals, and The Johns Hopkins University School of Medicine, Baltimore, Maryland*

SALLY P. SPRINGER, *Department of Psychology, State University of New York, Stony Brook, New York*

JOHN S. STAMM, *Department of Psychology, State University of New York, Stony Brook, New York*

HARRY VAN DER VLUGT, *Department of Psychology, Tilburg University, Tilburg, The Netherlands*

DONALD H. WILSON, *Department of Neurology, Department of Neurosurgery, Dartmouth Medical School, Hanover, New Hampshire*

DAVID L. WOODS, *Department of Neurosciences, University of California, San Diego, La Jolla, California*

Foreword

As the *Handbook of Behavioral Neurobiology* moves into a second volume, it is appropriate to take into general account the scope and content of this series. In its broadest sense, behavioral neurobiology is the study of the behaviors of animal organisms with reference to their neurological bases. The overall objective of this handbook series is to assemble, in ten volumes, a comprehensive and up-to-date treatment of the major areas that comprise behavioral neurobiology. Within such a framework, it is possible to provide the fundamental concepts, methods, and substantive advancements in these fields in a manner that will be useful to educational programs and that will also serve as a reference source for researchers who desire a well-balanced overview of the component areas of neurobiology.

The intent in each volume has been to bring together a spectrum of approaches and disciplines that focuses upon the topic at hand. The first volume presented and discussed the problems of sensory integration; the present work is concerned with the neurobiology of cognitive processes; and forthcoming volumes will include the topics of motor coordination, learning and memory, biological rhythms, motivation, sexual behavior, social behavior and communication, and the evolution of nervous systems and behavior. Thus the purpose of the editors in planning this series has been to offer a distinct handbook, employing the many varied and prevailing avenues of attack upon current problems in behavior and neurological processes, that should prove of unique value and usefulness to professionals and students alike.

FREDERICK A. KING
General Editor

Yerkes Regional Primate Research Center
Emory University
Atlanta, Georgia

Preface

I find myself writing this preface soon after attending the NATO seminar on the Neurobiology of Vision in Crete. As is typical of all meetings, there was a day off, and several of us visited the fascinating Minoan ruins at Phestos. Along with us was the irresistible Herb Killackey from the University of California, Irvine, dutifully reading through the guidebook about the King's palace. After several moments he sighed, "some of these visual scientists are just like the archaeologists. They make a supposition in one sentence based on recordings from one cell, then they treat it as a general fact for the entire visual system."

Now Herb, who has made brilliant studies of the somatosensory system, guided his finger to a fundamental truth. In a word, the study of brain and behavior is indeed still young, no matter what the level of inquiry might be. All of us are trying our best to impose order, often with a data base as small as the archaeologists or cellular neurophysiologists, on a sea of complex, at times seemingly impenetrable, mystery. The job of figuring out brain and behavioral relationships from a neuropsychological point of view is every bit as difficult. Yet, some fascinating and intriguing advances have been made and many of these are reported in this volume.

My apologies in advance for those ideas and those people who are not included. Everybody, it turns out, cannot possibly be set forth in one volume. Good reading.

New York, N.Y.   MICHAEL S. GAZZANIGA

Contents

PART II CORTICAL LOBES AND FUNCTION

PART III DEVELOPMENTAL NEUROPSYCHOLOGY

CHAPTER 6

Minimal Brain Dysfunction: Psychological and Neurophysiological
Disorders in Hyperkinetic Children 119

John S. Stamm and Sharon V. Kreder

PART IV LANGUAGE MECHANISMS AND THEIR DISORDERS

CHAPTER 7

Speech Perception and the Biology of Language 153
Sally P. Springer

PART VI DISORDERS OF PSYCHOLOGICAL PROCESSES FOLLOWING
BRAIN DAMAGE

CHAPTER 16

Long-Term Psychological Consequences of Cerebral Lesions 495

Freda Newcombe and Graham Ratcliff

PART VII TOWARD UNDERSTANDING THE MECHANISMS OF
CONSCIOUSNESS

CHAPTER 17

Beyond Commissurotomy: Clues to Consciousness 543

Jospeh E. LeDoux, Donald H. Wilson, and Michael S. Gazzaniga

PART I

Neuropsychological Assessment

Assessment of Cognitive Deficit in the Brain-Injured Patient

HAROLD GOODGLASS AND EDITH KAPLAN

INTRODUCTION

The cognitive abilities of the individual after brain injury are a consequence of a complex interaction between the premorbid anatomical organization of cerebral functions and the site or sites of damage to the brain, and are reflected by the strategies which the patient brings to bear on the tasks that we employ to probe these abilities. With respect to the first of these factors, some of the abilities which we conceptualize are readily defined in terms of a specific high-order sensory or motor function (e.g., "the ability to recognize faces"), and their loss corresponds to damage to well-defined structures (in the case cited, to bilateral damage in the visual association cortex). Other functions (e.g., new learning, abstract thinking) are not clearly localized, and their degree of deficit is more a function of lesion size than location, although increasing size of lesions may be more damaging in some zones than others. Moreover, the range of cognitive aftereffects of brain injury includes not only *deficits* in definable capacities but also "positive" symptoms (e.g., perseveration, confabulation, unilateral neglect). To ascribe these symptoms to a deficit in a preexisting capacity requires that we generate ad hoc normal processes whose disruption by brain damage is postulated.

The second of the interacting factors is the nature and site of the lesion—a

HAROLD GOODGLASS AND EDITH KAPLAN   Boston Veterans Administration Medical Center and Department of Neurology, Boston University, Boston, Massachusetts 02130. This work was supported in part by the Medical Research Service of the Veterans Administration and in part by NIH Grants NS 06209 and NS 07615.

consideration which immediately demands some knowledge of the types of destruction associated with various etiologies. For example, it is useful to know that the presenile dementias attack the association areas bilaterally without affecting the primary motor and sensory zones. Thus the examiner will look for behavioral indications as to whether the parietal or the frontal association areas are primarily involved. It is useful to know that a cerebral thrombosis is generally a unilateral event and that the initial effect is to produce extensive edema, with extensive functional impairment, but eventually leaving a lesion defined by the area of tissue dependent on the obstructed blood supply.

It is beyond the scope of this chapter to cover the physiological basis of the various recurring patterns of brain damage. However, we wish to stress the importance of being familiar with the various syndromes and their expected psychological concomitants. By the same token, the examiner should acquaint himself thoroughly with the case history so that he may select his tests appropriately and be alert to interpret his findings in the light of the previously known features of the disorder in question—to note either the presence or the absence of anticipated features. For example, patients who suffer an occlusion in the distribution of the left posterior cerebral artery may, because of the brain structures implicated by this occlusion, show an inability to match colors to their names, a marked recent memory defect, and an inability to read, in the presence of preserved writing. The sophisticated examiner will not fail to include tests of color naming when this syndrome is suspected. Moreover, he will be able to pick out the features critical for a particular syndrome from among other abnormalities which have less differential diagnostic value.

The possibility of failing to observe an expected deficit leads us to consider the general issue of negative psychological findings. Organic damage may be too slight to produce measurable psychological changes, or it may be located in an area which is relatively "silent" with respect to cognitive functions. Deficits which were originally present may abate with time so as to be undetectable. In brief, it is generally not possible to rule out organic brain damage on the basis of normal cognitive function. It is possible, however, to conclude that particular behavioral symptoms are not due to cerebral damage, as in the case of complaints of "forgetting" due to emotional causes.

On the other hand, certain configurations of normal and spared functions make it possible to infer the presence and locus of brain damage with a high degree of probability, even in the absence of confirmatory physical findings. For example, some forms of aphasia may appear as isolated linguistic deficits with no elementary neurological abnormalities.

The Nature of Neuropsychological Deficits

Localizing versus Nonlocalizing Deficits

On the hypothesis that psychological abnormalities are present in a test protocol, the examiner will look for those which are nonspecific indicators of impaired function at the same time that he scans for highly selective deficits or configurations of deficits which permit him to infer the laterality or even the region within a hemisphere which is implicated. It is the general rule that selective deficits occur on a background of some degree of nonspecific psychological dysfunction, although virtually "pure" defects may be encountered from time to time. Since nonspecific disorders may express themselves in all areas of performance (e.g., perceptual, motor, visuospatial, verbal, numerical), it may be difficult to identify selective deficits in the context of generally depressed performance, with impairment of attention, motivation, and effort. The examiner not only adjusts the interpretation of particular deficits to the expectations given the overall level of performance but also identifies qualitative error patterns which are virtually pathognomonic of specific deficit and not explicable by the generalized performance deficit.

THE NONSPECIFIC (NONLOCALIZING) DEFICITS

IMPAIRMENT IN CONCEPTUAL THINKING. One of the most common but not universal deficits following cerebral damage is more or less reduced ability to deal with the relationship between objects and their properties, especially those properties which are not sensorily obvious. First to suffer are abstract superordinate concepts, as in the ability to apply the term "furniture" when asked for the similarity between "table" and "chair." Descriptive attributes such as "They both have legs" or functional attributes such as "They are both for sitting and eating" are indicative of conceptual deficiency when given by adults. With more severe deficits, even this level of response to common properties is lost, and the patient provides contrasting associates for each term, such as "You sit on a chair and you eat at a table," and is persistently unable to grasp the idea of providing common properties.

There are many test techniques based on the requirement to abstract common features, among them the Object Sorting Test (Goldstein and Scheerer, 1953), the Color-Form Sorting Test (Weigl, 1941), numerous "cross-out" tests based on rejecting one of an array of pictures lacking a property common to the others, and the verbalization of similarities between two or more concepts.

A particularly sensitive task is proverb interpretation, where a total situation must be translated into the superordinate class of situations which it typifies metaphorically. In the case of proverbs, failure often takes the form of literal interpretation, e.g., "You should save for a rainy day because you should have money when it rains."

SLOWING AND "STICKINESS" OF IDEATIONAL PROCESSES. The brain-injured patient is commonly slow to orient himself to a new mental set and is impaired in his ability to shift from one set to another. It is difficult for him to produce ideas spontaneously, although he may respond appropriately to externally structured demands. When this deficiency exists in a mild degree, the patient is slow in serial tasks which require rapid reorientation from one step to the next and has difficulty in moving from one attempted solution of a problem to a new approach. The result is either complete failure or inability to perform within time limits on new problem-solving tests, while tasks calling on the evocation of old knowledge or requiring one-step solutions are little affected. At more severe levels of reduced rate of ideation and change of set, we encounter *perseveration*, or the persistence of a response determined by a previous stimulus which is inappropriate to the new stimulus. The patient who displays this degree of deficit in shifting is generally observed clinically to persist in the same activity or inactivity at his bedside until directed to do otherwise by another person. Frontal lobe damage, particularly when it is bilateral, is most notable for producing this form of deficit; however, it tends to be a correlate of size of lesion almost anywhere in the cerebral hemispheres.

REDUCED SCOPE OF ATTENTION. Not only is the brain-injured patient's cognition slowed down across time, but also his capacity to apprehend and manipulate multiple aspects of a stimulus situation at any moment in time is often reduced. This results in a simplified perception or a simplified response. Again, this tendency to behave in terms of a simplification of stimulus or response may manifest itself in any modality of behavior without impinging on the integrity of the elementary perceptual motor skills or memories within that modality. At more severe levels of impaired attention, the patient may have great difficulty focusing his attention on a salient aspect of a given stimulus and screening out irrelevant extraneous stimuli.

STIMULUS BOUNDNESS. Stimulus boundness is a qualitative feature in the failures of brain-injured patients. It can be defined as the propensity to respond to some salient property of the stimulus (e.g., its manipulability) while failing to grasp or remain oriented to the task set by the examiner. In the verbal sphere it is illustrated by providing common associations to the stimulus words when the task requires abstracting their similarity. For example, in response to a request for the similarity between eye and ear, a common failure is "Eye you see and ear you hear." In visuospatial tasks, it may be noted in such drawing tasks as the visual reproduction subtest of the Wechsler Memory Scale. A patient may successfully reproduce a design and then proceed to add components, losing sight of the original task requirement. In Fig. 1 we see on the left the model design and on the right a representation of the outcome of a stimulus-bound performance.

A form of stimulus boundness called "closing in" (Critchley, 1953) is noted particularly in conjunction with right parietal lobe disease. Closing in is manifested when the patient, required either to copy a figure in pencil or to reproduce a

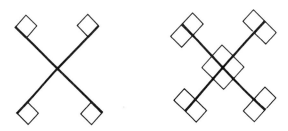

Fig. 1. Stimulus boundness in reproduction (right) of Wechsler Memory Test design. Original figure on left reproduced from the Wechsler Memory Scale by permission. Copyright 1945, renewed 1972 by the Psychological Corporation, New York, N.Y. All rights reserved.

design with blocks, attempts to execute his work directly on the model, by tracing on it or placing his block on it.

IMPAIRMENT OF MEMORY. Efficiency of recall has long been recognized as being particularly vulnerable to the effects of brain damage. Impaired memory is often the earliest presenting symptom of organic mental changes.

Although, quantitatively, memory loss has been treated as simply an absence of recall, the errors made are often of greater interest. Certain forms of distortion are extremely characteristic, if not pathognomonic, of organic damage. These may be classified as automatization, perseveration, and confabulation. Automatization interferes with memory when well-established associative habits conflict with the task set for the patient to recall. For example, the paired associates learning subtest of the Wechsler Memory Scale requires the patient to learn, among others, the associates "school-grocery" and "crush-dark." A typical automatized response of brain-damaged patients is "school-bus" and "crush-ice," which they may give on repeated trials in spite of correction by the examiner.

Defects of attention, perception, or encoding efficiency may underlie the reduced capacity to learn and remember new material, whereas defects in attention and retrieval may contribute to the degradation of long-term memory. Selective disorders of memory that have localizing value will be discussed in the following section.

LATERALIZING AND LOCALIZING SIGNS AND DEFICITS

LANGUAGE DISORDERS. With few exceptions, almost all of these exceptions being in left-handers, injury in the perisylvian zone of the left but not right hemisphere leads to impairment of language in one or more of its channels of input and output. In perhaps 30% of instances, not only do we have a clue as to laterality, but also the configuration among component deficits in the language sphere identifies the patient as having a particular aphasic syndrome, with localizing value within the left hemisphere. Up to this time it has not been possible to unravel which of the component deficits that co-occur repeatedly are psychologically interdependent as opposed to being vulnerable to anatomically contiguous lesions. Hence, in this brief summary, we will first treat the individual deficits and then review their common recurring configurations in relation to the usual lesion localizations.

WORD-FINDING DIFFICULTY (ANOMIA). Virtually all aphasics have reduced access to their vocabulary for oral production, as measured by naming to visual confrontation of object pictures. Detecting a deficit of this type will usually indicate some degree of aphasia, but not its type. Word-finding difficulty refers to the inability to evoke the names for substantives, principal verbs, and other highly information-loaded vocabulary elements in the stream of speech. Inability to produce the terms making up the grammatical matrix of the sentence (pronouns, articles, auxiliaries, common adverbs) does not constitute word-finding difficulty and may coexist with a good picture-naming vocabulary; preservation of the grammatical structure may appear with profound naming difficulty. Isolated word-finding difficulty in a context of fluent articulation and grammar is difficult to localize and may be the first behavioral deficit caused by a brain tumor remote from the language zone. When accompanied by a disturbance of reading and writing, with spared auditory comprehension, anomia is generally associated with a left temporoparietal lesion. When word-finding failures occur in a context of speech which is fluent but garbled in sound sequence, word choice, or sentence meaning, there is usually impaired comprehension as well, denoting the syndrome of Wernicke's aphasia (lesion in posterior-superior temporal lobe).

GRAMMAR AND SYNTAX. When aphasia is due to a lesion of the anterior portion of the anatomical speech zone, the capacity to express grammatical relationships is often lost or markedly reduced. Meaning is expressed through one- or two-word sentences or through the juxtaposition of words or sentence fragments. The small grammatical words or "functors," such as articles, pronouns, prepositions, auxiliaries, and inflectional endings, are dropped, producing the characteristic "telegram" style of speech. While, as observed above, access to the contentive or information-carrying words may be quite difficult, these words—nouns and principal verbs—predominate over grammatical terms in the total verbal output.

Grammar is often defective with aphasias of the posterior speech zones, but the defects are qualitatively very different. Sentences may be left dangling because of word-finding failure, words of the wrong part of speech may appear incongruously, and the semantic thread of the sentence may be lost. However, complex verb inflections and small grammatical words fall into place automatically, subordinating constructions are heard, and complex grammatical constructions may be present even though the total sentence may be semantically anomalous.

ARTICULATION. While articulation might be thought of as primarily a motor coordination skill, the clinical manifestations of aphasia show that articulatory errors are governed by linguistic principles and that their occurrence is often highly determined by the communicative intent of the speech act. Articulation difficulty may be absent in the recitation of memorized material or during repetition, but becomes severely disabling when the patient makes an effort at propositional speech. The pattern of effortful, distorted articulation is generally associated with anterior speech zone lesions, and thus is frequently accompanied by agrammatism. Aphasia with normal facility of articulation (as well as availability of grammatical formulation) generally denotes a lesion of the posterior speech zone.

DISORDERS INVOLVING WRITTEN LANGUAGE. Except for rare instances, aphasia always entails a disturbance of reading and writing which is commonly more severe than the corresponding aspect of oral language. Thus detection of a speech disorder whose aphasic nature is in question should always, as a rule of thumb, lead to a careful screening of written language. It is conjectured that, for the normally hearing individual, reading and writing are acquired as associative elaborations of the preexisting oral language system, which remains physiologically a part of the organic substrate of written language. Thus injury of the oral language substrate necessarily removes some of the basis for written language.

READING DISORDERS (ALEXIA). Severe impairment of reading ability may arise through several different mechanisms, all involving the posterior language zones. In the most severe instances, even letters cannot be matched, although more commonly alexia spares the recognition of letters and common words. Patients with predominantly anterior speech zone lesions usually preserve functional reading at a reduced level of complexity. Pure alexia is a well-documented but infrequent disorder involving occipital lobe structures, and may exist without any other language deficit. It usually involves loss of vision in the right visual field and disconnection at the callosal level of fibers carrying left visual field information to the left hemisphere.

WRITING. As it does speech, aphasia may affect writing at the level of mechanics (inability to recall letter-forming movements), at the level of symbol recall (inability to remember the spelling of words), or at the syntactic level (inability to combine isolated words into sentences). As the patient with any of these deficits attempts to write, his partial performance reflects the level of the disorder and his residual abilities.

Incomplete agraphia often mirrors the pattern of the patient's speech defect. Thus the agrammatic patient may produce a written agrammatic output, consisting of nouns and principal verbs without the small grammatical words or inflections. In contrast, the Wernicke aphasic may produce runs of repetitious, semantically nonsensical writing. Since the latter patients are usually free of paralysis in their writing hand, they often have perfectly preserved penmanship.

Isolated writing disturbances as a result of focal lesions are quite rare. However, severe agraphia without other evidence of aphasia is a usual feature of toxic confusional states (Geschwind and Chedru, 1972).

AUDITORY COMPREHENSION DISORDERS. Auditory comprehension may be selectively and severely impaired by injury which includes the left temporal lobe. In this event, individual words may be perceived and even repeated as familiar acoustic patterns but not recognized at a semantic level. However, comprehension is usually impaired with sizable lesions of the language zone, even outside of the temporal area. In nontemporal lesions, however, comprehension of common words usually approaches normal levels, while failures arise when messages are long or syntactically complex—particularly when meaning depends on grasping a relationship encoded in a single grammatical morpheme.

Careful examination has revealed that auditory comprehension cannot be treated as lying on a single continuum of difficulty. Some patients show highly selective disturbances affecting given classes of words such as numbers (Gardner *et al.*, 1975), body parts (Goodglass and Cohen, 1954), colors (Geschwind and Fusillo, 1966), or particular prepositional relationships (Goodglass *et al.*, 1970). Caramazza and Zurif (1976) have shown that even those patients whose comprehension is traditionally regarded as intact (pure Broca's aphasics) depend on semantic inferences from the key words, abetted by standard word order strategies. Even they fail when the fine points of syntax must be correctly interpreted.

PARAPHASIA. Injury to the mechanisms of articulation, word finding, and syntactic organization results in effortful, inaccurate articulation, omission or circumlocution, or, in the case of syntax, simplification and reduction to telegraphic speech. However, many aphasics are subject to another type of error—the inadvertent production of an off-target response—with facile articulation and often without the patients' awareness of error. "Paraphasia," as these productions are called, may be heard at any of the linguistic levels of speech. At the phonological level, sounds or syllables may be transposed ("ephalent" for "elephant") or ill chosen ("flair" for "chair"). This is termed "literal paraphasia" or "phonemic paraphasia." At the lexical level, words may be substituted, usually from the same semantic sphere (e.g., "my doctor" for "my lawyer"); at the grammatical level, a series of well-formed clauses may be strung together so that the entire sentence is formless and makes no semantic sense.

Paraphasia, particularly uncorrected paraphasia in the course of fluent verbal output, is most characteristic of the Wernicke aphasic, who has focal damage to the posterior portion of the upper temporal lobe. Paraphasia which is predominantly literal is characteristic of "conduction aphasics," produced in most cases by injury to the supramarginal gyrus of the parietal lobe and its underlying white matter.

SYNDROMES OF APHASIA. It is possible to identify at least six recurring patterns of aphasia, each associated with a different lesion within the language zone of the left hemisphere. The major features of each type are summarized here.

Broca's Aphasia. Output sparse and articulation effortful, often with simplified grammar; "telegraphic" or totally agrammatic speech. Auditory comprehension mildly impaired, often within normal limits. Reading mildly impaired and writing severely impaired. Lesion usually anterior to sylvian and rolandic fissues.

Wernicke's Aphasia. Fluent, paraphasic speech with impaired word finding and impaired auditory comprehension. Both reading and writing usually impaired. Lesion in posterior portion of superior temporal gyrus.

Anomic Aphasia. Fluent speech with word-finding difficulty and good auditory comprehension. Little or no paraphasia. Reading and writing variable; severely impaired when anomia is caused by temporoparietal lesion.

Conduction Aphasia. Output basically fluent in articulation and grammar, but marred by phonemic paraphasia and frequent blocking. Paraphasia and blocking particularly disabling during efforts to repeat. Reading mildly affected and writing often severely affected. Lesion either immediately above or below the sylvian fissure.

Transcortical Motor Aphasia. Perfectly preserved ability to repeat in a patient who has lost all spontaneity of output and responds to questions with brief, effortfully initiated replies. Object naming also well preserved. Reading mildly affected; writing severely. Lesion usually just anterior and superior to Broca's area.

Transcortical Sensory Aphasia. Remarkably well preserved repetition in a patient with very poor comprehension and grossly paraphasic speech, severe anomia, alexia, and agraphia. Usually produced by a lesion in the "border zone" concentric to, but sparing, Wernicke's area.

APRAXIA. The loss of ability to carry out purposeful movements that cannot be explained by comprehension, motor, or sensory deficity (apraxia) is often overlooked in the neuropsychological examination, although it is a strong lateralizing sign of left hemisphere damage. Limb apraxia is manifested by the inability to carry out pretended movements (saluting, brushing teeth, hammering a nail) on verbal request, with only partial improvement on imitation. Buccofacial apraxia (dissociable from limb apraxia) is impaired movements involving the face and respiratory organs in such actions as pretending to cough, sniff a flower, blow out a match, sip through a straw, or lick the lips. Allowing the patient to perform with a real object (e.g., hammer, lighted match) often produces a dramatic return to normal praxis, which breaks down when the real object is removed. Apraxia is rarely observed without some degree of aphasia, but its severity is not closely correlated with the severity of aphasia.

LEFT PARIETAL LOBE DISORDERS

LEFT-RIGHT DISORIENTATION. A left parietal lobe lesion may produce a marked confusion as to the meaning of "left" and "right" on one's own body, which may be even more severe as applied to the examiner's body. This disorder is rarely found without some degree of aphasia. It can be identified only if the patient points correctly to the body parts when side is not specified.

FINGER AGNOSIA. The impairment of the ability to discriminate among the fingers of the hand in response to various modes of testing is a strong lateralizing sign of left hemisphere damage in the parietal lobe. If the patient can name other body parts, he may be asked to name each finger (e.g., thumb, index, middle, ring, little finger); to show a finger on auditory request; to match two-finger gestures by the examiner; to match a finger touched on one hand to his other hand or to a drawing of a hand. Since aphasia is usually present, its effects on naming and comprehension must be considered in the testing of finger gnosis.

DISORDERS OF CALCULATION (DYSCALCULIA). The ability to do mental arithmetic beyond one- to two-step operations is sensitive to brain damage of any extent. However, left parietal lobe injury may produce a selectively severe disturbance affecting even elementary arithmetic operations. On the other hand, patients with right parietal lobe disease show a distinctive difficulty in confusing the spatial order of operations in written arithmetic. They attack multidigit additions, etc., from the wrong side, misplace column totals, and obtain incorrect answers in spite of good command of the basic arithmetic concepts. In general, attribution of localizing interpretation to disorders of calculation requires that they be disproportionately severe in the context of other cognitive functions.

The cooccurrence of left-right disorientation, finger agnosia, acalculia, and agraphia is thought to constitute the four major components of the Gerstmann syndrome (Gerstmann, 1940, 1957). Typically, patients who are observed to have this cluster of deficits are, in addition, more or less impaired in word finding and usually demonstrate significant impairment on visuospatial constructional tasks.

SYMPTOMS OF RIGHT HEMISPHERE DISORDER

Lesions lateralized in the right hemisphere usually express themselves through a severe breakdown in visuospatial performance, and less often through a unilateral neglect of the left side of personal or extrapersonal space.

Visuospatial Performance. The reproduction of drawings, geometric designs, or constructions with sticks or blocks is more often grossly impaired with right cerebral than left cerebral injuries, particularly in the case of right parietal disease. The patient characteristically focuses on individual elements of a design and may neglect or severely misrepresent the relation of elements to each other. In the case of the Wechsler (or Kohs) blocks, he may violate the squareness of the outer configuration.

As noted above, the right parietal patient is prone to demonstrate the "closing in" maneuver of making his reproduction as close to the model as possible.

Dressing Disorder. A common feature of right parietal lobe disease is the inability to orient articles of clothing with respect to one's body and limbs while attempting to put them on. The examiner may ask the patient to remove his bathrobe and then return the bathrobe for the patient to put back on. In attempting to do so, the patient may turn the robe about randomly, unable to put the sleeves in proper relation to his body, until aided.

Hemispatial Neglect (Hemi-inattention). Neglect of the side of the body or of external space contralateral to the lesion may be encountered with unilateral lesions of either hemisphere, but this neglect is much more often dramatic in the case of right cerebral lesions, particularly those involving parietal lobe. In the test situation, neglect may be manifested by the patient's ignoring test materials (e.g., blocks) lying in the left of his field of view. His drawings of familiar objects may leave the left side incomplete. For example, a daisy may be drawn with petals on the right side only. A clock may be drawn with the hours numbered entirely on the right side.

Hemi-inattention may also be manifested in the patient's unawareness of the left side of his own body. He may put his robe on the right arm only, leaving the left dangling. The patient with a left-sided paralysis may ignore that side completely and even deny that it is part of his body.

Frontal Lobe Signs

While injury to the frontal lobes does not produce a selective impairment of a particular sensorimotor skill, it does produce distinctive difficulties on neuropsychological tests as well as characteristic changes in personality. The personality change is chiefly affective in character, shown by lack of drive or spontaneity, unconcern with the future, and disregard for social amenities. It is typical of the frontal lobe patient to remain in bed, taking no initiative, but responding when addressed. In some instances, a tendency to socially inappropriate humor is prominent, ranging from silliness or vulgarity to subtle humorous jibes at the examiner. An inability to monitor the intensity of emotional response may result in outbursts of rage, which are very short lived and from which the patient may easily be distracted. It is not uncommon in patients with bilateral frontal disease to have lability of emotional expression. Such patients can be involuntarily provoked to laughter or tears by a minimally appropriate stimulus, and again the expression of emotion may be easily interrupted. On occasion, patients have reported that they cannot predict the onset of such expression and that they do not experience the corresponding emotion.

Tests sensitive to frontal lobe disturbance are those which demand establishing and shifting sets, particularly maintaining the capacity to shift between alternative responses in rapid serial presentation. This deficit is highlighted by tasks in which the patient must inhibit a dominant mode of response in favor of a more arbitrary one (see discussion of the Stroop Test and reciprocal tapping test later). The clinical observation that frontal patients lack the ability to plan sequential behavior can be demonstrated objectively by such tests as the Porteus Mazes.

SELECTIVE DISORDERS OF MEMORY (AMNESIC SYNDROMES)

The amnesic syndrome of Korsakoff's disease makes us aware of a sharp distinction between tasks requiring immediate reproduction (e.g., digit span), those involving the span from a few minutes to a few years back (recent memory), and those involving remote memories of childhood and early adulthood. Severe defects in recent memory may occur with little or no damage to other cognitive functions. When recent memory alone is impaired, the likelihood is that damage has occurred to certain subcortical structures, notably the dorsomedial nucleus of the thalamus in the case of Korsakoff's disease (Victor *et al.,* 1971) or the hippocampus in various other conditions such as the syndrome of occlusion of the posterior cerebral artery (Benson *et al.,* 1974). The patient is usually disoriented as to the year and day, and cannot recall recent public events or public figures (e.g., the current or preceding presidents). On testing, it is common to find that immediate reproduction (e.g., digit span test) is intact but the ability to learn material (e.g., word lists, paragraphs) longer than the immediate memory span is severely impaired. Memory loss extends to visually presented material, such as designs for reproduction. Patients with alcoholic Korsakoff's disease have a memory loss which is severe for the recent past and extends into the premorbid period, with better and better recall as one goes further back in time. Patients with presenile dementias more commonly have a patchy loss which is stable along the time dimension.

An important aspect of the examination of amnesic syndromes is the extent of retrograde amnesia associated with head trauma. Patients rendered unconscious by head injury commonly experience a loss of memory for events preceding the injury, sometimes extending to hours or days before the event. With recovery, memory returns, first for the events more remote in time, then for those nearer to the time of injury (shrinking retrograde amnesia). No standard tests for retrograde amnesis exist, and the clinician must probe by interview, in some cases obtaining a history from other sources to guide his questioning.

There is experimental evidence that verbal memory is most sensitive to left temporal damage, even without clinical evidence of aphasia (Milner, 1958), and visual, nonverbal memory is most sensitive to right temporal damage (Kimura, 1963). Nonverbal auditory memory (tonal patterns) is also reported as right temporal lobe dependent (Milner, 1962), while auditory verbal memory is found to be more sensitive than visual verbal memory to temporal lobe removals, right or left (Samuels *et al.,* 1972).

Agnosias

Lesions in the association areas adjacent to each of the three major primary sensory areas (i.e., visual, auditory, tactile) may result in failure to recognize familiar stimulus configurations in spite of normal primary sensory function in the corresponding modality.

Visual Agnosia. In visual agnosia, the patient is unable to recognize seen objects, although he can see and describe their visual features. He must pick up objects, recognizing them by touch, in order to realize what they are. The lesion involves destruction of the left occipital visual association cortex.

Prosopagnosia. Prosopagnosia, the loss of ability to recognize faces, is usually dependent on bilateral lesions of the visual association areas, and may leave intact all other visual perceptual skills. The patient recognizes people by voice only. These patients may perform normally on short-term matching tasks for new faces. However, they can no longer recognize friends and family members or remember the faces of new individuals in their hospital environment. They fail badly when shown pictures of famous personalities.

Tactile Agnosia. Tactile agnosia may be produced by a lesion of the parietal association cortex of the left hemisphere. The patient is unable to recognize objects by touch and naturally, therefore, is unable to name them through this modality. It is tested by requiring the patient to identify objects palpated in one hand. If the patient has sufficiently impaired tactile sensitivity and position sense loss, he will thereby lose his stereognosis, i.e., his capacity for tactile recognition. However, in order to diagnose tactile agnosia, one assumes the integrity of the primary sensory modalities of touch and position sense in the hand.

Auditory Agnosia. In auditory agnosia, the patient, in spite of normal audiometric performance, is unable to recognize the nature of the sounds which he perceives. It is examined by having the patient match environmentally produced noises (crumpling paper, jingling keys, clapping hands) to their source. For more formal examination, a tape recording of assorted sounds is used in conjunction with a multiple-choice picture display for each item.

Test Battery

A basic battery of tests is described here, and the reader is referred to Lezak's *Neuropsychological Assessment* (1976) for a fuller account of most of these and a considerable selection of additional tests.

Wechsler Adult Intelligence Scale (1955)

The Wechsler Adult Intelligence Scale, a universally used test of intelligence, serves in a variety of ways in the assessment of cognitive deficits in brain damage.

First, the overall level of performance is compared to expectation based on premorbid educational-occupational attainment. Second, the relation between the verbal and performance subscales is examined for major discrepancies. If the verbal score is severely depressed (by more than 15 points), the possibility of language impairment is considered and the qualitative adequacy of verbal expression is examined carefully in answers to the subtests of Comprehension, Similarities, and Vocabulary. If the performance scale is markedly lower, right hemisphere damage may be suspected, but, again, this depends on examination of the qualitative features of Block Design performance. In general, except in the presence of large verbal vs. performance discrepancies, inferences concerning lateralization cannot safely be made on the basis of scores alone; it is necessary to consider the qualitative features of performance.

There are a number of other special features of the WAIS which permit inferences concerning organic impairment. One is that it consists of subtests that tap established knowledge (Vocabulary, Comprehension, Information), which is relatively resistant to impairment, and of other subtests (Block Design, Arithmetic, Digit Symbol, Similarities) that involve new learning or problem solving, which is more susceptible to damage. Not all brain-damaged patients show marked discrepancies between these classes of operations, but when a disparity is found it is important to take note of it. The Similarities test, demanding some degree of verbal abstraction, may show marked concretization of verbal reasoning. The Digit Span subtest contrasts the immediate reproduction of a digit string with the mental manipulation entailed in giving digits in reverse order. A difference of more than two digits between the forward and backward portion of this subtest is strongly suggestive of organic involvement. Finally, the Digit Symbol subtest, with its demand for rapid serial matching of different digit-symbol pairs, is highly vulnerable to the slowing of associative processes in brain damage.

WECHSLER MEMORY SCALE (1945)

While no published test covers all the clinically important facets of memory, the Wechsler Memory Scale has proven to be a useful and sensitive instrument. It combines a brief survey of orientation in place and time and awareness of current public information with new learning of factual paragraphs, verbal paired associates, and memory for designs. A subtest tapping sustained attention (Mental Control) is included. Unfortunately, because of its predominantly verbal character, it provides an inadequate sampling of memory in the severely verbally impaired (e.g., aphasic) patient. The ability to recall information from the recent past is underrepresented (knowledge of president, governor, and mayor), while remote memory items are absent. Nevertheless, because of the correlation between new learning ability and retention of recent facts and events, it is likely that patients having difficulty with the latter are picked up by this test. Patients with amnesic states due to Korsakoff's disease, trauma, or postencephalitic conditions are usually identified, as are those whose memory problems are more evenly spread across immediate, recent, and remote time periods. Scoring is based on an age-corrected scale which takes account of the expected decline with age. The scale is such that the expected "memory quotient" is approximately the same as the IQ. A discrepancy of more than 15 points raises the possibility of an organically based memory loss.

A number of special performance characteristics of organic patients are worth noting. The orientation items, which ask for month, day, year, and location of the place of testing, are particularly sensitive to recent memory deficits, as seen in Korsakoff's disease. Patients with more generalized intellectual defects may pass these items while showing across-the-board drops in other subtests. The verbal paired associates—a list of ten word pairs to be learned in the course of three teaching presentations—consists of six "easy" (or semantically related, high transitional probability associates) and four "hard" (arbitrary) associates. It is common for impaired patients to learn the "easy" associates (which tap old learning) at once while failing all the "hard" associates.

TESTING LANGUAGE FUNCTION

The administration of the WAIS and Wechsler Memory Scale serves as a screening procedure to detect any clinically obvious impairment in speech production and comprehension. Aphasic word-finding difficulties will obstruct answers in all of the subtests of the verbal scale of the WAIS—most notably, Comprehension and Vocabulary—while sentence formulation difficulties interfere with replies to Comprehension and Similarities subtests. On the WMS, verbal memory is more severely impaired in aphasia even than in Korsakoff's disease (Cermak and Moreines, 1976), not only in retention of paragraphs and paired verbal associates but also in the immediate span for digits.

It is rare for writing to escape significant impairment even in the mildest aphasia, whose existence may be in doubt on the basis of the WAIS and WMS. Hence, a writing sample should always be included in any screening for organic language impairment. For this purpose, the patient should write a paragraph of at least three or four sentences on some readily available topic, such as an account of his stay in the hospital or a description of his work. An aphasic writing disturbance may be betrayed by malformations of letters, spelling errors, omissions of words (particularly the "small words" of grammar), undue simplification of sentence structure (taking into account patient's educational level), or extreme slowness and self-correction in completing the writing task.

When, on the basis of the foregoing tests, there is evidence of some aphasic difficulty, a more complete examination for aphasia is in order. Among the published tests which can be used are the Boston Diagnostic Aphasia Examination (BDAE) (Goodglass and Kaplan, 1972), the Porch Index of Communicative Abilities (PICA) (Porch, 1971), the Minnesota Diagnostic Test for Aphasia (Schuell, 1965), and Eisenson's *Examining for Aphasia* (1954). Any of these will provide a basic inventory of function in all the modalities of language. The PICA is the most rigorously quantified, particularly for the more severe aphasic, while the BDAE provides for evaluation of features of speech production which are important for diagnosis but not readily reduced to an objective score.

The simplest and most direct procedures for revealing deficits in visuospatial functions involve paper-and-pencil drawings of familiar objects and geometric forms. Commonly used objects include clock, daisy, house, elephant, bicycle. The most widely used set of geometric figures are those of the Bender Visual Motor Gestalt Test. We prefer to use a variant of this test, which provides more distinct contrast between the ability to cope with the outer configurations as opposed to inner details—a dimension of performance which often reveals distinctive differences in approach between left and right brain-damaged patients. Another highly recommended geometric drawing test is the well-known Rey-Osterrieth complex figure (Osterrieth, 1944) illustrated in Fig. 2.

Right cerebral damage produces the most glaring deficits in this function. Since the patient cannot deal at once with the organizing configuration of the figure, he tends first to seek out smaller units or visually codable details, and may then attempt unsuccessfully to link them into a whole. This contrasts with the approach of the left brain-damaged patient, which resembles the normal in initial response to the global configuration, although ultimately the left hemisphere subject simplifies by omitting significant details.

The second major (although not universal) deficit with right brain-damaged subjects is neglect of one side of space, as described earlier. Curiously, neglect of the right side following left brain damage is much less frequent. When it occurs, omissions of right side detail are less blatant than commonly seen in the case of right brain lesion-left field neglect.

"Frontal Lobe" Tests

Tests aimed at detecting frontal lobe dysfunction involve (1) the ability to initiate and maintain a series of directed associations, (2) the ability to maintain a set in the face of interference, (3) the ability to shift from one conceptual frame to

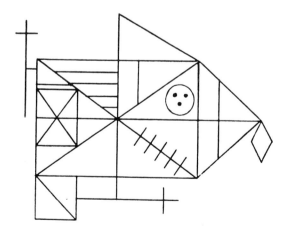

Fig. 2. Rey-Osterrieth Complex Figure (Osterrieth, 1944).

another, and (4) the ability to maintain a series of alternating motor activities. While these performances are vulnerable to severe brain damage in any of the association areas, they are most impaired by damage to the frontal lobes.

WORD LISTS. In word lists tests, the patient is asked to produce a series of words belonging to a particular category (e.g., flowers, animals, makes of cars) or beginning with a given letter of the alphabet. The average adult produces 18 animals in a minute. The Spreen-Benton Neurosensory Center Aphasia Test (1969) provides norms for words beginning with "F," "A," and "S."

STROOP TEST. The Stroop Test consists of three color-naming test cards: one in which color names are read from graphic representation, one in which randomly ordered colored squares are named in sequence, and one (the interference card) in which the names of colors are printed in ink of a different color, the subject being required to call off the color of the ink rather than to read the printed word. Left frontal patients are particularly prone to fail on the interference card.

WISCONSIN CARD SORTING TEST. The Wisconsin Card Sorting Test uses a series of 64 cards on which from one to four identical symbols appear in one of four colors. The symbols are triangles, stars, crosses, or circles. Each card is to be assigned to a category based on color, number, or shape, the guiding principle being deduced from the examiner's response of "right" or "wrong" to the patient's placement. As the patient demonstrates mastery of a given placement criterion, the criterion category is shifted, and the subject must again deduce the correct placement principle. Frontally damaged patients tend either to have great difficulty determining the first sorting principle or, once obtaining it, to shift to a second principle when required to.

INTERLEAVED SERIES. A number of frontal lobe tests require the patient to carry out a motor sequence involving alternating between two or three elements. An example is learning to tap once in response to two taps by the examiner and twice in response to one tap. Some patients are totally unable to respond correctly to random alternations by the examiner and fall into the dominant tendency to imitate his tap. Another task is to learn a series of three positions of the hand on the table and carry them out repeatedly in sequence (fingers extended together, palm flat; fist clenched, flat; hand on edge, fingers extended together).

CASE ILLUSTRATION

The following case* illustrates the quantitative and qualitative aspects of the performance of a patient with a relatively focal lateralized lesion on neuropsychological testing.

C. J., a 29-year-old, single, right-handed, high-school-educated fireman was in good health until 10 years ago, when he sustained a cerebrovascular accident. Current neurological examination reveals a left hemiparesis with face more affected than arm, arm more than leg, abnormal EEG activity over right hemi-

*Patient was examined by Dawn Bowers, clinical neuropsychology associate, and supervised by Edith Kaplan.

sphere, CT scan positive for lesion over right frontal, deep right parietal, and right anterior temporal regions.

TESTS ADMINISTERED. WAIS, WMS, and frontal lobe tests—motor sequencing, alternating programs, contrasting programs, go–no go, Wisconsin Card Sort, Porteus Mazes, Money Road Map Test, Stroop Test, FAS word fluency, Boston Diagnostic Parietal Battery, Hooper Visual Organization Test, Benton Test of Visual Recognition, Modified Bender-Gestalt Designs from memory, and, to copy, Rey-Osterreith Complex Figure.

BEHAVIORAL OBSERVATIONS. Appearance and attire were somewhat unkempt. Speech was a fluent, flat monotone and was never spontaneously initiated. C. J. appeared placid, never showed signs of overt frustration or irritation, and was not self-critical.

FINDINGS. Intellectually, the patient is functioning in the borderline range (WAIS FIQ = 79), with performance scale (PIQ = 72) considerably lower than verbal scale (VIQ = 86). Relatively good performance on Information and Vocabulary (scaled scores 12 and 11, respectively) suggests that the patient's current IQ scores represent a significant depression of his premorbid functioning. Overall, his general fund of knowledge and mathematical ability (arithmetic scaled score 11, Arithmetic in Parietal Lobe Battery 31/32) are good. The patient's ability to deal with more abstract material, however, is limited; e.g., proverb interpretations are extremely concrete (on "Strike while the iron is hot," he responded "Pressing clothes, it has to be hot to be effective").

Most dramatic were C. J.'s difficulties on visuomotor constructive tasks which required the analysis and synthesis of geometric designs or familiar figures. On Block Design he frequently broke the external configuration (even on the easier 2 × 2 designs). C. J. seemed to be pulled by the salient figural feature of the design. This type of error, notably associated with right frontal pathology, is best demonstrated in his attempt to recreate the model displayed on the left in Fig. 3.

One interesting aspect of C. J.'s performance was that however the blocks were initially randomly arranged at the beginning of a trial he rarely turned them over to expose another side. This same "inertia" was observed on Picture Arrangement, a finding that is considered pathognomonic of right frontal pathology (McFie, 1975).

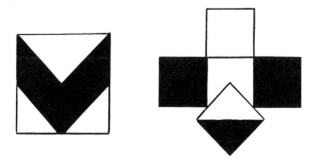

Fig. 3. Patient's reproduction (right) of block design from Wechsler Adult Intelligence Scale. Original figure on left reproduced from the Wechsler Adult Intelligence Scale by permission. Copyright 1947, © 1955 by the Psychological Corporation, New York, N.Y. All rights reserved.

In contrast to his poor performance on the above tasks, his scores on two other "visuospatial" tasks were good (Hooper Visual Organization Test and Gollin Figures). This may be accounted for by his marked tendency to make inferences on the basis of detail cues rather than perceptually integrating configurative spatial information.

All tests of verbal memory, both immediate and delayed, were well executed. His Wechsler Memory Quotient was 114. Visuospatial material, provided that construction was not required (e.g., Benton Visual Recognition from multiple choice), was similarly preserved. In sharp contrast, drawings of geometric figures from memory (WMS visual reproductions and Berea Designs) were poor, reflecting such errors as angle distortion, shape distortion, perseveration, segmentation, and aberrant sequence. It should be noted that drawing to copy reflected the same errors. C. J.'s constructional difficulties are most strikingly illustrated by the strategy he employed in copying the complex Rey-Osterrieth figure (Fig. 4). He correctly drew the individual components of the design, segment by segment, but their spatial relationships to one another were grossly distorted. Difficulty in "set shifting" was highlighted by poor performance on the Wisconsin Card Sort. Similarly, he was impaired on tasks associated with right frontal functioning, i.e., Porteus Mazes, continuous alternation in writing "mn" repeatedly (generating extra humps on "n," which were also noted in his written narrative of the BDAE cookie theft picture). However, on tasks that have been presumed to tap left frontal functions, e.g., Stroop Test and Money Road Map Test, he performed adequately. On motor tasks of frontal functioning, he made numerous perseverative errors. This pattern of deficits is most compatible with pathology involving right frontal parietal areas, with relative sparing of right temporal areas and of the entire left hemisphere.

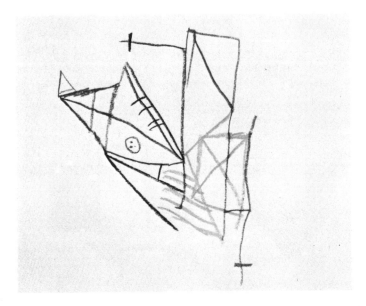

Fig. 4. Patient's reproduction of Rey-Osterrieth figure, showing rotation of design and overlapping of segments.

In this chapter, we have tried to convey the approach of the clinical neuropsychologist to the cognitive assessment of the brain-injured patient. The deficits associated with brain disease were reviewed. A distinction was drawn between defects associated with brain damage in general and those which are selective for a particular hemisphere or a lobe within a hemisphere, and a case summary illustrating a right frontal lesion was presented.

It should be emphasized that the development of tests for organic deficit is still an ongoing process and is closely linked to the continuing research on brain-behavior relationships.

REFERENCES

Benson, D. F., Marsden, C. D., and Meadows, J. The amnesic syndrome of posterior cerebral artery occlusion. *Acta Neurologica Scandinavica,* 1974, *50,* 133–145.

Benton, A. L. *Manuel du test de Rétention Visuelle: Applications Cliniques et Experimentales.* 2nd ed. Paris: Centre de Psychologie Appliquée, 1955.

Carmazza, A., and Zurif, E. B. Dissociation of algorithmic and heuristic processes in language comprehension: Evidence from aphasia. *Brain and Language,* 1976, *3,* 572–582.

Cermak, L. S., and Moreines, J. Verbal retention deficits in aphasia and amnesic patients. *Brain and Language,* 1976, *3,* 16–27.

Critchley, M. *The Parietal Lobes.* Baltimore: Williams and Wilkins, 1953.

Eisenson, J. *Examining for Aphasia.* New York: Psychological Corporation, 1954.

Gardner, H., Strub, R., and Albert, M. L. A unimodal deficit in operational thinking. *Brain and Language,* 1975, *2,* 333–344.

Gerstmann, J. Syndrome of finger agnosia, disorientation for right and left, agraphia, and acalculia. *Archives of Neurology and Psychiatry,* 1940, *44,* 398–408.

Gerstmann, J. Some notes on the Gerstmann syndrome. *Neurology,* 1957, *7,* 866–869.

Geschwind, N., and Chedru, F. Writing disturbances in acute confusional states. *Neuropsychologia,* 1972, *10,* 343–353.

Geschwind, N., and Fusillo, M. Color-naming defects in association with alexia. *Archives of Neurology,* 1966, *15,* 137–146.

Goldstein, K., and Scheerer, M. Tests of abstract and concrete behavior. In A. Weider (ed.), *Contributions to Medical Psychology.* Vol. 2. New York: Ronald Press, 1953.

Goodglass, H., and Cohen, M. L. Disturbance in body-part comprehension in aphasia. Paper presented at meeting of American Psychological Association, Washington, D.C., 1954.

Goodglass, H., and Kaplan, E. *The Assessment of Aphasia and Related Disorders.* Philadelphia: Lea and Febiger, 1972.

Goodglass, H., Gleason, J. B., and Hyde, M. R. Some dimensions of auditory language comprehension in aphasia. *Journal of Speech and Hearing Research,* 1970, *13,* 595–606.

Kimura, D. Right temporal lobe damage—Perception of unfamiliar stimuli after damage. *Archives of Neurology,* 1963, *8,* 264–271.

Lezak, M. *Neuropsychological Assessment.* New York: Oxford University Press, 1976.

McFie, J. *Assessment of Organic Intellectual Impairment.* London: Academic Press, 1975.

Milner, B. Psychological defects produced by temporal lobe excision. *Research Publication of the Association for Research in Nervous and Mental Diseases,* 1958, *36,* 244–257.

Milner, B. Laterality effects in audition. In V. B. Mountcastle (ed.), *Interhemispheric Relations and Cerebral Dominance.* Baltimore: Johns Hopkins Press, 1962.

Osterrieth, P. A. Le test de copie d'une figure complexe. *Archives de Psychologie,* 1944, *30,* 206–356.

Porch, B. *Porch Index of Communicative Ability.* Palo Alto, Calif.: Consulting Psychologists Press, 1971.

Samuels, I., Butters, N., and Fedio, P. Short term memory disorders following temporal lobe removals in humans. *Cortex,* 1972, *8,* 283–298.

Schuell, H. *Differential Diagnosis of Aphasia with the Minnesota Test.* Minneapolis: University of Minnesota Press, 1965.

Spreen, O., and Benton, A. L. *Neurosensory Center Comprehensive Examination for Aphasia.* Victoria, B.C.: Neuropsychology Laboratory, Department of Psychology, University of Victoria, 1969.

Stroop, J. R. Studies of interference in serial verbal reactions. *Journal of Experimental Psychology,* 1945, *18*, 643–662.

Victor, M., Adams, R., and Collins, G. *The Wernicke-Korsakoff Syndrome.* Philadelphia: F. A. Davis, 1971.

Wechsler, D. A. A standardized memory scale for clinical use. *Journal of Psychology,* 1945, *19*, 87–95.

Wechsler, D. *Wechsler Adult Intelligence Scale Manual.* New York: Psychological Corporation, 1955.

Weigl, E. On the psychology of so-called processes of abstraction. *Journal of Abnormal and Social Psychology,* 1941, *36*, 3–33.

PART II

Cortical Lobes and Function

2

The Frontal Lobes

Marc Jouandet and Michael S. Gazzaniga

Introduction: Past Obstacles to a Description of the Frontal Syndrome

It appears that the human prefrontal regions have emerged over the years to distinguish themselves among the cerebral cortical structures as those most elusively resistant to neurocognitive analyses. Although a very substantial number of clinical observations based on human patients suffering from severe prefrontal injury have accumulated in the literature within the last century, theories of prefrontal functioning proving consistently applicable and reasonably unifying have not, until relatively recently, evolved.

One great obstacle to the development of an adequate theory describing the functions of the prefrontal cortex has been the perplexing paradox presented by the basic "frontal syndrome": although massive, bilateral frontal lobe damage does not clearly and consistently result in any specific visual, auditory, somatosensory, motor, or verbal impairments, striking deterioration in general behavior is apparent. It has been from the attempts to characterize this rather amorphous psychological deterioration that confusion has sprung. In a great variety of earlier studies, the usual psychiatric categories and general terminology have proven insufficient. They have neither clearly described alternations in emotional states and personality nor explained the nature of the underlying dysfunctions. This failure has led Nauta (1971) to write that such descriptions must, for the present, "remain somewhat at the periphery of the search for common denominators in the frontal syndrome," and Luria (1973b) to concur by writing that "science is still faced with the task of explaining prefrontal lobe function in clear terms accessible to further analysis."

Marc Jouandet and Michael S. Gazzaniga · Department of Neurology, Cornell University Medical College, New York, New York 10021.

MARC JOUANDET AND
MICHAEL S.
GAZZANIGA

The symptom constellations manifesting themselves after prefrontal injury vary to an extent much greater than is ever observed when damage is confined to any of the more posterior areas of the cerebral cortex (Teuber, 1964; Hécaen, 1964; Nauta, 1971). If it could be assumed that frontal cortical tissue is equipotential, then the wide variation in clinical symptoms manifest after injury could be explained simply on the basis of effects related directly to the peculiar mechanical and biochemical consequences of various natural accidents. Tumors, cerebrovascular accidents, penetrating missile wounds, and surgical ablations of surface corical tissue all have, of course, radically different effects on cortical functioning. When such injuries appear in the posterior cortical regions, the intrinsic effects of these diseases and accidents are anchored by relatively specific sensory, verbal, or motor deficits consistently resulting from destruction in reasonably localized, differentially organized cortical areas. When such injuries appear in the prefrontal regions, however, their intrinsic effects obscure the more subtle prefrontal functions. If the injuries themselves are not too massive, the impaired functions are compensated for by the remaining frontal tissues, resulting, occasionally, in full recovery. The subtlety of the functional impairments and the capriciousness with which they appear are suggested by Milner (1971), who writes that "even minor variations in the testing procedures determine whether or not deficits are seen."

Because all these barriers obscuring the subtleties of frontal processing proved almost insurmountable to earlier investigators, widely diverging theories on the nature of frontal function have been formulated. In the 1930s and 1940s, many investigators attributed to the frontal cortex the most stupendous of cognitive capabilities, variously calling the prefrontal regions the seat of "abstract intelligence" and the "organs of civilization." A reaction against such viewpoints subsequently emerged in the 1950s, contending that no specifiable functions could be attributed to the prefrontal areas (Hebb, 1939; Mettler, 1949; Teuber, 1959). It was not that these authors held the presence of the frontal lobes to be superfluous, but simply that they were not aware of any undisputable evidence suggesting that there existed any cognitive processes subserved exclusively by the prefrontal regions or that these areas did not function physiologically in an equipotential manner. It is against this background that the clinical evidence accumulated since the early 1960s must be viewed in order to be most fully appreciated.

In this chapter, we will review some of the evidence available in the clinical literature that suggests how the prefrontal regions may function in an intergrative manner with other structures of the brain. Prefrontal experiments conducted upon rhesus monkeys will be occasionally mentioned in order to explicate more fully some current theories.

FUNCTIONAL CHARACTERISTICS OF THE POSTERIOR FRONTAL REGIONS

In order to orient ourselves to a discussion of human prefrontal functioning, let us first consider briefly some of the functional properties of the more caudal regions of the frontal lobes (see Figs. 1 to 7).

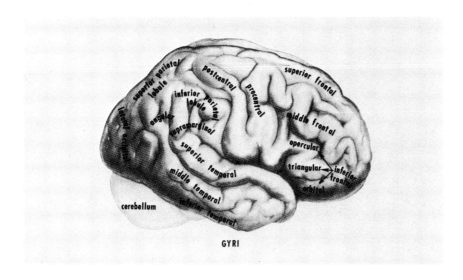

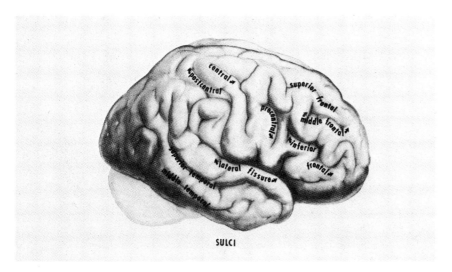

Fig. 1. Gyral and fissural pattern of the human frontal lobes. The frontal lobes encompass all those areas of the cerebral cortex anterior to the Rolandic fissure and dorsal to the sylvian fissure. (Reprinted with permission from Curtis, Jacobson, and Marcus. *An Introduction to the Neurosciences,* © 1972, W. B. Saunders Co., Philadelphia, Pa.)

As one moves rostrally from the Rolandic fissure, movements elicited by localized punctate electrical stimulation become less elemental, more organized in their patterning, yet less probable in their occurrence. Stimulation thresholds for the supplementary and premotor areas are higher than for the primary motor area 4, and movements are more coordinated. Ablation of both the premotor and supplementary areas is necessary to produce gait apraxia, for these two regions are sufficiently similar in the anatomical organization and versatile in their physiological functioning to assume the processing responsibilities of the other when

MARC JOUANDET AND
MICHAEL S.
GAZZANIGA

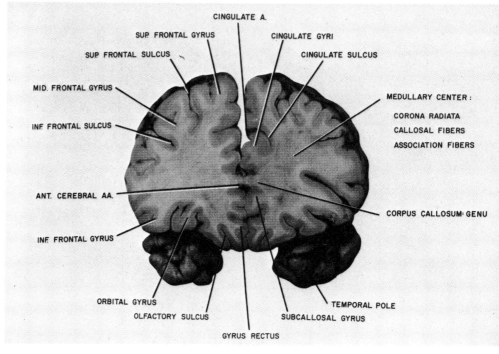

Fig. 2. Coronal section through the frontal regions. (Reprinted with permission from Curtis, Jacobson, and Marcus. *An Introduction to the Neurosciences,* © 1972, W. B. Saunders Co., Philadelphia, Pa.)

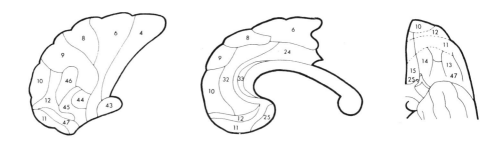

Fig. 3. Brodmann's cytoarchitectural designations of the lateral, medial, and orbital surfaces. On broadly defined anatomical and functional grounds, the frontal lobes have been generally viewed to be composed of three major subdivisions: the primary motor area (Brodmann's area 4), the premotor zone (areas 6, 8, 43, 44, and 45), and the frontogranular, or prefrontal, cortex (areas 9, 10, 11, 12, 46, 47, 13, 14, and 15). (Reprinted with permission from Robin and McDonald, © 1975, Henry Kimpton Publishers, London.)

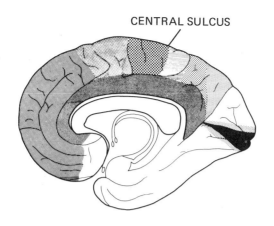

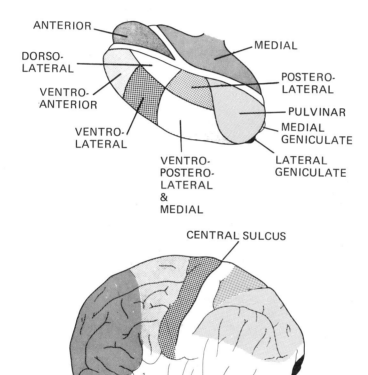

Fig. 4. Specific thalamocortical relationships of the frontal regions. The primary motor area receives afferents from the ventrolateral nucleus of the thalamus, the premotor regions are reciprocally interconnected with the medial ventroanterior nucleus, and the prefrontal cortex is connected with the mediodorsal thalamic nuclei. (Reprinted with permission from Curtis, Jacobson, and Marcus. *An Introduction to the Neurosciences,* © 1972, W. B. Saunders Co., Philadelphia, Pa.)

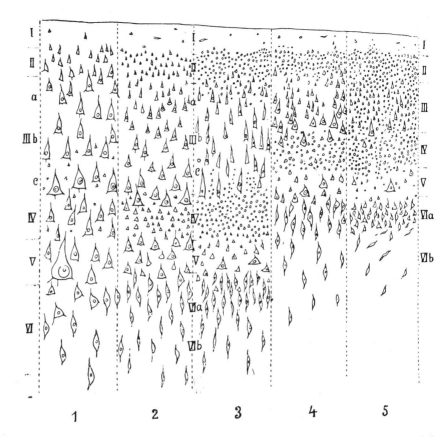

Fig. 5. The five fundamental types of cortical structure: type 1, agranular motor cortex; type 2, frontal homotypical (frontal-granular); type 3, parietal homotypical; type 4, polar; type 5, granular koniocortex (von Economo, 1929). The cytoarchitectural distinctions among the various areas of the frontal lobes basically reduce to three: the agranular primary motor zone, the granular prefrontal regions, and the transitional cortex between them. In the primary motor cortex, the external pyramidal layer III and the internal pyramidal layer V are fused into essentially one deep layer possessing a high concentration of large pyramidal cells and the giant pyramidal cells of Betz. The internal granular layer IV, which in other cortical regions consists mostly of stellate cells, is not present in the primary motor area. The premotor zone preserves the same laminar organization as the primary region, with the only exception that the Betz cells, among the large pyramidal cells, are no longer evident. The gradual reappearance of the granular layer IV in the rhesus monkey occurs in the depths of the arcuate sulcus and marks the border between the premotor and the prefrontal cortices. (From von Economo: *The Cytoarchitectonics of the Human Cerebral Cortex,* © 1929. Reprinted with permission from Oxford University Press.)

either is damaged. The opercular and triangular regions of the inferior frontal convolution (areas 44 and 45) of the dominant hemisphere, known for over a century as Broca's expressive speech area, are cytoarchitecturally continuous with area 6. Because the inferior frontal convolution is located immediately anterior to the primary motor region directly innervating the face, lips, tongue, and pharynx, damage to this premotor zone destroys neural circuits that have, in ontogeny, encoded information critical to the refined production of adaptive vocal patterns. The complex electrophysiological activity of the inferior convolution functions to spatially and temporally regulate activity in the region of the precentral gyrus directly responsible for varying the instantaneous configurations of the supra-pharyngeal vocal tract. Damage to this region in the dominant hemisphere, which by its intrinsic circuit organization and/or cellular biochemical properties is viewed to store "motor memories for speech patterns," can be seen to affect somewhat adversely an individual's ability to produce speech sounds.

This brief discussion has been necessarily superficial, for an adequate review of the functional properties of the primary and premotor cortices would easily fill volumes. Because such an undertaking is quite beyond the intended scope of this chapter, interested readers are referred to the excellent works of Denny-Brown (1951, 1966), Woolsey *et al.* (1950), Phillips (1966), and Pensfield and Jaspar (1954). The point to be made here is simply that as one moves rostrally from the Rolandic fissure, movements become more coordinated, yet less reliably elicited by electrical stimulation, until they disappear altogether on encountering the caudal border of the prefrontal cortex. This border region has remained a frontier for neurocognitive scientists since the pioneering experiments of Fritsch and Hitzig undertaken in the 1870s.

THE PREFRONTAL REGIONS

The prefrontal cortex may, in terms of gross anatomy, be seen to be composed of three subdivisions: the medial, lateral, and orbital surfaces. Apart from the cingulate and orbital cortices, the granular prefrontal regions are phylogeneti-

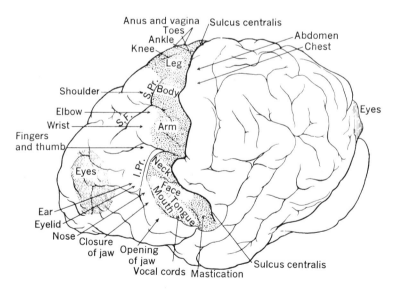

Fig. 6. All the skeletal muscles are somatotopically, although disproportionately, represented in the classical primary motor zone. In man, the thumb, fingers, lips, and tongue have by far the greatest area of motor cortex devoted to their control and, as a result, are capable of exquisitely fine motor movements. (From Bard, P., after Sherington, Motor functions of the cerebral cortex and basal ganglia. In V. B. Mountcastle (ed.), *Medical Physiology,* 12 ed., © 1968, Mosby, St. Louis, Mo.)

MARC JOUANDET AND
MICHAEL S.
GAZZANIGA

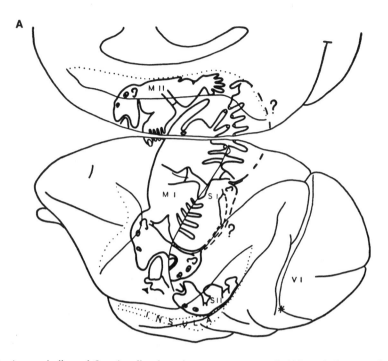

Fig. 7 A. Anatomically and functionally, the primary motor cortex is intimately integrated with the primary sensory zone located on the postcentral gyrus. Columnarly arranged cells of the primary motor cortex are interconnected, via the "U fibers" passing underneath the Rolandic fissure, with their somatotopic counterparts in the primary somatosensory receiving area. The primary motor and somatosensory areas function together such that the spatiotemporal patterns of electrophysiological activity in the motor zone directly activating movement are constantly modulated by the afferent feedback activity of the caudally adjacent primary somatosensory zone. The supplementary motor region, situated anterior to the classical motor area and extending from the upper bank of the cingulate sulcus to the superior convexity of the hemisphere, is cytoarchitecturally indistinguishable from the premotor areas 6 and 8. Like the primary motor area, the supplementary motor cortex represents, somatotopically but disproportionately, the musculature of the contralateral side of the body. The stimulation threshold for eliciting movement is higher for the supplementary area than for the primary region, and movements elicited from the supplementary region are longer lasting than the rapid, phasic contractions elicited by stimulation of the primary region. Unilateral ablation of the supplementary motor region produces no noticeable weakness, but biateral ablation does result in some spasticity. (From Woolsey, Settlage, Meyer, Spencer, Hamuy, and Travis, 1950*b*. Reprinted with permission from the Association for Research in Nervous and Mental Diseases.)

cally recent structures, achieving prominence only in primates and becoming quite formidable only in man. The lateral surface of the frontogranular cortex, like the inferior parietal area, is one of the last cortical regions to undergo myelination and appears to be, for the most part, cytoarchitecturally undifferentiated tissue (Nauta, 1971, 1974). Cytoarchitectural maps constructed by various investigators attempting to demarcate further subdivisions of the prefrontal regions (Brodmann, 1909; Vogt and Vogt, 1919; Walker, 1940; von Bonin and Bailey, 1947) have not always been found in concurrence (Akert, 1964) (see Fig. 8).

Only in negative findings have the traditional physiological techniques of ablation and stimulation provided some clues to the functional characteristics of the prefrontal regions. Noticeable changes in human behavior are not obvious if

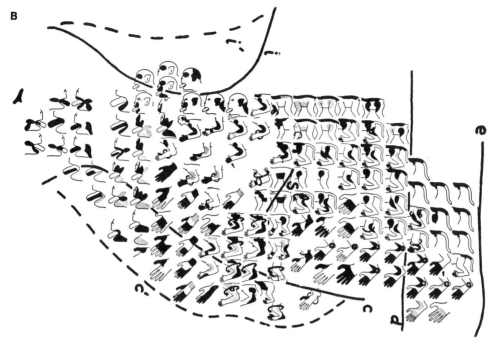

Fig. 7 B.   Figurine chart of primary motor zone demonstrating the specificity of muscular responding to stimulation of highly localized points in the primary motor zone. (From Woolsey, Settlage, Meyer, Spencer, Hamuy, and Travis, 1950*b*. Reprinted with permission from the Association for Research in Nervous and Mental Diseases.)

severe cortical damage is limited only to localized areas within the prefrontal region, but if a wide expanse of tissue is materially altered in a slight manner, observable alterations in behavior and mental processes will manifest themselves (Walter, 1973). Walter (1973) emphasizes that electrical stimulation applied to localized prefrontal areas does not readily spread to surrounding tissues and produces in humans

> no subjective or objective effects whatsoever . . . the waveforms of induced after discharges reproduce quite precisely all the appearances associated in conventional scalp EEG with epileptic seizures, but the patient shows no signs of any such disturbances: he continues to converse with attendants, to read a book, or even doze peacefully quite unaffected by the intense but strictly confined electrical tornado.

An awareness of afferent and efferent projections interconnecting cytoarchitecturally homogeneous, apparently equipotential tissues of the lateral prefrontal cortex with the more posterior sensory cortices, and of the orbitofrontal regions with the limbic system, might provide a background against which clinically observed cognitive processes subserved by these regions could perhaps be more logically or imaginatively viewed. However, such insights—gained from the clear visualization of a basic network pattern of cortical fiber systems serving to conduct sensory information from the primary areas to the phylogenetically more recent frontal structures recipient to and integrating bimodally and trimodally converging sensory input—are not easily arrived at for the human brain, simply because

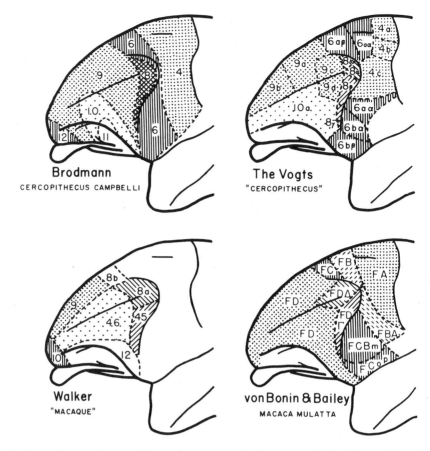

Fig. 8. Cytoarchitectural maps of rhesus frontal cortex by Brodmann (1909), Vogt and Vogt (1919), Walker (1940) and von Bonin and Bailey (1947). (From J. M. Warren and K. Akert (eds.), *The Frontal Granular Cortex,* copyright © 1964, McGraw-Hill Book Co., New York. Used with permission of the publisher.)

histochemical techniques currently available preclude the precise determination of these pathways in man. Current knowledge of these pathways is limited to, although quite extensive for, the rhesus monkey. Through the detailed and extensive investigation of many authors (Krieg, 1954, 1963; Akert, 1964; von Bonin and Bailey, 1947; DeVito and Smith, 1964; Pandya and Kuypers, 1969; Jones and Powell, 1970) and the excellent reviews of the field by Nauta (1971, 1972), a clear picture of the major interconnections has emerged, suggesting some outlines of qualitative patterns of information flow underlying the cognitive processes of the prefrontal regions of the rhesus monkey (see Fig. 9).

With the exception of the additional olfactory input, the prefrontal cortex rerepresents the external world first integrated in the inferoparietal regions (Nauta, 1971). The repetitiousness of this representation may explain why negligible sensory deficiencies appear with frontal ablations, whereas parietal, occipital, or temporal cortical damage, by cutting off information closer to the source, lead to more drastic sensory impairments.

The neural fiber systems integrating frontogranular and limbic activity are today widely believed responsible for regulating emotional states. In his landmark work, Papez (1937) proposed that the limbic circuit, interconnecting the septum, hippocampus, mammillary bodies, anterior thalamus, and cingulate gyrus, functions as the cerebral mechanism of emotion. In 1948, Yakolev extended this work by including the orbitofrontal and temporal cortices. These two circuits have come to be known, respectively, as the medial limbic and basolateral limbic circuits (Livingston and Escobar, 1973) (see Fig. 10).

The orbitofrontal cortex both monitors and modulates the activity of the telencephalic limbic system to an extensive degree. In summarizing the consensus of many neuroanatomists, Nauta (1971) has written that "it would seem justified to view the frontal cortex as the major neocortical representation of the limbic system." The only direct route from the neocortex to the hypothalamus arises from the prefrontal cortex: From the caudal orbital surface there descends a powerful projection to the preopticohypothalamic region (Nauta, 1962), and from the superior principal gyrus powerful projections descend to terminate in the lateral, posterior, and dorsal hypothalamic regions (Nauta, 1971). Afferents to the medial division of the mediodorsal thalamic nucleus, projecting specifically to the orbitofrontal cortex (Akert, 1964), arise from the septum, ventromedial mesencephalic tegmentum (Guillery, 1959), the interpeduncular nucleus, and the amygdala (Nauta, 1974). A large, ascending visceral sensory system terminates on the hypothalamus and on the medial thalamic nucleus relaying to the posterior orbital gyrus.

The orbitofrontal-hypothalamic connection partially subserves autonomic functions: stimulaton of the posterior orbital surface leads to changes in heart rate, respiratory movements, and blood pressure (Spencer, 1894; Kaada, 1951); when the hypothalamus is destroyed, blood pressure and cardial effects are no longer obtained from stimulation, but respiratory reactions remain unchanged (Wall *et al.*, 1951).

Trimodally integrated sensory information converges both on the lateral prefrontal cortex (Jones and Powell, 1970; Pandya and Kuypers, 1969; Chavis and Pandya, 1976) and on the anterior temporal pole (Powell, 1972; Livingston, 1977). The orbital cortex, interconnected with the adjacent lateral prefrontal cortex and, via the uncinate fasciculus, with the anterior temporal region, appears, according to Nauta (1971), as "the integrative site of two great functional realms": the rerepresentations of the external world in the lateral frontal and anterior temporal regions are integrated in the orbitofrontal cortex, with information ascending from the internal visceroendocrine environment.

Although the medial limbic and basolateral limbic circuits are not directly interconnected, both systems ramify powerful efferent projections that converge on the septal, hypothalamic, and midbrain nuclei. Therefore, the two circuits appear to function in a mutually antagonistic manner (Nauta, 1962; Livingston and Escobar, 1973), and normal emotional behavior appears to be regulated by the orbitofrontal cortices functioning to balance internal desires with external reality.

MARC JOUANDET AND
MICHAEL S.
GAZZANIGA

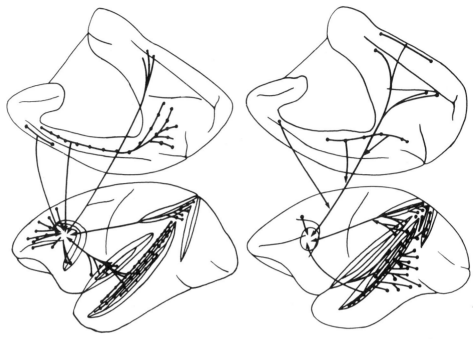

Fig. 9. Intrahemispheric cortical afferent projections to the lateral prefrontal cortex of the rhesus monkey. The regions rostral to the arcuate sulcus and dorsal and lateral to the principal sulcus receive afferents from the temporal, occipital, parietal, and cingulate cortices. Converging sensory inputs are thus bimodally and trimodally integrated in these prefrontal sites. (From Jacobson and Trojanowski, 1977. Reprinted with permission of the authors and Elsevier/North Holland Biomedical Press.)

Leucotomies, interrupting the orbitofrontal-limbic and thalamic fibers passing in the lower medial quadrant of the frontal lobes, and cingulectomies, involving the sectioning of the limbic circuits passing caudally in the anterior cingulate gyrus to terminate in the hippocampus, have been performed with the intention of establishing in emotionally unbalanced patients equilibrious, if not completely normal, states of emotional functioning.

PSYCHIATRIC SURGERY

The literature on psychosurgery is extensive. The *British Medical Journal* (1971) has reported that, since Moniz first performed his operations in 1936, as many as 100,000 psychosurgical interventions have been performed; half of these have occurred in the United States (Breggin, 1972; Chorover, 1974; Robin and McDonald, 1975). Dr. Walter Freeman, a leading proponent of psychosurgery, has performed more than 3500 operations (Freeman, 1971; Valenstein, 1977). A library computer search of the English language literature on psychosurgery from 1970 to the present, recently conducted by Valenstein for the National Commission for the Protection of Human Subjects of Biomedical and Behavioral Research, yielded approximately 700 articles dealing directly with psychosurgery

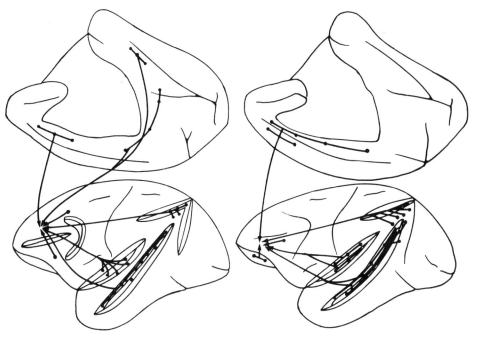

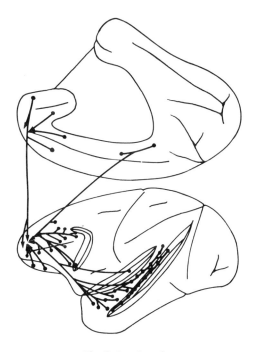

Fig. 9 (continued)

MARC JOUANDET AND
MICHAEL S.
GAZZANIGA

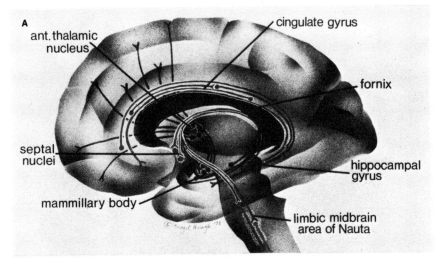

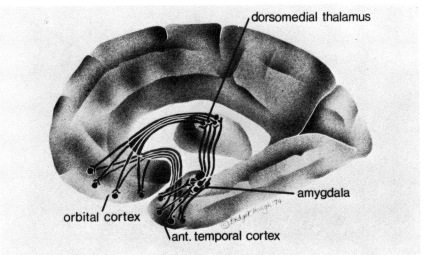

Fig. 10A. The medial limbic and basolateral limbic circuits. (Reprinted with permission from Living-ston,: Limbic system dysfunctioning induced by "kindling," In Sweet, Obrador, and Martin-Rodriguez (eds.), *Neurosurgical Treatment in Psychiatry, Pain, and Epilepsy,* © 1977, University Park Press, Baltimore, Md.)

and related scientific or ethical issues. The Commission estimates that as many as 414 psychosurgical operations have been performed annually in the United States during the period under study.

These operations have generally involved institutionally unmanageable, men-tally ill patients possessing, by every reasonable physiological and anatomical criteria, healthy brains. Indeed, the United States Senate Health Subcommittee on psychosurgery that convened in the spring of 1973 has, for the purpose of debate, defined psychosurgery as the "surgical removal or destruction of brain tissues to disconnect one part of the brain from another with the intent of altering behavior, even though there may be no direct evidence of structural disease or damage in

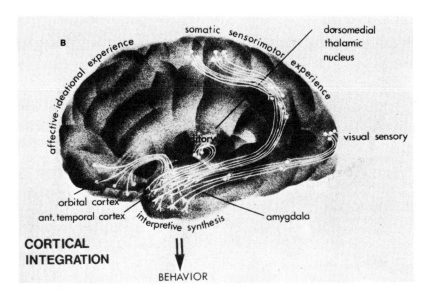

Fig. 10B. Tertiary sensory integration in the anterior temporal cortex and connections to the orbito-frontal cortex via the uncinate fasciculus. (Reprinted with permission from Livingston,: Limbic system dysfunctioning induced by "kindling." In Sweet, Obrador, and Martin-Rodriguez (eds.), *Neurosurgical Treatment in Psychiatry, Pain, and Epilepsy*, © 1977, University Park Press, Baltimore, Md.)

the brain." Let us now briefly consider the origins, direction, and current state of this field.

GENERAL HISTORY OF PSYCHOSURGERY. The Swiss psychiatrist Burckhardt was the first in modern times to execute frontal lobotomies on human patients with the intention of altering the emotional states of chronic, occasionally violent, schizophrenic patients. Relying almost exclusively on his own intuitions, Burckhardt performed the operations on six patients. In the article published in 1891, he praised the usefulness of the technique in rendering troublesome patients docile. This pioneer apparently elected to terminate further experimentation when his colleagues in the greater European medical community expressed some misgivings.

It was not until Fulton's address at the International Neurological Congress held in 1935 that interest in the potential usefulness of frontal lobotomies was again stimulated. Fulton reported on changes in the emotional behavior of chimpanzees following prefrontal ablation. The emotional behavior patterns of two normal chimpanzees to frustrating situations posed by complex discrimination problems were preoperatively assessed: to high failure rates the two chimpanzees expressed naturally their frustrations by engaging in temper tantrums. After having undergone bilateral prefrontal lobotomy, the chimpanzees no longer appeared anxious, and failed to engage in frustrational behaviors on making errors in discrimination (Fulton and Jacobsen, 1935; Fulton, 1952).

When Moniz reported in 1936 the beneficial effects of the prefrontal leuco-tomy operation he devised and tested on 20 severely impaired "schizophrenic" patients, modern psychosurgery was born, to eventually emerge as an almost

MARC JOUANDET AND
MICHAEL S.
GAZZANIGA

routine procedure in the battery of psychiatric therapies. Moniz's leucotomy did not involve cortical ablation but rather had as a target the underlying fiber systems deep within the frontal lobe. These operations involved the insertion of a hollow needle carrying within it a sharp wire functioning as a blade in sectioning these major connections. The relative selectivity of Moniz's innovative operation was, for that era, sufficient to secure the approval of the psychiatric community in light of his conclusions that seven patients improved to the extent that they were able to leave the institution, return to their families, and obtain productive employment (Moniz, 1937). In 1949, Egas Moniz won the Nobel Prize (*Nobel Lectures*, 1964).

In 1942, Freeman and Watts devised the surgical method that eventually succeeded in dominating the field for many years and that, as a consequence, came to be called the "standard prefrontal leucotomy." Although secondary cortical and vascular damage responsible for personality changes and intellectual blunting was unavoidably associated with the gross sectioning of the great majority of frontal thalamic fibers, the reduction in emotional volatility was sufficiently dramatic in a large number of cases reported by many authors to ensure the method's widespread utilization to the extent that it dominated as the preferred technique in the early to middle 1950s despite the availability of anatomically more selective surgical procedures.

Since that era, many neurosurgeons appear to have preferred devising and praising the merits of their own special approaches. A great number of new techniques have proliferated since the introduction of the standard leucotomy. In 1949, Scoville described the less traumatic technique of "orbital undercutting" to relieve the symptoms of obsessive-compulsive neurotics and has since claimed great success. Lindstrom (1960) has used an ultrasonic beam directed through trephine openings over the frontal lobes. Ballantine and his associates have performed numerous cingulectomies for manic depression, anorexia nervosa, obsessional neurosis, and intractable pain (Ballantine *et al.*, 1967) (see Fig. 11). Knight (1965) developed the technique of implanting radioactive yttrium-90 to destroy local tissue over time.

With the introduction of alternative strategies attempting to cure the symptoms of chronically disturbed mental patients—electroconvulsive therapy and psychotropic drugs in the late 1950s, and group, community, and behavior therapy in the 1960s—the popularity of psychosurgery ebbed and was for a time used only in chronic cases which proved insensitive to other therapies. However, with the introduction of stereotaxic procedures, with increased awareness of some of the functional properties of the limbic structures, and with the recognition of the limitations of drugs, ECT, and behavior therapy, the slight possibility of successfully treating debilitating psychotic behavior through more refined neurosurgical procedures once again presented itself as the final, unpromising, hope simply too enticing to resist (Rylander, 1973; Schvarcz, 1977; Scoville *et al.*, 1973; Ballantine *et al.*, 1967; Mark and Ervin, 1970; Valenstein, 1977).

FAILURE OF PSYCHIATRIC ASSESSMENT. The resurgence in psychosurgery has in this decade been met by vehement criticism on both scientific and ethical grounds. Annas and Glantz (1974) write:

Participants in the psychosurgery controversy generally espouse one of three competing points of view. First, there are surgeons who argue that psychosurgical procedures have developed beyond the experimental stage to the point where they may be considered therapeutic for certain types of patients. Second, there are those who support further research in the area in the hope of developing genuinely therapeutic procedures, but who recognize the importance of safeguarding against potential abuses in the course of this development. Finally, there are the antipsychosurgeons, who argue for the total prohibition of psychosurgery on ethical, spiritual, or political grounds, independent of its characterization as experimental or therapeutic.

The controversy reached up to the United States Senate Health Subcommittee in the spring of 1973 and resulted in U.S. Public Law 93-348, which created the National Committee for the Protection of Human Subjects of Biomedical and Behavioral Research. Although in its recommendations to the executive and legislative branches of the federal government the Commission did not feel it necessary to propose an extreme and complete moratorium on the performance of all psychosurgical interventions, the Commission did recommend the passage of strict legal guidelines regulating psychosurgery and patient selection in order to prevent the possibility of future abuses. The specific recommendations made by the Commission include the following:

1. Psychosurgery should be performed only at institutions having a DHEW-approved Institutional Review Board. The board evaluates the merits of performing surgery according to ethical, legal, medical, and psychiatric criteria outlined in the following recommendations.

2. Psychosurgical intervention can be applied for no other reason than to provide treatment to the individual.

3. The patient must give informed consent. If the patient is in no state of mind to give "informed" consent, another subset of very strict guidelines (not specified here) must be followed. In no case should psychosurgery be performed over the objections of an adult patient, even following adjudication of incompetence and with the consent of legal guardian. Prisoners, involuntarily committed mental patients, and children are not to be subjected to psychosurgery.

4. All surgery is to be carried out by neurosurgeons sufficiently familiar with the specific procedures to assure competent performance. The Commission reports that "approximately 25% of the total number of operations performed in the United States are performed by surgeons doing no more than three operations per year, and many surgeons who perform psychosurgery average only one per year."

5. A specific psychosurgical procedure must have had demonstrable benefit for the treatment of specific psychiatric symptoms.

6. Thorough pre- and postoperative psychiatric evaluations must be carried out in all cases. Comparable data are to be obtained from standardized, objective test batteries.

Such recommendations will, in all probability, lead to legislation regulating psychosurgical practice. Such legislation appears necessary, for it seems that in too many psychosurgical cases reported by psychiatrists and neurosurgeons having slightly more than an objective interest, glowingly optimistic conclusions have been

MARC JOUANDET AND
MICHAEL S.
GAZZANIGA

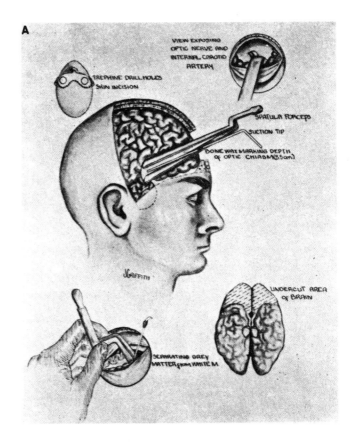

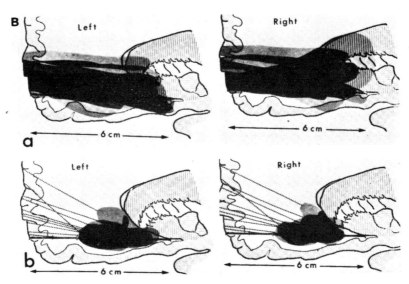

Fig. 11. A: Scoville's orbital undercutting (From Scoville: Surgical location for psychiatric surgery with special reference to orbital and cingulate operations. In Laitinen and Livingston (eds.), *Surgical Approaches in Psychiatry*, © 1973, University Park Press, Baltimore, Md. Reprinted with permission from Livingston.) B: Comparison between orbital undercutting and yttrium-90 implant techniques. (From Corsellis and Jack: Neuropathological observations on yttrium implants and on undercutting in the orbitofrontal areas of the brain. In Laitinen and Livingston (eds.), *Surgical Approaches in Psychiatry*, © 1973, University Park Press, Baltimore, Md. Reprinted with permission from Livingston.)

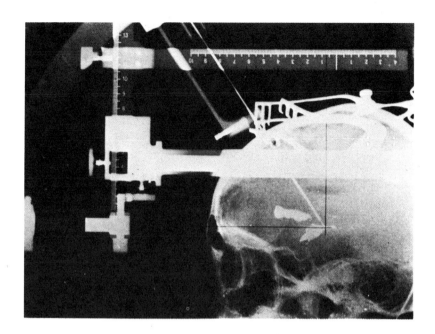

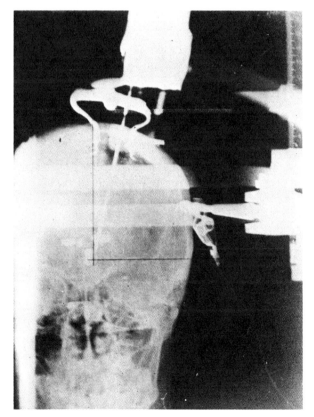

Fig. 12. Lateral and anteroposterior radiographs demonstrating the stereotaxic destruction of the posterior hypothalamus to control "aggressive behavior." (From Schvarcz: Stereotactic cryohypothalamotomy in aggressive behavior. In Sweet, Obrador, and Martin-Rodriguez (eds.), *Neurosurgical Treatment in Psychiatry, Pain, and Epilepsy,* © 1977, University Park Press, Baltimore, Md. Reprinted with permission from the author and the publisher.)

MARC JOUANDET AND
MICHAEL S.
GAZZANIGA

drawn without comparison to adequate control data. Annas and Glantz (1974) write:

> Psychosurgeons reporting their own results in their own scales have claimed amazing rates of success. Although these self-evaluated "before and after" studies reveal some of the danger involved [in psychosurgery], their anecdotal nature destroys their utility for the purpose of determining whether psychosurgery is a therapeutic medical procedure.

The National Commission provides some insight into the pervasiveness of this inadequate psychiatric evaluation:

> 54% of the articles published worldwide contained no information from objective tests. Of the 70 articles [out of 152] which reported the results of any objective tests, 16 referred only to an I.Q. test. In the United States, 56% of the published articles mentioned no objective tests, 11% reported only one, 8% only two, and approximately 25% reported from three or more.

The pervasive application of the "schizophrenia" diagnosis has produced much disagreement and not a little confusion within the psychiatric community as to the efficiency of psychosurgical intervention in the treatment of that malady. The majority of psychosurgical operations, however, have come in recent years to be applied in cases of fear, anxiety, obsessive-compulsive disorders, and neurotic depression (Valenstein, 1977).

However, in retrospective studies comparing leucotomized patients with control patients adequately matched for age, sex, marital status, educational and occupational levels, age on hospitalization, and duration of hospitalization, the differences in long-term recovery between the leucotomized and control patients are statistically insignificant when not entirely absent (Robin, 1958, 1959; Pollitt, 1960; Witton and Ellsworth, 1962; McKenzie and Kaczanowski, 1964; Tan *et al.*, 1971; Breggin, 1972; Robin and McDonald, 1975).

Rigorous statistical comparisons of the effectiveness of the therapeutic strategies of various psychoanalytic or behavioral schools, in general, have not been encouraging (Grinker, 1969). Mark (1974) admits that there are "no valid statistical data indicating that any particular form of psychotherapy is more effective in treating seriously ill mental patients than any other form of treatment or even chance alone." In the absence of clear neurophysiological and anatomical disease, current methods of psychological assessment are alone clearly inadequate in arriving at diagnoses justifying surgery (Robin and McDonald, 1975; Chorover, 1974; Annas and Glantz, 1974). Tragically, the operations performed on thousands of humans have not yielded a consistently applicable theory aiding in the a-priori selection of patients most likely to benefit from surgery because of inconsistencies in methods of data collection. It appears that elegant surgical technology has far surpassed psychological understanding.

Attempts to approximate successively the goal of eradicating symptoms of certain forms of mental illness while simultaneously preserving the personality, appropriate emotional responsiveness, and intellect of the patient, through the elegant refinement of surgical techniques producing more precise damage to specific anatomical structures, are completely gratuitous without correlation to accurate psychological data. But such attempts imply the adoption of assumptions that there are, in Scoville's (1973) words, "specific areas in the brain linked to depression, schizophrenia, or neurosis," as if there were particular centers in the brain solely associated with holistic psychological functions. The theoretical framework guiding the selection of certain tissues over others for destruction has remained as obscure as current knowledge remains limited on the exact functional role of specific target fibers within the limbic system and frontal lobes. But whatever the precise functions of these systems, it might safely be suggested that they will not ultimately be described in psychodynamic terms. Discrete lesions or arrays of lesions placed in various brain structures will never alleviate particular symptoms of a constellation; they will only succeed in decreasing the versatility of behavioral or emotional responding.

Because of the great proliferation of surgical methodologies, the utilization of inadequate diagnostic procedures, and the paucity of control or follow-up data, it is difficult to see how the occasional theoretical conclusions on the nature of physiological dysfunctioning of the orbitofrontal regions can be looked on without some skepticism. But even if such conclusions were based on rigorous statistical analyses, it should not be forgotten that the patients chosen for psychosurgery had been institutionalized for emotional or behavioral instability. Conclusions, therefore, on the functional properties of particular brain structures of specific patient samples can only with great care be generalized to the normal population.

LATERAL SURFACE OF THE PREFRONTAL CORTEX

It was because the lateral prefrontal cortex was believed responsible for subserving "intellectual" processes that psychiatric surgeons refined their techniques. In fact, a major inducement for refining the surgical procedures of leucotomy was to minimize or avoid completely secondary damage to the lateral surface. Because few psychosurgical papers report damaging these areas, theories of lateral prefrontal function do not arise from the psychosurgical literature. Much of what is currently known of the cognitive processing capabilities of the lateral surface is based on cases involving patients who were otherwise psychiatrically normal before the development of brain disease or before suffering accidents resulting in head injuries.

Patients suffering from cerebrovascular accidents, penetrating missle wounds, brain tumors, and other neural diseases in and around the lateral prefrontal regions were assessed by psychiatrists and neurologists who felt little need to justify, on psychological grounds, surgical interventions requiring debridement, the removal of tumors, or the excision of epileptogenic cortex or other diseased tissues. Such surgical interventions have often been straightforwardly justified in life-or-death terms. Neurocognitive analyses of these patients might be viewed to be somewhat more objective. Control data are often available in the form of comparison with patients suffering from cortical damage restricted to the parietal, temporal, or occipital lobes. Let us consider, then, some of the results and theoretical conclusions of researchers assessing cognitive dysfunctioning produced from damage restricted to the lateral prefrontal cortex and the insight into possible normal functioning that these studies provide.

MARC JOUANDET AND
MICHAEL S.
GAZZANIGA

VISUAL PROCESSES OF THE LATERAL PREFRONTAL CORTEX. Brodmann's area 8, although cytoarchitecturally agranular cortex, is, because of mediodorsal thalamic ramification (Akert, 1964), generally considered prefrontal cortex (von Bonin, 1949; Nauta, 1971, 1974). This region, located in the rhesus monkey anterior to the arcuate sulcus, has been popularly known as the "frontal eye fields" ever since Ferrier's (1886) discovery that conjugate horizontal or vertical eye movements could be evoked by the application of electrical stimulation to different portions of this region. Ablation, surprisingly, fails to cause long-lasting visual or oculomotor impairments (Pasik and Pasik, 1964). Earlier suggestions that the "frontal eye fields" function as a motor area for the ocular musculature have, over the years, been found incongruous with empirically determined facts.

Anatomical Connections of the "Frontal Eye Fields." There is no anatomical evidence for a direct connection between the frontal eye fields and the oculomotor nuclei (Astruc, 1971). The frontal termination field in the rhesus monkey for fibers arising from the visual association cortex (areas 18 and 19 of Brodmann) extends primarily from the rostral bank of the lower limb of the arcuate sulcus to the caudal tip of the principal sulcus (Chavis and Pandya, 1976). The gyrus immediately rostral to the arcuate sends fibers to the somatosensory regions of the inferior parietal region (Pandya and Kuypers, 1969; Nauta, 1971). There is some physiological evidence for direct frontal lobe influence on occipital functioning. Chusid *et al.* (1948) have indicated the presence of long fiber connections from the frontal to the occipital lobes; McCulloch (1947) suggested their presence by electrophysiologically identifying connections from area 8 to the homolateral areas 18, 31, and 32 and to the contralateral area 18. There is some evidence that these fibers from area 8 effecting the contralateral area 18 do so via the splenium of the corpus callosum (Yoshimura, 1909; Doty, 1973).

Ocular Movements and Corollary Discharge. The role of the prefrontal zones with respect to ocular movements is indirect, complex in the focusing of visual attention, and generally believed responsible for making visual perception a dynamically active process. Bizzi (1968), on the strength of electrophysiological recordings, has identified two cell types in the frontal eye fields of rhesus monkeys. Type I cells fire only during saccadic eye movements to one or the other side, whereas Type II cells fire only during smooth pursuit movements to one side or the other. Bizzi and Schiller (1970) have also reported a third cell type firing when the head is turned to one side or the other. All these cells, it should be emphasized, fire only *after* the initiation of eye or head movements. Because these experiments were carried out in a completely darkened room, afferent sensory information from the occipital lobes was eliminated as a possible source of the heightened activity; somatosensory afferent feedback from the proprioceptors of the ocular musculature was also ruled out on logical grounds because of the differential responding of the two cell types for different movement velocities. The authors suggest that their results support Teuber's (1960, 1964) corollary discharge theory, which states that the central initiation of voluntary movement consists of a primary efferent discharge to the appropriate musculature and a corollary discharge to the sensory systems which need to be set for anticipated changes in sensory input that may result from the voluntary movement. This hypothesis has been used to explain why a visual scene appears to remain stable despite naturally occurring voluntary eye movements, and also why apparent shifts of scene occur when the eyeball is moved passively in its orbit by some external object. Teuber (1964) has elegantly investigated the extent to which frontal lobe activity influences perceptual processes. When their heads were held upright, normal human subjects, as well as frontal and posteriorly lesioned patients, made few errors in vertically positioning a luminous straight line in a darkened room. However, when their heads were tilted as little as 30°, errors of overcompensation by the frontal patients were dramatically worse than those errors made by the posteriorly lesioned patients and normal subjects. The overcompensation seen for normal and posterior patients, Teuber suggests, is kept minimal because of the corollary discharge that presets the central receptor structures for sensory activity that is predictable given certain activity in the motor areas.

It might also be interesting to note at this point that a gradual accommodation to scotomata resulting from a lesion in area striata is permanently dissipated after frontal eye field extirpation (Weiskrantz and Cowey, 1970; Chow *et al.*, 1951; Doty, 1973).

Contralateral Visual Field Neglect, Visual Search, and Cognition. One consequence of frontal eye field ablation, first reported by Munk (1881), is a temporary contralateral visual field neglect (Bianchi, 1895; Hitzig, 1904; Minkowski, 1911; Lashley, 1921; Clark and Lashley, 1947; Morin *et al.*, 1951). Because this neglect has been reported to disappear between 2 and 6 weeks after the ablation, its observation in man has not often occurred (Doty, 1973). Jenkner and Kutschera (1965) report that their patient suffered a frontally produced "pseudohemianopia" involving a lack of attention to objects and persons in the contralateral visual field despite an intact visual field perimeter. This phenomenon might then be viewed to be one related to dysfunctions resulting from interruptions in corollary discharge. Teuber *et al.* (1960) also report that, in a visual search task, bifrontal patients exhibit significant reductions in speed and efficiency of search; in unilateral cases, disproportionately long searching times for correct stimuli located in the visual field contralateral to the lesion are reported.

Consistent with all this work are the findings of Luria and his fellow workers (Luria *et al.*, 1966; Luria, 1973*b*), who have observed that bifrontal patients suffer an "inertia of gaze" in which attention focuses persistently on only one aspect of the visual field. In addition, patients suffering massive bifrontal lesions fail to arrive at logical hypotheses on a thematic pictures test because oculomotor impairments preclude systematic visual exploration organized by the structure of the picture (see Fig. 13). The disturbances reported by Luria *et al.* (1966) are of a higher cognitive nature than the primary impairment of ocular movements. Although the patient could fixate on a point as well as visually trace a moving object, active control of eye movements by the patient was structured neither by thematic pictures nor by questions posed by the examiners on the thematic context of the pictures. The visual exploration patterns of normal subjects would, in contrast, differ greatly given different questions. Luria reports that frontal

MARC JOUANDET AND
MICHAEL S.
GAZZANIGA

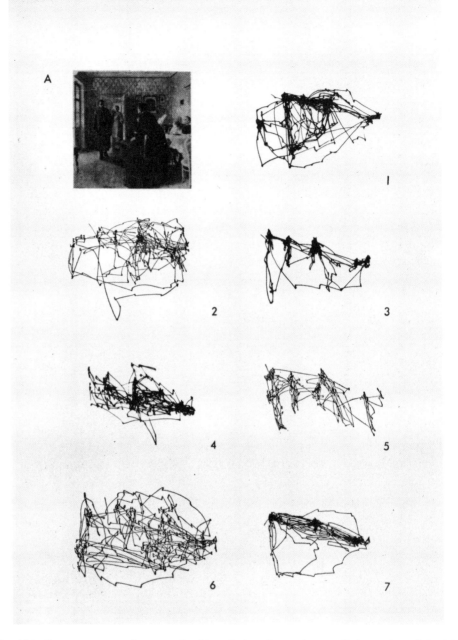

Fig. 13A. Eye movements of a normal subject during three minutes of observation of Repin's "Unexpected Return." Eye movement patterns change systematically in the analysis of particular details providing information relevant to the formation of answers to questions posed by the investigator. (From Luria, A. R. *Higher Cortical Functions in Man,* © 1966, Basic Books, New York. Reprinted with permission of the publisher.)

patients base their answers on isolated details rather than on details from initially given task features. Failure in this stage can render the issue of subsequent cognitive processing rather moot.

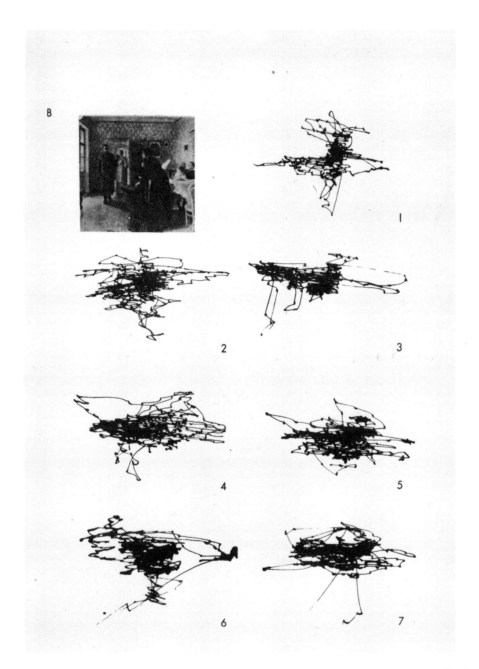

Figure 13B. Observations by frontal lobe patients. Eye movement patterns appear unstructured by the investigator's questions. (From Luria, A. R. *Higher Cortical Functions in Man,* © 1966, Basic Books, New York. Reprinted with permission of the publisher.)

Perhaps this brief discussion on the frontal eye fields begins to convey the level of complexity at which the prefrontal regions process information removed by several cognitive stages from the source of primary sensory input and the organization of primary motor output.

MARC JOUANDET AND
MICHAEL S.
GAZZANIGA

LANGUAGE PROCESSES OF THE LATERAL SURFACE. In the previous section on visual process, clinical observations have been able to rest on a fairly extensive literature based on experimental findings obtained with rhesus monkeys. When considering language impairments resulting from frontal lobe damage, no such rigorous experimental foundation exists—the clinical findings on language dysfunction, with all their potential for extreme variability among subjects, must stand alone.

The reports of language impairments resulting from frontal lobe damage discussed in subsequent sections of this chapter have been reported not to involve Broca's area, but rather regions anterior to it.

Teuber (1964) first drew attention to Feuchtwanger's (1923) study of 200 World War I veterans suffering frontal destruction resulting from cranial gunshot wounds. Zangwill (1966) highlighted Feuchtwanger's findings of "cerebral language disorders" in approximately 21% of those veterans with left frontal wounds anterior to Broca's area. This figure contrasts dramatically with the findings of only 2% language disorders for the veterans having right frontal destruction.

Verbal Fluency. A good deal of evidence has more recently accumulated that appears to suggest that there might be some lateralized differences in frontal functioning. Milner (1964) utilized a test of verbal paired associate learning and the Thurstone word fluency test to assess the verbal capacities of prefrontally excised patients. In the verbal learning test, she found no differences among subjects having left or right excisions; bilateral patients proved inferior to the two unilateral groups. She concluded that the verbal learning was equally subserved by the frontal regions of each hemisphere. On the Thurstone verbal fluency test, the patient is required to write down in 5 min as many words as possible that begin with a letter proposed by the experimenter. On this test, patients with left frontal excisions well anterior to Broca's area performed significantly worse than right frontal patients.

Benton (1968) confirmed these findings on the paired associate verbal learning test and on an oral version of the Thurstone verbal fluency test. There were no significant differences between the left and right unilateral groups on the verbal learning test. Each unilateral group performed much better than the bifrontal patients. Taken together, the Milner and Benton studies suggested that learning deficits were roughly proportional to the amount of frontal cortical damage incurred, whereas the verbal fluency deficits appeared attributable largely to damage in the left frontal lobe. Because the verbal fluency disability resulting from left frontal disease manifested itself independently of the mode of expression, whether oral or written, Benton suggested the existence of "a generalized higher language impairment in these non-aphasic patients." In addition to the verbal task results, Benton found some evidence indicating that right frontally damaged patients are equivalent to bifrontals and worse than left frontals on tasks involving block constructions and design copying. On the basis of these results, the attribution of spatial deficits exclusively to the parietooccipital regions of the right hemisphere was questioned.

Decay in verbal fluency performance after left frontal lesions was also observed by Ramier and Hécaen (1970). In an experiment involving 76 frontal and posteriorly damaged patients, left frontals were inferior to right frontals on verbal fluency tests. In addition to this finding, however, the authors were able to demonstrate that the right frontals were inferior to patients suffering right posterior lesions. These results led Ramier and Hécaen to postulate that performance on verbal fluency tasks depends on the interaction and integrity of two realms of cognitive processing: a general frontal lobe function responsible for regulating "spontaneity and initiative" and the classically recognized hemispheric specialization of the left cerebral hemisphere for verbal processes.

By correlating results obtained from oral verbal fluency tests with results from a modified version of the Stroop Test, Perret (1974) succeeded in demonstrating that the deficiency in verbal fluency following left frontal lesions is, in actuality, a manifestation of a more fundamental dysfunction. The Stroop Test applied consisted of three parts: in the first, patients were to identify the color (red, blue, yellow, green) in which an array of dots was printed; in the second, they were to identify the color in which words (conjunctions and adverbs) were printed, without saying the word; in the third, they were to identify the color in which different color names were printed. In order to perform the last portion of the test quickly and accurately, the patient must be able to categorize the separate features of the stimuli into ink color and verbal content, suppress the latter category, and respond only in accordance with the former. Among the six groups consisting of left and right frontal, temporal, and posterior lesioned patients, only the left frontals showed sharp deterioration in performance in the face of increasing categorical conflict. The results of the oral verbal fluency test administered to the six groups were completely consistent with those of Milner (1964), Benton (1968), and Ramier and Hácaen (1970). Correlation of the time taken to orally respond to the Stroop stimuli with the verbal fluency scores obtained on all groups yielded extremely significant product-moment correlation coefficients. Perret concludes by maintaining that the poor performance of left frontal patients on the Stroop Test and verbal fluency test stems from an inability to suppress the "normal habit of using words according to their meaning," and likened this difficulty to the "inertia of initial sets" displayed by the bifrontal rhesus monkeys in Mishkin's experiments (Mishkin, 1964; Mishkin *et al.*, 1969). Fluency decay, therefore, may be only a surface manifestation of deeper dysfunctioning: general response spontaneity and initiative (Ramier and Hécaen, 1970) or flexibility in switching cognitive sets (Perret, 1974) may be impaired.

Dissociation between Language and Behavior. In several of his excellent publications, Luria (1966*a*, 1973*b;* Luria and Homskaya, 1964; Luria *et al.*, 1964) has reported that some of his frontal patients exhibited poor abilities to "regulate their motor behaviors by speech." Although such patients exhibit no obvious motor dysfunctions and are quite capable of comprehending and repeating task instructions, they are nevertheless unable to carry out task instructions. Luria's views on the regulative functions of speech are clearly supported by Milner's findings demonstrating that the great majority of errors committed on a stylus maze task by patients having undergone frontocortical excision resulted from a failure to "follow the rules"—that is, they were unable to regulate their motor behaviors in accordance with comprehended verbal instructions. Awareness of task requirements is an end product of language processing. Presumably, consciousness of environmental contingencies remains through the functioning of the intact posterior cortical regions. However, either because this awareness is "disconnected" from frontal processors or because the processors themselves are destroyed, the awareness is ineffectual in patterning appropriate motor sequences. Language and motor behavior are therefore viewed to be dissociated, each functioning independently.

In a rather interesting case study, Konow and Pribram (1970) have described the symptoms of a patient who not only understood the task requirements well enough to repeat the instructions but also did so sufficiently well to detect and comment on her own errors as well as those purposely committed by the investigators when they demonstrated the task. These findings led the authors to distinguish between error recognition and error utilization: although frontal patients recognize their own errors and those of others, they are unable to use this higher-order error feedback information to improve their own motor performances. This inability to utilize error feedback is consistent with findings of high perseverative error rates on the relatively nonverbal Wisconsin Card Sorting Test. For one of our own frontal patients, it was quite apparent that he was puzzled and concerned about his perseverative errors that persisted even after he discerned and verbalized to us the requirements of the task. He exhibited, in Milner's (1964) words, the "curious dissociation between the ability to verbalize the requirements of the task and the ability to use this verbalization as a guide to action." Because language and speech in these frontal patients appear to be largely intact, as hinted at in Perret's (1974) findings, the "dissociation of language and behavior" may also really be only one manifestation of a deeper dysfunction. It is not that motor behavior is dissociated from speech but simply that there is a breakdown in the system that sequences or guides motor behaviors toward the attainment of some immediate or distant goal.

PREFRONTAL ORGANIZATION OF BEHAVIOR. That prefrontal damage leads to an impairment in the planning of future behavioral activities has been suspected ever since publication of Harlow's (1868) classical report of Phineas Gage's unfortunate mishap: "The passage of an iron bar through the head." Harlow writes that Mr. Gage was "obstinate yet capricious and vacillating in devising many plans of future operations which are no sooner arranged than they are abandoned in turn for others appearing more feasible." Bianchi's (1895, 1922) observations on frontally ablated dogs and monkeys led him to conclude that the coordination and fusion of various sensorimotor elements into more complex goal-directed activities breaks down as a result of such damage.

Performance Errors and Flexible Noticing Orders. More recently, Luria and his colleagues (Luria, 1966a, 1973b; Luria *et al.,* 1964) have proposed that successful problem-solving behavior involves several stages of processing. These stages have been succinctly reduced to four by Lhermitte, Derouesne, and Signoret (1972): (1) systematic orientation to and analysis of initially presented task features, (2) generation of several alternative hypothetical solutions, (3) flexible formulation of appropriate motor programs for each of those solutions, and (4) evaluation of result adequacy through comparison of the programs with higher-order error feedback.

Some frontal patients fail problem-solving tasks because they cannot, for various reasons, extract information-rich details from initially given task features. The failure of some frontal patients on Luria's thematic pictures task, for example, precludes subsequent hypothesis formulation.

Other prefrontal patients capable of understanding the task requirements and analyzing relevant stimuli, as exhibited by their verbal description of appropriate action programs, appear to suffer a dysfunctioning in the process of comparing response feedback information with the planned action of the program. Although some of these patients are capable of verbally expressing task requirements, they may not sense or express dissatisfaction with the inappropriate results of their actions. The goal-oriented action programs lose their regulating influence on behavior because of a breakdown in neural systems utilizing error feedback information in comparator processes. This breakdown in the comparison between programmed action and behavioral feedback results in errors that express themselves in two ways that on the surface appear strikingly contradictory: susceptibility to distraction by irrelevant stimuli; and perseverative tendencies in responding. Pribram (1973) argues that frontal monkeys fail delayed-response tasks because they fail to inhibit responding to irrelevant stimuli. Pribram further suggests that this failure may be due to an inability to "register novelty," which would otherwise be an aid to inhibition through habituation.

Although perseveration, the stereotyped repetition of motor patterns no longer appropriate, appears to be contradictory to distraction, it may be that perseveration results from the "influence of irrelevant *associations*"—the dominating influence of prior associations over the contingencies presented by the current situation (Luria, 1966*a*). Luria *et al.* (1964) have suggested that the "inability to inhibit impulsive reactions" to irrelevant stimuli and the "tendency toward a fixed repetition of movement" both stem from the subject's "inability to organize and reorganize behavior when flexibility is demanded."

Pribram (1973) theorizes that, in situations in which appropriate behaviors are incompletely specified by the environmental situation, the frontal lobes normally function to keep interference at a minimum through a context-dependent "flexible noticing order" system regulating information flow and processing. The flexible noticing order system functions by assigning processing time and space priorities to a multitude of simultaneously noticed and weighted sensory events so that each event impinging on the system is processed in turn of importance while other events are held back to avoid overloading. It is believed that in this way the appropriate focusing of attention is facilitated, interference by irrelevant stimuli and associations is inhibited, and higher-order error feedback is effectively utilized. When the frontal lobes are functioning properly, goal-directed, problem-solving behaviors need not be deterred from their more excellent, long-range pursuits.

Contingent Negative Variation. Pribram finds neurophysiological support for the existence of a flexible noticing order in Walter's (Walter *et al.*, 1964*a,b*, 1965) discovery of the contingent negative electrical variation (CNV), or expectancy wave, recorded from scalp electrodes over the human frontal cortex. The CNV appears during the anticipatory intervals preceding motor responses whose timing of occurrence is not completely specified by current environmental contingencies

(Walter *et al.*, 1964*a,b*, 1965, 1966). This wave-form is believed to function as a "marker or flag" necessary to prevent distracting interference in a flexible noticing order system.

Since Walter's discovery, an entire literature has flourished to demonstrate the reality of the phenomenon. Stamm and Rosen (1969) found negative electrical shifts in the occipital cortex when conditioning and reinforcement lights were presented, in the prefrontal cortex during the delay period, and in the motor cortex during the instrumental response. The degree of motivation to perform the expectancy task is proportionally reflected by the amplitude of the CNV (Irwin *et al.*, 1966; Rebert *et al.*, 1967; Borda, 1970). Walter (1973) discusses some phenomenal findings indicating the sensitivity of the expectancy wave to social influences. Expectancy wave amplitude increases slowly during the initial training trials of the delayed-response task and, once established, persists for as long as the subject remains motivated to accurately perform the task. Twenty to fifty extinction trials are necessary to return the amplitude of the contingent negative variation back to zero. However, when the subject is told by the experimenter that the operant response is no longer necessary, the change in electrophysiological activity is dramatic: Walter (1973) writes that

> the CNV subsides at once. One can say that a single accurate trustworthy social instruction is equivalent in probability to 20 to 50 direct experiences of associations of extinction. This "figure of merit" naturally depends on the social relation between the experimenter and the subject, because instructions from a stranger or anyone likely to tease or trick the subject have an adverse effect on the CNV.

Quantitative Examination of the Theory. Although the data obtained from the Wisconsin Card Sorting Task and from the verbal and spatial fluency exams have been rigorously quantitative, the greatest drawback to Luria's and Pribam's theories lies in the largely qualitative, anecdotal nature of the case reports. Only recently have quantitative tests of these theories appeared (Drewe, 1974; 1975*a,b*). On go–no go, go left–go right, compatible and incompatible conditional discrimination tasks, Drewe (1975*a*) reported data somewhat inconsistent with the theories proposed by Luria and his colleagues. Drewe's tests have been those fairly commonly used in the past to map the cognitive capabilities of rhesus monkeys (Rosvold and Mishkin, 1961; Mishkin, 1964; Brutokowski, 1964). Although consistent with the results obtained on nonhuman primates, they are, however, greatly reductionistic measures of human cognitive processes.

Conclusion

The various functions of the lateral prefrontal cortex appear to converge in suggesting that these tissues contribute a special feature to human imagination. We might speculate that, just as the left parietal region evolved the capability of analyzing the external environment verbally, and as the right parietal cortex came to analyze the external world in three spatial dimensions, so may the frontal lobes have come to contribute in their later stages of phylogenic evolution to the limitless analytic powers of the human psyche by superimposing on the three spatial dimensions a profound mastery of the fourth dimension of time.

Aimard, G., Devic, M., Lebel, M., Trouillas, P., and Boisson, D. Agraphie pure (dynamic?) d'origine frontale. *Revue Neurologique (Paris),* 1975, *31(7),* 505–512.

Akert, K. Comparative anatomy of frontal cortex and thalamofrontal connections. In J. M. Warren and K. Akert (eds.), *The Frontal Granular Cortex and Behavior.* New York: McGraw-Hill, 1964, p. 372.

Annas, G. J., and Glantz, L. H. Psychosurgery: The law's response. In *Psychosurgery.* Boston University Law Review and Center for Law and Health Sciences, Boston University School of Law. Lexington, Mass.: Lexington Books, 1974, pp. 33–51.

Astruc, J. Corticofugal connections of area 8 (frontal eye field) in *Macaca mulatta. Brain Research,* 1971, *33,* 241.

Bailey, P., and von Bonin, G. *The Isocortex of Man.* Urbana: University of Illinois Press, 1951.

Ballantine, H. T., Cassidy, W., Flanagan, N. B., and Marino, R. Stereotaxic anterior cingulectomy for neurpsychiatric illness and untractable pain. *Journal of Neurosurgery,* 1967, *26,* 488.

Barbizet, J. Role du lobe frontal dans les conduites Mnesique. *La Press Medicale,* 1971, *79,* 2033–2037.

Barbizet, J., Duizabo, P., and Flavigmy, R. Role des lobe frontaux dans le langage. *Revue Neurologique (Paris),* 1975, *131(8),* 525–544.

Benton, A. L. Differential behavioral effects in frontal lobe disease. *Neuropsychologia,* 1968, *6,* 53–60.

Bianchi, L. The functions of the frontal lobes. *Brain,* 1895, *18,* 497–522.

Bianchi, L. *The Mechanism of the Brain and the Function of the Frontal Lobes.* New York: Livingstone, 1922.

Bizzi, E. Discharge of frontal eye field neurons during saccadic and following eye movements in unanesthetized monkeys. *Experimental Brain Research,* 1968, *9,* 69.

Bizzi, E., and Schiller, P. H. Single unit activity in the frontal eye fields of unanesthetized monkeys during eye and head movements. *Experimental Brain Research,* 1970, *10,* 151.

Borda, R. P. The effects of altered drive states on the contingent negative variation in rhesus monkeys. *Electroencephalographic Clinical Neurophysiology,* 1970, *29,* 173–180.

Breggin, P. R. The return of the lobotomy and psychosurgery. *Congressional Record,* 1972, *118,* 26, Feb. 24.

Brodmann, K. *Vergleichende Lokalisationslehre der Grosshirnrinde.* Leipzig: Barth, 1909.

Brutokowski, S. Prefrontal cortex and drive inhibition. In J. M. Warren and K. Akert (eds.), *The Frontal Granular Cortex and Behavior.* New York, McGraw-Hill, 1964.

Burckhardt, G. Ueber Rindenexcisionen, als Beitrag zur operativen Therapie der Psychoen. *Allgemeine Zeitschrift für Psychiatrie und Ihre Grenzigebriete,* 1891, *47,* 463–548.

Chavis, D. A., and Pandya, D. N. Further observations on corticofrontal connections in the rhesus monkey. *Brain Research,* 1976, *117,* 3, 369–386.

Chorover, S. L. Psychosurgery: A neurophysiological perspective. In *Psychosurgery.* Boston University Law Review and Center for Law and Health Sciences, Boston University School of Law. Lexington Mass.: Lexington Books, 1974, pp. 15–32.

Chow, K. L., Blum, J. S., and Blum, R. A. Effects of combined destruction of frontal and posterior "associative areas" in monkeys. *Journal of Neurophysiology,* 1951, *14,* 59–71.

Chusid, T. G., Sugar, O., and French, J. D. Corticortical connections of the cerebral cortex lying within the arcuate and lunate sulci of the monkey *(Macaca mulatta). Journal of Neuropathology and Experimental Neurology,* 1948, *7,* 439–446.

Clark, G., and Lashley, K. S. Visual disturbances following frontal ablations in the monkey. *Amatomical Record,* 1947, *97,* 326.

Corsellis, J., and Jack, A. B. Neuropathological observations on yttrium implants and on undercutting in the orbitofrontal areas of the brain. In L. Laitinen (ed.), *Surgical Approaches in Psychiatry.* Baltimore: University Park Press, 1973, pp. 96–100.

Curtis, B. A., Jacobson, S., Marcus, E. M. *An Introduction to the Neurosciences.* Philadelphia: Saunders, 1972.

Denny-Brown, D. The frontal lobes and their functions. In A. Feiling (ed.), *Modern Trends in Neurology.* London: Butterworth, 1951, pp. 13–89.

Denny-Brown, D. *The Cerebral Control of Movement.* The Sherrington Lectures VII. Springfield, Ill.: Thomas, 1966.

DeVito, J. L., and Smith, O. E. Subcortical projections of the prefrontal lobe of the monkey. *Journal of Comparative Neurology,* 1964, *123,* 413–424.

Doty, R. W. Ablation of visual areas in the central nervous system. In R. Jung (ed.), *Handbook of Sensory Physiology.* Berlin: Springer-Verlag, 1973.

Drewe, E. A. The effect of type and area of brain lesion on Wisconsin Card Sorting Test performance. *Cortex,* 1974, *10,* 159–170.

Drewe, E. A. An experimental investigation of Luria's theory on the effects of frontal lobe lesions in man. *Neuropsychologia*, 1975a, *13*, 421–429.

Drewe, E. A. Go–no go learning after frontal lobe lesions in humans. *Cortex*, 1975b, *11*, 8–16.

Ferrier, D. *The Functions of the Brain*. London: Smith, Elder and Co., 1886.

Feuchtwanger, E. Die Funktioner des Stirnhirns. In O. Forster and K. Willmanns (eds.), *Monographien aus dem Gesamtgebiete der Neurologie und Psychiat*. Berlin: Springer, 1923.

Freeman, W. Frontal lobotomy in early schizophrenia. *British Journal of Psychiatry*, 1971, *119*, 621–622.

Freeman, W., and Watts, J. W. *Psychosurgery*. Springfield, Ill.: Thomas, 1942.

Fritsch, G. T., and Hitzig, E. Über die electrische erregbarkeit des Grosshirns. *Archiv für Anatomie und Physiologie, Physiologische Abteilung*, 1870, *37*.

Fulton, J. H. *The Frontal Lobes and Human Behavior*. Sherrington Lectures II. Springfield, Ill.: Thomas, 1952.

Fulton, J. F., and Jacobsen, C. F. The functions of the frontal lobes, a comparative study in monkeys, chimpanzees, and man. *Abstracts of the Second International Neurological Congress*. London, 1935, pp. 70–71.

Grinker, G. Emerging concepts of mental illness and models of treatment: The medical point of view. *American Journal of Psychiatry*, 1969, *125*, 865–866.

Guillery, R. W. Afferent fibers to the dorsomedial thalamic nucleus in the cat. *Journal of Anatomy (London)*, 1959, *93*, 403–419.

Harlow, J. M. Recovery from the passage of an iron bar through the head. *Publications of the Massachusetts Medical Society*, 1868, *2*, 327.

Hebb, D. O. Intelligence in man after large removals of cerebral tissue: Report on four left frontal lobe cases. *Journal of Genetic Psychology*, 1939, *21*, 73–87.

Hécaen, H. Mental symptoms associated with tumors of the frontal lobe. In J. M. Warren and K. Akert (eds.), *The Frontal Granular Cortex and Behavior*. New York: McGraw-Hill, 1964, pp. 335–351.

Hitzig, E. Physiologische und klinische Untersuchunger über des Gehirn. *Gessammelte Abhandlungen*, I, II, 1904.

Irwin, D. A., Knott, J. R., McAdam, D. W., and Rebert, C. S. Motivational determinants of the "contingent negative variation." *Electroencephalographic Clinical Neurophysiology*. 1966, *21*, 584–543.

Jacobson, S., Trojanowski, J. Q. Prefrontal granular cortex of the rhesus monkey. I: Intrahemispheric cortical afferents. *Brain Research*, 1977, *132*, 209–233.

Jenkner, F. L., and Kutschera, E. Frontal lobes and vision. *Confinia Neurologica*, 1965, *25*, 63–78.

Jones, E. G., and Powell, T. P. S. An anatomical study of converging sensory pathways within the cerebral cortex of the monkey. *Brain*, 1970, *93*, 793.

Kaada, B. R. Somatomotor autonomic and electrocorticographic responses to electrical stimulation of rhinencephalic and other structures in primates, cat and dog. *Acta Physiologica Scandinavia*, 1951, *23*, Suppl. 83.

Krieg, W. J. S. *Connections of the Frontal Cortex of the Monkey*. Springfield, Ill.: Thomas, 1954.

Krieg, W. J. S. *Connections of the Cerebral Cortex*. Evanston, Ill.: Brain Books, 1963.

Knight, G. C. Stereotaxic tractotomy in surgical treatment of mental illness. *Journal of Neurology, Neurosurgery, and Psychiatry*, 1965, *28*, 304.

Konow, A., and Pribram, K. H. Error recognition and utilization produced by injury to the frontal cortex in man. *Neuropsychology*, 1970, *8*, 489–491.

Lashley, K. S. Studies of cerebral functioning in learning. III. The motor areas. *Brain*, 1921, *44*, 3, 255–285.

Lhermitte, F., Derouesne, J., and Signoret, J. L. Analyse neuropsychologiques du syndrome frontale. *Revue Neurologique*, 1972, *127*, 415–440.

Lindstrom, P. Psychosurgery. In Speigel (ed.), *Progress in Neurology and Psychiatry*. New York: Grune and Stratton, 1960, p. 15.

Livingston, K. E. Limbic system dysfunctioning induced by "kindling." Its significance for psychiatry. In W. H. Sweet, S. Obrador, and J. G. Martin-Rodriguez (eds.), *Neurosurgical Treatment in Psychiatry, Pain, and Epilepsy*. Baltimore: University Park Press, 1977, p. 245.

Livingston, K. E., and Escobar, A. Tentative limbic system models for certain patterns of psychiatric disorders. In L. V. Laitinen and K. E. Livingston (eds.), *Surgical Approaches in Psychiatry*. Baltimore: University Park Press, 1973, p. 245.

Luria, A. R. *Higher Cortical Functions in Man*. New York: Basic Books, 1966a.

Luria, A. R. *Human Brain and Mental Processes*. New York: Harper and Row, 1966b.

Luria, A. R. *The Working Brain*. New York: Basic Books, 1973a.

Luria, A. R. The frontal lobes and the regulation of behavior. In K. H. Pribram and A. R. Luria (eds.), *Psychophysiology of the Frontal Lobes*. New York: Academic Press, 1973b, pp. 3–26.

Luria, A. R., and Homskaya, E. D. Disturbances in the regulative role of speech with frontal lobe lesions. In. J. M. Warren and K. Akert (eds.), *The Frontal Granular Cortex and Behavior.* New York: McGraw-Hill, 1964, p. 352.

Luria, A. R., Pribram, K. H., and Homskaya, E. D. An experimental analysis of the behavioral disturbances produced by a left frontal arachnoidal endothelioma (meningioma). *Neuropsychologia,* 1964, *2,* 280.

Luria, A. R., Karpov, B. A., and Yarbuss, A. L. Disturbances of active visual perception with lesions of the frontal lobes. *Cortex,* 1966, *2,* 202–212.

Luria, A. R., Homskaya, E. D., Blinkov, S. M., and Critchley, M. Impaired selectivity of mental processes associated with a lesion of the frontal lobe. *Neuropsychologia,* 1967, *5,* 105–117.

Mark, V. H. Psychosurgery versus anti-psychiatry. In *Psychosurgery.* Boston University Law Review and Center for Law and Health Sciences, Boston University School of Law. Lexington, Mass.: Lexington Books, 1974, pp. 1–14.

Mark, V. H., and Ervin, F. *Violence and the Brain.* New York: Harper and Row, 1970.

McCulloch, W. S. Modes of functional organization of the cerebral cortex . *Federation Proceedings,* 1947, *6,* 448–452.

McKenzie, K. G., and Kaczanowski, G. Prefrontal leucotomy: A five year controlled study. *Canadian Medical Association,* 1964, *91,* 1193.

Mettler, F. A. *Selective Partial Ablation of the Frontal Cortex.* New York: Hoeber, 1949.

Meyer, A. The frontal lobe syndrome, the aphasias, and related conditions. *Brain,* 1974, *97,* 565–600.

Milner, B. Effects of different brain lesions on card sorting. The role of the frontal lobes. *Archives of Neurology,* 1963, *9,* 90–99.

Milner, B. Some effects of frontal lobectomy in man. In J. M. Warren and K. Akert (eds.), *The Frontal Granular Cortex and Behavior.* New York: McGraw-Hill, 1964, pp. 313–331.

Milner, B. Interhemispheric differences in the localization of psychological processes in man. *British Medical Bulletin,* 1971, *27,* 272–277.

Minkowski, M. Zur Physiologie der Sehsphäre. *Pfluegers Archiv Gesamte für die Physiologie des Menschen und der Tiere,* 1911, *141,* 171.

Mishkin, M. Perseveration of central sets after frontal lesions in monkeys. In J. M. Warren and K. Akert (eds.), *The Frontal Granular Cortex and Behavior.* New York: McGraw-Hill, 1964, pp. 219–237.

Mishkin, M., Vest, B., Waxler, M., and Rosvold, H. E. A re-examination of the effects of frontal lesions on object alternation. *Neuropsychologia,* 1969, *7,* 357–363.

Moniz, E. Prefrontal leucotomy in the treatment of mental disorders. *American Journal of Psychiatry,* 1937, *93,* 1379.

Morin, G., Donnet, V., Maffre, R., and Naquet, R. Sur les troubles de la vision consécutifs aux décortications frontale chez le chien. *Journal of Physiology (Paris),* 1951, *43,* 825–826.

Munk, H. *Über die Funktion der Groshirnrinde: Gerammelte Mitteilunger aus den Jahren.* Berlin: Hirschwald, 1881.

Nauta, W. J. H. Neural associations of the amygdaloid complex in the monkey. *Brain,* 1962, *85,* 505.

Nauta, W. J. H. Some efferent connections of the prefrontal cortex in the monkey. In J. M. Warren and K. Akert (eds.), *The Frontal Granular Cortex and Behavior.* New York: McGraw-Hill, 1964, p. 397.

Nauta, W. J. H. The problem of the frontal lobe: A reinterpretation. *Journal of Psychiatric Research,* 1971, *8,* 167–187.

Nauta, W. J. H. Neural associations of the frontal cortex. *Acta Neurologica Experientia,* 1972, *32,* 125–140.

Nobel Lectures for Physiology and Medicine: 1942–1962. New York: Elsevier, 1964.

Pandya, D. N., and Kuypers, H. G. J. M. Cortico-cortical connections in the rhesus monkey. *Brain Research,* 1969, *13,* 13.

Papez, J. W. A proposed mechanism of emotion. *Archives of Neurological Psychiatry,* 1937, *38,* 725.

Pasik, P., and Pasik, T. Oculomotor functions in monkeys with lesions of the cerebrum and superior colliculus. In M. B. Bender (ed.), *The Oculomotor System.* New York: Harper and Row, 1964.

Penfield, W., and Jasper, H. *Epilepsy and the Functional Anatomy of the Human Brain.* Boston: Little, Brown, 1954.

Perret, E. The left frontal lobe of man and the suppression of habitual responses in verbal categorical behavior. *Neuropsychologia,* 1974, *12,* 323–330.

Phillips, G. C. Changing concepts of the precentral motor area. In J. C. Eccles (ed.), *Brain and Conscious Experience.* New York: Springer-Verlag, 1966.

Pippard, J. Leucotomy in Britain today. *British Journal of Psychiatry,* 1962, *108,* 249.

Pollitt, J. D. Natural history studies in mental illness. *Journal of Mental Science,* 1960, *106,* 93.

Powell, T. P. S. Sensory convergence in the cerebral cortex. In L. V. Laitinen and K. E. Livingston (eds.), *Surgical Approaches in Psychiatry*. Proceedings of the Third International Congress of Psychosurgery. Baltimore: University Park Press, 1973, pp. 266–281.

Powell, T. P. S., Cowan, W. M., and Raisman, G. The central olphactory connections. *Journal of Anatomy (London)*, 1965, *99*, 791.

Pribram, K. H. Theprimate frontal cortex—Executive of the Brain. In K. H. Pribram and A. R. Luria (eds.), *Psychophysiology of the Frontal Lobes*. New York: Academic Press, 1973.

Ramier, A. M., and Hécaen, H. Role respectif des atteintes frontales et de la lateralisation lesionelle dans les deficits de la "fluence verbale." *Revue Neurologiques*, 1970, *123*, 17–22.

Rebert, C. S., McAdam, D. W., Knott, J. R., and Irwin, D. A. Slow potential change in human brain related to level of motivation. *Journal of Comparative and Physiological Psychology*, 1967, *63*, 20–23.

Robin, A. A. A controlled study of the effects of leucotomy. *Journal of Neurology, Neurosurgery, and Psychiatry*. 1958, *21*, 262.

Robin, A. A. The value of leucotomy in relation to diagnosis. *Journal of Neurology, Neurosurgery, and Psychiatry*, 1959, *22*, 132.

Robin, A. A., and McDonald, D. *Lessons of Leucotomy*. London: Kimpton, 1975.

Rosvold, H. E., and Mishkin, M. Nonsensory effects of frontal lesions on discrimination learning and performance. In J. F. DeLafresnaye (ed.), *Brain Mechanisms and Learning*. Oxford, Blackwell, 1961.

Rylander, G. The renaissance of psychosurgery. In L. V. Laitinen and K. E. Livingston (eds.), *Surgical Approaches in Psychiatry*. Baltimore: University Park Press, 1973, pp. 3–12.

Schvarcz, J. R. Stereotactic cryohypothalamotomy in aggressive behavior. In W. H. Sweet, S. Obrador, and J. G. Martin-Rodriguez (eds.), *Neurosurgical Treatment in Psychiatry, Pain, and Epilepsy*. Baltimore: University Park Press, 1977, pp. 429–428.

Scoville, W. B. Selective cortical undercutting as a means of modifying and studying frontal lobe functions in man. *Journal of Neurosurgery*, 1949, *6*, 65.

Scoville, W. B. Surgical location for psychiatric surgery with special reference to orbital and cingulate operations. In L. V. Laitinen and K. E. Livingston (eds.), *Surgical Approaches in Psychiatry*. Baltimore: University Park Press, 1973, pp. 29–36.

Scoville, W. B., and Bettis, D. B. Results of orbital undercutting today: A personal series. *Neurosurgical Treatment in Psychiatry, Pain, and Epilepsy*, 1977, pp. 189–202.

Spencer, W. G. The effect produced upon respiration by faradic excitation of the cerebrum in the monkey, dog, and cat. *Philosophical Transactions of the Royal Society of London*, 1894, *185b*, 609–657.

Stamm, J. S., and Rosen, S. C. The locus and crucial time of implication of prefrontal cortex in the delayed response task. In K. H. Pribram and A. R. Luria (eds.), *Psychophysiology of the Frontal Lobes*. New York: Academic Press, 1973, pp. 139–153.

Tan, E., Marks, E. M., and Marset, P. Bimedial leucotomy in obsessive compulsive neuroses. A controlled serial inquiry. *British Journal of Psychiatry*, 1971, *118*, 115.

Teuber, H. L. Some alterations in behavior after cerebral lesions in man. In A. D. Bass (ed.), *Evolution of Nervous Control from Primitive Organisms to Man*. Washington, D.C.: American Association for the Advancement of Science, 1959, p. 157.

Teuber, H. L. The riddle of frontal lobe function in man. In J. M. Warren and K. Akert (eds.), *The Frontal Granular Cortex and Behavior*. New York: McGraw-Hill, 1964, p. 311.

Teuber, H. L., Battersby, W. S., and Bender, M. B. *Visual Field Defects After Penetrating Missle Wounds of the Brain*. Cambridge, Mass.: Harvard University Press, 1960.

Valenstein, E. S. The practice of psychosurgery: A survey of the literature (1971–1976). In *Psychosurgery*. The National Commission for the Protection of Human Subjects of Biomedical and Behavioral Research, 1977.

Vogt, C., and Vogt, O. Allgemeinere Ergebnisse unserer Hirnforschung. *Journal of Psychology and Neurology*, 1919, *25*, 279–461.

Von Economo, C. *The Cytoarchitectonics of the Human Cerebral Cortex*. New York: Oxford University Press, 1929.

von Bonin, G. Architecture of the precentral motor cortex and some adjacent area. In P. C. Bucy (ed.), *The Precentral Motor Cortex*. Urbana: University of Illinois Press, 1949.

von Bonin, G., and Bailey, P. *The Neocortex of Macaca mulatta*. Urbana: University of Illinois Press, 1947, 1–91.

Walker, A. E. A cytoarchitectural study of the prefrontal area in the macaque monkey. *Journal of Comparative Neurology*, 1940, *73*, 59–86.

Wall, P. D., Glees, P., and Fulton, J. F. Corticofugal connections of posterior orbital surface in rhesus monkey. *Brain*, 1951, *74*, 66–71.

Walter, W. G. Expectancy waves and intention waves in the human brain and their application to the direct cerebral control of machines. *Electroencephalographic Clinical Neurophysiology*, 1966, *21*, 616.

Walter, W. G. Human frontal lobe function in sensory motor association. In K. H. Pribram and A. R. Luria (eds.), *Psychophysiology of the Frontal Lobes*. New York: Academic Press, 1973, pp. 109–122.

Walter, W. G., Cooper, R., Aldridge, V. J., and McCallum, W. C. The contingent negative variation: An electrocortical sign of sensorimotor association in man. *Electroencephalographic Clinical Neurophysiology*, 1964a, *17*, 441.

Walter, W. G., Cooper, R., Aldridge, V. J., McCallum, W. C., and Winter, A. L. Contingent negative variation: An electric sign of sensory motor association and expectancy in the human brain. *Nature (London)*, 1964b, *23*, 380–384.

Walter, W. G., Cooper, R., McCallum, C., and Cohen, J. The origin and significance of the contingent negative variation on "expectancy wave." *Electroencephalographic Clinical Neurophysiology*, 1965, *18*, 720.

Weiskrantz, L., and Cowey, A. Filling in the scotoma: A study of residual vision after striate cortex lesions in monkeys. In E. Stellar and J. M. Sprague (eds.), *Progress in Physiological Psychology*. New York: Academic Press, 1970, p. 3.

Witton, K., and Ellsworth, R. B. Social and psychological (MMPI) changes 5–10 years after lobotomy. *Diseases of the Nervous System*, 1962, *23*, 440.

Woolsey, C. N., Settlage, P. H., Meyer, D. R., Pinto, T., and Travis, A. M. Patterns of localization in precentral and supplementary motor areas and their relation to the concept of a premotor area. *Research Publications, Association for Research in Nervous and Mental Disease*, 1950a, *30*, 238.

Woolsey, C. N., Settlage, P. H., Meyer, D. R., Spencer, W., Hamuy, T. P., and Travis, A. M. Patterns of localization in precentral and "supplementary" motor areas and their relation to the concept of a premotor area. *Annual Research of Nervous and Mental Disease, Proceedings*, 1950b, *30*, 238–264.

Yakolev, P. I. Motility, behavior, and the brain: Stereodynamic organization and neural coordinates of behavior. *Journal of Nervous Mental Diseases*, 1948, *107*, 313.

Yoshimura, K. Über des Benziehunger des Balkens zum Sehakt. *Pfluegers Archiv für die Gesamte Physiologie des Menschen und der Tiere*, 1909, *129*, 425–469.

Zangwill, C. L. Psychological deficits associated with frontal lobe lesions. *International Journal of Neurology*, 1966, *5*, 395–402.

3

Parietooccipital Symptomology: The Split-Brain Perspective

JOSEPH E. LeDoux

INTRODUCTION

During the period in which Lashley was promoting the view that cortical functions in the rat defied localization, clinical observations of humans with focal brain lesions were painting quite a different picture of cerebral organization. Localized damage to specific cortical regions was found to result in specific behavioral disturbances. Moreover, the behavioral disorders that emerged seemed to be dependent on the hemisphere damaged as well as on the intrahemispheric location of the pathology. This approach to brain and behavior caught on, and the field of neuropsychology was the result.

In the early 1960s, a series of reports appeared concerning observations of patients having undergone cerebral commissurotomy in an effort to manage otherwise intractable epileptic seizure activity. In these "split-brain" patients, it was possible to study hemispheric functions directly, rather than by inference of functions from capacities lost following lateralized damage. This was an important methodological breakthrough, for the symptoms produced by brain pathology do not necessarily coincide with the normal function of the damaged tissue. Although the split-brain approach is naturally limited in its potential for contributing to functional localization within a hemisphere, it can suggest hypotheses that are testable in a more general clinical setting, and, in addition, it can, to a large extent,

JOSEPH E. LeDoux   Department of Neurology, Cornell University Medical College, New York, New York 10021.

set some limiting conditions for interpreting the results of lesion studies of localization.

The goal of this chapter is to show how the results of split-brain and lesion studies can be integrated into a general clinical approach to brain and behavior. The discussion focuses on what split-brain data say about a variety of neuroclinical syndromes resulting from damage to the parietal lobes, the occipital lobes, or the fringe area in between.

CONSTRUCTIONAL APRAXIA

Constructional apraxia is a disturbance of formative activities in which the spatial part of the task is missed, although there is no apraxia for individual movements (Kliest, 1934). The syndrome is commonly elicited by having the patient manually reproduce a visually presented pattern by drawing or copying, or by arranging patterned cubes or matchsticks.

The nature of constructional apraxia has been the subject of speculation and debate. When Kliest (1934) first described constructional apraxia, he viewed it as an inability to translate visual perceptions into the appropriate motor activity. A similar position was adopted by Lhermitte *et al.* (1925), Lange (1936), Marie *et al.* (1922), and Mayer-Gross (1935, 1936), the last of whom viewed constructional apraxia as an executive disorder related to complex manipulative activities. Others have suggested that the disturbed function in constructional apraxia is visuospatial perception (Paterson and Zangwill, 1944; McFie *et al.*, 1960).

While the early observations stressed the importance of left hemisphere lesions (Kliest, 1934; Lhermitte *et al.*, 1925), the current consensus is that constructional apraxia can result from parietooccipital lesions of either hemisphere, although it is seen more frequently following right damage (McFie *et al.*, 1960; Hécaen *et al.*, 1951; Critchley, 1953; Piercy *et al.*, 1960; McFie and Zangwill, 1960; Piercy and Smyth, 1962; Warrington *et al.*, 1966). It has been suggested that the more frequent occurrence of the syndrome following right hemisphere pathology may reflect larger lesions of the right half-brain (Woolf, 1962; Arrigoni and DeRenzi, 1964).

Several reports have emphasized the qualitative differences between the left and right hemisphere syndromes (McFie *et al.*, 1960; Critchley, 1953; Piercy *et al.*, 1960; Piercy and Smyth, 1962; Warrington *et al.*, 1966; Arrigoni and DeRenzi, 1964; Duensing, 1953). With right lesions, the reproduced patterns frequently lack the left side, undoubtedly because of unilateral neglect (see below) which typically accompanies right hemisphere constructional apraxia. In addition, right lesions tend to produce a preoccupation with detail. With left lesions, the designs are sometimes completed, but in a simplified form. Moreover, while left-damaged patients can give better structure to their reproductions of patterns by repeatedly consulting the sample, right-damaged patients are unable to improve their design, even with repeated reference to the sample. In general, the left syndrome is characterized as less severe than the right syndrome.

An important problem that has pervaded constructional apraxia literature is that the right hand alone has generally been tested, regardless of the hemispheric locus of the lesion. Yet observations of split-brain patients have pointed out how important a factor hand use is when the separate capacities of the hemispheres are being evaluated. For example, the left hand of split-brain patients performs in a more or less normal fashion on constructive tasks, but the preferred right hand does not (Bogen and Gazzaniga, 1965; LeDoux *et al.,* 1977; Gazzaniga and LeDoux, 1978). These observations suggest that spatioconstructive skills are minimally represented in the left hemisphere, and the question naturally arises as to why left hemisphere damage produces deficits on constructive tasks.

This paradox is best approached by first considering how the constructive skills of the right hand are normally mediated. After all, neurologically intact right-handed persons are at worst equally efficient with the left and right hands on constructive tasks and at best more efficient with the right hand. Because the right hand loses much of this capacity following brain bisection, it would seem that the spatioconstructive skills of the right hand are highly dependent on commissural connections.

The right parietooccipital region would thus appear to contribute significantly to the constructive skills of both hands. That is, it is as if the syndrome resulting from left hemisphere damage goes beyond a simple lesion effect, and, instead, the lesion serves to callosally disconnect the right parietooccipital cortex from the left hemisphere. In this context, the lesion of the posterior left hemisphere is viewed as breaking a critical link in the circuit between the right parietooccipital region and the motor cortex of the left hemisphere, which, of course, controls the right hand. That the left hemisphere syndrome has been described as a "mild" version of the right syndrome suggests the possibility that the right hemisphere is homolaterally directing the spatioconstructive activities of the right hand. It could well be the inefficiency of homolateral control that gives the appearance of mild apraxia.

These ideas are subject to experimental evaluation. The prediction is that patients with right hemisphere lesions should show signs of constructional apraxia with either hand, whereas left damage should give rise to apraxic symptoms with the right but not the left hand. Such a finding would not only be of great value in clarifying some of the confusion in the constructional apraxia literature but would also be of practical use to clinical neurologists and neurosurgeons, as it would provide a quick and noninvasive index of the hemispheric locus of parietooccipital disease.

ASTEREOGNOSIA

The classic view of the way that the brain manages object recognition (stereognosis) is that there is a primary sensory cortex, the excitation of which results in elementary sensations, and an adjacent association cortex, which combines the sensations into perceptions and integrates the perceptions with past experiences, thereby generating the idea of an object (Semmes, 1965). With regard to somesthesis, the primary sensory region is thought to be the postcentral gyrus, with the posterior parietal cortex (which includes the superior and inferior parietal lobules) serving as the association areas. This suggests that damage to the postcentral gyrus should produce "sensory" defects, but that damage to the posterior parietal regions should result in an inability to recognize objects by touch, a disorder known as "astereognosia."

As it turns out, damage to the postcentral gyrus does, in fact, result in sensory loss in the contralateral hand (Head, 1920; Lewin and Phillips, 1952; Hécaen *et al.*, 1956; Krueger *et al.*, 1954; Corkin *et al.*, 1970). However, posterior parietal lesions do not seem to lead to astereognosia, which is seen only after postcentral gyrus lesions in man (Corkin *et al.*, 1970). Although there have been reports suggesting sensory and stereognostic disturbances following damage to areas other than the postcentral gyrus, and failures to find deficits following postcentral gyrus lesions (Evans, 1935; Semmes *et al.*, 1960), the discrepancies have been attributed to difficulties in specifying the locus of damage in these studies (Corkin *et al.*, 1970).

Observations such as these lead one to question the concept of stereognosis, which is based on the assumption that object recognition has a neural reality of its own. Suppose we forego this assumption and instead turn to a more contemporary view of touch.

Gibson (1962) has suggested a distinction between active and passive touch. He views active touch as the process of "touching," while passive touch involves "being touched." In a less restrictive sense, passive touch involves recognizing or discriminating stimuli by the initial contact of the hand with the item, but active touch involves the exploratory manipulations necessary to identify the features of complex or unfamiliar stimuli. Thus both stereognosis (the recognition of familiar objects) and the more basic sensory functions (as measured by point-localization tests, two-point discriminations, and the like) are within the processing capacity of the passive touch mechanism.

Let us backtrack for a moment and consider why posterior parietal lesions in monkeys (Ettlinger *et al.*, 1966) but not in humans produce deficits in tactile object discriminative ability. While humans are usually familiar with and will thus have had experience with the common objects used in tests of stereognosis, monkeys are, in all likelihood, unfamiliar with the objects employed to test their discriminative capacities following posterior parietal damage. This suggests that while the human experiments have evaluated passive touch, animal studies have, at least in part, employed active touch tests. Moreover, when monkeys are trained preoperatively on these tests and subsequently undergo bilateral posterior parietal lesions, they are able to perform the discrimination. This suggests that while the posterior parietal regions play a critical role in mediating active manual exploration, which is necessary for tactually discriminating unfamiliar stimuli, once the animal is familiar with the test items, the posterior parietal cortex is no longer necessary.

It thus seems reasonable to speculate that the posterior parietal region might play an important role in active exploratory touch, with the postcentral area being more important for passive touch. This idea is consonant with the types of deficits (astereognosia, sensory loss) seen after damage to the postcentral gyrus in man, as well as with the results of animal lesion studies. Moreover, recent studies of the physiological response properties of cells in the monkey posterior parietal cortex suggest that the posterior parietal region of each hemisphere is critically involved in the active, manual exploration of extrapersonal space with the contralateral hand (Mountcastle *et al.*, 1975; Semmes, 1965). Finally, it is of interest to note that the posterior parietal areas are ideally wired to mediate active manual exploration.

They receive somatotopic projections from the postcentral gyrus and project to the premotor region of the frontal cortex (Jones and Powell, 1970). It is as if this pattern of circuitry provides a corticocortical sensory-motor loop for active touch.

In split-brain humans, the left hemisphere falls short, relative to the right, on tasks requiring active touch (LeDoux *et al.*, 1977; Gazzaniga and LeDoux, 1977; Levy-Agresti and Sperry, 1968; Nebes, 1971, 1972, 1973; Zaidel and Sperry, 1973; Milner and Taylor, 1972; Franco and Sperry, 1977). While common objects and simple shapes that are routinely encountered can be tactually processed by either hemisphere, more complex or unfamiliar items find the left hemisphere deficient. For example, it has recently been shown that while both hemispheres can tactually apprehend the spatial features of Euclidean geometry (which involves the spatial relations with which we are most familiar), the left hemisphere performs poorly on tests involving the more complex and less familiar relations, as in topological geometry (Franco and Sperry, 1977). In this regard, it is interesting to note that most of the "spatial" perceptual tests that have elicited a right hemisphere advantage over the left in split-brain patients have required active manual exploration of haptic stimuli. Moreover, we have recently shown that the dramatic right hemisphere advantage on a representative subset of these tests is either eliminated or severely diluted by circumventing the manipulative mode in the test design while holding the stimulus material constant (LeDoux *et al.*, 1977; Gazzaniga and LeDoux, 1977). Since normal individuals do not show such dramatic differences in the perceptual capacities of the two hands, it would seem that the right posterior parietal regions and their commissural connections normally play an important role in mediating the active touch functions of both hands.

The active-passive dichotomy thus provides a fresh view of touch mechanisms. It would not be too surprising if different cortical areas were involved, for, on the spinal level, it appears that active and passive touch utilize separate ascending pathways (Semmes and Mishkin, 1965; Wall, 1970; Azulay and Schwartz, 1975). However, the simple approach of tracing these separate spinal projections through the thalamus and to the cortex won't provide the answer, as the active pathway (dorsal column-medial lemniscus) and the passive pathway (spinothalamic tract) project, at least in part, to the same thalamic nuclei. It thus seems that the cortical contributions to active and passive touch will have to be teased apart using the standard neuropsychological approach—correlating behavioral observations with lesion data. It might be expected that postcentral gyrus lesions will result in both active and passive deficits since the posterior parietal regions are functionally dependent on the postcentral gyrus (Jones and Powell, 1970). We might also expect to see active deficits in the absence of passive deficits following damage of the posterior zones; moreover, the split-brain data give us reasons to expect hemispheric differences in the extent to which posterior parietal lesions will result in active deficits.

FINGER AGNOSIA

Finger agnosia is a disturbance in the ability to name, select, indicate, and orient as to the individual fingers of either hand (Gerstmann, 1924). It sometimes extends beyond the patient's own hand and can involve an inability to perform such activities relative to someone else's hand. The syndrome is generally bilateral (involves both hands) and is usually seen only after left hemisphere (parietooccipital) damage in right-handed patients (Lunn, 1948; Fredericks, 1969; Hécaen and de Ajuriaguerra, 1963; Benton, 1959).

The exact nature of the disorder in finger agnosia is not fully understood. It is generally agreed, however, that finger agnosia is a special case of autotopagnosia (disorder of the body schema). In fact, finger agnosia seems to be the only localized form of autotopagnosia (Piercy *et al.*, 1960). Usually, autotopagnosia involves either the fingers alone or the entire body. This observation has led to speculation concerning the special role of the hands and fingers in human ecology and evolution (Piercy *et al.*, 1960; Klien, 1931; Fredericks, 1969). In this regard, Fredericks (1961, 1969) notes that no other part of the body is verbally differentiated to the extent that the hand is, thus making the hand especially susceptible to autotopagnosia, particularly verbal autotopagnosia (Wright, 1956; Selecki and Herron, 1965). Moreover, Fredericks notes that in his own as well as in other finger agnosia cases in the literature, amnesic aphasia is frequently present, suggesting that finger agnosia is a linguistic disturbance (Fredericks, 1969). Similarly, Benton's (1959) observations point to a disorder of linguistic symbolism involving the hands. While Kinsbourne and Warrington (1962) attempted to rule out language disturbances in their study of finger agnosia, it is not clear that this was accomplished.

Observations on brain-bisected humans are more in line with the view that the basic disturbance in finger agnosia is in verbal symbolism involving the hands. Finger agnosia is usually a consequence of left hemisphere lesions. This suggests that, in neurologically intact persons, the left hemisphere mediates the "finger schema" of the left hand either through descending ipsilateral pathways or by commissural connections to the right hemisphere. When split-brain patients are asked to verbally identify which finger is being touched or are verbally asked to move certain fingers in a particular way, correct responding is observed only with regard to the right hand (Gazzaniga *et al.*, 1967). In addition, if line drawings of complex finger postures are presented to either hemisphere, the contralateral but not the ipsilateral hand is able to accurately mimic the finger positions; this holds regardless of which hemisphere is tested (Gazzaniga and LeDoux, 1977; Gazzaniga *et al.*, 1967, 1977). Taken together, these observations suggest that the only apparent hemisphere difference in what might be called a schematic representation of the fingers is on the verbal dimension, because a nonverbal finger schema seems to be present in each hemisphere. In addition, the idea that the verbal-symbolic awareness and use of the left hand are normally mediated by descending ipsilateral connections from the left hemisphere is ruled out, thus suggesting that, in the normal brain, the cerebral commissures make it possible for the left hemisphere to use and appreciate the left hand in a verbal-symbolic context.

Consequently, it would seem that the finger agnosia syndrome seen after left hemisphere damage involves the loss of the capacity to use the hands in a verbal-symbolic context. In this regard, it is of interest to note that dysgraphia (an inability to write) and dyscalculia (an inability to perform arithmetic calculations on paper), as well as left-right confusion, are frequent concomitants of finger agnosia. Dysgraphia and dyscalculia clearly involve disorders of hand use in a verbal-symbolic context, and how else do we know left and right but by naming spatial direction relative to our verbally labeled hands?

Unilateral Spatial Agnosia

Unilateral spatial agnosia involves the inattention to or the neglect of one-half of visual space. In the vast majority of cases reported, the disorder occurs as a consequence of lesions in the posterior parietal region of the right hemisphere, and it is the left half of space that is ignored (McFie *et al.,* 1960; Hécaen *et al.,* 1951, 1956; Brain, 1941; Battersby *et al.,* 1956). Occasionally, however, neglect of the right side of space is seen following damage to the left posterior hemisphere, (Brain, 1941; Hécaen *et al.,* 1956; Denny-Brown and Banker, 1954).

Patients manifesting neglect will often bump into objects that are unattended to on the left side of their paths. They will frequently be unable to find their way around the corridors of the hospital, always making right turns, acting as though left turns do not exist. When performing simple constructive tasks such as drawing patterns or arranging items in a systematic way, they frequently ignore the left side of the pattern, completing only the right side. When reading, they will start in the middle of a line, again ignoring the left side. If asked to point to the middle of a horizontal line, they will invariably point somewhere in the middle of the right side, which is probably very close to the middle of the line that is actually perceived.

Thus neglect actually accounts for the poor performance of right-damaged patients on a variety of "spatial" tasks. In many cases, it is not that the patient has really lost the capacity to perceive spatial relations, but instead that the patient neglects part of space and thus performs poorly on tasks requiring the use of the neglected space, while still manifesting intact visuospatial skills in the unneglected space.

A variety of theories have surfaced to explain unilateral spatial agnosia. Because neglect generally occurs in homonymous hemianopic half-fields, the question immediately arises as to whether sensory defects account for the disorder. Battersby *et al.* (1956) note several reasons why unilateral spatial agnosia cannot be attributed entirely to simple sensory loss. In the first place, many patients that show neglect have some intact vision in the defective homonymous half-fields, and many others that have homonymous half-field defects fail to show neglect. A second and related point is that the unilateral inattention does not correspond to the areas of anopia, as revealed by perimetry tests. Finally, neglect is sometimes not restricted to vision, but can also involve an agnosia for one-half of auditory space, as well as neglect of one-half of the body. In spite of these reservations, Battersby *et al.* concluded that sensory defects (in conjunction with general mental deterioration) contribute substantially to unilateral spatial agnosia.

Critchley (1953) views unilateral spatial agnosia as a disregard for objects in one-half of space rather than as a disregard for space itself. Denny-Brown and his colleagues have put forward a similar notion, treating neglect as a disorder of form recognition (morphosynthesis) (Denny-Brown and Banker, 1954; Denny-Brown and Chambers, 1958). Thus damage to the posterior parietal areas produces "amorphosynthesis," a loss or reduction in the spatial summation of stimuli from one-half of external space, or one-half of the body. While they suggest that lesions of either parietal lobe can produce contralateral amorphosynthesis, the rarity of neglect following left hemisphere damage has been difficult to resolve.

Still others view unilateral inattention as an "associational" disturbance. This theory, which was originally suggested by Holmes (1918) and later supported by Riddoch (1935), is based on the idea that the parietal lesion disrupts the association pathways between the visual association areas and the rest of the brain.

Most theorists agree that neglect represents a disturbance in the mechanism by which one-half of space is attended to. This suggests that attention to one side of space requires such a mechanism. If this is so, we are then faced with the problem of explaining how the right side of space is normally attended to, because neglect usually involves the left side of space.

Since the left hemisphere of split-brain patients can and does attend to the right half of space, we have no choice but to accept the conclusion that each hemisphere has its own mechanisms for attending to the contralateral half of space. A reasonable hypothesis is that the parietooccipital junction plays an important role in this attentional mechanism by mediating between the cortical sensory and association areas and various subcortical attentional mechanisms, including the tectum, which has, for some time been implicated in multimodal attentional processes (Schneider, 1969; Stein and Arigbede, 1972; Trevarthen, 1968).

Given this model, consider possible explanations for the rarity of unilateral inattention following left hemisphere lesions. Perhaps neglect of the right half of space is seldom seen because damage to the left parietooccipitotemporal junction produces such severe distortions of consciousness (due to extensive linguistic losses) that it becomes difficult, if not impossible, to assess more subtle disturbances such as neglect. Alternatively, the invasion of the left parietooccipitotemporal region by linguistic functions in humans may force the visual attentional mechanisms to occupy more posterior cortical areas. The lesion leading to neglect of the right half of space would thus be in or close to the occipital cortex. As occipital lesions are far more likely than more anterior lesions to render the patient blind in the opposite half-field, and the difficulty in assessing neglect escalates with the degree of visual field defect, left-lesioned patients would be less likely to show unilateral spatial agnosia.

VISUAL AGNOSIAS: APPERCEPTIVE, ASSOCIATIVE, AND FACE AGNOSIA

Visual agnosia was first described by Lissauer (1890), who suggested that the disorder could be classified into two forms, depending on which phase of visual recognition was disturbed. Lissauer distinguished the act of conscious perception of sensory information from the process by which visual perceptions are linked with memory images stored in other modalities, and, in addition, are provided with verbal labels (Warrington and James, 1967; DeRenzi *et al.*, 1969). The first stage of visual recognition was termed "apperception" and the second "association." According to Lissauer, disorders involving the first stage lead to defective perceptual processing, whereas disorders of association involve an inability to visually recognize objects in the absence of perceptual defects. In other words, in associative agnosia, objects lose their meaning.

In general, the clinical literature has focused on associative agnosia, which usually results from left hemisphere lesions involving the occipitoparietal region (Lissauer, 1890; Lange, 1936; Brain, 1941; Ettlinger and Wyke, 1961; Hécaen and Angelergues, 1963; Geschwind, 1965; DeRenzi and Spinnler, 1965, 1966; Bisiach *et al.*, 1976; Kimura, 1966). It would, on the surface, seem that the capacity to visually recognize objects, then, is localized to the left hemisphere. Yet, Geschwind (1965) points out that while (associative) agnostic patients are unable to verbally identify objects, they are frequently able to respond to the object in a nonverbal fashion. For example, a patient with left occipitoparietal damage may be unable to verbally identify a glass of water, but a few minutes later might pick up the glass and drink the water. This capacity to respond nonverbally is not uncommon in such patients. Most probably, the intact visual mechanisms of the right hemisphere allow for these nonverbal responses, and Geschwind suggests that a naming defect, due to a disconnection between the right posterior cortex and the speech regions of the left hemisphere, is the simplest explanation for the disorder.

Observations of split-brain patients are consonant with the view that the right hemisphere has the capacity to recognize objects and respond appropriately to them. If a line drawing of an object, for example, an apple, is lateralized to either hemisphere of a split-brain patient, the patient can, with the contralateral hand, retrieve the apple from a group of several objects. Such an act requires that the visual sketch be recognized as an apple before the apple can be recognized in another modality. Clearly, then, each hemisphere is capable of recognizing objects, and this is a fact that must be accounted for by any theory of visual agnosia where the syndrome results from unilateral left hemisphere damage.

Interest in the apperceptive form of agnosia has recently been stimulated by the observation that patients with posterior right hemisphere damage show greater deficits than left-damaged patients on some tests of visual perception (Warrington and James, 1967; DeRenzi *et al.*, 1969; Lange, 1936; Brain, 1941; Ettlinger and Wyke, 1961; Hécaen and Angelergues, 1963; Geschwind, 1965; DeRenzi and Spinnler, 1965, 1966; Bisiach *et al.*, 1976). These data have led to the idea that perceptual processing is the business of the right hemisphere, a view that is consistent with the interpretation given to normal and split-brain data showing hemisphere differences in perceptual skills. However, the hemisphere differences in normal studies of perceptual processing, when such differences are found, are small and statistical, and thus fail to justify the conclusion that the right hemisphere is unique in any qualitative sense. Similarly, the lesion data actually point out that the hemisphere differences are mainly seen at the upper limits of perceptual discrimination and integration. Moreover, when split-brain patients are tested on purely visual perceptual tasks where there is no tactual involvement, either both hemispheres perform at equivalent levels or the right proves to have a relative, statistical advantage (LeDoux *et al.*, 1977; Nebes, 1973). All things considered, it would appear that both hemispheres have a considerable capacity for perceptual processing, with the right possessing a relative advantage when the upper perceptual limits are tested.

These observations are important because they point out the relative nature of hemisphere differences in visual capacity. All too often, such differences are treated in absolute terms. The right hemisphere is viewed as doing the perceiving and the left as assigning meaning to the perception. Such a compartmental view of cerebral functioning is at best an oversimplification.

One factor that has no doubt contributed significantly to the idea that the hemispheres differ qualitatively in perceptual capacity is the syndrome called "prosopagnosia," or face agnosia. Prosopagnosic patients, as the theory goes, selectively lose the capacity to recognize faces following occipitoparietal damage in the right hemisphere. As a consequence, the view has emerged that the right hemisphere is the face perceiver.

While this conclusion may be based on a real clinical phenomenon, it is inconsistent with a variety of other lines of evidence. In the first place, although the clinical disorder involves the inability to recognize familiar faces, experimental evidence from normal subjects suggests a left hemisphere advantage on a familiar face recognition test (Berlucchi, 1974). Second, split-brain patients have no trouble associating familiar faces with names (all of which must be done in their left hemisphere). Third, when unfamiliar faces are used in recognition tests, unselected brain-damaged patients show more of a deficit following right hemisphere lesions (DeRenzi and Spinnler, 1966). These results, however, mirror the results seen on other recognition tests—a relative right hemisphere advantage. Finally, we administered a match-to-sample test to a split-brain patient, where unfamiliar faces were lateralized to one hemisphere or the other, and he was required to select the same face from a group of three faces of the same sex. On this simple test, both hemispheres performed at high levels (Gazzaniga and LeDoux, 1977).

Prosopagnosia thus remains a clinical mystery. As with so many other syndromes resulting from lateralized damage, it is difficult to use the behavioral defect as a valid index of functional localization, particularly when the syndrome is as rare and little understood as prosopagnosia.

All things considered, when the data are carefully examined, there seems to be little evidence to support the idea that the hemispheres differ qualitatively in perceptual capacity. While there is some evidence for a right hemisphere relative advantage over the left, especially on difficult visuoperceptual tests, the idea that the hemispheres differ in absolute terms in visual capacities is untenable.

ALEXIA WITHOUT AGRAPHIA

In alexia without agraphia, patients lose the capacity to read, while retaining the ability to write. Such patients, when asked to write their name, can do so with no problem. Moments later, however, they are unable to read what they have just written. This syndrome, which typically occurs as a consequence of damage to the left occipital lobe, is generally interpreted as a disconnection syndrome (Geschwind, 1965). The left occipital lesion essentially renders the left hemisphere blind (hemianopic). Although the visual functions of the right hemisphere remain intact, the lesion frequently destroys the splenium, the visual part of the corpus callosum. As a consequence, according to the disconnection hypothesis, the visual activity of the right hemisphere is isolated from the language areas of the left hemisphere. So, while words are visually perceived, they are not processed linguistically.

An important problem with the disconnection interpretation of alexia without agraphia is that while the patients are unable to name words, they can name objects. Geschwind (1965) suggests that this is so because objects arouse tactile associations when visually observed, and, as a consequence, the critical information flows from the right somatosensory areas to the homologous regions in the left hemisphere (by way of the intact callosal fibers anterior to the splenium) where naming occurs. This interpretation, however, is not in line with recent observations concerning the nature of the callosal code.

In the case of J. K. N., visual but not tactual information transferred between the hemispheres (see below). Thus he was unable to find an object with one hand that was felt by the other. However, if the object was shown to his left hemisphere, he could find it with the left hand, because the visual information transferred over to the right hemisphere, which, of course, mediates the touch functions of the left hand. If, instead of the object's being shown to the left hemisphere, the object was placed in his right hand and he was told to imagine a picture of it, the left hand was unable to find the object (Gazzaniga and LeDoux, 1977; Risse et al., 1976). Here, we see a distinction between cross-modal associations of internal and external origin. The information from both modalities must be externally perceived for transfer to occur. Thus it appears unlikely that, in alexia, object naming survives because the visual object arouses internal tactual associations.

Another problem with the disconnection theory involves recent observations of several patients with complete surgical sections of the corpus callosum, which leaves the anterior commissure intact (Risse et al., 1977). These patients are, in general, capable of naming and reading information presented in their left visual field (right hemisphere), thus confirming the results of studies of nonhuman primates that show that the anterior commissure is a viable pathway for interhemispheric visual transfer (Sullivan and Hamilton, 1973). Why, then, is the anterior commissure unable to sustain the transfer of words in the alexic cases? Although Geschwind has suggested the possibility that the anterior commissure might transfer nonverbal, but not verbal, visual information (Geschwind, 1974), we have not found this to be the case in our patients.

One possible explanation is that the anterior commissure does transfer objects and words in alexics, and the problem instead involves a selective disconnection within the left hemisphere subsequent to successful transfer. It does not seem unreasonable that verbal and nonverbal visual messages en route to the language areas might utilize distinct pathways within the left hemisphere.

Thus alexia continues to be an interesting and unresolved problem. Although we are not yet at the point of developing a comprehensive theory of alexia, the transfer capacity of the anterior commissure must be accounted for when such a theory emerges.

CONCLUSIONS

We have considered a variety of behavioral disorders due to parietooccipital pathology from the split-brain point of view. While, in some instances, it was possible to offer explanations and hypotheses, in others it was possible only to point out how split-brain data add new complexities that must be accounted for to explain the disorder in question. The main point is, however, that when split-brain and lesion data are considered together, rather than separately, we find ourselves a bit farther along in the endless task of relating mind to brain.

REFERENCES

Arrigoni, G., and DeRenzi, E. Constructional apraxia and hemispheric focus of lesion. *Cortex (Milano),* 1964, *1*, 170–197.

Azulay, A., and Schwartz, A. S. The role of the dorsal funiculus in tactile discrimination. *Experimental Neurology,* 1975, *46*, 315–332.

Battersby, N. S., Bender, M. B., Pollack, M., and Kahn, R. L. Unilateral spatial agnosia. *Brain,* 1956, *79*, 68–93.

Benton, A. L. Right-Left Discrimination and Finger Localization:*Development and Pathology.* New York: Hoeber-Harper, 1959.

Berlucchi, G. Cerebral dominance and interhemispheric communication in normal man. In F. O. Schmitt (ed.), *The Neurosciences: Third Study Program.* Cambridge, Mass.: MIT Press, 1973.

Berlucchi, G. Some features of interhemispheric communication of visual information in brain dam-aged cats and normal humans. In F. Michel and B. Schott (eds.), *Les Syndromes de Disconnexion Calleuse chez l'Homme.* Lyon: Colloque International de Lyon, 1974.

Bisiach, E., Nichelli, P., and Spinnler, H. Hemispheric functional asymmetry in visual discriminations between invariant stimuli. *Neuropsychologia,* 1976, *14*, 335–342.

Bogen, J. E., and Gazzaniga, M. S. Cerebral commissurotomy in man: Minor hemisphere dominance for certain visuo-spatial functions. *Journal of Neurosurgery,* 1965, *23*, 394–399.

Brain, R. Visual disorientation with special reference to lesions of the right cerebral hemisphere. *Brain,* 1941, *64*, 244–272.

Corkin, S., Milner, B., and Rasmussen, T. Somatosensory thresholds: Contrasting of postcentral-gyrus and posterior parietal-lobe excisions. *Archives of Neurology (Chicago),* 1970, *23*, 41–58.

Critchley, M. *The Parietal Lobes.* London: E. Arnold, 1953.

Denny-Brown, D., and Banker, B. Amorphosynthesis from left parietal lesions. *Archives of Neurology and Psychiatry,* 1954, *71*, 302–313.

Denny-Brown, D., and Chambers, R. A. The parietal lobe and behavior. *Research Publications, Association for Research in Nervous and Mental Disease,* 1958, *36*, 36–117.

DeRenzi, E., and Spinnler, H. Visual recognition in patients with unilateral cerebral damage. *Journal of Nervous and Mental Disease,* 1965, *142*, 515.

DeRenzi, E., and Spinnler, H. Facial recognition in brain damaged patients—An experimental approach. *Neurology,* 1966, *6*, 145–153.

DeRenzi, E., Scotti, G., and Spinner, H. Perceptual and associative disorders of visual recognition. *Neurology,* 1969, *9*, 634–642.

Duensing, F. Raumagnostische und ideatorischapraktische Störung des gestaltenden handelns. *Deutsche Zeitschrift für Nervenheilkunde,* 1953, *170*, 72–94.

Ettlinger, G., Warrington, E., and Zangwill, O. L. A further study of visuo-spatial agnosia. *Brain,* 1957, *80*, 335–361.

Ettlinger, G., Morton, H. B., and Muffett, A. Tactile discrimination in the monkey. *Cortex*, 1966, *2*, 5–29.

Evans, J. P. A study of the sensory defects resulting from excision of cerebral substance in humans. *Publication of the Association for Research in Nervous and Mental Disease*, 1935, *15*, 331–370.

Franco, L., and Sperry, R. W. Hemisphere lateralization for cognitive processing of geometry. *Neuropsychologia*, 1977, *15*, 107–113.

Fredericks, J. A. M. *Het Lichaamsschema*. Amsterdam: Van Rossen, 1961.

Fredericks, J. A. M. Disorders of the body schema. In P. J. Vinken and G. W. Bruyn (eds.), *Handbook of Clinical Neurology*. Amsterdam: North-Holland, 1969.

Gazzaniga, M. S., and LeDoux, J. E. *The Integrated Mind*. New York: Plenum, 1978.

Gazzaniga, M. S., Bogen, J. E., and Sperry, R. W. Dyspraxia following division of the cerebral commissures. *Archives of Neurology (Chicago)*, 1967, *16*, 606–612.

Gazzaniga, M. S., LeDoux, J. E., and Wilson, D. H. Language, praxis, and the right hemisphere. *Neurology*, 1977, *27*, 1140–1147.

Geffen, G., Bradshaw, J. L., and Wallace, G. Interhemispheric effects on reaction time to verbal and non-verbal stimuli. *Journal of Experimental Psychology*, 1971, *87*, 415–422.

Gerstmann, J. Fingeragnosie. Eine umschriebene Störung der Orientierung am eigenen Körper. *Wiener Klinische Wochenschrift*, 1924, *37*, 1010–1012.

Geschwind, N. Disconnexion syndromes in animals and man. *Brain*, 1965, *88*, 237–294, 584–644.

Geschwind, N. Discussion No. 5. In F. Michel and B. Schutt (eds.), *Les Syndromes de Disconnexion Calleuse chez l'Homme*. Lyon: Colloque International, 1974.

Gibson, J. J. Observations on active touch. *Psychological Review*, 1962, *69*, 477–491.

Gross, M. M. Hemisphere specialization for processing of visually presented verbal and spatial stimuli. *Perception and Psychophysiology*, 1972, *12*, 357–363.

Head, H. *Studies in Neurology*. London: Oxford University Press, 1920.

Hécaen, H., and Angelergues, R. *La Cécité Psychique*. Paris: Masson et Cie, 1963.

Hécaen, H., and de Ajuriaguerra, J. *Les Gauchers: Prévalence Manuelle et Dominance Cérébrale*. Paris: Presses Universitaires de France, 1963.

Hécaen, H., de Ajuriaguerra, J., and Massonet, J. Les troubles visuoconstructifs par lésion pariéto-occipitale droite: Rôle des perturbations vestibulaires. *Encéphale*, 1951, *40*, 122–179.

Hécaen, H., Penfield, W., Bertrand, C., and Malmo, R. The syndrome of apractognosia due to lesion of the minor cerebral hemisphere. *Archives of Neurology and Psychiatry (Chicago)*, 1956, *75*, 400–434.

Holmes, G. Disturbances of visual orientation. *British Journal of Ophthalmology*, 1918, *2*, 449–468.

Hyvarinen, J., and Poranen, A. Function of the parietal associative area 7 as revealed from cellular discharges in alert monkeys. *Brain*, 1974, *97*, 673–692.

Jones, E. G., and Powell, T. P. S. An anatomical study of converging sensory pathways within the cerebral cortex of the monkey. *Brain*, 1970, *93*, 793–820.

Kimura, D. Dual functional asymmetry of the brain in visual perception. *Neuropsychologia*, 1966, *4*, 275–285.

Kimura, D., and Durnford, M. Normal studies on the function of the right hemisphere in vision. In S. J. Dimond and J. G. Beaumont (eds.), *Hemisphere Function in the Human Brain*. New York: Halsted Press, 1974.

Kinsbourne, M., and Warrington, E. K. A study of finger agnosia. *Brain*, 1962, *85*, 47–66.

Klien, R. Zur Symptomatologie des Parietallappens. *Nervenartz*, 1931, *6*, 1–7, 67–74.

Kliest, K. *Gehirnpathologie*. Leipzig: Barth, 1934.

Krueger, E. G., Price, P. A., and Teuber, H. L. Tactile extinction in parietal lobe neoplasms. *Journal of Psychology*, 1954, *38*, 191–202.

Lange, J. Agnosien and Apraxien. In O. Bunke and O. Foerster (eds.), *Handbusch der Nerrologie*. Berlin: Springer, 1936.

LeDoux, J. E., Wilson, D. H., and Gazzaniga, M. S. Manipulo-spatial aspects of cerebral lateralization: Clues to the origin of lateralization. *Neuropsychologia*, 1977, *15*, 743–750.

Levy-Agresti, J., and Sperry, R. W. Differential perceptual capacities in minor and major hemispheres. *Proceedings of the National Academy of Sciences*, 1968, *61*, 1151.

Lewin, W., and Phillips, C. G. Observations on partial removal of the post-central gyrus for pain. *Journal of Neurology, Neurosurgery, and Psychiatry*, 1952, *15*, 143–47.

Lhermitte, J., Levy, G., and Kyriaco, N. Les perturbations de la représentation spatiale chez les apraxiques. *Revue Neurologique*, 1925, *2*, 586–600.

Lissauer, H. Ein Fall von Seelenblindheit nebst einem Beitrag zur Theorie derselben. *Archiv fuer Psychiatrie und Nervenkrankheiten*, 1890, *21*, 222.

Lunn, V. *Om Legemsbevidsthdenen.* Copenhagen: E. Munksgard, 1948.

Marie, P., Bouttier, H., and Bailey, P. La planotopokinésie: Etude sur les erreurs d'exécution de certains mouvments dans leurs rapports avec la représentation spatiale. *Revue Neurologique,* 1922, *1,* 505–512.

Mayer-Gross, W. Some observations on apraxia. *Proceedings of the Royal Society of Medicine,* 1935, *28,* 1203–1212.

Mayer-Gross, W. The question of visual impairment in constructional apraxia. *Proceedings of the Royal Society of Medicine,* 1936, *29,* 1396–1400.

McFie, J., and Zangwill, O. L. Visual constructive disabilities associated with lesions of the left cerebral hemisphere. *Brain,* 1960, *83,* 243–260.

McFie, J., Piercy, M. F., and Zangwill, O. L. Visual spatial agnosia associated with lesions of the right cerebral hemisphere. *Brain,* 1960, *73,* 167–190.

Milner, B., and Taylor, L. Right hemisphere superiority in tactile pattern recognition after cerebral commissurotomy: Evidence for nonverbal memory. *Neuropsychologia,* 1972, *10,* 1–15.

Mountcastle, V. B., Lynch, J. C., Georgopoulos, A., Sakata, H., and Acuna, C. Posterior parietal association cortex of the monkey: Command functions for operations within extrapersonal space. *Journal of Neurophysiology,* 1975, *38,* 871.

Nebes, R. Superiority of the minor hemisphere in commissurotomized man for the perception of part-whole relations. *Cortex,* 1971, *7,* 333–349.

Nebes, R. Dominance of the minor hemisphere in commissurotomized man on a test of figural unification. *Brain,* 1972, *95,* 633–638.

Nebes, R. Perception of spatial relationships by the right and left hemispheres of commissurotomized man. *Neuropsychologia,* 1973, *11,* 285–289.

Paterson, A., and Zangwill, O. L. Disorders of visual space perception associated with lesions of the right cerebral hemisphere. *Brain,* 1944, *67,* 331–358.

Piercy, M., and Smyth, V. O. G. Right hemisphere dominance for certain non-verbal intellectual skills. *Brain,* 1962, *85,* 775–790.

Piercy, M., Hécaen, H., and de Ajuriaguerra, J. 1960. Constructional apraxia associated with unilateral cerebral lesions. Left and right sided cases compared. *Brain,* 1960, *83,* 225–242.

Riddoch, G. Visual disorientation in homonymous half-fields. *Brain,* 1935, *58,* 376–382.

Risse, G., LeDoux, J., and Gazzaniga, M. Unpublished observation, 1976.

Risse, G., LeDoux, J., Springer, S., Wilson, D., and Gazzaniga, M. The anterior commissure in man: Functional variation in a multisensory system. *Neuropsychologia,* 1977, *16,* 23–31.

Schneider, G. Two visual systems. *Science,* 1969, *163,* 895–902.

Selecki, B. R., and Herron, J. T. Disturbances of the verbal body image: A particular syndrome of sensory aphasia. *Journal of Nervous and Mental Disease,* 1965, *141,* 42–52.

Semmes, J. A non-tactual factor in astereognosis. *Neuropsychologia,* 1965, *3,* 295–315.

Semmes, J., and Mishkin, M. 1965. Somatosensory loss in monkeys after ipisilateral cortical ablations. *Journal of Neurophysiology,* 1965, *28,* 473–486.

Semmes, J., Weinstein, S., Ghent, L., and Teuber, H. L. *Somatosensory Changes after Penetrating Brain Wounds in Man.* Cambridge, Mass.: Harvard University Press, 1960.

Stein, B. E., and Arigbede, M. O. Unimodal and multimodal properties of neurons in cat superior colliculus. *Experimental Neurology,* 1972, *36,* 179–196.

Sullivan, M., and Hamilton, C. Interocoular transfer of reversed and non-reversed discriminations via the anterior commissure in monkeys. *Physiology and Behavior,* 1973, *10,* 355–359.

Trevarthen, C. Two mechanisms of vision in primates. *Psychologische Forschung* 1968, *31,* 299–337.

Wall, P. D. The sensory and motor role of impulses traveling in the dorsal columns. *Brain,* 1970, *93,* 505–524.

Warrington, E., and James, M. Disorders of visual perception in patients with localized cerebral lesions. *Neuropsychologia,* 1967, *5,* 253–266.

Warrington, E. K., James, M., and Kinsbourne, M. Drawing disability in relation to laterality of lesion. *Brain,* 1966, *89,* 53–82.

Woolf, H. G. Discussion of Teuber's paper. In V. B. Mountcastle (ed.), *Interhemispheric Relations and Cerebral Dominance.* Baltimore: Johns Hopkins Press, 1962.

Wright, G. H. The names of the parts of the body. *Brain,* 1956, *79,* 188–210.

Zaidel, E., and Sperry, R. W. Performance on Raven's colored progressive matrices tests by commissurotomy patients. *Cortex,* 1973, *9,* 34.

4

The Temporal Lobes: An Approach to the Study of Organic Behavioral Changes

DAVID M. BEAR

SELECTION OF VARIABLES FOR SCIENTIFIC STUDY OF ORGANIC BEHAVIORAL CHANGES

From a clinical perspective, alterations in the emotions or behavior of an individual primarily present a problem in differential diagnosis. For this reason, a simple rule or generalization has long been sought to distinguish behavioral syndromes of organic causation from functional—idiopathic or learned—psychiatric disorders.

However, it would be most surprising if a variety of pathological processes, independent of their locus of effect within the brain, resulted in a nonspecific "organic brain syndrome." Despite the retention of this simplistic concept in the current standard psychiatric nomenclature (*Diagnostic and Statistical Manual of Mental Disorders,* 1968), it is clear, in fact, that there are multiple, discrete syndromes of behavioral change associated with specific pathological processes (Geschwind, 1975). Thus the paranoid psychosis of anticholinergic intoxication is accompanied by attentional deficits and agitation typical of a confusional state; acute paranoia with neologistic speech and loss of verbal comprehension may follow infarction of the dominant temporal lobe (Wernicke's aphasia); and paranoid delusions in the absence of cognitive impairment mark the syndrome of chronic amphetamine ingestion (Adams and Victor, 1974; Benson and Geschwind, 1971; Connell, 1958; Ellinwood, 1967; Bear, 1976c).

DAVID M. BEAR   Research Fellow, Massachusetts General Hospital, Boston, Massachusetts 02114.

Knowledge of specific organic syndromes refines the diagnostic search for the cause of a particular psychotic disorder. It is the purpose of differential diagnosis to proceed from clinical description of a patient's presenting status to a list of possible causative processes. Each of these must then be evaluated—ruled in or out—by further observations and laboratory procedures. Since such rules serve highly pragmatic functions in medicine, they tend to be formulated in the most generally utilized, clinical language.

Organic psychoses, physically caused syndromes which often first come to psychiatric attention, have thus been traditionally characterized in terms of nineteenth-century psychiatric nosology. From previous example, the organic differential diagnosis of "paranoid psychosis" would be said to include scopolamine overdose, emboli in the distribution of the left middle cerebral artery, and chronic amphetamine ingestion (Bear, 1976c).

There is, of course, clinical utility in correlating standard psychiatric presentations with possible organic etiologies, since the psychiatric clinician is most likely to describe his patient first using such a term as "psychosis," "paranoia," "mania," or "neurosis." He is then alerted by rules of differential diagnosis to consider physical disease processes as etiological alternatives to the functional syndromes.

This diagnostic approach has often been generalized to an epidemiological one in the attempt to extend knowledge of brain function relating to emotion and affective behavior. As an example of this common methodology, Davison and Bagley (1969), in an extensive review, summarized the coincident diagnosis of schizophrenia with physical processes occurring both outside the central nervous system and at discrete cerebral loci. While the comprehensive list of physical processes which have been associated with schizophrenialike psychosis (metabolic, vascular, neoplastic, infectious, autoimmune, degenerative) greatly extends the breadth of functional-organic differential diagnosis, the scientific conclusions from this global review are rather limited: that schizophrenia is an idiopathic, multifactorial illness which may be precipitated by genetic loading, environment, physical disease, or their interactions.

In general, it would seem that few, if any, new facts concerning structure-function relations have resulted from over a century of attempts to correlate specific psychiatric diagnoses with organic precipitants. This may reflect the fact that the logic of psychiatric-organic differential diagnosis has serious limitations when applied to the scientific study of neuroanatomical mechanisms.

I believe that the fundamental difficulties in generalizing the clinical approach result from the use of psychiatric diagnoses as independent variables. "Schizophrenia," for example, is neither a simple nor an objective description of behavior; it is a complex concept which continues to be applied inconstantly by different observers at different times and places (Everitt et al., 1971). To attempt to correlate objective physical parameters with such a poorly defined descriptive term is methodological suicide, since the psychiatrically defined index groups will be neither standard nor homogeneous. Recent attempts to operationalize psychiatric diagnoses by specifying inclusion and exclusion criteria (Feighner et al., 1972) may facilitate communication, but there can be no guarantee that such "committee-defined syndromes" are biologically heuristic. Since these complex definitions

77

THE TEMPORAL
LOBES: AN APPROACH
TO THE STUDY OF
ORGANIC
BEHAVIORAL
CHANGES

are generally derived from observations of functional psychoses in groups from which known organic conditions have been excluded, they are most unlikely to correlate meaningfully with specific organic processes.

Psychiatric variables, whether descriptive (psychosis, delusion) or diagnostic (schizophrenia), have the additional serious drawback that they may not be readily observed or reproduced in animals. Most so-called animal models of psychosis rely on highly inferential analogies of behavior (Ellinwood *et al.,* 1973). In fact, much more would be lost by way of description than gained by summarizing the effects of bilateral temporal lobectomy in monkeys (Kluver and Bucy, 1939) as an animal psychosis. The specification of emotional behavior in primarily psychiatric terms thus greatly limits cross-fertilization between clinical and animal studies of emotionality.

The primary goal in scientific investigation of organically produced behavior changes is an understanding of mechanism. Yet it is just here that the construction of studies in terms of psychiatric diagnosis is most limiting, since functional psychoses like schizophrenia remain idiopathic. While it is diagnostically relevant that a state resembling paranoid schizophrenia may appear in Huntington's disease (Dewhurst *et al.,* 1969), this correlation of a genetically identified, neuroanatomically localized disease process with an idiopathic condition can lead to no clarification of the underlying biological mechanism.

A scientific alternative to studies of "schizophrenialike" organic psychoses, in which the psychiatric state becomes the independent variable (Davison and Bagley, 1969; Slater and Beard, 1963; Slater, 1969; Slater and Moran, 1969), is to specify a physical variable (neuroanatomical, physiological, pharmacological) and to treat the behavioral state as the dependent variable to be described. For each disadvantage of the previous approach, there then appear to be resolutions. This simple reversal allows for precisely defined index groups: rather than patients judged schizophrenic by arbitrary criteria, patients with identifiable neuropathology. In many cases, the physical process under study may be directly reproduced, rather than inferentially modeled, in appropriate laboratory animals. If the process is structurally localized, hypotheses about the nature of behavioral effects may be suggested from knowledge of functional neuroanatomy. As well, emotional changes most readily detected in human clinical syndromes—i.e., behavioral effects of prefrontal lobe damage—may lead, *mutatis mutandis,* to appropriate animal observations.

Of course, these advantages of designing investigation around a physically defined independent variable are largely vitiated if the description of human behavior is restricted to such psychiatric terms as "depression," "schizophrenia," "psychosis," and "personality disorder." The mechanisms relating an organic process to behavior may produce—and be most clearly illuminated by—behaviors which are socially disapproved, neutral, or praiseworthy; in fact, the latter categories are the more likely to have been overlooked by previous clinical observers. For investigative purposes, therefore, behavior associated with an organic process might best be described in specific, objective terms. Relationships among disparate behaviors and the homogeneity of behavior change associated with a particular process may then be determined statistically. It would seem that such an investigative approach to elucidating the mechanism of organic behavior changes is more likely to clarify the basis of functional psychosis, by analogy, than the current Procrustean application of psychiatric nosology.

Behavioral Effects of a Localized Neurological Process: Temporal Lobe Epilepsy

I should like to illustrate these principles in the study of a specific, localized neurological process: an epileptic focus in the temporal lobe. Temporal lobe epilepsy is clearly a physical process, resulting in abnormal electrical activity in a delimited area of the brain which may be documented by electroencephalography (Gibbs and Gibbs, 1964). The process is most commonly associated with structural pathology in the temporal lobe (Falconer et al., 1964). At the same time, this condition has been observed by multiple investigators during the last century to produce changes in behavior which resemble major functional psychoses (Slater and Beard, 1963; Davison and Bagley, 1969).

Drawing on traditional psychiatric diagnostic labels and epidemiology, much investigation has then centered on the degree of association between the neurological diagnosis of temporal epilepsy and the psychiatric diagnosis of paranoid schizophrenia. In fact, all possible logical outcomes—lower than, equal to, and higher than population prevalences of schizophrenia—have, at some time, been reported by differing investigators (Yde et al., 1941; Guerrant et al., 1962; Stevens, 1966; Flor-Henry, 1972). While this divergence underscores the imprecision inherent in studies based on psychiatric variables, it is now generally accepted that temporal epileptics do experience schizophrenia more often than unselected members of a population, but that the majority of patients do not warrant such a diagnosis (Tizard, 1962; Stevens, 1966; Davison and Bagley, 1969). Careful descriptions of patients with "schizophreniclike" psychosis point up distinctions from as readily as similarities to schizophrenia: intense rather than flattened affect, preserved social relationships, and coherent associations (Slater and Beard, 1963). It seems clear, therefore, that "schizophrenia" is neither an explicit nor a comprehensive description of the behavioral changes produced by a temporal focus; the application of this psychiatric label provides no insight into structure-function relationships within the temporal lobe which might account for a behavioral mechanism.

For this reason, my colleagues and I, first at the National Institutes of Health and now at the McLean Hospital, have studied temporal epileptic patients by focusing on specific features of interictal* behavior. Multiple case reports suggest, for example, that patients may undergo frequent religious conversions (Dewhurst and Beard, 1970), keep extensive diaries and autobiographic texts (Waxman and Geschwind, 1974, 1975), or develop pervasive moralistic feelings (Blumer, 1975).

---

*This discussion is concerned throughout with behavior occurring between, not during, clinical seizures.

79

THE TEMPORAL
LOBES: AN APPROACH
TO THE STUDY OF
ORGANIC
BEHAVIORAL
CHANGES

These behaviors need not be seen as psychopathogical and would not necessarily lead to psychiatric attention, but a cluster of such features, if shown to occur regularly in association with temporal lobe foci, might elucidate the nature of an underlying neuropsychological process. In the studies summarized below, we have assessed 18 behavioral features which were drawn from literature review and pilot clinical testing. These are listed, with the clinical sources of the observations, in Table 1; they have been described in detail elsewhere (Bear, 1976a).

In general, we have approached temporal epileptic patients, not from the point of view of psychiatric nosology or psychodynamic postulates as incorporated in standard test batteries (Meier and French, 1965; Mignone et al., 1970; Donnelly et al., 1972), but with questions suggested by functional neuroanatomy. There is now extensive evidence that destructive lesions within the temporal lobe of primates may act to disconnect emotion-mediating, limbic structures such as the amygdaloid complex and hippocampus from sensory association cortices (Weiskrantz, 1956; Schwartzbaum, 1960; Downer, 1962; Geschwind, 1965a). Surgical disconnection appears to both disrupt established emotional bonds and inhibit formation of new sensory-limbic or stimulus-reinforcement linkages (Jones and Mishkin, 1972). In temporal lobe epilepsy, similar limbic structures and adjacent association cortex are repetitively stimulated by an active epileptic focus. Therefore, we speculated that changes in emotional association were a possible consequence, perhaps reflecting formation of new, adventitious emotional bonds (Bear, 1976a).

A second mechanistic question suggested by functional neuroanatomy was based on the established structural asymmetry of right and left temporal lobes in man (Geschwind and Levitzky, 1968; Lemay and Culebras, 1972). It has been demonstrated that there is a corresponding functional asymmetry in cognition, in which the left temporal lobe appears to be specialized for linguistic perception and memory, the right for spatial or geometric processing (Milner, 1971a,b, 1974). A differential role of the hemispheres in affect has also been proposed, in which the hemispheres exert competing mood biases (Rossi and Rosadini, 1967; Terzian, 1964) or the right hemisphere possesses a dominance for emotionality (Galin, 1974; Schwartz et al., 1975). Previous evidence from temporal lobe epilepsy which might bear on affective asymmetry has been based on a small fraction of patients who were diagnosed as psychotic. Within this group, right hemisphere foci were associated with manic-depressive illnesses, left hemisphere foci with paranoid schizophrenia (Flor-Henry, 1969a,b). We were thus interested in contrasting specific behavior profiles of right temporal with left temporal epileptics in a sample of predominantly nonpsychotic patients.

Following the considerations outlined above, we attempted to define the independent variable, an epileptic focus in the temporal lobe, in terms of objective, physical observations. Strict inclusion requirements for the temporal epileptic groups were that a patient demonstrate a spike focus confined to one temporal lobe in multiple electroencephalograms (Gibbs and Gibbs, 1964) as well as an unambiguous history of psychomotor seizures (Van Buren et al., 1975). Clinically, this would be too restrictive a criterion for the diagnosis of temporal epilepsy since

TABLE 1. CHARACTERISTICS ASCRIBED TO INTERICTAL BEHAVIOR IN TEMPORAL LOBE EPILEPSY

	Behavioral characteristic	Prior clinical observations	Investigators
I.	Affect Emotionality	Deepening of all emotions, sustained intense affect	Davison and Bagley (1969) Glaser (1964) Hill (1953a,b) Slater (1969) Slater and Beard (1963) Waxman and Geschwind (1975)
	Elation, euphoria	Grandiosity, exhilarated mood; diagnosis of manic-depressive disease	Flor-Henry (1969a,b) Slater and Beard (1963)
	Sadness	Discouragement, tearfulness, self-deprecation; diagnosis of depression; suicide attempts	Dominian et al. (1963) Glaser (1964) Slater and Beard (1963) Williams (1956)
	Anger	Increased temper, irritability	Falconer (1973) Sweet et al. (1969) Taylor (1969) Treffert (1964)
	Aggression	Overt hostility, rage attacks, violent crimes, murder	Davidson (1947) Mark and Ervin (1970) Mark et al. (1968) Serafetinides (1965)
	Altered sexual interest	Loss of libido, hyposexualism; fetishism, transvestism, exhibitionism, hypersexual episodes	Blumer (1970a,b) Blumer and Walker (1967) Davies and Morgenstern (1960) Gastaut and Collomb (1954) Hierons (1971) Hooshmand and Brawley (1970) Mitchell et al. (1954)
II.	Behavior Circumstantiality	Loquaciouness, pedantry, tendency to be overly detailed, peripheral	Bear (1976a) Slater and Beard(1963) Waxman and Geschwind (1975)
	Obsessionalism	Ritualism; orderliness; compulsive attention to detail	Bear (1976b) Blumer (1975) Bruens (1969) Waxman and Geschwind (1975)
	Viscosity	Stickiness; tendency to repetition	Blumer (1975) Glaser (1964)
	Hypermoralism	Attention to rules, with inability to distinguish significant from minor infraction; desire to punish offenders	Blumer (1975) Mark and Ervin (1970) Waxman and Geschwind (1975)
	Guilt	Tendency to self-scrutiny and self-recrimination	Bear (1976a) Blumer (1975) Dominian et al. (1963) Waxman and Geschwind (1975)
	Dependence, passivity	Cosmic helplessness, "at hands of fate"; protestations of helplessness	Bear (1976a) Blumer (1975) Slater and Beard (1973)

Table 1. *(continued)*   **81**

	Behavioral characteristic	Prior clinical observations	Investigators
III.	Thought		
	Philosophical interest	Nascent metaphysical or moral speculations, cosmological theories	Bear (1976a) Slater and Beard (1963) Waxman and Geschwind (1975)
	Sense of personal destiny	Events given highly charged, personalized significance; divine guidance ascribed to many features of patient's life	Glaser (1964) Slater and Beard (1963) Waxman and Geschwind (1975)
	Humorlessness, sobriety	Overgeneralized ponderous concern; humor lacking or idiosyncratic	Bear (1976a) Ferguson *et al.* (1969) Waxman and Geschwind (1975)
	Religiosity	Holding deep religious beliefs, often idiosyncratic; multiple conversions, mystical states	Dewhurst and Beard (1970) Ervin (1967) Hill (1953a) Slater (1969) Slater and Beard (1963)
	Hypergraphia	Keeping extensive diaries, detailed notes; writing auto-biography or novel	Blumer (1975) Waxman and Geschwind (1974, 1975)
	Paranoia	Suspicious, overinterpretative of motives and events; diagnosis of paranoid schizophrenia	Bruens (1969) Hill (1953a) Pond (1957, 1962, 1969) Slater and Beard (1963)

a temporal focus may lie outside the range of EEG electrodes and escape detection; there are, as well, patients with electroencephalographic abnormalities who do not experience seizures (Stevens, 1966). Rigorous inclusion criteria ensure, however, that the index groups represented well-established temporal epilepsy.

Much controversy over behavior in temporal epilepsy has concerned bias in sampling of patients (Tizard, 1962; Herrington, 1969; Stevens, 1966). Even if psychiatric diagnoses are not used as variables, it would seem probable that patients taken exclusively from psychiatric institutions have been preselected for particular behavioral features. On the other hand, to exclude the significant fraction of temporal epileptics who reach psychiatric attention (Weir, 1976) would admit an opposite bias. We therefore selected temporal epileptic patients without regard to psychiatric history, drawing subjects from outpatient clinics where the medical aspects of epilepsy were under treatment. If bias were thereby introduced, it would reflect an undersampling of those patients confined to psychiatric hospitals.

Another vexing point of methodology has been the choice of appropriate control or comparison groups. Again, the issue of differential diagnosis has often been confounded with the determination of a causal association between the temporal epileptic focus and behavior. The investigation of mechanism requires an objective account of regularly appearing, interictal behaviors. Many of these behaviors are unlikely to be unique to temporal lobe epilepsy. There are certain to be more common reasons for strong religious feeling (Dewhurst and Beard, 1970) than possessing a temporal focus. Yet this does not diminish the mechanistic interest of the possible association. To consider a medical analogy, hypertension occurs with both renal artery stenosis and pheochromocytoma, although the mechanisms producing it are quite different. It would therefore be misleading to choose pheochromocytoma as the control condition for a study of renal artery stenosis and to dismiss the finding of hypertension because it did not differ significantly between groups. We believe it would be an equivalent error to begin by contrasting the temporal epileptic sample with, for example, paranoid schizophrenic patients. For this reason, four groups of subjects were contrasted in an initial study completed at the National Institutes of Health: 15 patients with right temporal (RT) and 12 patients with left temporal (LT) epileptic foci; 12 normal sujbects equivalent in age, education, and geographic and socioeconomic distribution (C); and 9 patients with neuromuscular diseases (N). Research continuing at the McLean Hospital includes additional comparison groups of nontemporal epileptics.

Quantitative methods of testing and data processing have been presented elsewhere (Bear, 1976b). Briefly, each of the 18 behavioral characteristics of Table 1 was measured by five true-false questionnaire items. Ten buffer questions were modified from the Lie Scale of the Minnesota Multiphasic Personality Inventory to provide a means of assessing the diagnostic specificity of trait-derived items. One-hundred-item questionnaires were completed by each subject and by his rater, a long-time friend, relative, or professional. Items on the subject and rater were first- and third-person equivalents, allowing the explicit comparison of patient-rater divergence in each group.

The behavioral results can be summarized in terms of two outcomes: the discrimination of the temporal epileptic from the contrast groups, and the differentiation of the right from left temporal samples. On the basis of the analysis of variance of average scores for the 18 behavioral traits, temporal groups scored very significantly higher ($p < 10^{-6}$) than either the neurological or control samples, which did not differ reliably from each other. Rater scores were as dramatic in confirming that the interictal characteristics of Table 1 were specifically found within the epileptic groups ($p < 10^{-5}$). The buffer questions had no ability, either among subjects or among raters, to differentiate the epileptic subjects from neurological patients or controls.

We next examined the specificity of the individual behavioral characteristics. On the basis of subjects' scores, each of the 18 categories appeared to a greater extent ($p < 0.05$) in the epileptic group; the traits of humorless sobriety, dependence, and circumstantiality most powerfully differentiated the epileptic sample ($p < 10^{-4}$). Raters also stressed circumstantiality and dependence among the epileptic groups, including the related observation of obsessionalism ($p < 10^{-4}$). On the basis of average scores, 14 of the traits appeared significantly more often among temporal subjects.

While particular traits were thus shown to occur more frequently among the temporal groups, the univariate analysis of variance of average scores did not determine whether the same or different epileptic patients possessed these traits.

83

THE TEMPORAL
LOBES: AN APPROACH
TO THE STUDY OF
ORGANIC
BEHAVIORAL
CHANGES

For example, some patients might have manifested obsessional characteristics, others aggressive behavior, and a different subgroup religious concerns. Furthermore, a small number of "severe" patients might have elevated mean scores, while many temporal epileptic patients were scoring indistinguishably from normals. These possibilities would have differing implications for the generality of the mechanism of behavioral changes.

A multivariate statistic was employed to resolve these questions. The technique of stepwise discriminant analysis (Lachenbruch, 1975) seeks to derive a profile of the typical temporal epileptic patient based on the shortest combination of nonredundant behavioral traits which characterizes the largest number of subjects. The success of the procedure is reflected in a percentage of accurate classification.

Based on subject scores, the "typical" temporal epileptic described himself as humorless, dependent, and obsessional. Ninety percent accurate discrimination between epileptic and contrast subjects was possible with this profile. Raters saw a typical patient as circumstantial, philosophical, and angry, allowing for 92% successful classification.

To increase the precision of these descriptions of the temporal epileptic subject, stepwise discriminant analysis was utilized to construct profiles based on the most discriminant combination of individual items. Separate profiles were constructed from self-descriptions and rater assessments. From subject responses, a six-item profile was generated. The discriminant function was 98% accurate, misclassifying only one epileptic subject in the sample of 48 individuals. The seven-item rater profile was equally effective in that only one neurological patient was incorrectly classified.*

The discriminant items, all endorsed more frequently by temporal epileptics than by neurological patients or controls, are listed in Table 2. In the self-report profile, items selected at steps 1 and 4 reflect a sense of personal meaning and humorless sobriety with which many events are viewed, item 3 reflects dependency, and items 2 and 5 reflect the obsessive concern with details. The rater description includes obsessional and circumstantial preoccupation with detail (1, 4), religious and philosophical concerns (3, 5), and several examples of deepened emotionality (2, 6, 7). The discriminant profiles identify clustered features of behavior, thought, and emotion which, appearing together, distinguish temporal epileptic subjects from either contrast group.

With this evidence that temporal epilepsy was regularly associated with characteristic behavioral features, we proceeded to consider differential effects of a focus in the right vs. the left temporal lobe. While the temporal lobe groups scored and were rated equivalently overall, significant differences in trait profiles appeared. In self-descriptions, right temporals described more elation, and left temporals more anger, paranoia, and dependence. Item analysis confirmed that left temporal subjects consistently described themselves more severely, emphasizing the characteristics of anger and paranoia ($p < 0.004$).

Rater descriptions also differentiated the groups, but suggested very different

*The probability that these discriminations are the result of chance is less than 0.001.

TABLE 2. DISCRIMINANT PROFILES OF TEMPORAL EPILEPTIC SUBJECTS

Step	Self-report
1.	I am sure there is a significant meaning behind suffering.
2.	Sometimes my mind gets stuck on so many different things that I cannot make a decision or do anything.
3.	I have gotten people angry by asking them to do so much for me.
4.	There is too much foolishness in the world these days.
5.	People sometimes tell me that I have trouble getting to the point because of all the details.
6.	I try to keep track of special details about my life and thinking.

Step	Rater description
1.	Rarely tells people something without giving them all the details.
2.	Subject to big shifts in mood—from very happy to very sad.
3.	Believes the bible has special meaning which he can understand.
4.	Tends to get bogged down with little details.
5.	More preoccupied than most people with the order and purpose of life.
6.	Talks about ripping some people to shreds.
7.	Feels that the future is hopeless.

distinctions. Right temporals were differentiated by unusual sexual behavior, remonstrations of helplessness, periods of sadness, emotional arousability, or moralistic fervor; obsessional concerns were also characteristic. By contrast, left temporal patients were concerned with personal destiny, philosophical exploration, and sober intellectual and moral self-scrutiny ($p < 0.001$).

To clarify these disparate profiles, principal component factor analysis was performed separately on subject and rater scores, employing all 48 subjects in the

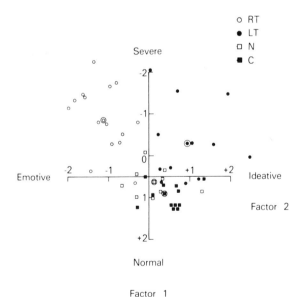

Fig. 1. Scattergram of all the subjects as evaluated by raters' standardized factor scores. Circled symbols indicate group means. Epileptic subjects (RT, LT) are separated from both controls (C) and neurological patients (N) by severity scores ($p < 0.001$). Right temporal (RT) are separated from left temporal (LT) patients by the emotive-ideative factor ($p < 0.001$).

85

THE TEMPORAL
LOBES: AN APPROACH
TO THE STUDY OF
ORGANIC
BEHAVIORAL
CHANGES

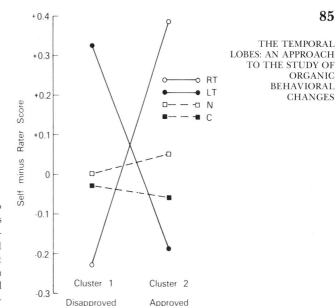

Fig. 2. Discrepancies between subjects and raters. Zero indicates patient-rater agreement, positive scores patient overreport, negative scores patient underreport of clustered items. Cluster 1: socially disapproved items. Cluster 2: socially approved items. Contrast groups (N, neurological; C, control) agreed closely with raters on both types of items, while right temporal (RT) and left temporal (LT) epileptics diverged selectively ($p < 0.001$).

sample (Harris, 1975). Details of this analysis are supplied elsewhere (Bear, 1976b). The first two principal components, accounting for greater than 55% of the total variance and strongly replicated in subject and rater analyses ($p < 0.001$), represented, respectively, a general severity factor on which all traits loaded, and a qualitative factor which separated externally directed, emotive characteristics (anger, aggression, emotionality, sadness) from introspective, ideative traits (philosophical concern, religiosity, humorlessness, personal destiny, hypergraphia).

Based on rater evaluations, factor scores were calculated for each subject. Figure 1, a scattergram of all subjects located by their rater factor scores, demonstrates a twofold separation. Epileptic patients were generally rated severer than contrast subjects ($p < 0.001$). Right temporals were more emotive ($p < 0.001$) and left temporals more ideative ($p < 0.005$) than the contrast groups, resulting in a double dissociation. Qualitatively, every right temporal subject fell on the emotive side of the ordinate and every left temporal on the ideative.

Right and left temporal subjects could thus be distinguished from each other either by self scores or by rater scores. However, the bases of discrimination were quite different, suggesting that the epileptic groups gave a different profile of themselves from that supplied by raters. Analysis of variance disclosed that significant patient-rater discrepancies occurred only in the temporal epileptic groups. These differences were qualitatively opposite in right and left subsamples ($p < 0.005$).

To identify areas of patient-rater discrepancy, difference scores were constructed by subtracting rater responses from corresponding patient items. Thus patient-rater agreement led to zero, patient overreport to positive, and patient underreport to negative scores. From trait and item analysis of these difference scores, right temporal subjects were seen to underreport sadness and agression, traits which were overreported by left temporal subjects. Conscientious-ness, however, was overreported by right subjects and underreported by left subjects ($p < 0.001$).

To generalize the basis of these group-specific discrepancies, individual items were identified which, by patient-rater discrepancy, separated right from left temporal patients. The 12 significant items ($p < 0.001$) were then cluster-analyzed (McKeon, 1967) on the basis of responses by all 48 subjects. Two compact clusters emerged. Cluster 1 was composed of items involving depression, suicidal feeling, explosive temper, peevish anger to irritation, and inappropriate dependence. We interpreted these as socially disapproved feelings or tendencies. By contrast, items of cluster 2 dealt with self-worth, the ability to see meaning behind suffering, exceptional personal etiquette, prompt attention to obligations, and minimal sexual demands. These qualities tend to be socially valued.

The mean responses of all groups to these clusters are summarized in Fig. 2. While the contrast groups agreed closely with raters on all items, temporal epileptics showed opposing discrepancies. Right temporals underreported disap-proved tendencies, greatly overreporting desirable qualities; left temporals showed a strongly opposite pattern ($p < 0.001$).

In principal component analysis of these data, the first principal component algebraically summed the tendency to overreport approved and underreport disapproved items. Positive scores thus indicate an overall embellishment or "polish" of the behavioral description; negative scores indicate the opposite bias of making the assessment overly severe or "tarnishing." Near-zero scores are consis-tent with patient-rater agreement. Figure 3 illustrates sharp differences among the groups in terms of this dimension. The right and the left temporal samples

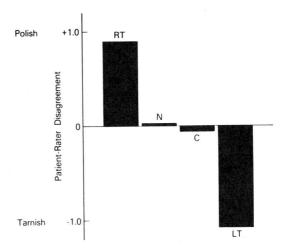

Fig. 3. Principal component analysis of patient-rater differences. Positive scores indicate overall "polish" to description, negative scores "tarnish" (see text). Near-zero score is consistent with close patient-rater agreement. Each epileptic group is significantly different from either contrast group (N, neurological; C, control). Right temporal (RT) vs. left temporal (LT) patients demonstrate qualitatively opposite patterns of disagreement ($p < 0.001$).

were significantly different from either of the contrast groups ($p < 0.005$), displaying qualitatively opposite patterns of divergence from raters ($p < 0.001$).

87

THE TEMPORAL
LOBES: AN APPROACH
TO THE STUDY OF
ORGANIC
BEHAVIORAL
CHANGES

IMPLICATIONS FOR THE STUDY OF THE NEUROANATOMY OF EMOTION

The results of this study allow for some tentative suggestions concerning the mechanism of interictal behavior characteristics in temporal lobe epilepsy. As well, this approach to the behavioral effects of a localized neurological process may shed light on two more general aspects of the functional neuroanatomy of emotion: hemispheric asymmetry in affective expression and perception, and a hierarchical sequence of emotional processing in the primate brain.

As noted previously, the present behavioral findings were based on epileptic outpatients unselected for prior psychiatric history. Retrospectively, it was found that 33% of the patients had at one time received psychiatric treatment, in good agreement with recent findings from a large midwestern epilepsy clinic (Weir, 1976). However, it is as important to stress that the majority of the temporal epileptic patients had never received psychiatric attention and were gainfully employed. It would therefore be inaccurate to describe the sample of 27 patients as schizophrenic, manic-depressive, or even personality disordered. The exclusive use of psychiatric diagnoses would have obscured the generality of behavioral description. In fact, we conclude that the specific behaviors of Table 1 occurred far more frequently among temporal epileptic patients. The discriminant behavioral profiles of Table 2—a combination of circumstantial concern with details, religious and philosophical interests, and intense, sober affect—were characteristic of virtually every patient, distinguishing them on an individual basis from each of the contrast subjects.

The most discriminating traits (humorless sobriety, circumstantiality, religiosity) tend to be stable, dispositional characteristics of interictal behavior. The most typical pattern of aggressive behavior, as well, involved characterologically worsening temper, exacerbated by environmental provocation, leading to consciously expressed and remembered anger. Because the intensity of most of the behavioral parameters correlated positively with duration of the epileptic illness, but not with seizure frequency, and because the behaviors lack episodic or paroxsymal quality, it seems improbable that they are direct expressions of subclinical seizures (Bear, 1976*b*).

Rather, we have proposed that the mechanism of interictal behavior change involves progressive physiological modification of limbic function secondary to the temporal lobe focus. We have suggested that the characteristics of Table 1 are derived from enhanced affective association to previously neutral stimuli, events, or concepts. Thus objects and events shot through with affective coloration may be incorporated into a mystical or religious view of the world. As immediate actions and thoughts are similarly charged with emotion, the patient experiences a heightened sense of personal destiny. Events dismissed by others are perceived as affectively relevant, allowing for paranoid interpretations or the conviction that the patient is a pawn in the hands of powerful forces which structure his experiences. Feeling fervently about rules and laws may lead him to a punitive type of hypermoralism. Sensing emotional importance in even the smallest acts, the patient is likely to perform these ritualistically and repetively. Since details bear the imprimatur of affective significance, many will be mentioned in lengthy, circumstantial speech or writing.

The interictal behavior syndrome of temporal lobe epilepsy may, then, be the converse of the Kluver-Bucy syndrome (Gastaut and Collomb, 1954), in which stimuli are dissociated from learned emotional associations. Experimental evidence points to the amygdaloid complex as a critical link in the pathway of sensory, particularly visual, limbic association (Weiskrantz, 1956; Jones and Mishkin, 1972; Sunshine and Mishkin, 1975). As well, this temporal limbic structure is the most readily involved in the physiological process of kindling (Goddard *et al.*, 1969), which has many parallels with normal learning (Goddard and Douglas, 1975). In contrast to the sensory limbic disconnection produced by amygdalectomy (Weiskrantz, 1956) or anterior temporal lobectomy (Kluver and Bucy, 1939; Geschwind, 1965*a*), an active epileptic process in the temporal lobe may bring about new connections through a process of physiological learning. While the electrophysiological mechanism remains undetermined, it has recently been demonstrated that an epileptic focus potentiates the use of alternate anatomical pathways for information transfer (Hunter *et al.*, 1976). Based on the neuroanatomy of the anterior temporal lobe, we have, then, interpreted the extensive affective associations as an expression of new functional connections between limbic structures and sensory association neocortices, "hyperconnections" (Bear, 1976*a*).

The behavioral data are consistent with this physiological interpretation, but certainly do not establish it. Necessary links to support this mechanism would be direct evidence of increased spurious "superstitious" emotional associations in temporal epileptic man or animal, in addition to the lesionlike deficits in emotional reversal learning which have been demonstrated (Stamm and Pribram, 1961; Stamm and Rosen, 1971). To construct a bridge from the physiological side, my colleagues and I at the Massachusetts General Hospital are employing a radioactive metabolite (Kennedy *et al.*, 1975) to attempt to map functional limbic connections and follow their evolution during creation of a neighboring epileptic focus.

An unanticipated feature of the current results was the clarity of the behavioral distinction between right and left temporal patients. In terms of profile, right temporal epileptics were seen as more overtly or externally emotive: aggressive, depressed, emotionally labile. Patients with left temporal foci developed an introspective, ideational pattern of behavioral traits: religiosity, philosophical interest, personal destiny, hypergraphia. These findings are qualitatively consistent with the previously reported association of right temporal foci with disorders of mood and left foci with thought disturbance (Flor-Henry, 1969*b*).

It would thus appear that foci in either hemisphere may modify emotional associations. If the temporal epileptic process leads to primarily intrahemispheric sensory limbic hyperconnections, these contrasting patterns of altered behavior

89

THE TEMPORAL
LOBES: AN APPROACH
TO THE STUDY OF
ORGANIC
BEHAVIORAL
CHANGES

may reflect the characteristic mode of affective expression of each of the hemispheres. The consequence of an active irritative process may, then, be opposite to that of lateralized anesthesia (Rossi and Rosadini, 1967; Terzian, 1964) or tissue-destroying lesions (Gainotti, 1972).

From this perspective, the right hemisphere process leads to nonverbal, behavioral reactions: emotive, impulsive, dispositional. The pattern of left hemisphere response—contemplative, ideative—suggests a logical, verbal representation of affect as reflected in cosmological or religious conceptualizations.

Contrasting discrepancies between patients and raters in the right vs. the left temporal epileptic groups raise additional mechanistic questions concerning the self-perception of emotional behavior. We have implicitly assumed in this presentation that raters, on the average, provided an objective account of behavior, and that patients were the distorting medium. This proposition has been statistically justified elsewhere (Bear, 1976b), but perhaps the most telling point in its favor is that clinically observed discrepancy—denial of documented criminal aggression by right temporal patients—was the initial motivation to examine patient-rater divergences.

Patients with right temporal foci tended to deny dysphoric, socially disapproved behaviors, simultaneously exaggerating valued qualities, "polishing." Left temporal epileptics, emphasizing negative behavioral features and minimizing conscientious behavior, "tarnished" their images. These contrasting distortions in self-reported behavior parallel observations concerning reactions to neurological deficit following lateralized cerebral lesions. Anosagnosia, as reflected in the denial or minimization of hemiplegia, for example, is selectively associated with lesions of the right hemisphere (Babinski, 1914; Weinstein and Kahn, 1955; Weinstein *et al.*, 1964). In general, the reactions of patients with right hemisphere injury have been characterized as facetious and inappropriately indifferent (Gainotti, 1972). By contrast, a "catastrophic reaction" of paralyzing anxiety and despair in the face of demonstrated deficits is a more common consequence of left hemisphere lesions (Goldstein, 1939; Gainotti, 1972).

Explanations proposed for these differential reactions have often drawn on the concept of right hemisphere emotional dominance (Hécaen and Angelergues, 1963; Gainotti, 1972). However, it would seem that during verbal interrogation of a patient—by examiner or questionnaire—it is the left hemisphere which ultimately surveys the situation and formulates responses. The left hemisphere may receive no report of associations established in the right hemisphere if there has been intrahemispheric injury (left hemiplegia) or callosal disconnection (commissurotomy or lesion of the genu of the corpus callosum), or if new limbic associations are established exclusively and nonverbally within the right hemisphere (right temporal epileptic focus; Babinski, 1914; Sperry, 1974; Laitenan, 1972; Bear, 1976b). In these cases, the denial of physical deficit or emotional excess may reflect a confabulatory response of the left hemisphere in the absence of reports—sensory or affective—from right hemisphere structures. Confabulation concerning unobserved stimuli has been observed frequently among patients with split-forebrain commissures (Gazzaniga, 1970; Sperry, 1968, 1974).

Within the left hemisphere, deficits in lateralized cognitive functions (language, calculation) or new affective associations will be directly accessible to verbal inquiry. The availability of emotional associations in "verbal format" may lead the left temporal epileptic to exaggerate the actual behavioral consequences of his affects. One may propose, somewhat facetiously, that he becomes verbally "hyperconscious" of emotional associations (Bear, 1976b).

While these possibilities remain speculative, there is a testable implication of the right-left differences in verbal self-report. Among the patients who reach psychiatric attention because of interictal behavior (aggression, hypermoralism, viscosity, guilt), it would be predicted that left temporal patients are more likely to self-report these difficulties and right temporals are more likely to be referred for treatment by others. This is supported by the relationship, within our sample, between self vs. rated scores of overall severity and the history of psychiatric hospitalization.

PROLEGOMENA

The goal of this chapter has been to suggest alternative investigative approaches to the phenomena of emotional and behavioral changes produced by physical processes. Using the example of temporal lobe epilepsy, we have attempted to select a neuroanatomically localized physical process as the independent variable and to treat specific features of behavior as the resultant dependent variables. The findings, of course, raise additional mechanistic questions, but these may be translated back into further neuroanatomical and physiological investigations.

In proposing that a similar approach may be productively applied to the understanding of additional emotional mechanisms, I should like to locate the current results within a highly schematic neuroanatomical and functional model of three heirarchical levels of affective processing within the primate brain. In the functional organization of appetitive behavior, for example, a first level of control involves the question of how much the organism must eat to maintain body weight. Dependent on neuroendocrine monitoring of the internal milieu, the final common pathway for the initiation of eating and satiety requires the integrity of distinct hypothalamic centers, the lateral and ventromedial nuclei (Marshall *et al.*, 1955; Olds, 1955). When these centers are destroyed by neoplasia in patients, marked aberrations of drive control regularly develop (Reeves and Plum, 1969).

A second level of control, which reflects the independent evolutionary development of neocortical perceptual systems, turns on the question of selecting an appropriate food object from its visual appearance. It is this level of integration which anatomically requires sensory-limbic connections. The destruction of these connections in the anterior temporal lobe does not disrupt maintenance of body weight but does lead to inappropriate decisions of edibility based on visual appearance (Kluver and Bucy, 1939; Geschwind, 1965a; Marlowe *et al.*, 1975). We have proposed that an active physiological alteration at this level of sensory limbic associations underlies emotional changes in temporal lobe epilepsy.

91

THE TEMPORAL
LOBES: AN APPROACH
TO THE STUDY OF
ORGANIC
BEHAVIORAL
CHANGES

If the first level of control concerns how much to eat, and the second level which object to eat, the third level may involve when to eat, rather then fight, flee, or copulate. To fulfill this complex function requires the construction of temporal contingencies governing which positive reinforcers will be sought and which negative ones avoided in the face of changing discriminative stimuli from the physical and social environments. The granular prefrontal cortex is the limbic association area which receives the necessary limbic, sensory, and sensory-limbic inputs to achieve this integration (Nauta, 1971). I believe that many features of the human frontal lobe syndrome of deficits (Luria, 1969; Hécaen and Albert, 1975) can be understood as a breakdown of this "later" stage of organization. An investigative approach guided by functional neuroanatomy, analogous to that which we attempted to apply to temporal epilepsy, may lead to mechanistic clarification of frontal emotional changes more readily than the frequent clinical deliberation over whether such patients are best described as "depressed," "psychopathic," or "manic."

Acknowledgment

The writer would like to acknowledge the very diligent secretarial assistance of Miss Laurie Bilger in preparing this chapter.

REFERENCES

Adams, R. D., and Victor, M. Delirium and other confusional states. In M. W. Wintrobe, T. Thorn, R. A. Adams, E. Braunwald, K. Isselbacher, and R. G. Petersdorf (eds.), *Principles of Internal Medicine*, 7th ed. New York: McGraw-Hill, 1974.

Babinski, J. Contribution a l'étude des troubles mentaux dans l'hémiplégie cérébrale (anosagnosia). *Revue Neurologie*, 1914, *27*, 845–487.

Bear, D. Temporal lobe epilepsy: A syndrome of sensory-limbic hyperconnection. *Cortex*, 1976a, in press.

Bear, D., and Fedio, P. Quantitative analysis of interictal behavior in temporal lobe epilepsy. *Archives of Neurology* 1976b, *34*, 454– 467.

Bear, D. Personality change associated with organic processes. In A. Lazare (ed.), *Textbook of Outpatient Psychiatry*. Baltimore: Williams and Wilkins, 1976c, in progress.

Benson, D. F., and Geschwind, N. Aphasia and related cortical disturbances. In A. B. Baker and L. M. Baker (eds.), *Clinical Neurology*. New York: Harper and Row, 1971.

Blumer, D. Changes in sexual behavior related to temporal lobe disorder in man. *Journal of Sexual Research*, 1970a, *6*, 173–180.

Blumer, D. Hypersexual episodes in temporal lobe epilepsy. *American Journal of Psychiatry*, 1970b, *126*, 1099–1106.

Blumer, D. Temporal lobe epilepsy and its psychiatric significance. In D. F. Benson and D. Blumer (eds.), *Psychiatric Aspects of Neurologic Disease*. New York: Grune and Stratton, 1975.

Blumer, D., and Benson, D. F. Personality changes with frontal and temporal lobe lesions. In D. F. Benson and D. Blumer (eds.), *Psychiatric Aspects of Neurologic Disease*. New York: Grune and Stratton, 1975.

Blumer, D., and Walker, A. E. Sexual behavior in temporal lobe epilepsy. *Archives of Neurology*, 1967, *16*, 37–43.

Bruens, J. H. Psychoses in epilepsy. In P. J. Vincken and A. W. Gruyn (eds.), *Handbook of Clinical Neurology,* Vol. 15, New York: Wiley, 1969, pp. 593–610.

Connell, P. H. *Amphetamine Psychosis.* London: Chapel Hill, 1958.

Davidson, G. A. Psychomotor epilepsy. *Canadian Medical Association Journal,* 1947, *56*, 410–414.

Davies, B. M., and Morgenstern, F. S. A case of cysticercosis, temporal lobe epilepsy and transvestism. *Journal of Neurology, Neurosurgery and Psychiatry,* 1960, *23*, 247–249.

Davison, K., and Bagley, C. Schizophrenia-like psychoses associated with organic disorders of the central nervous system: Review of literature. *British Journal of Psychiatry,* 1969, *4*, 113–184.

Dewhurst, K., and Beard, A. W. Sudden religious conversions in temporal lobe epilepsy. *British Journal of Psychiatry,* 1970, *117*, 497–507.

Dewhurst, K., Oliver, J., Trick, K. L. K., and McKnight, A. L. Neuropsychiatric aspects of Huntington's chorea. *Confinia Neurologia,* 1969, *31*, 258–268.

Diagnostic and Statistical Manual of Mental Disorders, 2nd ed. Washington, D.C.; American Psychiatric Association, 1968.

Dominian, J., Serafetinides, E. A., and Dewhurst, M. A follow-up study of late onset epilepsy. II. Psychiatric and social. *British Medical Journal,* 1963, *1*, 428–435.

Donnelly, E. F., Dent, J. K., Murphy, D. L., and Mignone, R. J. Comparison of temporal lobe epileptics and affective disorders on the Halstead-Reitan test battery. *Journal of Clinical Psychology,* 1972, *28*, 61–62.

Downer, J. L. Interhemispheric integration in the visual system. In V. Mountcastel (ed.), *Interhemispheric Relations and Cerebral Dominance.* Baltimore: Johns Hopkins Press, 1962.

Ellinwood, E. R. Amphetamine psychosis: Description of the individuals and process. *Journal of Nervous and Mental Disease,* 1967, *144*, 273–283.

Ellinwood, E. R., Sudilovsky, A., and Nelson, L. M. Evolving behavior in the clinical and experimental amphetamine (model) psychosis. *American Journal of Psychiatry,* 1973, *130*, 1088–1093.

Ervin, F. R. Brain disorders associated with convulsions (epilepsy). In A. M. Freedman and H. I. Kaplan (eds.), *Comprehensive Textbook of Psychiatry.* Baltimore: Williams and Wilkins, 1967, pp. 795–816.

Everitt, B. S., Gourlay, A. J., and Kendall, R. E. An attempt at validation of traditional psychiatric syndromes by cluster analysis. *British Journal of Psychiatry,* 1971, *119*, 399–412.

Falconer, M. A. Reversibility by temporal lobe resection of the behavioral abnormalities of temporal lobe epilepsy. *New England Journal of Medicine,* 1973, *289*, 451–455.

Falconer, M. A., Serafetinides, E. A., and Corsellis, J. A. Etiology and pathogenesis of temporal lobe epilepsy. *Archives of Neurology,* 1964, *10*, 233–248.

Feighner, J. D., Robins, E., Guze, S. B., Woodruff, R. A., Winokur, G., and Monore, R. Diagnostic criteria for use in psychiatric research. *Archives of General Psychiatry,* 1972, *26*, 57–63.

Ferguson, S. M., Schwartz, M. L., and Rayport, M. Perception of humor in patients with temporal lobe epilepsy: A cartoon test as an indicator of neuropsychologic deficit. *Archives of General Psychiatry,* 1969, *21*, 363.

Flor-Henry, P. Psychosis and temporal lobe epilepsy: A controlled investigation. *Epilepsia,* 1969a, *10*, 363–395.

Flor-Henry, P. Schizophrenic-like reactions and affective psychoses associated with temporal lobe epilepsy: Etiological factors. *American Journal of Psychiatry,* 1969b, *126*, 400–403.

Flor-Henry, P. Ictal and interictal psychiatric manifestations in epilepsy: Specific or nonspecific? *Epilepsia,* 1972, *13*, 773–783.

Gainotti, G. Emotional behavior and hemispheric side of the lesion. *Cortex,* 1972, *8*, 41–55.

Galin, D. Implications for psychiatry of left and right cerebral specialization. *Archives of General Psychiatry,* 1974, *31*, 572–583.

Gastaut, H., and Collomb, K. Etude du comportement sexuel chez les épileptiques psychomoteurs. *Annales Médico-Psychologiques,* 1954, *112*, 657–696.

Gazzaniga, M. S. *The Bisected Brain.* New York: Appleton-Century, 1970.

Geschwind, N. Disconnexion syndromes in animals and man. Part I, *Brain,* 1965a, *88*, 237–294.

Geschwind, N. Disconnexion syndromes in animals and man. Part II. *Brain,* 1965b, *88*, 585–644.

Geschwind, N. The borderland of neurology and psychiatry. In D. F. Benson and D. Blumer (eds.), *Psychiatric Aspects of Neurologic Disease.* New York: Grune and Stratton, 1975.

Geschwind, N., and Levitsky, W. Human brain: Left-right asymmetries in temporal speech area. *Science,* 1968, *161*, 186–187.

Gibbs, F. A., and Gibbs, E. L. *Atlas of Electroencephalography.* Cambridge Mass.: Addison-Wesley, 1964.

Glaser, G. H. The probelm of psychosis in psychomotor temporal lobe epileptics. *Epilepsia*, 1964, *5*, 271–278.

Goddard, G. V., and Douglas, R. M. Does the engram of kindling model the engram of normal long-term memory? *Le Journal Canadian des Sciences Neurologiques*, 1975, 385–394.

Goddard, G. V., McIntyre, D. C., and Leech, C. K. A permanent change in brain function resulting from daily electrical stimulation. *Experimental Neurology*, 1969, *25*, 295–330.

Goldstein, K. *The Organism: A Holistic Approach to Biology*. New York: American Book, 1939.

Guerrant, J., Anderson, W. W., Fischer, A., Weinstein, M. R., Jaros, R. M., and Deskins, A. *Personality in Epilepsy*. Springfield, Ill.: Thomas, 1962.

Harris, R. J. *A Primer of Multivariate Statistics*. New York: Academic Press, 1975.

Hécaen, H., and Albert, M. Disorders of mental functioning related to frontal lobe pathology. In D. F. Benson and D. Blumer (eds.), *Psychiatric Aspects of Neurologic Disease*. New York: Grune and Stratton, 1975.

Hécaen, H., and Angelergues, R. *La Cecite Psychique*. Paris: Masson, 1963.

Herrington, R. N. The personality in temporal lobe epilepsy. *British Journal of Psychiatry*, Special Publication 4, 1969, 70–76.

Hierons, R. Impotence in temporal lobe lesions. *Journal of Neurovisceral Relations*, Supplement X, 1971, 477–481.

Hill, D. Psychiatric disorders of epilepsy. *Medical Press*, 1953a, *20*, 473–475.

Hill, D. Clinical study and selection of patients in discussion on the surgery of temporal lobe epilepsy. *Proceedings of the Royal Society of Medicine*, 1953b, *46*, 965–976.

Hooshmand, H., and Brawley, B. W. Temporal lobe seizures and exhibitionism. *Neurology*, 1970, *19*, 1119–1124.

Hunter, M., Maccabe, J. J., and Ettlinger, F. Transfer of training between the hands in a split-brain monkey with chronic parietal discharges. *Cortex*, 1976, *12*, 27–30.

Jones, B., and Mishkin, M. Limbic lesions and the problem of stimulus-reinforcement associations. *Experimental Neurology*, 1972, *36*, 362–377.

Kennedy, C., Des Rosiers, M., Jehle, J., Reivich, M., Sharpe, F., and Sokolov, L. Mapping of functional neural pathways by autoradiographic survey of local metabolic rate with ^{14}C deoxyglucose. *Science*, 1975, *187*, 850–853.

Kluver, H., and Bucy, P. C. Preliminary analysis of functions of the temporal lobes in man. *Archives of Neurology and Psychiatry*, 1939, *42*, 979–1000.

Lachenbruch, P. *Discriminant Analysis*. New York: Haffner Press, 1975.

Laitenan, L. V. Stereotactic lesions in the knee of the corpus callosum in the treatment of emotional disorders. *Lancet*, 1972, *7748*, 472–475.

Lemay, M., and Culebras, A. Human brain-morphologic differences in the hemispheres demonstrable by carotid arteriography. *New England Journal of Medicine*, 1972, *287*, 168–170.

Luria, A. R. Frontal lobe syndromes. In P. J. Vinchen and G. W. Bruyn (eds.), *Handbook of Clinical Neurology*. Amsterdam: North-Holland, 1969.

Mark, V. H., and Ervin, F. R. *Violence and the Brain*. New York: Harper and Row, 1970.

Mark, V. H., Ervin, F. R., Geschwind, N., Solomon, P., and Sweet, W. H. The neurology of behavior: Its applications to human violence. *Medical Opinion Review*, 1968, *4*, 26–31.

Marlowe, W. V., Mancall, E. L., and Thomas, J. J. Complete Kluver-Bucy syndrome in man. *Cortex*, 1975, *11*, 53–59.

Marshall, N. B., Barnett, R. J., and Mayer, J. Hypothalamic lesions in gold-thioglucose injected mice. *Proceedings of the Society of Biology and Medicine of New York*, 1955, *90*, 240–244.

McHugh, P. R., and Folstein, M. Psychiatric syndromes of Huntington's chorea. In D. F. Benson and D. Blumer (eds.), *Psychiatric Aspects of Neurologic Disease*. New York: Grune and Stratton. 1975.

McKeon, J. J. *Hierarchial Cluster Analysis—Computer Program*. Washington, D.C.: George Washington University Biometric Laboratory, 1967.

Meier, M. J., and French, L. A. Changes in MMPI scale scores and an index of psychopathology following unilateral temporal lobectomy for epilepsy. *Epilepsia*, 1965, *6*, 263–273.

Mignone, R. J., Donnelly, E. F., and Sadowsky, D. Psychological and neurological comparisons of psychomotor and nonpsychomotor epileptic patients. *Epilepsia*, 1970, *11*, 345–359.

Milner, B. Interhemispheric differences in the localization of psychological processes in man. *British Medical Bulletin*, 1971a, *27*, 272–277.

Milner, B. Memory and the medial temporal regions of the brain. In K. H. Pribram and D. F. Broadbent (eds.), *Biology of Memory*. New York: Academic Press, 1971b, pp. 29–50.

93

THE TEMPORAL
LOBES: AN APPROACH
TO THE STUDY OF
ORGANIC
BEHAVIORAL
CHANGES

Milner, B. Hemispheric specialization: Scope and limits. In F. O. Schmitt F. G. Warden (eds.), *The Neurosciences—Third Study Program.* Cambridge, Mass. MIT Press, 1974, pp. 75–89.

Mitchell, W., Falconer, M. A., and Hill, D. Epilepsy with fetishism relieved by temporal lobectomy. *Lancet,* 1954, *2,* 626–636.

Nauta, W. J. H. The problem of the frontal lobe—A reinterpretation. *Journal of Psychiatric Research,* 1971, *9,* 167–187.

Olds, J. Physiological mechanisms of reward. In M. Jones (ed.), *Nebraska Symposium on Motivation.* Lincoln. University of Nebraska Press, 1955.

Pond, D. A. Psychiatric aspects of epilepsy. *Journal of the Indian Medical Profession,* 1957, *3,* 1441–1451.

Pond, D. A. The schizophrenia-like psychoses of epilepsy—Discussion. *Proceedings of the Royal Society of Medicine,* 1962, *55,* 316.

Pond, D. A. Epilepsy and personality disorders. In P. J. Vincken and A. W. Gruyn (eds.), *Handbook of Clinical Neurology,* Vol. 15. New York: Wiley, 1969, pp. 576–592.

Reeves, A. G., and Plum, F. Hyperphagia, rage, and dementia accompanying a ventromedial hypothalamic neoplasm. *Archives of Neurology,* 1969, *20,* 616–624.

Rossi, G. F., and Rosadini, G. Experimental analysis of cerebral dominance in man. In C. H. Milikan and F. L. Darley (eds.), *Brain Mechanisms Underlying Speech and Language.* New York: Grune and Stratton, 1967, pp. 167–184.

Schwartz, G. E., Davidson, R. J., and Maer, F. Right hemisphere lateralization for emotion in the human brain: Interactions with cognition. *Science,* 1975, *190,* 286–288.

Schwartzbaum, J. S. Changes in reinforcing properties of stimuli following ablation of the amygdaloid complex in monkeys. *Journal of Comparative and Physiological Psychology,* 1960, *53,* 388–395.

Serafetinides, E. A. Aggressiveness in temporal lobe epileptics and its relation to cerebral dysfunction and environmental factors. *Epilepsia,* 1965, *6,* 33–42.

Slater, E. The schizophrenia-like illnesses of epilepsy. *British Journal of Psychiatry,* 1969, *4,* 77–81.

Slater, E. , and Beard, A. W. Schizophrenia-like psychoses of epilepsy: Relations between ages of onset. *British Journal of Psychiatry,* 1963, *109,* 95–150.

Slater, E., and Moran, P. A. P. The schizophrenia-like psychoses of epilepsy: Relation between ages of onset. *British Journal of Psychiatry,* 1969, *115,* 599–600.

Sperry, R. W. Hemisphere deconnection and unity in conscious experience. *American Psychologist,* 1968, *23,* 723–733.

Sperry, R. W. Lateral specialization in the surgically separated hemispheres. In F. O. Schmitt and F. G. Warden (eds.), *The Neurosciences—Third Study Program.* Cambridge, Mass.: MIT Press, 1974, pp. 5–20.

Stamm, J. S., and Pribram, K. H. Effects of epileptogenic lesions of inferotemporal cortex on learning and retention in monkeys. *Journal of Comparative and Physiological Psychology,* 1961, *54,* 614–618.

Stamm, J. S., and Rosen, S. C. Learning of a somesthetic discrimination and reversal tasks by monkeys with epileptogenic implants in anteromedial temporal cortex. *Neuropsychologia,* 1971, *9,* 185–194.

Stevens, J. R. Psychiatric implications of psychomotor epilepsy. *Archives of General Psychiatry,* 1966, *14,* 461–471.

Sweet, W. H., Ervin, F., and Mark, V. H. The relationship of violent behavior to focal cerebral disease. In S. Garattini and E. B. Sigg (eds.), *Agressive Behavior.* Amsterdam: Excerpta Medica, 1969, pp. 336–352.

Sunshine, J., and Mishkin, M. A visual-limbic pathway serving visual associative functions in rhesus monkeys. *Federation Proceedings,* 1975, *34,* 440.

Taylor, D. C. Aggression and epilepsy. *Journal of Psychosomatic Research,* 1969, *13,* 229–236.

Terzian, H. Behavioral and EEG effects of intracarotid sodium amytal injections. *Acta Neurochirurgica,* 1964, *12,* 230–240.

Tizard, B. The personality of epileptics: A discussion of the evidence. *Psychological Bulletin,* 1962, *59,* 196–210.

Treffert, D. A. The psychiatric patient with an EEG temporal lobe focus. *American Journal of Psychiatry,* 1964, *120,* 765–771.

Van Buren, J. M., Ajmone-Marsan, C., Matsuga, N., and Sadowsky, D. Surgery of temporal lobe epilepsy. In D. P. Purpura, J. K. Penry, and R. D. Walter (eds.), *Advances in Neurology,* Vol. 8. New York: Raven Press, 1975, pp. 155–196.

Waxman, S. F., and Geschwind, N. Hypergraphia in temporal lobe epilepsy. *Neurology,* 1974, *24,* 629–636.

Waxman, S. F., and Geschwind, N. The interictal behavior syndrome of temporal lobe epilepsy. *Archives of General Psychiatry,* 1975, *32,* 1580–1586.

95

THE TEMPORAL
LOBES: AN APPROACH
TO THE STUDY OF
ORGANIC
BEHAVIORAL
CHANGES

Weinstein, E. A., and Kahn, R. C. *Denial of Illness: Symbolic and Physiologic Aspects.* Springfield, Ill.: Thomas, 1955.

Weinstein, E. A., Mitchell, M., and Lyerly, O. G. Anosagnosia and aphasia. *Archives of Neurology,* 1964, *10*, 376–386.

Weir, W. Psychosis in temporal lobe epilepsy. Unpublished retrospective study at University of Illinois Epilepsy Clinic, 1976.

Weiskrantz, L. Behavioral changes associated with ablation of the amygdaloid complex in monkeys. *Journal of Comparative and Physiological Psychology.* 1956, *49*, 381–391.

Williams, D. The structure of emotions reflected in epileptic experiences. *Brain,* 1956, *79*, 28–67.

Yde, A., Edel, L., and Feurbye, A. On the relation between schizophrenia, epilepsy, and induced convulsions. *Acta Psychiatrica,* 1941, *16*, 325–388.

PART III
Developmental Neuropsychology

5

Aspects of Normal and Abnormal Neuropsychological Development

Harry van der Vlugt

Introduction

Research in developmental neuropsychology has emphasized empirical methods and differences in methodology have probably restricted broader conceptual understanding. Moreover, attention has too often been focused on isolated tests purporting to measure left-right discrimination, form perception, writing, and calculation. This state of affairs has generated a plethora of studies into specific developmental disorders, but these are often based on unrepresentative cases, inadequate design, and isolated behaviors. Theory development has been slow, thus preventing the conceptual integration of findings which appear unrelated or discrepant with specific hypotheses.

The following section will attempt to provide a theoretical frame of reference in which underlying neurophysiological mechanisms are postulated and a number of developmental hypotheses are generated which might predict specific behavioral patterns expected to occur as a function of the disorder and the age of the child.

The Theoretical Frame of Reference

The human mind needs a theoretical structure for understanding the diverse facts of nature and science. A conceptual framework for thinking about the brain

Harry van der Vlugt   Department of Psychology, Tilburg University, Tilburg, The Netherlands. This research was supported in part by funds from The Netherlands Organization for the Advancement of Pure Research (Z.W.O.).

is a prerequisite for guiding research. One should be aware of the fact that each theoretical frame of reference is an abstraction and a simplification of reality.

The great contribution to philosophy by Descartes left us with a dualistic world concept. Many philosophical developments based on this two-world concept did and still do (Bruyn, 1976) provide an explanation of our experience and knowledge in terms of inner and outer world. Recently, Eccles (1970, 1973), formerly a dualist, converted to a trialist as a consequence the philosophical achievements of Popper (1968*a,b*). Earlier, trialism based on the evolutionary view was proposed. Preceding Darwin, Herbert Spencer developed an evolutionary view of the nervous system emanating from the concepts of organization and function of the brain. In the first edition of his *Principles of Psychology* (1855), and thus 4 years before Darwin's *Origin of Species,* Spencer (1899, 4th ed.) stated "that Life in its multitudinous and infinitely varied embodiments has risen out of the lowest and simplest beginnings, by steps as gradual as those which evolve a homogeneous, microscopic germ into a complex organism, by progressive unbroken evolution. . . ." Spencer accounted for the more complex aspects of neural evolution primarily in Lamarckian terms: "Regarding as superimposed, each on the preceding, the structural effects produced generation after generation and species after species, we have formed a general conception of the manner in which the most complex nervous systems have arisen out of the simplest."

Hughlings Jackson was enormously influenced by Spencer and took over his evolutionary view of the nervous system (Taylor, 1958). He proposed that a given function is represented several times at different levels of the nervous system. The higher levels of the nervous system—having evolved later—mediate a given function in a more finely tuned fashion than the lower levels. Furthermore, they are more easily excited, and they may have an inhibitory influence on the lower levels. Damage at a higher level releases the lower ones from inhibition. The lower levels continue to subserve the function as best they can. Jackson thus held that hierarchical representation underlies what he called the "principle of compensation" in neural functioning. This hierarchical representation is the basis of the triality which is shown, among others, in Table 1. In my opinion, two recent trialist

TABLE 1. EVOLUTIONARY CONCEPTS OF THE ORGANIZATION AND FUNCTION OF THE BRAIN

Jackson (in Taylor, 1958)	Pavlov (1955)	Yakovlev and Lecours (1967)	Luria (1973)	Eccles (1973)	MacLean (1970, 1972)	Isaacson (1974)	
Highest level	Second signal system	Supralimbic zone	Programming, regulating, verifying mental activity	Conscious self	Neomammalian brain	Guru	Level III
Middle level	Conditioned reflex	Paramedian or limbic zone	Obtaining, processing, storing of information	Memory stores	Paleomammalian brain	Lethe	Level II
Lowest level	Unconditioned reflexes	Median zone	Regulating tone or waking	Sensorimotor brain stem	Protoreptilian brain	Graven Image	Level I

approaches deserve serious consideration. Their conceptual framework, as a guide in our research, might show aspects relevant to neuropsychological development which are easily overlooked.

101

ASPECTS OF NORMAL
AND ABNORMAL
NEUROPSYCHO-
LOGICAL
DEVELOPMENT

The Triune Brain

Based on comparative anatomy, neurochemistry, and evolutionary theory, MacLean (1970) proposes that neural as well as behavioral evidence suggests three types of systems in the brains of mammals. MacLean distinguishes in the brain a protoreptilian, a paleomammalian, and a neomammalian brain (see Table 1). The protoreptilian brain consists of systems in the upper spinal cord and parts of the midbrain, diencephalon, and basal ganglia. The paleomammalian brain corresponds to the limbic system. The neomammalian brain is thought to consist of the neocortical structures.

The related trialist approach is advocated by Isaacson (1974). In the final chapter of his book *The Limbic System*, he distinguishes the following three types of systems: the Graven Image, Lethe, and the Guru. These three divisions must be considered as speculative, because no animals with a pure protoreptilian or paleomammalian brain are known. The triune brain approach is significant because it provides a model for relating behavioral data to more or less specific anatomical systems. Particularly, the triune brain model deserves serious consideration as a metaphor for the hierarchical structures of the brain as it relates to behavior.

Protoreptilian Brain—Graven Image—Level I

MacLean considers the protoreptilian brain as responsible for instinctive and well-trained behaviors based on "ancestral learning and ancestral memories." It plays a crucial role in the establishment of home territories, the finding of shelter, hunting, homing, mating, breeding, and other activities necessary for survival. Isaacson's Graven Image is fairly well in agreement with MacLean's protoreptilian brain.

Paleomammalian Brain—Lethe—Level II

The paleomammalian or limbic brain is thought to be nature's tentative first step toward providing self-awareness. It is supposed to play a basic role in the integration of emotional expression because of its strong connections with the hypothalamus. To MacLean, the paleomammalian brain is still a "visceral brain" (MacLean, 1949, 1955). It has, however, some role related to neocortical formation. It is hierarchically superior and has the ability to override the ancestral basis of behavior found in the protoreptilian brain. All memories, according to MacLean's view, depend on a mixture of information from the inner and the outer world. This mixture is supposed to occur in the hippocampus, which receives "internal information" from the septal area and "external information" from the sensory systems projecting to the nearby transitional cortical areas (MacLean, 1972). According to Isaacson (1974), the limbic system (Lethe, the river of forgetting) acts to produce forgetfulness by inhibiting the ancient memories of the protoreptilian brain. Isaacson considers the limbic system basically as the regulator, primarily in an inhibitory fashion, of the reptilian core brain. The limbic system is responsible for the suppression of previously learned behavioral sequences. It provides the basis of forgetting of ancient memories, the graven images, and opens the way for new, temporary associations. Stimulation of the limbic system often produces a suppression of ongoing behaviors. Lesions within the limbic system can produce an intensification of activities in systems representative of activities of the protoreptilian brain.

NEOMAMMALIAN BRAIN—THE GURU—LEVEL III

The role of the neocortex is not greatly discussed in MacLean's writings. He seems to consider it to be responsible for the cold (nonemotional) and fine-grain analysis of the external environment. It operates "unhindered by signals and noise generated in the internal world." Its nice differentiating ability is emphasized, and it is thought to have "the propensity to subdividing things into smaller and smaller entities" (MacLean, 1970). The primary motor areas of the neocortex impose a rapidly conducting system controling fine-grain movements of the extremities on a reasonably effective motor apparatus largely based in subcortical and brain stem regions (Isaacson, 1974). Damage to the primary motor cortex of mammals results in a loss of the rapid, fine-grain movements of the digits (Haaxma and Kuypers, 1975).

The neocortex seems to be especially capable of the quick and efficient processing of information which has many fine details. Its adjustive contributions are those which require a delicacy beyond the capabilities of the lower centers. It provides man with the highest standard of motor skill which is reached in the art of speaking and in the development of fine finger movements. In 1 sec man can perform as many as 32 different isolated consecutive flexions or extensions using ten digits while playing the piano (Zülch, 1975).

The major characteristic that distinguishes man from other animals is language. This capability is related to certain regions of the left hemisphere. Language gives man the opportunity to override the demands of his internal world and those of the outer world. Directly or indirectly, the neocortex suppresses the habits or memories of the past. The neocortex looks into the future. Like a Guru, it pleads to give up old habits, to give up the sin of excessive "attachment" to the past (Isaacson, 1974).

IMPLICATIONS OF THE TRIUNE BRAIN MODEL FOR DEVELOPMENTAL NEUROPSYCHOLOGY

Although it is heuristically helpful to categorize different aspects of brain function, it would be a mistake to imagine that each of these units can carry out a

103

ASPECTS OF NORMAL
AND ABNORMAL
NEUROPSYCHO-
LOGICAL
DEVELOPMENT

certain form of activity completely independently. Behavior appears to be dependent on the combined working of all three brain systems, each of which makes its own contribution. "It is clear that all three principal functional brain units work concertedly" (Luria, 1973, p. 101).

For developmental neuropsychology, the triune brain model has several implications. As a child grows older, the development of both brain and behavior will follow an orderly, predictable, interrelated sequence. Each developmental step is in some way dependent on a certain degree of maturation of the previous steps. "The formation of higher nervous activity in children is determined by the degree of maturity of the cortex and the subcortical formations" (Sarsikov, 1964). The model implies also that during maturation the brain retains some of the organization of the previous steps. Encephalization is not substitutional but additional control. The same kinds of functions are repeated at several levels of the brain. The higher levels, as they develop, also remain dependent on the lower structures.

Green (1958) stated that "The impression is gained that by surgery one can somewhat reverse the evolutionary tide of development" by sectioning the brain at progressively more caudal levels. Green's suggestion is that the evolutionary past is still reflected in successively lower levels of the brain. Other authors hold similar positions (Penfield, 1954; Denny-Brown, 1960).

A basic error in the mainstream of developmental neuropsychology has been in the direction of considering all sensation, perception, and cognition as exclusively neocortical, overlooking the probability that some subcortical function may still be critical. As the brain evolved, adding more complex structures to deal with the environment more effectively, a change in the potential for motor output also occurred. The brain stem is primarily concerned with total massive patterning involving overt responses of the entire body, determined by a relatively simple integration. The interesting aspect of the hierarchical organization lies as well in the sequential appearance of successively more refined adaptive mechanisms in human development, as in the later complex interactions among systems of different degrees of complexity.

The advent of the cerebral hemispheres allowed more discrete, individualistic motor patterns based on more precise interpretation of sensory information. While evolution has favored increased localization of functions of the brain, it has not eliminated the dependence of each part of the central nervous system on other parts, especially on lower or more caudal structures. The primary sensory areas of the brain have become highly competent, and this competence has been enhanced with increasing localization. By the same evolutionary process, the capacity for interaction among the localized areas has been increased through the association areas, which overlap association areas of other sensory modalities. The overlapping topography presumably facilitates coordination and totality of function. "In man the zones in which there is 'overlapping' of the cortical boundaries of different analyzers comprise 43% of the total mass of the cortex, so that it appears that the evolution of the cortex proceeds mainly on the basis of formations responsible for this integrative activity of the central nervous system" (Luria, 1966).

In cases in which the development of the brain deviates from the norm, the resultant behavior is often reminiscent of lower levels, with interference in the sequential expression of the developmental patterns. For example, primitive reflexes often are present, the sense of touch is apt to be diffuse rather than well differentiated, and some children are overly ready with a fight-or-flight reaction in response to some tactile stimuli.

This theory is consonant with those positions in developmental psychology which postulate that the child goes through consecutive stages of behavior (Gessel and Amatruda, 1948) and thought (Hunt, 1961; Piaget, 1926; Bruner, 1974) during development, each of which incorporates the processes of the preceding stage into a more complex and hierarchically integrated form of adaptation.

DEVELOPMENTAL NEUROLOGY

The neuroanatomical development of the human brain cannot be studied by the precise methods employed in animal research. Lack of information on the developing human brain leads to relying on basic brain research on lower vertebrates. Being aware of the multitude of limitations of applying animal research data to human beings, one might say that generalizations from lower animals applied to man are probably safest where the brains of the two species are most similar. Of the brain's structures, the interspecies difference will increase from the protoreptilian brain (Graven Image) to the neomammalian brain (Guru).

LEVEL I

Animals with lesions limited to the basal ganglia suffer disturbances of posture and postural control, locomotion, equilibrium, and righting as the most important part of the syndromes recorded. The brain stem reticular system and the various motor nuclei of this level constitute a system for coordinating gross body movements, for example, innate mechanisms for bilateral coordination of head, eyes, and trunk. Present also are more discrete stimulus-response systems such as the sucking reflex, rooting reflex, and pupillary reflex. Although the newborn baby is able to move the proximal joints of arms and legs and can suck and swallow in a very skillful manner, it cannot use its fingers in any skillful act. If it receives an injury to the cortex, there may be little or no evidence of disability until it passes its first year of life. Only when skillful employment of the hand and foot normally appears will the defect first become apparent. In the adult, when the precentral gyrus has been removed, dexterous employment of fingers and toes is not possible, but skillful use of the subcortical motor mechanisms of swallowing, vocalizing, and looking is still possible, as is gross movement of the extremities (Penfield, 1954).

LEVEL II

The hippocampal formation occupies a central position within the limbic system. Adequate stimulation of the hippocampus (cornu ammonis and the

105

ASPECTS OF NORMAL
AND ABNORMAL
NEUROPSYCHO-
LOGICAL
DEVELOPMENT

fornix) produces ipsilateral movement, and the contralateral movement added to this results in a bilateral movement (Votaw, 1959). The well-known observation in young children of identical and mass-associated movements possibly has its origin in an "extrapyramidal" pathway. If these associated movements are still present in older children, it might be indicative of a lack of suppression of these movements by the higher cortical functions. This lack of suppression may be the resultant of a cortical lesion or an immature, undifferentiated state of the neocortex.

Animals with hippocampal lesions exhibit hyperactive behavior in open-field situations (Douglas, 1967; Kimble, 1968). The descriptive characterization of hippocampectomized animals as "exuberant," "reckless," and "unobservant" suggest that the hippocampus has a role in behavioral maturation. The significance of this activity is unknown (Isaacson, 1974). However, hyperactive behavior has never been observed in human adults with hippocampal lesions. A possible relationship might exist with hyperactivity in children. The hyperactivity might be the behavioral resultant of a deficiency in hippocampal function, probably in combination with a lack of differentiated cortical control.

The spontaneous alternation paradigm is closely related to hippocampal function (Douglas, 1975) and is a way to "measure" hippocampal development. Spontaneous alternation is usually studied by placing an animal in a T-shaped maze. The tendency of the subject is to alternate visits to the two goal boxes of the T-maze on consecutive trials without a reward for the response. If the choices on the two consecutive trials were independent, the animal would enter the opposite goal box about 50% of the time by chance. The young rat performs this way, showing total lack of spontaneous alternation behavior. An adult rat showing the spontaneous alternation behavior does not choose randomly, but instead visits opposite alleys about 85% of the time. Bilateral lesions to the hippocampal system result in a loss of spontaneous alternation behavior. Another important aspect of spontaneous alternation behavior is the fact that this behavior is resistant to lesions outside the hippocampal system. Finally, it should be noted that removal of one side of the hippocampus in adulthood has no effect on alternation, whereas the same unilateral lesion in infancy has a drastic effect on alternation in adulthood. This might indicate that lesions in the hippocampal system at a younger age have a more devastating effect on behavior than those at an older age. Douglas *et al.* (1972) were able to develop an alternation test suitable for human subjects and capable of individual analysis. By means of a slide test, they were able to show the shift from the nonalternation (below 49 months of age) to the alternation (above 49 months of age) strategy. Pate and Bell (1971), using giant mazes, found alley alternation rates of 41%, 70%, 83%, and 83% for children aged 3, 4, 5, and 6 years, respectively. Lack of alternation might be called perseveration. Jones (1970) found that nursery school children under 4 years of age perseverated in their guesses, while children over 4 years of age alternated guesses. The above studies suggest that the hippocampal system shows a functional development which can be measured by behavioral changes in man as well as in subhuman species (Douglas, 1975).

Pribram and Isaacson (1975), summarizing the two volumes of *The Hippocampus,* state: "The suggestion emerges that the hippocampus functions to determine whether appetitive-consumatory processes should proceed in their habitual manner (a well-integrated habitual behavior which depends among others on the basal ganglia), or whether novel, unfamiliar inputs have occurred which must be attended to." By emphasizing the *attentional-intentional* (voluntary) behavior hypothesis of hippocampal function, Pribram and Isaacson (1975) offer a possible solution to the irreconcilability of the human long-term memory loss with the animal disinhibition literature. Possibly, consolidation (memory) deficiencies have to be explained as a failure in attention, and disinhibition can be seen as the consequence of a loss of intentional (voluntary) capability. The association between hippocampal functions and memory is usually inferred through observations of memory impairment in patients with hippocampal damage (Grunthal, 1947; Glees and Griffith, 1952). Weiskrantz and Warrington (1975), analyzing memory disturbances due to bilateral medial temporal lobe lesions, point out that there are defects in retrieval rather than in storage. The human amnesic subject has difficulty in controlling and restraining the influence of prior learning on present performance (Weiskrantz, 1971). The subject is not capable of discriminating new information from older information. Gaffan (1972, 1974) has suggested that amnesic patients may be impaired in discriminating degrees of familiarity of an item. He cites Talland's comment on search cycles in memory: "each phase [of the search] being terminated by an implicit act of recognition. . . . Our patients were apt to terminate their search with an incorrect match" (Talland, 1965, pp. 304–305). This implies that for the amnesic patient all items tend to appear more nearly equally familiar (or unfamiliar) than for the normal subjects. It is as if the temporal organization of the memory load is disturbed. Associative memory is intact, recognition memory is disturbed. If the experimental situation, however, is such that the amnesic patients are presented with relevant contextual information, their memory performance is much better. One may assume that the retention of an item depends on associations acquired or used during learning. Successive similar learning experiences will be deficient, so that one event is confused with another event that occurred before or after it. The ability to discriminate between successive sets of material seems to be lost.

LEVEL III

The representation of higher functions such as speech and language evolves from a state of diffuse and bilateral representation to one of increased differentiation and lateralization within the left hemisphere. When the maturational process has reached its mature state, cerebral lateralization is firmly established (Basser, 1962; Lenneberg, 1967). The establishment of the representation of language might optimize the acquisition of conceptual or formal operations.

Anatomical (Geschwind and Levitsky, 1968; Witelson and Pallie, 1973; Wada *et al.*, 1975) and neurophysiological (Molfese *et al.*, 1975) studies reveal a difference between right and left cerebral hemispheres as early as the 29th gestational week. Studies on the developing pyramidal tract show projections from the left hemisphere crossing before those on the right (Yakovlev and Rakic, 1966). Autopsy data indicate that the size of the left temporal planum increases over that of the right as a function of age (Wada *et al.*, 1975). This anatomical increase in

107

ASPECTS OF NORMAL
AND ABNORMAL
NEUROPSYCHO-
LOGICAL
DEVELOPMENT

magnitude is in agreement with developmental neuropsychological reports of an increase in magnitude of ear asymmetry using the dichotic listening paradigm (Satz *et al.*, 1975). Hammer and Turkewitz (1974) demonstrated lateral differences in sensitivity. Cardiac acceleration occurred significantly more frequently to stimulation of the right than to stimulation of the left side of the body in 38-hr-old girls. Studies of the myelinization of the cerebral cortex (Flechsig, 1901) show a sequential and hierarchical development. "Early myelinating zones, or 'primordial' zones include all of the classic motor and sensory zones, and the primary somesthetic, visual and auditory cortices" (Geschwind, 1968, p. 183). These "primordial" zones have the most efferent and afferent connections with the subcortical structures, in contrast to later-myelinating or "terminal" zones (i.e., left angular gyrus), which have mostly corticocortical connections. These terminal zones are important for the mediation of more complex language skills. Studying the myelinization of the developing brain, Yakovlev and Lecours (1967) discovered that the hemispheres and the brain stem exhibit three zones which mature at different rates; these zones are more or less comparable with the three levels of the triune brain (see Table 1). The median zone myelinates over two to three decades, the paramedian zone myelinates during the first decade until puberty, and the supralimbic zone has a maturational cycle which extends to old age.

Semmes (1968) expanded the concept of sequential and hierarchical development in order to account for the phenomenon of hemispheric lateralization of speech. Based on studies of sensory and motor capacities (e.g., primordial zones) of the hand in brain-injured subjects, she observes that the sensorimotor organization is more focally represented in the left hemisphere and more diffusely represented in the right hemisphere. According to Semmes (1968, p. 11), "it is proposed that focal representation of elementary functions in the left hemisphere favors integration of similar units and consequently specialization of behaviors which demand fine sensori-motor control, such as manual skills and speech." She suggests that each of the milestones in motor, somatosensory, and language development depends on the integrity and growth of the left cerebral hemisphere. Gross and fine motor functions differentiate and lateralize first, followed by lateralization of somatosensory functions, and, finally, lateralization of speech and language functions. Thus Semmes provides a neurophysiological basis for bridging the developmental milestones in motor, somatosensory, and language functions.

Developmental Psychology

According to the concept of maturation, the organism develops in an orderly sequence from an undifferentiated to a highly differentiated level. During this process of differentiation, an increase in integration takes place. Functions significant at earlier periods are in subsequent periods incorporated into functions with a higher level of differentiation and a higher integrative power.

Between the ages of 5 and 9 years, the primary development of perceptual-motor and perceptual-spatial skills takes place (Elkind *et al.*, 1962; Hunt, 1961;

Piaget, 1926). There is a hierarchical development in motor functions, and it has also been shown that there is a hierarchical development within the process of perception. Piaget (1952) has long advocated an orderly sequence in the structural development of intelligence in children. The sensorimotor and preconceptual stages precede and influence the development of language and formal operations in later stages (see Table 2). Thurstone (1955) demonstrated that perceptual and spatial abilities develop ontogenetically earlier than verbal abilities. He also demonstrated a slower development of the verbal abilities. Bruner (1968) suggests that the child goes through three stages in cognitive development. It consecutively constructs models of its world through action (enactive representation), through imagery (iconic representation), and through language (symbolic representation). The appearance of these representations in the life of the child is in that order, each depending on the previous one for its development, yet all of them remaining more or less intact throughout life (Bruner, 1968). According to Bruner, the transition to symbolic representation marks the final and most important stage in cognitive development. This stage frees the child from dependence on the concrete and immediate aspects of perceptual representation. This verbalization by Bruner is clearly in consonance with the verbalization of Isaacson of the Guru, the third level of the triune brain. The internalization facilitates a so-called second-signal system (Luria, 1966) in which experience can be both represented and transformed. The writings of Piaget (1926), Vygotsky (1962), Luria (1961), and Kendler and Kendler (1962) all suggest that an important change takes place during the 5- to 7-year age shift. This shift gives way to higher mental processes. According to White (1965), "the 5–7 period is a time when some maturational development, combining perhaps with influences in the model environment, inhibits a broad spectrum of first level function in favor of a new, higher level of function" (p. 213). During this period, the undifferentiated and impulsive behavior of the infant will be inhibited.

Studies have shown that visual orientation and localization change in such a way that in 7-year-old children fewer perceptual rotations and position reversals occur (Wechsler and Hagin, 1964; Lyle and Goyen, 1968) than in younger children. Our own findings are in accord with this view. In a visual attention-discrimination task, we had children cross the "q" from the alternatives "p," "d," "b," and "q." Table 3 illustrates the drastic decrease in rotation errors between the ages of 6 and 8 years. Vernon (1958) and Piaget and Inhelder (1956) suggested that form is independent of orientation in the young child. The visuospatial orientation skill improves as the child matures and will be fully developed by the age of 6 or 7 years according to Ingram (1970), Vernon (1937), and Wechsler and

TABLE 2. ONTOGENETIC STAGES OF THE DEVELOPMENT OF HUMAN BEHAVIOR

	Piaget	Bruner
Stage 3	Formal operations, cognitive thought	Symbolic representation
Stage 2	Concrete operations, conceptual thought	Iconic representation
Stage 1	Preoperational stage, sensorimotor phase	Enactive representation

109

ASPECTS OF NORMAL
AND ABNORMAL
NEUROPSYCHO-
LOGICAL
DEVELOPMENT

TABLE 3. TOTAL AMOUNT OF ERRORS IN A "q" DISCRIMINATION TASK BY 40 CHILDREN IN EACH AGE GROUP

6 year		8 year		10 year	
q	p 950	q	p 261	q	p 184
d 91	b 27	d 64	b 34	d 49	b 22

Hagin (1964), or by the age of 9 or 10 years according to Piaget and Morf (1956). White (1965) suggested that some of these changes complete themselves between 5 and 7 years of age, whereas others, such as verbal mediation, are just beginning to develop. White referred to this later process as the "cognitive layer." This "cognitive layer" is supposed to inhibit lower-level associative responses and develops later and at a relatively slower rate. Language, a characteristic of this "cognitive layer," evolves from a state of diffuse and bilateral representation to one of increased differentiation and lateralization within the left hemisphere. Language development in normal children goes through an orderly sequence. Gibson (1968) distinguished three sequential phases in the learning-to-read process: (1) learning to differentiate graphic symbols, (2) learning to decode letters to sounds, and (3) learning to utilize higher-order units of linguistic structure. This indicates that in the learning-to-read process each phase is characterized by its own reading strategy, which might be related to the maturational level of the underlying neurological structures. Satz and Sparrow (1970) and Satz and Van Nostrand (1973) state that the process of development, characterized by different stages of thought, is facilitated by experience and by the increased maturation and differentiation of the central nervous system.

ABNORMAL NEUROPSYCHOLOGICAL DEVELOPMENT

It is emphasized above that the age variable has to be considered as a critical factor in both developmental neurology and developmental psychology. The two disciplines recognize an increased maturation of the brain with age and a corresponding differentiation and growth of cognitive functions. The process of continuous change implies that the same underlying disturbance can manifest itself at different age levels in different behavioral abnormalities. Instead of a multiple-etiology explanation for the multitude of functional deviations observed in the child with abnormal neuropsychological development, this variety of disturbances may be explicable in terms of more basic mechanisms.

"Maturational lag" has been offered as one of the basic explanations for abnormal neuropsychological development, i.e., developmental dyslexia (Critchley, 1967, 1968, 1970; Cohn, 1961; Satz and Van Nostrand, 1973; de Hirsch *et al.*, 1966; Money, 1966; Bakker, 1973, 1976). The keynote in these studies is the hypothesis that the behavioral patterns observed in dyslexic children resemble the behavioral patterns of chronologically younger normal children. Satz and Van Nostrand (1973) regard dyslexia as more than a reading disorder *per se*. Depending on the age of the child, the lag manifests itself as a delay in sensorimotor abilities (at 6 years) or as a delay in conceptual-linguistic abilities (at 10 years). Leong (1976) recently confirmed these findings of Satz and associates. Both studies validate the earlier suggestion by Benton (1962) that perceptual deficiencies are found more in younger dyslexics and that conceptual deficiencies are found in older dyslexics. This implies that when early prediction of learning disabilities is desired, we should focus our attention toward tests assessing skills which are primarily developed at younger ages. Visual perception and perceptual-motor tests are particularly sensitive in terms of maturation and predictive validity (Satz and Friel, 1973; Sapir and Wilson, 1967; Galante *et al.*, 1972). It has been shown by Chissom (1971) that early-developing skills (e.g., balance and motor coordination) correlate with academic achievement in younger boys (first grade) but not in older boys (third grade).

Satz and Friel (1973) suggested that, since no brain damage is postulated in the maturational lag model, children with reading disabilities may eventually "overcome" their problem. It is well known, however, that many dyslexics never "overcome" their problem. In a large-scale study, Kuipers (1976) compared normal gifted students with dyslexic gifted students at the Delft University of Technology. Many dyslexics met a considerable delay or never finished their study. Rourke (1976) believed that if some dyslexics do not overcome their problem, it necessarily means that for them the maturational lag hypothesis is wrong. However, it is quite conceivable to suppose that the lag prevented the child from acquiring essential skills during the critical periods of its development, resulting in a persisting handicap. Thus the statement of Rourke (1976) that the query of "lag" vs. "defect" may be answered by means of outcome studies is not necessarily true. Another possibility is that the maturational lag is caused by a biochemical defect which usually is hard to detect (Wender, 1973, 1976).

Although the maturational lag hypothesis does not explain the basic cause of dyslexia, the major advantage of Satz's approach is that he does not accept the static disease model. Instead, Satz describes a dynamic, continuously changing process. Satz and Sparrow (1970) hypothesized that whereas damage to the left hemisphere in adults may produce temporary loss of a function, a delay in the physical maturation of the left hemisphere in children may retard the acquisition of the same function, rather than cause its loss. In this way, Satz and associates limited their maturational lag theory to the maturation of the left hemisphere, the third level of the triune brain. Recently, Satz (1976), reviewing the magnitude of the problem concerning hemispheric dominance and reading disabilities, concluded that "reading disability and ear asymmetry appear not to be related. The fact is that developmental differences in ear asymmetry (dichotic listening) seem more related to handedness than to reading disability" (Satz, 1976, p. 293).

A possible explanation for this seemingly discouraging conclusion can be found in the work of Bakker and associates (Bakker, 1973; Bakker *et al.*, 1973). They suggested that there is a relationship between cerebral dominance and the learning-to-read process. Every stage is characterized by its own optimal lateralization pattern. At an advanced stage, proficient reading goes with left hemisphere dominance only (Bakker, 1973; Bakker *et al.*, 1973; Satz and Sparrow, 1970). At an earlier stage, proficient reading may go with either left or right hemisphere dominance, depending on the reading strategy (Bakker *et al.*, 1976). Older dyslexic children might still rely on a right hemisphere reading strategy that was appropriate in the early stage only. In concordance with this hypothesis are reports indicating a high incidence of left ear advantage (in dichotic listening) in older dyslexic children (Witelson and Rabinovitch, 1972; Zurif and Carson, 1970). The flexibility of normal readers to switch from one reading strategy to the other might be a characteristic of incomplete lateralization. This incomplete lateralization in childhood is a generally accepted idea (Brown and Hécaen, 1975). Aphasia in childhood shows a very distinctive picture which depends on age and is different from aphasia in the adult (Guttmann, 1942; Basser, 1962; Alajouanine and Lhermitte, 1965; Collignon 1968; Brown and Hécaen, 1975). The idea of incomplete lateralization of the language function in childhood is supported by the fact that aphasia in early childhood might be caused by lesions in the left as well as in the right hemisphere and the fact that recovery from aphasia goes faster and is more complete than in the adult, indicating a possible takeover of function by the other hemisphere. Regarding motor functions, it is also known that the earlier the destruction of the pyramidal pathway occurs, the better developed and less rigid the synergies are (Zülch, 1974). Even in the adult, destruction of the pyramidal pathways does not result in a complete loss of motor function. The same holds for the primary sensory areas of the neocortex. Lesions in the primary auditory neocortex do not alter auditory thresholds for frequency or intensity (e.g., Diamond and Neff, 1957). Destruction of the primary visual areas does not eliminate some forms of pattern discriminative capacities, even in primates (Humphrey and Weiskrantz, 1967).

Cortical damage (level III) in the neonate often does not become apparent before the age of 6 months. A special neurological examination of the newborn is necessary (Prechtl, 1968; Touwen and Prechtl, 1970). In this examination, special attention is paid to the "lower" functions. A diagnosis in terms of lateralization and localization of the lesion is often impossible. A general impression of the functional integrity of the nervous system of the newborn can be obtained. This is possibly due to the fact that "it seems possible that when the baby first moves he may not employ his cortex at all" (Penfield, 1954). Or as Zülch (1975) postulates: "Immediately after birth, the motor patterns are initiated by an 'archaic' apparatus which is later suppressed by the higher 'voluntary' functions of the pyramidal pathway."

During maturation, the association cortex and the commissures become more elaborate. This process is considered to be essential for the hemispheric lateralization of function at a later stage. However, in case of agenesis of the corpus callosum, a remarkable degree of brain compensation becomes evident. The remaining commissures at a lower level are apparently capable of cross-transmission (Ettlinger *et al.*, 1974). This study and evidence from split-brain studies (Gazzaniga, 1975*a,b*) illustrate the capacity of the vertical pathways between hemispheres and the lower brain levels. Throughout life, but especially during

111

ASPECTS OF NORMAL
AND ABNORMAL
NEUROPSYCHO-
LOGICAL
DEVELOPMENT

infancy, these vertical pathways play a major role in the integration of functions (Trevarthen, 1974).

Another example of a more basic approach not incompatible with the maturational lag hypothesis could be the "attention process" hypothesis. Sheer (1976) referred to it as a primary deficit in "focused arousal," Douglas (1974, 1976) as "sustained attention and impulsivity," Dykman *et al.* (1971) as "attentional deficit," Kinsbourne (1973) as "selective attention," and Wender (1971) as "poor modulated activation." Many observers noticed the shortness of attention span and poor concentration ability as major characteristics of abnormal neuropsychological development (Wender, 1976; Kinsbourne, 1973; Conners, 1971; Douglas, 1974, 1976). Depending on the chronological age of the child, a deficit in "attention" might be a symptom of a maturational lag. Some children achieve cortical control over attention at an unduly slow rate. Possibly the brain stem reticular formation incorporates a rigid pattern of attentional shift, which gradually comes under cortical control (Hutt and Hutt, 1965). Kinsbourne (1974) attempted to integrate the attention process hypothesis and the problem of hemispheric asymmetry. "In the early years of life the asymmetry in hemisphere function is probably attentional rather than one of differing competences of the hemispheres" (p. 269). The left hemisphere is supposed to pay attention to speech, and, by doing so, inhibits the right hemisphere for this function. Over time, this suppression of the right hemisphere by the left hemisphere results in the left hemisphere dominance for language (Kinsbourne, 1974).

The way each hemisphere drives attention toward the contralateral space might in Gazzaniga's (1974) opinion be based on decision-processing systems in both left and right hemispheres. "If the dominance of a hemisphere is not properly established, which is widely suggested to be the case in children with dyslexia, if information fluctuates between the decision-making networks, the overall behavioral result would be disastrous" (Gazzaniga, 1974). Learning disabilities, motor clumsiness, and continuous shifting of attention might be the resultant of two cognitive systems continually competing for the control of behavior.

Abnormal neuropsychological development may be the resultant of a dysfunction on each of the three levels of the triune brain, manifesting itself in one or more stages of psychological development. Studying the neuropsychological development of the child, we should not look at it as a miniature adult, but as a rapidly developing subject, functioning at a certain level depending on the maturational status of its nervous system. One of the practical implications is that a child will execute the "same" task with different strategies, depending on the child's maturational level. A free quotation of a statement by Otfried Spreen (1976) in his postconference review regarding the neuropsychology of learning disorders might be: "Just for speculation's sake, one can imagine a level of general arousal and resulting general difficulties related to the reticular activating system (level I) and a more focused deficit resulting from malfunction at a higher level, e.g., the midbrain (level II), and one can assume that deficits may result from disorders in the functional development of the neocortex, right or left or specific areas of each (level III)" (p. 454).

References

113

ASPECTS OF NORMAL
AND ABNORMAL
NEUROPSYCHO-
LOGICAL
DEVELOPMENT

Alajouanine, T., and Lhermitte, F. Acquired aphasia in children. *Brain,* 1965, *88,* 653–661.

Bakker, D. J. Hemispheric specialization and stages in the learning-to-read process. *Bulletin of the Orton Society,* 1973, *23,* 15–27.

Bakker, D. J. Development of asymmetric perception and proficiency in written language. Paper presented to the Orton Society International Symposium on Dyslexia, New York, November 1976.

Bakker, D. J., Smink, T., and Reitsma, P. Ear dominance and reading ability. *Cortex,* 1973, *9,* 301–312.

Bakker, D. J., Teunissen, J., and Bosch, J. Lateralization in severely disabled readers in relation to functional cerebral development and synthesis of information. In R. M. Knights and D. J. Bakker (eds.), *The Neuropsychooogy of Learning Disorders: Theoretical Approaches.* Baltimore: University Park Press, 1976.

Basser, L. S. Hemiplegia of early onset and the faculty of speech with special reference to the effects of hemispherectomy. *Brain,* 1962, *85,* 427–460.

Benton, A. L. Dyslexia in relation to form perception and directional sense. In J. Money (ed.), *Reading Disability: Progress and Research Needs in Dyslexia.* Baltimore: Johns Hopkins Press, 1962.

Brown, J. W., and Hécaen, H. Lateralization and language representation: Observations on aphasia in children, left-handers and "anomalous" dextrals. Paper presented to the Boerhaave Conference on Lateralization of Brain Functions, Leiden, The Netherlands, June 1975.

Bruner, J. S. The course of cognitive growth. In N. S. Endler, L. R. Boulter, and H. Osser (eds.), *Contemporary Issues in Developmental Psychology.* New York: Holt, Rinehart and Winston, 1968.

Bruner, J. S. *Beyond the Information Given.* London: George Allen & Unwin, 1974.

Bruyn, G. W. *Neurologie Tussen Buiten- en Binnenwereld.* Amsterdam: B. V. Noord-Hollandsche Uitgeversmaatschappij, 1976.

Chissom, B. S. A factor-analytic study of the relationship of motor factors to academic criteria for first- and third grade boys. *Child Development,* 1971, *42,* 1133–1143.

Cohn, R. Delayed acquisition of reading and writing abilities in children. *Archives of Neurology (Chicago),* 1961, *4,* 153–164.

Collignon, R., Hécaen, H., and Angelèrgues, R. A propos de 12 cas d'aphasie acquise de l'enfant. *Acta Neurologica Belgica,* 1968, *68,* 245–277.

Conners, C. K. Recent drug studies with hyperkinetic children. *Journal of Learning Disabilities,* 1971, *9,* 476–483.

Crichley, M. Some observations upon developmental dyslexia. In D. Williams (ed.), *Modern Trends in Neurology,* No. 4. London: Butterworths, 1967.

Critchley, M. Minor neurologic defects in developmental dyslexia. In A. H. Keeney and V. T. Keeney (eds.), *Dyslexia, Diagnosis and Treatment of Reading Disorders.* St. Louis: Mosby, 1968.

Critchley, M. *The Dyslexic Child.* London: Heinemann, 1970.

de Hirsch, K., Jansky, J., and Langford, W. S. *Predicting Reading Failure.* New York: Harper and Row, 1966.

Denny-Brown, D. Motor mechanisms—Introduction: The general principles of motor integration. In J. Field (ed.), *Handbook of Physiology,* Section I: *Neurophysiology,* Vol. II. Washington D.C.: American Physiological Society, 1960.

Diamond, I. T., and Neff, W. D. Ablation of temporal cortex and discrimination of auditory patterns. *Journal of Neurophysiology,* 1957, *20,* 300–315.

Douglas, R. J. The hippocampus and behavior. *Psychological Bulletin,* 1967, *67,* 416–422.

Douglas, R. J. The development of hippocampal function: Implications for theory and for therapy. In R. L. Isaacson and K. H. Pribram (eds.), *The Hippocampus,* Vol. II. *Neurophysiology and Behavior.* New York and London: Plenum, 1975.

Douglas, R. J., Packouz, K., and Douglas, D. Development of inhibition in man. *Proceedings: APA,* 1972, 839–840.

Douglas, V. I. *Sustained Attention and Impulse Control: Implications for the Handicapped Child,* Vol. 6. Washington D.C.: U.S. Department of Health, Education, and Welfare, Office of Education, 1974, pp. 149–164.

Douglas, V. I. Perceptual and cognitive factors as determinants of learning disabilities: A review chapter with special emphasis on attentional factors. In R. M. Knights and D. J. Bakker (eds.), *The Neuropsychology of Learning Disorders: Theoretical Approaches.* Baltimore: University Park Press, 1976.

Dykman, R. A., Ackerman, P. T., Clements, S. D., and Peters, J. E. Specific learning disabilities: An attentional defect syndrome. In H. R. Myklebust (ed.), *Progress in Learning Disabilities*, Vol. II. New York: Grune and Stratton, 1971.

Eccles, J. C. *Facing Reality: Philosophical Adventures by a Brain Scientist*. New York: Springer-Verlag, 1970.

Eccles, J. C. *The Understanding of the Brain*. New York: McGraw-Hill, 1973.

Elkind, D., Koegler, R. R., and Go, E. Effects of perceptual training at three age levels. *Science*, 1962, *137*, 755–756.

Ettlinger, G., Blakemore, C. B., Milner, A. D., and Wilson, J. Agenesis of the corpus callosum: A further behavioral investigation. *Brain*, 1974, *97*, 225–234.

Flechsig, P. Developmental (myelogenetic) localization of the cortex in human subjects. *Lancet*. 1901, Oct. 19, 1027–1029.

Gaffan, D. Loss of recognition memory in rats with lesions of the fornix. *Neuropsychologia*, 1972, *10*, 327–341.

Gaffan, D. Recognition impaired and association intact in the memory of monkeys after transsection of the fornix. *Journal of Comparative and Physiological Psychology*, 1974, *86*, 1100–1109.

Galante, M. B., Fley, M. E., and Stephens, L. S. Cumulative minor deficits: A longitudinal study of the relation of physical factors to school achievement. *Journal of Learning Disabilities*, 1972, *5*, 75–80.

Gazzaniga, M. S. Determinants of cerebral recovery. In D. G. Stein, J. J. Rosen, and N. Butters (eds.), *Plasticity and Recovery of Function in the Central Nervous System*. New York: Academic Press, 1974.

Gazzaniga, M. S. Partial commisurotomy and cerebral localization of function. In K. J. Zülch, O. Creutzfeldt, and G. C. Galbraith (eds.), *Cerebral Localization*. Berlin: Springer-Verlag, 1975*a*.

Gazzaniga, M. S. Brain mechanisms and behavior. In M. S. Gazzaniga and C. Blakemore (eds.), *Handbook of Psychobiology*, New York: Academic Press, 1975*b*.

Geschwind, N. Neurological foundations of language. In H. R. Myklebust (ed.), *Progress in Learning Disabilities*, Vol. I. New York and London: Grune and Stratton, 1968.

Geschwind, N., and Levitsky, W. Human brain: Left-right asymmetries in temporal speech region. *Science*, 1968, *161*, 186–187.

Gessel, A. *The Embryology of Behavior*. New York: Harper and Row, 1945.

Gessel, A., and Amatruda, C. S. *Developmental Diagnosis: Normal and Abnormal Child Development*, 2nd ed. New York: Hoeber, 1948.

Gibson, E. J. Learning to read. In N. S. Endler, L. R. Boulter, and H. Osser (eds.), *Contemporary Issues in Developmental Psychology*. New York: Holt, Rinehart and Winston, 1968.

Glees, P., and Griffith, H. B. Bilateral destruction of the hippocampus (cornu ammonis) in a case of dementia. *Monatsschrift für Psychiatrie und Neurologie*, 1952, *123*, 193–204.

Green, J. D. The rhinencephalon and behavior. In G. E. W. Wolstenholme and C. M. O'Connor (eds.), *Ciba Foundation Symposium on the Neurological Basis of Behavior*. London: J. & A. Churchill, 1958.

Grunthal, E. Ueber das klinische Bild nach umschriebenem beiderseitigem Ausfall der Ammonshorn-rinde: Ein Beitrag zur Kenntnis der Funktion des Ammonshorns. *Monatsschrift für Psychiatrie und Neurologie*, 1947, *113*, 1–16.

Guttmann, E., Aphasia in children. *Brain*, 1942, *65*, 205–219.

Haaxma, R., and Kuypers, H. G. J. M. Intrahemispheric cortical connections and visual guidance of hand and finger movements in the rhesus monkey. *Brain*, 1975, *98*, 239–260.

Hammer, M., and Turkewitz, G. A sensory basis for the lateral difference in the newborn infant's response to somesthetic stimulation. *Journal of Experimental Child Psychology*, 1974, *18*, 304–312.

Humphrey, N. K., and Weiskrantz, L. Vision in monkeys after removal of the striate cortex. *Nature (London)*, 1967, *215*, 595–597.

Hunt, J. M. *Intelligence and Experience*. New York: Ronald Press, 1961.

Hutt, C., and Hutt, S. J. The effect of environmental complexity upon stereotyped behavior in children. *Animal Behavior*, 1965, *13*, 1–4.

Ingram, T. T. S. The nature of dyslexia. In F. A. Young and D. B. Lindsley (eds.), *Early Experience and Visual Information Processing in Perceptual and Reading Disorders*. Washington D.C.: National Academy of Sciences, 1970.

Isaacson, R. L. *The Limbic System*. New York: Plenum, 1974.

Isaacson, R. L., and Pribram, K. H. (eds.), *The Hippocampus. Vol. II, Neurophysiology and Behavior*. New York and London: Plenum Press, 1975.

Jones, S. J. Children's two-choice learning of predominantly alternating and predominantly non-alternating sequences. *Journal of Experimental Child Psychology*, 1970, *10*, 344–362.

Kendler, T. S., and Kendler, H. H. Inferential behavior in children as a function of age and subgoal constancy. *Journal of Experimental Psychology*, 1962, *64*, 406–466.

Kimble, D. P. Hippocampus and internal inhibition. *Psychological Bulletin*, 1968, *70*, 285–295.

115

ASPECTS OF NORMAL
AND ABNORMAL
NEUROPSYCHO-
LOGICAL
DEVELOPMENT

Kimble, D. P. C hoice behavior in rats with hippocampal lesions. In R. L. Isaacson and K. H. Pribram (eds.), *The Hippocampus.* New York: Plenum, 1975.

Kinsbourne, M. Minimal brain dysfunction as a neurodevelopmental lag. *Annals of the New York Academy of Science,* 1973, *205,* 268–273.

Kinsbourne, M. Mechanisms of hemispheric interaction in man. In M. Kinsbourne and W. L. Smith (eds.), *Hemispheric Disconnection and Cerebral Function.* Springfield Ill.: Thomas, 1974.

Klapper, Z. S. Reading retardation. II. Psychoeducational aspects of reading disabilities. *Pediatrics,* 1966, *37,* 366–376.

Kuipers, C. G. *Dyslexia bij Begaafden* (Dyslexia in the Gifted). den Haag, the Netherlands: Koninklijke Drukkerij de Swart, 1976.

Lenneberg, E. H. *Biological Foundations of Language.* New York: Wiley, 1967.

Leong, C. K. Lateralization in severely disabled readers in relation to functional cerebral development and synthesis of information. In R. M. Knights and D. J. Bakker (eds.), *The Neuropsychology of Learning Disorders: Theoretical Approaches.* Baltimore: University Park Press, 1976.

Luria, A. R. *The Role of Speech in Regulation of Normal and Abmormal Behavior.* London: Pergamon, 1961.

Luria, A. R. *Higher Cortical Functions in Man.* New York: Basic Books. 1966.

Luria, A. R. *The Working Brain: An Introduction to Neuropsychology.* London: Penguin Press, 1973.

Lyle, J. G., and Goyen, J. Visual recognition, developmental lag, and strephosymbolia in reading retardation. *Journal of Abnormal Psychology,* 1968, *17,* 25–29.

MacLean, P. D. Psychosomatic disease and the "visceral brain": Recent developments bearing on the Papez theory of emotion. *Psychosomatic Medicine,* 1949, *11,* 338–353.

MacLean, P. D. The limbic system ("visceral brain") and emotional behavior. *Archives of Neurology and Psychiatry,* 1955, *73,* 130–134.

MacLean, P. D. The triune brain, emotion, and scientific bias. In F. O. Schmitt (ed.), *The Neurosciences: Second Study Program.* New York: Rockefeller University Press, 1970.

MacLean, P. D. Cerebral evolution and emotional processes. *Annals of the New York Academy of Sciences,* 1972, *193,* 137–149.

Molfese, D. L., Freeman, R. B., and Palermo, D. S. The ontogeny of brain lateralization for speech and nonspeech stimuli. *Brain and Language,* 1975, *2,* 356–368.

Money, J. *The Disabled Reader, Education of the Dyslexic Child.* Baltimore: Johns Hopkins Press, 1966.

Palermo, D. S., and Molfese, D. L. Language acquisition from age five onward. *Psychological Bulletin,* 1972, *78,* 409–428.

Pate, J. L., and Bell, G. L. Alternation behavior in children in a cross-maze. *Psychonomic Science,* 1971, *23,* 431–432.

Pavlov, I. P. *Selected Works.* K. S. Koshtoyants (ed.). Moscow: Foreign Languages Publishing House, 1955.

Penfield, W. Mechanisms of voluntary movement. *Brain,* 1954, *77,* 1–17.

Piaget, J. *Judgement and Reasoning in the Child.* New York: Harcourt and Brace, 1926.

Piaget, J. *The Origins of Intelligence in Children.* New York: International Universities Press, 1952.

Piaget, J. Piaget's theory. In R. H. Mussen (ed.), *Carmichael's Manual of Child Psychology,* 3rd ed. New York: Wiley, 1970.

Piaget, J., and Inhelder, B. *The Child's Concept of Space.* New York: Humanities Press, 1956.

Piaget, J., and Morf, A. Recherches sur le développement des perceptions. XXX. Les comparaisons verticale a faible intervalle. *Archives de Psychologie (Genève),* 1956, *35,* 289–319.

Popper, K. R. Epistemology without a knowing subject. In Van Rootselaar and Staal (eds.), *Logic, Methodology and Philosophy of Sciences,* Vol. III. Amsterdam: North-Holland, 1968*a.* In Eccles (1970).

Pooper, K. R. On the theory of the objective mind. *Akten des XIV Internationalen Kongresses für Philosophie,* Vol. I. Wien, 1968*b.* In Eccles (1970).

Prechtl, H. F. R. Neurological findings in newborn infants after pre- and paranatal complications. In J. H. P. Jonxis, H. K. A. Visser, and J. A. Troelstra (eds.), *Aspects of Praematurity and Dysmaturity.* Leiden: Leiden University Press, 1968.

Pribram, K. H., and Isaacson, R. L. Summary. In R. L. Isaacson and K. H. Pribram (eds.), *The Hippocampus.* New York: Plenum, 1975.

Rourke, B. P. Reading retardation in children: Developmental lag or deficit? In R. M. Knights and D. J. Bakker (eds.), *The Neuropsychology of Learning Disorders: Theoretical Approaches.* Baltimore: University Park Press, 1976.

Sapir, S. G., and Wilson, B. M. A developmental scale to assist in the prevention of learning disability. *Educational and Psychological Measurement,* 1967, *27,* 1061–1068.

Sarsikov, S. The evolutionary aspects of the integrative function of the cortex and subcortex of the brain. In D. P. Purpura and J. P. Schade (eds.), *Growth and Maturation of the Brain*, Vol. 4 of *Progress in Brain Research*. Amsterdam: Elsevier, 1964.

Satz, P. Cerebral dominance and reading disability: An old problem revisited. In R. M. Knights and D. J. Bakker (eds.), *The Neuropsychology of Learning Disorders: Theoretical Approaches*. Baltimore: University Park Press, 1976.

Satz, P., and Friel, J. Some predictive antecedents of specific learning disability: A preliminary one-year follow-up. In P. Satz and J. J. Ross (eds.), *The Disabled Learner*. Rotterdam: Rotterdam University Press, 1973.

Satz, P., and Sparrow, S. Specific developmental dyslexia: A theoretical reformulation. In D. J. Bakker and P. Satz (eds.), *Specific Reading Disability: Advances in Theory and Method*. Rotterdam: Rotterdam University Press, 1970.

Satz, P., and Van Nostrand, G. K. Developmental dyslexia: An evaluation of a theory. In P. Satz and J. Ross (eds.), *The Disabled Learner*. Rotterdam: Rotterdam University Press, 1973.

Satz, P., Bakker, D. J., Teunissen, J., Goebel, R., and van der Vlugt, H. Developmental parameters of the ear asymmetry: A multivariate approach. *Brain and Language*, 1975, *2*, 171–185.

Semmes, J. Hemispheric specialization: A possible clue to mechanism. *Neuropsychologia*, 1968, *6*, 11–26.

Sheer, D. E. Focussed arousal and the 40-Hz EEG. In R. M. Knights and D. J. Bakker (eds.), *The Neuropsychology of Learning Disorders: Theoretical Approaches*. Baltimore: University Park Press, 1976.

Spencer, H. *The Principles of Psychology*, 4th ed., 3 vols. London, 1899.

Spreen, O. Neuropsychology and learning disorders: Post-conference review. In R. M. Knights and D. J. Bakker (eds.), *The Neuropsychology of Learning Disorders: Theoretical Approaches*. Baltimore: University Park Press, 1976.

Talland, G. A. *Deranged Memory*. New York: Academic Press, 1965.

Taylor, J. (ed.) *Selected writings of John Hughlings Jackson*, 2 vols. London: Staples, 1958.

Thurstone, L. L. *The Differential Growth of Mental Activities*. Chapel Hill: University of North Carolina Psychometric Laboratory, No. 14, 1955.

Touwen, B. C. L., and Prechtl, H. F. R. *The Neurological Examination of the Child with Minor Nervous Dysfunction*. London: Heinemann, 1970.

Trevarthen, C. Cerebral embryology and the split brain. In M. Kinsbourne and W. L. Smith (eds.), *Hemispheric Disconnection and Cerebral Function*. Springfield Ill.: Thomas, 1974.

Vernon, M. D. *Visual Perception*. London: Cambridge University Press, 1937.

Vernon, M. D. *Backwardness in Reading*. Cambridge: Cambridge University Press, 1958.

Votaw, C. L. Certain functional and anatomical relations of the cornu ammonis of the macaque monkey. *Journal of Comparative Neurology*, 1959, *112*, 353–382.

Vygotsky, L. S. *Thought and Language*. Edited and translated by E. Haufmann and G. Vakar. Cambridge, Mass., and New York: MIT Press and Wiley, 1962.

Wada, J. A., Clarke, R., and Hamm, A. Cerebral hemispheric asymmetry in humans. *Archives of Neurology (Chicago)*, 1975, 239–245.

Wechsler, D., and Hagin, R. A. The problem of axial rotation in reading disability. *Perceptual and Motor Skills*, 1964, *19*, 319–326.

Weiskrantz, L. Comparison of amnestic states in monkey and man. In L. E. Jarrard (ed.), *Cognitive Processes of Nonhuman Primates*. New York: Academic Press, 1971.

Weiskrantz, L., and Warrington, E. K. The problem of the amnestic syndrome in man and animals. In R. L. Isaacson and K. H. Pribram (eds.), *The Hippocampus*. New York: Plenum, 1975.

Wender, P. H. *Minimal Brain Dysfunction in Children*. New York: Wiley-Interscience, 1971.

Wender, P. H. Some speculations concerning a possible biochemical basis of minimal brain dysfunction. In F. F. de la Cruz, B. H. Fox, and R. H. Roberts (eds.), Minimal Brain Dysfunction. *Annals of the New York Academy of Sciences*, 1973, *205*, 18–28.

Wender, P. H. Hypothesis for a possible biochemical basis of minimal brain dysfunction. In R. M. Knights and D. J. Bakker (eds.), *The Neuropsychology of Learning Disorders: Theoretical Approaches*. Baltimore: University Park Press, 1976.

White, S. H. Evidence for a hierarchical arrangement of learning processes. *Advances in Child Development and Behavior*, Vol. 2. New York: Academic Press, 1965, pp. 187–220.

Witelson, S. F., and Pallie, W. Left hemisphere specialization for language in the newborn: Neuroanatomical evidence of asymmetry. *Brain Research*, 1973, *96*, 641–646.

Witelson, S. F., and Rabinovitch, M. S. Hemispheric speech lateralization in children with auditory-linguistic deficits. *Cortex*, 1972, *8*, 412–426.

Yakovlev, P. I., and Lecours, A. R. The myelogenetic cycles of regional maturation of the brain. In A. Minkowski (ed.), *Regional Development of the Brain in Early Life*. Oxford, Blackwell, 1967.

Yakovlev, P. I., and Rakic, P. Patterns of decussation of bulbar pyramids and distribution of pyramidal tracts on two sides of the spinal cord. *Transactions of the American Neurology Associations*, 1966, *91*, 366–367.

Zülch, K. J. Motor and sensory findings after hemispherectomy: Ipsi- or contralateral functions? *Clinical Neurology and Neurosurgery*, 1974. *1*, 3–14.

Zülch, K. J. Pyramidal and parapyramidal motor systems in man. In K. J. Zülch, O. Creutzfeldt, and G. C. Galbraith (eds.), *Cerebral Localization*. Berlin: Springer-Verlag. 1975.

Zurif, E. F., and Carson, G. Dyslexia in relation to cerebral dominance and temporal analysis. *Neuropsychologia*, 1970, *8*, 351–361.

117

ASPECTS OF NORMAL
AND ABNORMAL
NEUROPSYCHO-
LOGICAL
DEVELOPMENT

Minimal Brain Dysfunction: Psychological and Neurophysiological Disorders in Hyperkinetic Children

JOHN S. STAMM AND SHARON V. KREDER

INTRODUCTION

Minimal brain dysfunction (MBD) has become an important diagnostic label for the disorders in many children who exhibit certain constellations of learning and behavior problems. There remains, however, considerable misunderstanding about the meaning and the applicability of this term. The disagreements about MBD result from differing views regarding evidence for brain disorders and the significance of the many symptoms that have been attributed to the children with this diagnosis. In order to clarify these issues and establish an acceptable definition for MBD, a national task force was convened (Clements, 1966). The definition, which still lacked simplicity and clarity, stated that MBD should only be applied to describe those children with at least near-average intelligence whose learning and behavioral disabilities are the consequence of certain perceptual, cognitive, and attentive dysfunctions. A review of the symptoms and signs that had been used for

JOHN S. STAMM AND SHARON V. KREDER   Department of Psychology, State University of New York, Stony Brook, New York 11794. Preparation of this chapter was supported by a grant from The Grant Foundation.

MBD diagnosis resulted in a list of 99 items; these were reduced to ten major characteristics. The author cautioned that this "sign" approach should be employed only as a guideline for identification and diagnosis, because any one MBD child exhibits only some of these symptoms, with varying degrees of severity. The efforts by this task force resulted in clarification of several issues: the MBD diagnosis requires the exclusion of other disorders such as mental retardation, sensory impairments, "major" neurological disorders (e.g., cerebral palsy, epilepsy, and aphasia), and psychiatric disturbances. Also, evaluations of children have indicated that the symptoms tend to occur in clusters and that, for diagnostic purposes, only a few are of major importance. Thus Ross *et al.* (1973) state: "the child usually assigned this label has one or more of the following symptoms: short attention span, motor impulsivity, hyperactivity, emotional lability, poor eye-hand coordination, motor clumsiness, and defective use of language" (p. 154). The issue of whether brain dysfunction can or should be inferred from this diagnosis may be considered only in the context of symptomology.

Among the clusters of symptoms that were suggested by the task force (Clements, 1966) are those related to hyperkinesis (HK). Since substantial progress has been made in the identification of HK, as well as in delineations of the underlying dysfunctions and their neurophysiological correlates (e.g., Cantwell, 1975a; Ross and Ross, 1976), this chapter will focus on the HK syndrome. The incidence of hyperkinesis is substantial, with conservative estimates of 4–10% among elementary-school-aged children (Stewart *et al.*, 1966), which would correspond to 1.4–3.5 million children in the United States. Also, the sizable literature on MBD indicates that at least 60% of the children with this diagnosis meet the criteria for the HK syndrome. This chapter will describe the main characteristics of this syndrome and will then review research findings of the specific psychological dysfunctions in HK, namely those of attention and impulse control. Evidence for possible neurophysiological dysfunctions will then be presented according to two lines of investigations, pharmacological studies and electrophysiological studies. Our evaluations of these findings provide indications for specific frontal lobe dysfunctions. Consequently, a conceptual model will be proposed for brain disorders that may account for the hyperkinetic syndrome and the children's responses to drugs.

In our review of the literature, each clinical sample is indicated by the term used by the investigator. Many clinicians object to the "MBD" label and prefer that of "learning disability" (LD). These terms are associated with differing conceptual views of childhood disorders by medically and educationally oriented professional persons, and the diagnosis of LD is not equivalent to that of MBD. However, the disorders in many LD children have also been diagnosed as MBD. Other investigators have designated their samples as "hyperactive." Since hyperactivity is only one of the symptoms in the HK syndrome, we limit the use of the term "hyperactivity" to the behavioral description of the child. For the present review, only studies were selected in which the clinical children appeared to have met the criteria for the HK syndrome, regardless of the diagnostic label that was used by the investigators.

MINIMAL BRAIN
DYSFUNCTION:
PSYCHOLOGICAL AND
NEUROPHYSIO-
LOGICAL DISORDERS
IN HYPERKINETIC
CHILDREN

The HK Syndrome

Although hyperactive behavior in otherwise healthy children has long been recognized, clinical descriptions were first presented in 1902 by the English pediatrician Still (cited by Ross and Ross, 1976), who found this condition initially in children with demonstrable brain lesions and subsequently in children without known brain injury. In recent years, the concept of the hyperkinetic child syndrome, first proposed by Stewart *et al.* (1966) and described by many clinicians, has become widely accepted. This syndrome, which occurs in 4 times as many boys as girls, has been delineated by Cantwell (1975*b*) as consisting of four core and several secondary symptoms. The main symptoms are as follows: (1) Hyperactivity, which is manifested not necessarily by the amount of excessive activity *per se* but rather by its frequent occurrence in situations where this behavior is inappropriate, such as the child's inability to sit still and remain quiet when these are required. (2) Distractibility, which is indicated by parent and teacher reports that the child is unable to persevere with his work in school and at home, unable to listen to a story, or unable to take part in games. (3) Impulsivity, which is typically expressed by inappropriate motor responses and by tactless statements. (4) Excitability, which is indicated by temper tantrums, fighting over trivial matters, and the tendency to become overexcited and more active in stimulating situations. These symptoms are among the top six characteristics that the task force (Clements, 1966) found to be most frequently cited in the literature. Cantwell (1975*b*) considers antisocial (aggressive) behavior as a secondary symptom, because it is seen in only a minority of HK children and becomes pronounced primarily during adolescence. Therefore, this symptom seems to develop as a reaction to continuing failures of academic achievement and social relations. Other emotional symptoms, such as depression and low self-esteem, have been found in HK adolescents (Dykman *et al.,* 1973; Weiss *et al.,* 1971). Of further importance to the HK syndrome are the child's frequent difficulties and failures in the acquisition of academic skills (Cantwell, 1975*b*).

The clinical diagnosis for HK occurs most frequently during the children's primary school years, because the symptoms are manifested in the classroom settings. Considerable evidence has also been obtained, especially from interviews with parents, for the existence of this disorder since early childhood. Many HK children have been reported as "difficult" since infancy and as delayed in their development of motor and language functions and their control over emotional expressions. Also, their performance on many standardized tests has been found to be equivalent to that of younger normal children. These findings have led to the interpretation of HK, and MBD in general, as the consequence of neurodevelopmental lag (Kinsbourne, 1973; Satz and Van Nostrand, 1973). This concept is also supported by the diminution of hyperactivity during the children's pubescent years and by their ability to acquire basic skills in reading, spelling, and arithmetic. Consequently, many professional persons have considered HK as a transitory childhood disorder that will subside during the course of maturational development. However, contrary evidence has been obtained from the few reports of retrospective and prospective studies.

In their 5-year follow-up study of 64 HK and control boys who were 10–18 years old, Weiss *et al.* (1971) found that double-blind observations of classroom behavior revealed significantly more disorganized activity by the HK boys, such as fidgeting, playing with pencils, and working on the wrong assignment. Also, their academic performance was still below normal; 80% of this group had repeated at least one grade, compared with 15% of the controls. The mothers' reports indicated that 70% of the boys were emotionally immature, aggressive, and distractible, and 30% had no steady friends. A different follow-up study (Dykman *et al.*, 1973) was conducted with 22 normal and 31 LD boys (14 years of age) who had previously been examined when they were 8–13 years old. The LD boys showed considerable progress in many academic abilities, improvements on tests for impulsivity and reaction time, and better behavioral control, as indicated by teachers' and parents' rating scales. Nonetheless, they remained deficient, in comparisons to the controls, on all of these measures. In addition, their responses on personality inventories indicated that they had many problems, especially those related to self-image. These studies showed that, although the high activity levels in the clinical boys had diminished, many problems remained, especially disorders of attention and chronic underachievement.

Their review of retrospective and follow-up studies led Ross and Ross (1976) to conclude that "there is now evidence that hyperactivity may span the major developmental stages, often being apparent in the last trimester of pregnancy and continuing well into adulthood. . . . It [hyperactivity] is now conceptualized as the tip of the iceberg, a catalytic agent which . . . can trigger off a chain of secondary problems in childhood" (p. 289). This conclusion raises serious questions about the adequacy of the "developmental lag" explanations of the HK disorders and strengthens the view that the HK symptoms are expressions of underlying brain dysfunctions. However, objections to this interpretation have been raised by professionals who maintain that there is insufficient evidence for neurological impairment and/or specifiable brain damage. These objections may be based on misunderstandings regarding the requirements for "adequate evidence." An analogous situation was faced by nineteenth-century neurologists in determining the cause of epilepsy, which has long been considered as a major brain disorder. At that time, the diagnosis of epilepsy was derived solely from behavioral signs, namely, episodic manifestations of motor, sensory, or psychic dysfunctions, with or without unconsciousness, and motor convulsions that occurred less frequently. Neurologists such as Hughlings Jackson recognized the significance of these diverse signs, which appeared in differing forms and severity in the patient population, and they made meaningful inferences about the nature and often the cerebral locus of the brain disorder. More direct confirmations of these diagnoses with recordings of abnormal electrocortical activity and surgical techniques were not possible until the technological advances in the middle of this century (Penfield and Jasper, 1954). Also, effective anticonvulsant medications had been used for a long time, although their modes of action on the nervous system were not understood. Finally, it should be noted that, in spite of the extensive investigations of this disease, the etiology of epilepsy is as yet not well understood and many cases are still designated as idiopathic.

Likewise, the inference for brain disorders in HK requires systematic evaluations of its symptomology, as well as an understanding of the underlying psychological dysfunctions. These have been identified by systematic investigations conducted in several laboratories.

ATTENTION AND IMPULSE CONTROL

The series of investigations by the Montreal group (Douglas, 1972, 1974) have been concerned with analyses of dysfunctions in attention and impulse control by HK children. The children for these studies were carefully selected according to several criteria: (1) hyperactive behavior had to be present since early childhood, sustained throughout the day, and the major complaint of both parents; (2) the child had to be of normal intelligence, attending regular school classes, and living at home with at least one parent; (3) every child was screened by a psychiatrist, and those with signs of emotional disturbance, epilepsy, or gross brain damage were excluded. For each study, a group of 6- to 12-year-old HK children was compared with normal controls matched for age, sex, and WISC full-scale IQ. The resulting ratio of boys to girls was about 6:1. An extensive battery of psychological and educational tests was individually administered to each child. Douglas (1972, 1974) stresses the importance of determining those functions on which the HK child is unimpaired as well as those that differentiate him from normals. On the WISC, the HK children were not unlike normals in differences between Verbal and Performance IQ, nor were there consistent patterns among subtests, although subtest variability was greater for HK children. These children also responded as well as controls on items measuring short-term memory, language ability, abstract reasoning, and reading ability. The HK group responded consistently more poorly than the normal group on tests of perceptual-motor and motor abilities: the Bender Visual Motor Gestalt, the Lincoln-Oseretsky Motor Development Schedule, the Eye-Motor Coordination Subtest of the Frostig Test, and the Goodenough-Harris Draw-a-Person Test. Evaluation of the kinds of responses HK children make on these measures indicate not only motor but also attentional deficits, and provide strong evidence for close associations between attentional and fine-motor disorders.

Although the inference of attentive disorders in HK children has been made from psychological test results, it has proved difficult to delineate the specific dysfunctions and obtain quantitative measures. The difficulty in studying attentional disorders in HK stems from our imprecise understanding of the phenomenon of attention. As Worden (1966) pointed out, the experimental investigation of attentional processes presents conceptual and methodological problems which are peculiarly difficult for the psychologist to resolve. The various components of attention operate at all psychological levels, from sensation through cognition to response. Moreover, these attentional processes, many of which are "psychologically silent," overlap and fuse into seemingly inseparable aspects of functionally integrated behavior. The term itself denotes a number of differing psychological events, including such phenomena as alertness, selection, effort, vigilance, and focusing. In order to obtain a better understanding of attentional processes, Douglas (1974) attempted to delineate the demands that are made on the child when he must attend, e.g., he has to remain selectively alert toward certain stimuli and maintain this state for long periods of time, sometimes in the presence of other competing stimuli. These demands are made whether the child finds the task interesting or boring and whether or not he is given aids in directing and maintaining his attention. Also, differential demands are often made on the child—stimuli have direct signal value or the child has to search out and react to more subtle or abstract aspects of the stimuli. For some tasks, the child has to delay his response, but in all cases he is required to inhibit any tendency to respond to incorrect stimuli. Thus the demands of the tasks always include impulse control. Experimental analyses of attentive disorders have been investigated with paradigms that permit evaluations of the child's responses to each of the specific requirements.

The paradigm that has been used most extensively is that of the reaction time task, because it allows for the controlled variations of several independent variables and provides quantitative measures of the child's responses. In one study by the Montreal group, Sykes et al. (1973) selected 20 HK and 20 control children (mean ages 8.2 and 8.3 years) who were tested in random order on several different tasks and task variations. For the Choice Reaction Time, the child had to respond to a series of visual stimuli: two stimuli, four stimuli, or four stimuli with different color backgrounds. Each trial was presented as a separate unit and was initiated by the experimenter only when the child was considered ready to perform the task. The results, as expressed by analysis of variance, indicated no significant group differences, e.g., the RTs for the HK children were equivalent to those of the controls, with both groups having longer RTs as the stimulus display became more complex. For the Serial Reaction Time task, the stimuli were five lights, each associated with its own pushbutton. For each trial, one light was turned on, and the child was instructed to tap the appropriate button which turned off that light and immediately activated a second light which he then had to turn off. This procedure continued with random presentations of 100 stimuli (lasting 3 min) and the series was repeated three times. Analysis of variance showed no significant group differences either in mean correct responses or in deteriorations of performance during time on task. However, the HK group made significantly more incorrect responses than the normal group, with means of 29.15 and 18.11 errors, respectively. The results indicate that HK children can perform adequately on a RT task, provided that discrete trials are presented and trial duration is relatively brief. However, the demands of experimenter-paced trials prove more difficult for HK children and result in significantly poorer performance.

For the second of two studies reported by Dykman et al. (1971), 82 LD boys (8–12 years of age) from a children's clinic in Arkansas and 34 controls of the same age were selected. The LD boys were classified as hyperactive, normoactive, or hypoactive on the basis of teacher ratings. The procedure entailed eight phases in which several forms of the RT paradigm were used and certain variations were

125

MINIMAL BRAIN
DYSFUNCTION:
PSYCHOLOGICAL AND
NEUROPHYSIO-
LOGICAL DISORDERS
IN HYPERKINETIC
CHILDREN

introduced, such as distraction, differing foreperiods (1–5 sec), and reversals between relevant and irrelevant stimuli. The results indicated significantly greater error scores of all types by the LD than by the normal group. The hyperactive subgroup made the highest error scores (9.0 per child), followed in order by hypoactive (8.0 per child), normoactive (4.8 per child), and control (4.0 per child). Response latencies were longest for hypoactive, intermediate for normo- and hyperactive, and shortest for control.

The RT paradigm, utilizing visual (Czudner and Rourke, 1972) and auditory (Rourke and Czudner, 1972) stimuli, was also employed with children having "relatively mild, chronic cerebral dysfunctions" as determined from neuropsychological tests. The experiments were self-paced in that the child pressed a key to activate the warning signal and released it when the imperative stimulus occurred. Interstimulus intervals of 2–8 sec were used, with either a regular or an irregular procedure (random ISIs). The clinical and matched controls were each divided into two age groups, with means of 7.5 and 11.6 years. For the two age groupings, mean RTs were longer for the MBD than for the control subgroups, but significant differences were obtained only between the young-MBD and both its control and the old-MBD subgroup. The lack of significant RT difference between the two older subgroups seems to be the consequence of the parameters of the task. Since the mean RT of the older controls was not significantly shorter than that of the younger controls, the task seemed too easy for the 11-year-olds and therefore insensitive to possible differences between them and the older MBD children. The signaled RT paradigm has also been employed with HK children in investigations of their arousal responses and evaluations of the reactions to medication. A review of these studies, presented in subsequent sections, has shown consistent deficits in the performance of clinical groups as expressed by longer and more variable RTs. The analyses of response times by several investigators have indicated that the outstanding characteristic of HK children is their erratic response behavior; i.e., although they are capable of producing responses which are as fast as those of their controls, many of their responses are substantially longer than those of normal agemates.

Another paradigm for the assessment of attentive functions is the Continuous Performance Task (CPT). In the study by Sykes *et al.* (1973) the children were also tested on visual and auditory CPTs. The stimuli for each series consisted of 12 letters, with each letter presented for 0.2 sec and ISIs of 1.5 sec. The child was instructed to press a button only when the letter "X" was preceded by the letter "A." For each series, 100 stimuli were presented in a pseudorandom sequence (15 significant stimuli) which lasted 2.5 min. The results indicated that the HK group made significantly fewer correct and more incorrect responses than the controls and that their performance deteriorated significantly with time, while that of the controls remained stable. The HK group made significantly more error responses of all types than the controls: namely, anticipatory, random (to nonsignificant stimuli), and slow responses. They also made more multiple presses and more nonobserving responses (as recorded by the experimenter). Similar findings were reported by Anderson *et al.* (1973), who tested 30 LD boys and matched controls (mean age of 9.3 years) on a 30-min CPT task that consisted of 900 visual stimuli.

The LD group made significantly fewer correct and more incorrect responses than the controls. Furthermore, comparisons among LD subgroups according to activity criteria indicated that the performance of the hyperactive subgroup was poorer than that of the normoactive or hypoactive children.

In the field of developmental psychology there has been increasing interest in the differing approaches that children employ in problem solving. The resulting research has delineated several cognitive styles, among which are the dimensions of reflectivity-impulsivity and field dependence-independence. Reflectivity, according to Kagan *et al.* (1964), depicts "the tendency to reflect over alternative solutions or classifications in which several response alternatives are available simultaneously." This cognitive style has been assessed in normal children by the Matching Familiar Figures (MFF) Test, in which the child is presented with the picture of a familiar object and is required to match this with one of six alternative pictures. Only one of these is identical to the sample, while the other five differ in some small detail. Measures of response latencies and errors distinguish between reflective and impulsive styles. It has been found that the normal impulsive child differs from the reflective child by his greater physical activity, higher distractibility, and poorer control of attentive and motor processes (Kagan *et al.*, 1964). Field dependence-independence refers to the differences seen in individuals in their ability to separate an item from the context or field in which it is embedded (Witkin *et al.*, 1962), and is most frequently tested by the Embedded Figures Test. While an analytical approach is apparently taken by the field-independent subject, the field-dependent individual is believed to operate within a more global or diffuse perceptual mode and to be more influenced by these global aspects in problem-solving situations. Both impulsivity and field dependence have been found to decrease with age and to be unrelated to verbal intelligence (Kagan, 1966; Witkin *et al.*, 1962).

In their research, the Montreal group has investigated a number of cognitive styles in HK children (Campbell *et al.*, 1971). The results obtained with 19 HK and 19 matched control children (mean age 8.3 years) showed greater impulsivity by the HK children as indicated by significantly shorter response latencies and higher error scores on the MFF. Their greater field dependence was seen in their isolation of fewer embedded figures. However, when assessed on two additional cognitive dimensions (automatization and constricted-flexible control), significant group differences were not found on the measures employed. These findings provide evidence for distinct cognitive styles in HK, namely, impulsivity and field dependence. Support for the persistence of these styles into adolescence was obtained in a follow-up study of Montreal children, with mean age of 15.0 years (Cohen *et al.*, 1972). The responses on the MFF test indicated significantly greater impulsivity for the HK group than for the control group. On the Embedded Figures Test, the HK group's errors were only insignificantly higher than those of the controls, but their response latencies were significantly longer. The usefulness of the MFF test as a diagnostic instrument is supported by the findings of Keogh and Donlon (1972), who tested 27 boys with severe and prolonged learning problems and 25 boys with moderate learning difficulties (mean ages of 10.4 and 9.0 years, respectively). The severe LD boys were substantially more impulsive as

127

MINIMAL BRAIN
DYSFUNCTION:
PSYCHOLOGICAL AND
NEUROPHYSIO-
LOGICAL DISORDERS
IN HYPERKINETIC
CHILDREN

indicated by significant group differences in scores of errors and response latencies. The Rod and Frame Test (Witkin *et al.*, 1962), which was used for assessing
field dependence, showed no significant group difference for upright errors, but
the severe LDs had significantly faster response times. The latter test was also
employed by Zahn *et al.* (1975), who found significantly greater field dependence
in their clinical group of 42 MBD children (mean age of 10 years) compared to
controls.

Several authors have also suggested the important role which eye movements
play in the child's style of responding. Keogh (1971) and Douglas (1974) cite a
number of studies which indicate that impulsive children make fewer appropriate
eye movements to the experimental stimuli than do reflective children. On the
MFF test, the reflective child scans more systematically, showing a greater number
of comparison movements between the sample and the choice figures. As Douglas
(1974) comments, "such an approach demands sustained, well-organized attention
as well as inhibition of the inclination to settle for a less than perfect alternative. It
seems likely that similar processes enable the field-independent child to withstand
the influence of a confounding context and to differentiate the designs on the
Embedded Figures Test into their component parts, rather than treating them in
a diffuse, global manner." Although eye movements in HK children have not been
measured under such problem-solving situations, there are suggestions in the
literature of disturbed oculomotor functioning in this population (Cantor, 1971).
One recent study (Bala, 1976) found significant differences in the manner in
which normal and HK children visually follow a moving target. Saccadization of
pursuit occurred in both the normal and HK groups. However, the HK children
made larger saccades than normals during pursuit and also showed many saccades
distant to the pursuit path.

These research findings provide substantial support for specific dysfunctions
of attention and impulse control in HK children. Deficits were obtained not only
with the paradigms for selective and sustained attention, but also with tests for
cognitive processes.

Effects of Stimulant Medication

The 1937 report by Bradley concerning the beneficial effects of benzedrine in
children with behavior problems served as the impetus for the use of central
nervous system stimulants in the treatment of MBD. The most widely used drugs
are now methylphenidate and amphetamine sulfate, with the former considered
"the treatment of choice in the control of hyperactive behavior" (Millichap, 1973).
Millichap's review (1973) of reports between 1958 and 1968 indicated that, for 367
children given methylphenidate medication, clinical improvement occurred in
83% and exacerbated hyperactivity in 5%, while the effects for dextroamphetamine with 610 children were improvement in 69% and increased hyperactivity in
11%. Since dextroamphetamine has some undesirable side reactions, its effectiveness has been compared with that of levoamphetamine (Arnold *et al.*, 1972). Both
of these isomers were found significantly more effective than placebo, but dex-

troamphetamine had somewhat better results, and no differences in side effects were found. A weaker CNS stimulant, pemoline, has been found to be almost as effective as amphetamine, but the onset of clinical improvement is considerably slower (Conners *et al.,* 1972). Tranquilizers and sedatives have also been used, but with limited success. Clinical improvement was reported (Millichap, 1973) for 60% of the children with chlordiazepoxide, for 57% with thioridazine, and for 55% with chlorpromazine. These medications, however, have the undesirable side effect of drowsiness, and further investigations of these drugs have found them to be of little benefit. Among antidepressants, imipramine has been beneficial in the treatment of enuretic children and has also resulted in improvements for some MBD children (Millichap, 1973; Gross, 1975; Conners *et al.,* 1972), but serious side effects have been observed. Anticonvulsants have been used primarily with children whose behavior problems are complicated by seizures. Although some beneficial effects have been reported with diphenylhydantoin medication, a systematic evaluation with delinquent boys and with children having severe temper outbursts indicated no benefits with this drug (Conners *et al.,* 1972). Finally, caffeine, which had been reported to reduce hyperactivity (Schnackenberg, 1973), has been found ineffective with more systematic investigations (Garfinkel *et al.,* 1975; Gross, 1975). In the latter study, methylphenidate and *d*-amphetamine resulted in marked improvements, and imipramine produced minor benefits, whereas caffeine had generally negative effects on hyperactive behavior.

The findings from these studies have provided strong support for the effectiveness of dextroamphetamine and methylphenidate in alleviating the clinical signs of hyperactivity. More systematic investigations have been conducted for obtaining objective measures of these drugs on specific behavioral and psychological functions. Among the instruments that have been used for quantitative evaluations of drug effects are batteries of standardized psychological tests and several objective rating scales for behavioral categories. The results of such studies and their significance are obviously dependent on the methodology employed. An adequate design for drug evaluations requires placebo controls, double-blind procedures for drug administration and behavioral evaluations, and sequential drug administrations with pretreatment and balanced crossover procedures. These requirements raise the questions of appropriate dosage levels and duration of treatment under each condition. In view of the individual differences in drug responses, optimal dosage levels are usually determined for each child by gradually administering increasing dosages until the parents recognize signs of behavioral improvements without serious side effects. Clinical reports indicate that 70–80% of HK children are positive drug responders, while nonresponders exhibit increased hyperactivity and irritability. The aim for the assessment of long-term medication effects is difficult to meet, because the balanced crossover procedure places practical limits on the duration of each drug condition, and each medication should be administered for several weeks. The criteria for subject selection are also important experimental vaiables. Although most clinicians give stimulants only to children who exhibit hyperactive and/or attentive disorders, and who appear as positive drug responders, other criteria vary greatly among different investigators. Thus some studies exclude children with equivocal neurological and

129

MINIMAL BRAIN
DYSFUNCTION:
PSYCHOLOGICAL AND
NEUROPHYSIO-
LOGICAL DISORDERS
IN HYPERKINETIC
CHILDREN

EEG signs, while others report considerable incidence of these signs in their samples (e.g., Gross and Wilson, 1974; Satterfield *et al.*, 1973; Wender, 1971), and still others give no information about these signs. Finally, the inclusion of normal control groups is virtually impossible with these investigations, and there are only fragmentary reports on the effects of stimulants in healthy children.

In an early study (Millichap *et al.*, 1968), a battery of psychological tests was administered to 30 MBD children before and following methylphenidate or placebo administration. The drug resulted in significantly greater improvements than placebo on tests of visual and auditory perception, visual-motor coordination, and motor activity. However, the beneficial drug effects were diminished by the improved test scores with placebo. Knights and Hinton (1969) selected 40 LD children, 17 of whom had hyperactivity and poor attention span as the major complaint. After initial neurological and psychological assessment, the children were randomly assigned to methylphenidate or placebo treatment for 6-week periods. Teacher and parent ratings with several scales indicated substantial behavioral improvements with both treatments, but significantly greater drug than placebo improvements were found for only one of the scales (Werry, 1968). The overall scores on five psychological tests showed no significant drug-related improvements between pre- and on-medication testing. However, scores for several subtests indicated greater drug than placebo improvements. These were found on three performance subtests of the WISC and on two special tests for motor coordination. The better motor performance was attributed to the child's increased ability to attend to the demands of the task. Side effects of the drug were small weight loss (mean of 2%) and increased heart rate (mean of 20%). The EEG recordings indicated predrug abnormal patterns in 33% of the children (mainly excessive slow activity) and no significant changes with medication.

Gross and Wilson (1974) reported on a study involving 1056 outpatient children between 2 and 18 years of age. A diagnosis of MBD was made for 817 children, of whom 78.2% were boys. The sequence of medication was 1–2 weeks of placebo, then generally three types of drugs, each with increasing dosage, and finally medication with one of these drugs for at least 6 months. Both parents and teachers provided periodic (weekly) records of the child's behavior, and behavioral changes were then scored by an investigator on an 8-point scale ranging from "considerably worse" (−2) to "almost total relief from symptoms" (+5). A double-blind procedure was followed for drug administration and scoring of behavior items. Of 618 children who were given placebo, either no or very mild changes were found for 98.7% and this group's mean improvement score was 0.01. By contrast, active medication resulted in substantial behavioral improvements in 78% of these children, with mean improvement scores of 2.88 (moderate) for methylphenidate, 2.59 for *d*-amphetamine, and 2.97 for imipramine. This study was unusual because psychoactive medication was also given to healthy children, namely, 19 siblings of MBDs. The mean improvement score for this group was −0.15, and the reports for several boys indicated that they became irritable, cranky, and touchy.

In a study by the Montreal investigators (Weiss *et al.*, 1968), 36 HK children were selected according to multiple criteria (Douglas, 1972). Following predrug testing, they were randomly assigned to *d*-amphetamine or placebo groups for 3- to 5-week periods. In general, ratings by the mothers indicated greater improvements in the drug group than in the placebo group, and analysis of covariance of their ratings for four behavior categories showed significant drug effects for hyperactivity and distractibility but not for aggressivity and excitability. The results for 32 measures on five psychological tests, as evaluated by analysis of covariance (for pretest scores), showed no significant change on any of the tests, but did show near-significant ($p < 0.10$) drug-related improvements on WISC Vocabulary and Digit Symbol and on the Primary Mental Abilities Test. These findings were compared with an earlier investigation of chlorpromazine medication, which indicated significant improvements only on the mothers' ratings for hyperactivity. An extensive psychological evaluation was conducted by Conners *et al.* (1969) with 45 LD children from an outpatient clinic, most of whom had behavioral problems. The children were randomly assigned to *d*-amphetamine or placebo medication for a 4-week period. Impressive and significant drug-related improvements in behavior were found with the rating scales for teachers (Conners, 1969) and for parents (Conners, 1970). The results from psychological tests indicated significantly better performance with drug than with placebo for the Porteus Maze, CPT, and paired associate learning, and less pronounced improvements on tests for visual perception, auditory synthesis, and arithmetic achievement. Marked group differences were not obtained for the Bender and Draw-a-Person tests, or for measures of intelligence (WISC), oral reading, auditory discrimination and memory, and motor inhibitions.

These reports provide little support for the utility of standard psychological tests either for the identification of HK children or for evaluation of drug effects. Even those tests that have been frequently used in diagnostic procedures, such as the Bender-Gestalt, Frostig battery, or Draw-a-Person tests, appear inappropriate for research purposes. More impressive results have been obtained with behavioral rating scales, which are easy to administer and can be used in double-blind evaluations of drug effects. The scales that have been found most useful are those developed by Conners for teachers (1969) and parents (1970). However, normative data had not been reported in these early studies.

Rating scales have been included in the systematic research on the effects of stimulant medication conducted at Illinois by Sprague and his colleagues. In one study (Sprague *et al.*, 1974), Conners (1969) teachers' rating scale was used with 291 normal children who attended public schools and 64 HK children, some of whom were their classmates. Factor analysis of the normative ratings on the 39-item scale yielded the factors of conduct problems, inattentive-passive, hyperactivity, and tension-anxiety. The HK sample differed significantly from the normals on the first three factors, but not on the fourth. In investigations of dosage effects (Sprague *et al.*, 1974), 37 HK children received placebo and methylphenidate, at levels of 0.1, 0.3, and 1.0 mg/kg. A double-blind crossover procedure was followed, with dosage order varying in Latin square designs, during the 16-week period of the study. The results indicated beneficial drug effects regardless of time of medication, with significant improvements on the three factors of the teacher scale but not on the tension-anxiety factor. Ratings by teachers and physicians on the NIMH scale of Global Improvement also showed significant drug-related improvements, but these were not found with the Conners (1970) parent rating scale, or for WISC scores. All three dosage levels were more effective than placebo, and maximal improvements were obtained with 0.3 and 1.0 mg/kg methylphenidate. A slight increase in anxiety scores with the highest dosages indicates that 0.3 mg/kg would produce optimum effects. Evaluations of side effects, mostly anorexia, weight loss, and stomachaches, indicated that these were a direct function of dosage, but these symptoms were generally mild and associated only with the first 2 weeks of drug administration.

131

MINIMAL BRAIN
DYSFUNCTION:
PSYCHOLOGICAL AND
NEUROPHYSIO-
LOGICAL DISORDERS
IN HYPERKINETIC
CHILDREN

In an earlier study (Sprague *et al.*, 1970), the effects of two drugs were evaluated with 12 "emotionally disturbed" children, many of whom exhibited the HK syndrome. A counterbalanced design was followed for six conditions involving placebo, thioridazine, and methylphenidate, each at low and high dosage levels. On a task for recognition of familiar pictures, significantly more correct responses and shorter response latencies were obtained under methylphenidate medication than under the two other conditions. This drug also resulted in significantly lower scores of activity level, as measured with a stabilimetric cushion, and on teacher ratings for the child's activity, attention, and cooperation, but not for deviant behavior. The lack of differential findings between the two methylphenidate dosages (0.25 and 0.35 mg/kg) seems related to the small dosage difference. No indications were obtained for beneficial effects of thioridazine, which actually resulted in poorer performance than placebo on the picture recognition task. Differential dosage effects have been found (Sleator and Sprague, 1974) for measures of activity and task performance. An unspecified number of HK children were evaluated with a double-blind crossover procedure involving placebo and methylphenidate at dosages of 0.1, 0.3, and 0.7 mg/kg. The results show that dosage levels were related by linear functions to teacher ratings on the Conners (1969) and NIMH Global Improvement scales and to activity measures on the stabilimetric cushion, with the best scores obtained for the highest dosage. However, correct responses on the picture recognition test reached optimal levels at 0.3 mg/kg methylphenidate and were slightly lower for the higher dosage. These findings indicate that the commonly recommended therapeutic dosages, as determined by behavioral observations, may be excessive for attaining optimal levels of cognitive functions in HK children.

A 2-year follow-up study (Sleator *et al.*, 1974) on the need for continuing medication was conducted with HK children who were considered as good drug responders. Monthly teacher ratings (Conners, 1969) were obtained while the children were on either placebo or methylphenidate, with a mean dosage of 0.66 mg/kg. The preliminary findings for 42 children indicate that during the month of placebo administration the behavior of 17 children deteriorated markedly, while the ratings for 11 children (26%) did not change from those obtained during medication. These subgroups did not differ in mean age or IQ. Thus it seems important to continue long-term evaluations of drug responses for identification of those children for whom medication can be terminated.

The reports reviewed thus far have provided evidence that stimulant drugs lead to reductions in those undesirable behaviors that are included in the HK syndrome. Other studies have been designed for the assessment of drug effects on functions of attention and impulse control. The RT paradigm has been used in

JOHN S. STAMM AND
SHARON V. KREDER

investigations of autonomic responses in HK children, as reviewed in the following section (Cohen *et al.*, 1971; Porges *et al.*, 1975; Sroufe *et al.*, 1973; Zahn *et al.*, 1975). These studies showed that stimulant medications resulted in improved RT performance, as indicated by decreased response latencies and variabilities. Stimulants have also been found to result in better performance on the CPT by a group of LD boys (Anderson *et al.*, 1974). The effects of methylphenidate on cognitive styles were determined in a double-blind, crossover study (Campbell *et al.*, 1971) with 20 HK children from the Montreal clinic. After pretesting, the children were placed in random order on 2-week periods of drug and placebo. Significantly better performance under drug than placebo conditions was obtained on the Matching Familiar Figures (MFF) Test, with lower error scores and longer response times, and on a special Color Distraction Test, with fewer errors of commission. However, no significant treatment differences were found on the Embedded Figures and Naming Repeated Animals tests. Eighteen of these HK children had also participated in an earlier study (Campbell *et al.*, 1971) in which their performance on these four tests compared unfavorably to that of normal controls, with the most marked deficiencies on the MFF. The MFF test was also used in a double-blind, crossover study with methylphenidate, caffeine, and placebo (Garfinkel *et al.*, 1975). Although only eight HK boys were selected, the results seem impressive. Significantly better performance was found with methylphenidate than placebo on the MFF, as well as on Reitan's Motor Steadiness Test and on daily teacher ratings (Conners, 1969), especially for items of hyperactivity and inattention. By contrast, caffeine had no significant effects on any of the test scores and resulted in somewhat poorer ratings than placebo. Performance on the Rod-and-Frame Test was also found to improve significantly with stimulant medication (Zahn *et al.*, 1975), i.e., the responses of the MBD children became less field dependent.

Furthermore, the effects of medication have been compared with several alternative methods for the management of HK children. In one study (Conrad *et al.*, 1971), a rating scale was used to assess hyperactive behavior in 1350 elementary-grade children in a public school system. From this group, the 68 most hyperactive children were assigned to one of four conditions involving the administration of either amphetamine or placebo, and either special tutoring or no tutoring. During the 4- to 6-month-long study, those subjects who received tutoring were given two 90-min sessions every week by trained volunteers. An extensive test battery involving 34 variables was administered before and at the end of treatment. Parent and teacher ratings indicated significant improvements with the drug on measures of hyperactivity, motor coordination, and visual perceptual functions, while no marked gains were found with the tutoring. Both treatments resulted in improvements on the WISC and a visual tracking task. Thus the medication alone was clearly superior to the extensive tutoring remediation, which may have been of secondary benefit when combined with the drug. A different study (Sprague *et al.*, 1974) compared the effects of drugs with those of a conditioning procedure on the reduction of seat activity, as measured with a stabilometric cushion. Twelve HK boys (mean age 9.5 years) were selected and placed into methylphenidate (0.30 mg/kg) or placebo groups. Thirteen sessions

133

MINIMAL BRAIN
DYSFUNCTION:
PSYCHOLOGICAL AND
NEUROPHYSIO-
LOGICAL DISORDERS
IN HYPERKINETIC
CHILDREN

were given (20 min duration) while the boys were viewing filmstrips. The sequence of sessions consisted of baseline recordings, conditioning procedures, and postconditioning. With the conditioning method, a white light signaled reduced seat activity. During the conditioning phase, seat activity by both groups declined significantly from baseline levels, but the reduction for the drug group was over 3 times greater than that for the placebo group. Moreover, during the three postconditioning sessions, seat activity for the placebo group returned to baseline level, while that for the drug group remained significantly below its preconditioning level. These results indicate that conditioning methods are most effective when used in combination with stimulant medication.

This review of scientific studies provides strong evidence for the beneficial effects of methylphenidate and amphetamine in HK children. The drugs result in improvements of those specific behavioral symptoms and psychological functions that have been identified for the HK syndrome, namely, selective and sustained attention, impulse control, and restless behavior. The findings that lower drug dosages are required for optimal improvements of cognitive functions than for reductions in behavioral signs have implications for the determinations of the appropriate dosage for each child. It is possible that some of the 20–30% of HK children who do not show behavioral improvements with drugs (i.e., "nonresponders") may nonetheless perform better on cognitive tasks with low dosages of medication. There is also evidence that some of the nonresponders had been incorrectly diagnosed as HK or MBD. Conners's (1972) findings, derived from factor analyses of test scores obtained with a large group of LD children, identified a subgroup of children whose tests gave no indications of marked attentive, perceptual, or cognitive dysfunctions and who were nonresponders to drugs.

The delineation of attentive dysfunctions in HK children and the improvements of these functions with medication suggest that related neurophysiological disorders may be detected by appropriate electrophysiological techniques.

ELECTROPHYSIOLOGICAL SIGNS IN HYPERKINETIC CHILDREN

ELECTROENCEPHALOGRAPHY

The success of clinical EEG investigations in relating abnormal EEG patterns to differing forms of epileptic disorders has suggested the applicability of this technique to the identification of EEG pathologies in MBD. Although EEG recordings have been obtained from many MBD children, only a few systematic studies have been conducted with substantial groups of clinical children and normal controls. Capute *et al.* (1968) selected 106 MBD children from a medical clinic, who had no known neurological or psychiatric disorders, but neurological soft signs were found for all children. The age range was 2.3–16.3 years, and a control group was selected of 33 normal children of corresponding ages. Independent evaluations by four clinicians indicated EEG abnormalities in 50% of the MBD group and 15% of the control group. The type of abnormality in the MBD children was nonspecific in 24 children, 6/sec and 14/sec positive spike in 18 children, and paroxysmal patterns in 14 children. The degree of abnormality was judged as slight or moderate for 85% of the abnormal recordings and as marked in only 15%. Within the broad MBD age span, the incidence of abnormal recordings was 63% for the 8- to 11-year range, 31% for the younger subgroup, and 52% for the older subgroup. Also, the pediatric, neurological, and psychological evaluations showed no differences between MBD children with normal and with abnormal EEGs. In the study by Gross and Wilson (1974), EEGs were evaluated for 817 MBD children and for 160 normal controls who were their classmates. Abnormal EEG recordings were found in 53.8% of the MBD children and in 3.8% of the control children. The types of abnormal recordings were 14/sec and/or 6/sec positive spikes, 27%; abnormal fast patterns, 14%; negative spikes, 9%; and excessive slow waves, 4%. A small age trend was found, with the highest incidence of abnormal recordings (58%) in the 7- to 11-year age range. In their group of 57 HK children (6–9 years old), Satterfield *et al.* (1973) recorded abnormal EEGs in 32%, with excessive slow activity as the most frequent abnormality.

A carefully designed EEG study was conducted by Hughes (1971), who selected 8- to 11-year-old children from suburban schools. Each of the 214 underachievers, as determined by IQ above 89 and Learning Quotient below 90, was matched with a normal control for sex, age, and classroom. EEGs were evaluated by three independent clinicians, who found abnormalities in 41% of the underachievers and 30% of the normal group, with the following respective incidences: slow waves, 22% and 13.3%; sharp waves (epileptiform), 4.8% and 6.0%; positive spike, 19.9% and 15.2%; and extreme spindles, 1.9% and 0.9%. Significant group difference was found only for the incidence of slow waves. The severity of EEG abnormality, as judged on a 5-point scale from mild to marked, was mild in 83% and marked in only 15% of the underachievers.

The low incidence of epileptoid signs in the large clinical samples provides support for the differential diagnoses of MBD and epilepsy. However, the EEG evaluations contribute little toward our understanding of putative brain dysfunctions in MBD. The lack of consistent relationships between EEG abnormalities and MBD symptoms may be the consequence of the inadequacy of the clinical EEG procedure. Recordings are obtained while the subject is relaxed or asleep, a condition that is advantageous for the detection of epileptic signs. By contrast, the symptoms and psychological dysfunctions in MBD are clearly identified only when the child is active, responding to stimuli, and performing tasks.

Among the few studies in which EEGs were recorded while HK children performed a task is that by Grünewald-Zuberbier *et al.* (1975). Two groups of 11 boys each were selected from an institution for maladjusted children on the basis of diagnostic and observational signs of motor activity and restlessness. Children whose scores fell in the upper and lower third on these measures were placed, respectively, in the hyperactive and hypoactive groups. EEGs were obtained while the subjects performed a signaled RT task. Recordings of the hyperactive group differed from those of the hypoactive group in that (1) during resting periods and ITIs there were more α and fewer β wave epochs, with larger amplitudes for both types of waves; (2) in response to the warning signal the reductions in amplitudes developed more slowly and were less pronounced; (3) the EEG arousal responses to the imperative signal were shorter. Also, the hyperactive children had longer reaction times. These findings were considered to indicate that the hyperactive children had lower states of EEG arousal during resting conditions and poorer, more sluggish arousal responses to the stimuli. This interpretation seems consistent with the findings of investigations on autonomic nervous system measures of arousal in HK children.

135

MINIMAL BRAIN
DYSFUNCTION:
PSYCHOLOGICAL AND
NEUROPHYSIO-
LOGICAL DISORDERS
IN HYPERKINETIC
CHILDREN

Autonomic Measures of Arousal Responses

The excessive motor activity and short attention span commonly observed in HK children have suggested disorders in the neurophysiological regulation of arousal (Laufer and Denhoff, 1957; Wender, 1971). Consequently, investigations have been conducted with psychophysiological procedures that involve recordings of skin conductance (SC) or resistance (SR), heart rate (HR), and finger blood volume pulse (BVP). The findings from differing studies are sometimes inconsistent because they depend not only on the criteria for selection of the experimental and control subjects but also on the specific autonomic measures that are recorded and the experimental paradigms that are followed. Recordings can be obtained during periods of rest, when brief auditory or visual stimuli may or may not be presented, or during periods of task performance. The RT task permits optimal control over the subject's state of arousal and attention and is useful in the comparison of electrophysiological and behavioral measures, as well as for evaluations of drug effects. Stimulus presentations elicit arousal or orienting reactions (OR), which are normally indicated by increased SC and brief HR deceleration. The adequate assessment of ORs requires the measurement of deviations from baseline levels in response to stimuli for each subject, because prestimulus levels vary widely among individuals. However, many investigators have used other methods for evaluating ORs.

In spite of these methodological complexities, an evaluation of the research reports provides evidence for deficiencies in autonomic arousal responses in HK children. In an early investigation with 24 clinically diagnosed HK children (6–12 years old) and 12 normal boys, Satterfield and Dawson (1971) found that the HK group had significantly lower baseline SC levels (during rest) and fewer spontaneous SC responses to nonattended tones. Their conclusion of hypoarousal in MBD was, however, only partially supported by their results, because only 12 HK children had baseline SC levels below the range of the normals, while two others were above normal range.

A carefully controlled experiment was conducted in the Montreal laboratory with 20 HK boys (mean age 8.1 years) and their matched controls (Cohen and Douglas, 1972). The experimental sequence consisted of relaxation, nonsignal tone presentation, and a signaled RT task in which the subject was instructed to press a key to a warning tone and release it to a light flash. The criterion for an OR was a SC change of at least 0.1 μmho, occurring within 0.5–4.0 sec of stimulus onset. No significant group differences were found in baseline SC levels during rest or nonsignal tone presentations, in the incidence of ORs to these tones, or in the rates of habituation for the ORs. However, during RT performance the frequency of ORs to the warning signal increased significantly for the control subjects but did not change appreciably for the HK group. The RTs for the HK group were also significantly longer and more variable than those for the controls. These findings suggest that the warning tone for the RT task did not adequately alert the HK subject and prepare him to respond to the imperative stimulus. This task was also used for evaluating the effects of different reinforcement conditions on RTs of 27 HK boys and normal controls (Firestone and Douglas, 1975). At the start of the experiment, mean RTs were determined, without feedback for response times. Three subgroups were then tested with differing reinforcement conditions, which consisted of informing each boy when his responses were faster (reward) or slower (punishment) than his baseline RT, or both types of feedback were given. For HK and control children, mean RTs were shorter for every reinforcement than nonreinforcement condition, but RTs remained longer for the HK group. An unexpected finding was the fivefold increase in interstimulus responses from baseline to reinforcement conditions by the HK but not by the control group. Thus the improved RT performance by the HKs occurred at the cost of greater impulsivity. Electrodermal recordings indicated increasing basal SC levels in both groups during the course of the experiment, with no significant effects of group or reinforcement conditions. However, the frequency of phasic ORs to the warning signal was significantly less for the HK group than for the normal group.

These results of lower autonomic reactivity by HK children to meaningful stimuli are in general agreement with those reported by Dykman *et al.* (1971). In their first of two studies, they recorded SC, HR, and muscle potentials in 26 MBD children who showed a "high incidence of hyperactivity" and in normal controls. The recordings were obtained after completion of a behavioral experiment so that all subjects were acquainted with the experimental procedure and presumably were relaxed. During the first 5-min resting period, no significant group differences were obtained on any of the autonomic measures. However, during task performance, when the children responded differentially to one of two tones, the overall results indicated greater autonomic reactivity by the normal group than by the MBD group. Reactivity was determined by *T* scores that measured differences between pre- and poststimulus periods. These scores showed significantly higher ST, lower HR, and lower muscle potentials for the MBD group than for the normal group. The MBD children also responded significantly more poorly on behavioral measures of the task.

The effects of stimulant medication on autonomic responses have been evaluated in several investigations. For most of the investigations, each HK child received the drug dosage that had been determined as optimal by clinical judgments. In their first study, Satterfield and Dawson (1971) also administered methylphenidate to some of the HK children and found higher baseline SC levels and more spontaneous SC responses than in HK children who were off medication. In a subsequent study (Satterfield *et al.*, 1974), comparisons were made between subgroups of HK children who had been classified on the basis of their clinical response to medication. The best responders had lower baseline SC levels

137

MINIMAL BRAIN
DYSFUNCTION:
PSYCHOLOGICAL AND
NEUROPHYSIO-
LOGICAL DISORDERS
IN HYPERKINETIC
CHILDREN

before treatment and greater SC increases with medication than did the poor drug responders. Spring *et al.* (1974) selected 38 HK boys (mean age 10 years) who, from physician's reports, had shown positive responses to methylphenidate medication. Subjects were randomly assigned to an on-drug or off-drug group, with the boys continuing their daily medication or being taken off medication for 72 hours before testing. Placebo was not used, but 20 normal boys constituted a control group similar to the clinical children in age and IQ. Recordings of SR were obtained during 10-min periods each of rest and presentation of 40 nonsignaled tones. No significant group differences were found for baseline SR levels. However, the frequency of ORs to the tones was significantly greater for the normal group than for the off-drug group, but not for the on-drug group. Furthermore, trials to habituation were significantly greater for the normal group than for the off-drug group, and tended to be more for the on-drug than off-drug group.

The experimental procedure of Cohen and Douglas (1972) was followed with 20 HK boys (Cohen *et al.*, 1971). A double-blind, crossover method was used, with half the group first receiving methylphenidate and the other half placebo. The drug resulted in significantly higher SC and HR basal levels than the placebo during relaxation and tone presentations. A differential effect was also found for tonic SC changes. The baseline SC levels for both groups increased significantly during the course of the experiment, with highest levels during the RT phase, but this increase was significantly less for the drug group than for the placebo group. This result was attributed to the "law of initial values," which states that the response to a stimulus decreases in amplitude as the prestimulus or basal level increases. Habituation rates of ORs to both types of stimuli were about equal for both groups. The RT responses were faster and less variable under methylphenidate than under placebo.

Sroufe *et al.* (1973) tested 21·MBD children from a pediatric clinic and 17 normal controls on a signaled RT task. Two testing sessions were given at 6-week intervals: both groups were tested first without medication; only the MBD children were tested for the second session, either on methylphenidate or on placebo. HR deceleration (HRD), as determined by the difference between HR for the beat occurring at onset of the imperative stimulus and the third beat prior to the stimulus, showed significant predrug differences between MBD and controls, with HRDs of 2.61 and 7.51 beats/min, respectively. RT measures obtained during the first session showed no significant group differences between mean latencies, but did show significantly greater variability by the MBD group. Comparisons between the two sessions indicated significant increase in HRD and decrease in mean RT for the drug, but no significant changes for the placebo subgroup. Significant correlations between HRD and RT were obtained for the normal and drug subgroups, but not for the predrug MBD and placebo subgroups. These findings were interpreted as indicating beneficial effects of methylphenidate on the MBDs' attentive functions, specifically on the "maintenance of set." More detailed analyses of HR changes were obtained with 16 HK boys from the Urbana laboratory (Porges *et al.*, 1975). Each child was tested on a special RT task, with variable ISIs, while either on methylphenidate (0.3 mg/kg) or on placebo medication. Comparisons of HR changes between 5-sec pretrial and the first 5-sec ISI periods indicated no significant group differences in either the initial HRD or the subsequent HR acceleration. However, mean pretrial HR levels were significantly higher for the drug group than for the placebo group, while the reverse relation was found for the final 5-sec period of the ISI. This tonic increase in HR for the placebo group was considered as an "abnormal" autonomic response. Mean reaction times were somewhat shorter for the drug group than for the placebo group.

The inconsistent findings among some of these studies were recognized by Zahn *et al.* (1975), whose experiment was designed for clarification of the issues. They tested 42 MBD children (6–12 years old) who had been referred to a psychiatrist for their persistent hyperactivity and inattention. Fifty-four normals of equivalent age served as controls. Recordings of SC, HR, and skin temperature (ST) were obtained during conditions of rest, presentations of tones, and a signaled RT task. Control children were tested once; each MBD child was tested twice at 10-week intervals, under off- and on-drug (either *d*-amphetamine or methylphenidate) conditions, with 25 children first tested off drug. Comparisons between normal and off-drug MBD groups showed no reliable differences for baseline levels of SC, HR, or ST during the resting phase or between trials. However, the gradual decrease of SC levels during the course of the experiment was slower for the off-drug MBD group, which indicated poorer adaptation to the demands of the task. OR indicators, obtained by analysis of covariance for prestimulus levels, showed lower autonomic reactivity in the off-drug MBDs than in the normal children to all kinds of stimuli. The SC measures of the off-drug MBDs indicated smaller amplitudes and slower rates of change for both the increase to maximum levels and the return to baseline. Similar group differences were found with HR measures, which showed slower deceleration to tone onset and slower rates of recovery for the MBDs. With regard to drug effects, which were the same for both stimulants, baseline levels of SC and HR were significantly higher, and ST levels lower, for on-drug than for off-drug conditions. The drug effects on ORs to tones appeared paradoxical in that more sluggish SC measures were obtained. But analysis of covariance, which took into account prestimulus levels and changes in ST, substantially reduced these group differences, so that the SC changes could be explained by peripheral drug effects in lowering ST. Off-drug RT responses by the MBD group compared to normals showed longer mean latencies and greater variabilities; both of these measures decreased significantly with medication.

In spite of the differing results reported by some of these investigators, several consistent findings emerge from this review. The evidence obtained with baseline recordings provides no convincing support for views of either over-arousal or underarousal in HK children. However, their deficient autonomic reactivity is indicated by their smaller and slower responses to brief stimuli, especially under the demands of the RT task, and their slower rates of change from baseline levels during the course of the experiment. Thus both phasic and tonic processes of autonomic reactivity appear impaired. Stimulant medication has been found to raise autonomic base levels and to improve performance on the RT task. Therefore, these improvements appear to be the consequence of heightened autonomic base levels. The evidence supports the conclusion (Zahn *et al.*, 1975) that optimal task performance by HK children occurs when they are at above-normal levels of autonomic arousal.

139

MINIMAL BRAIN
DYSFUNCTION:
PSYCHOLOGICAL AND
NEUROPHYSIO-
LOGICAL DISORDERS
IN HYPERKINETIC
CHILDREN

The pronounced behavioral aberrations in HK children cannot be readily explained by autonomic dysfunctions, because their baseline levels are generally within normal range. The evidence for attentive disorders suggests dysfunctions in the neuronal processes subserving attention, which have been found to involve cerebral cortex (Luria, 1973). The inadequate autonomic reactivity might be the consequence of deficient modulation on the neuronal arousal system via descending pathways from the cortex. More direct evidence for cortical dysfunctions in attention has been obtained by recordings of cortical evoked potentials.

CORTICAL EVOKED POTENTIALS (EPs)

The electrical response in the brain to a brief stimulus consists of a complex pattern of low-voltage fluctuations which are difficult to detect with scalp recordings because of the higher amplitudes of the ongoing EEG activity. Therefore, a series of stimuli are presented and averages are obtained of responses that are time locked on stimulus onset. The emerging averaged EP consists of a sequence of positive and negative deflections from prestimulus baseline that are identified by their latencies from stimulus onset. Early investigators (e.g., Chapman and Bragdon, 1964; Davis, 1964; Haider *et al.*, 1964; Satterfield, 1965; Spong *et al.*, 1965) found that manipulations of experimental variables could affect the amplitudes of some of the late components, i.e., those with latencies longer than 50 msec. Presentations of series of flashes and/or clicks, with instructions to the subject to count or respond motorically to certain stimuli and ignore others, resulted in larger amplitudes to the relevant than to the irrelevant stimuli. This enhancement of amplitudes has been interpreted as an expression of selective attention. The experimental paradigms, however, provided inadequate control over attentive states. Since relevant and irrelevant stimuli had been presented in predictable sequences, the enhanced components could also be considered to reflect heightened states of arousal (Naatanen, 1969). Furthermore, it has been difficult to compare the findings from different investigations because the EP pattern depends on the stimulus modality and electrode location. Each component's latency and amplitude are also affected by the experimental paradigm and by the time constants of the apparatus.

Recent investigators have agreed to designate each positive (P) and negative (N) component by its latency from stimulus onset. For experiments on attention, EP recordings are generally obtained from vertex with reference to ear or mastoid, and the different types of stimuli are presented in nonpredictable sequences. With simultaneous presentations of two independently timed series of flashes, Donchin and Cohen (1967) found an enhancement of a late positive component (P_{300}) to the relevant stimuli. Eason *et al.* (1969), who presented relevant stimuli to one visual half-field and irrelevant ones to the other half-field, found enhanced amplitudes of negative components at 120–220 msec latencies. Presentations of both types of stimuli to the same retinal region (Harter and Salmon, 1972) resulted in enhancement of the N_{220} and P_{300} components. For the auditory modality, random presentations of two series of tones (Wilkinson and Lee, 1972) resulted in enhancements to the relevant stimulus of the N_{80}–P_{160} amplitude and of the P_{300} component. These carefully designed studies indicate that relevant stimuli result in enhanced amplitudes of late components in two latency ranges, namely, 80–220 msec (negative) and around 300 msec (positive). It should be noted that the subjects for the difficult discrimination tasks had been sophisticated adults, often the coinvestigators.

The investigations of EPs in MBD children have frequently been designed for the evaluation of medication and the identification of good drug responders. Satterfield *et al.* (1972) recorded EPs to auditory clicks (0.1 msec) from 31 HK (6–9 years old) and 21 normal boys. Their finding of smaller late-component amplitudes for the HK group than for the normal group seems questionable, because the recordings were obtained while the boys watched interesting cartoons. In a different investigation, Buchsbaum and Wender (1973) tested 24 MBD children (21 boys) and 24 controls (12 boys) of the same age. EP recordings to the onset of 500-msec light stimuli of differing intensities indicated a greater mean voltage change between the N_{140} and P_{200} peaks for the MBD (21.4 μV) than for the control (17.5 μV) group. The further finding of higher amplitudes of this measure by the younger (6–9 years) than the older (10–12 years) controls led to the authors' conclusion that EPs provide indications for maturational lag in MBD. The effects of increasing flash intensity on amplitude of N_{140}–P_{200} were also determined. The slope of this function was steeper for the MBD group than for the control group and it became smaller in drug responders with amphetamine medication, but not in nonresponders.

A more systematic investigation of visual EPs was conducted by Hall *et al.* (1976). Twenty-six HK boys (7–11 years old) were selected according to multiple criteria, including the absence of abnormal EEG signs, and 16 normals served as controls. Flashes (15 msec) of white light at four intensities were presented under two conditions: first attention, when the boy pressed a button to an interspersed dim green light, and then inattention, when this light and the button press did not occur. Five testing sessions were given over a 5- to 6-week period: after pretesting, the boys were randomly assigned to amphetamine or placebo medication, which was reversed for the third session, and testing under the drug was repeated after intervals of 1 and 5 weeks. The controls received placebo. The results indicated no pretreatment differences between the HK and control groups for any late EP component or for the slopes of the flash intensity vs. EP amplitude functions, no differences in EPs between attention and inattention conditions, no effects of the drug on any of these measures, and no correlations between clinical drug responses and EPs. However, ratings of hyperactive behavior (Conners, 1969, 1970) showed significant negative correlations between severity of the HK symptoms and EP amplitude of N_{150}–P_{200}. Also, evaluations of EPs by a computer-derived measure of "stability" provided positive correlations between EP stability and the degree of behavioral improvement with drugs. This stability measure appears related to the index of variability (Halliday *et al.*, 1976) that was determined from 250 points in each EP sample. These investigators selected 42 children (mean age of 9½ years) who had a history of HK and no sensory or EEG abnormality. EPs were recorded to randomly presented flashes (40 msec) and clicks (50 msec), first under an attention condition, when the subject pressed a button to an interspersed light that was dimmer than the test flash, and then under a passive condition, when this light and the press did not occur. Three sessions were given at 1-week intervals, initially for pretreatment and then under methylphenidate (10 mg) or placebo medication, which were administered in a counterbalanced order. The effects of the drug on EPs to visual stimuli were different for groups of drug responders and nonresponders, who were identified with Conners', (1969) rating scale. For the responders, EP variability increased from the attention to the passive task, whereas EP variability decreased for nonresponders in the transition between these tasks. Also, for the drug responders, only the N_{140}–P_{190} amplitude under attention conditions increased from placebo to methylphenidate treatment.

141

MINIMAL BRAIN
DYSFUNCTION:
PSYCHOLOGICAL AND
NEUROPHYSIO-
LOGICAL DISORDERS
IN HYPERKINETIC
CHILDREN

These investigations did not provide convincing evidence for EP indicators of attentive dysfunctions in MBD. The experiments were not designed for adequate control over differing states of attention, especially under the "inattentive" conditions, when the subjects were not prevented from continuing to attend to the demands of the task. A further limitation is the lack of control over the sensory input to the receptors. This is especially important with HK children who are restless in the experimental situation and have excessive eye movements. The amplitudes of EPs to visual stimuli have been found to be affected by position of the eyes, eye rotation, and whether eyes are open or closed (Tecce, 1970). Testing with closed eyes results in excessive activity, which may be time locked to stimulus onset. When auditory stimuli are presented by loudspeakers, the subject's body and head movements will affect the sensory input to the ear, and consequently will also affect the EPs. Therefore, the use of headphones is preferable. The following investigations have attempted to control these important experimental variables.

Prichep *et al.* (1976) randomly presented single or double clicks (950 msec interval) via loudspeakers under two conditions: uncertainty, when the subject guessed prior to each trial whether a single or double click would be presented, and certainty, when this information was given before stimulus presentation. In order to minimize movement artifacts, the trial was initiated by the subject's pressing of a key. Sixteen HK boys (8–11 years old) were selected from a clinic on the basis of their history and high HK ratings (Conners, 1969). Eight normal boys served as controls. The results showed no significant group differences under certainty conditions in EP amplitudes to the first or second click. However, under uncertainty, the HK group responded to the second click with significantly smaller P_{200} and larger N_{250} ampltiudes (baseline to peak) than the controls, regardless of correct or wrong guesses. The effects of methylphenidate, as determined with repeated sessions and placebo controls, were indicated by increased P_{200} and decreased N_{250} amplitudes, but these still differed from those of the control group. Since the authors considered the uncertain condition to require greater attention than the certain condition, they interpreted their EP findings as indicative of attentive deficits in the HK boys. This view, however, does not seem well founded, because these EP components have not been related to attentive states in normal subjects. The alternative interpretation of hypoarousal seems more likely, in view of the findings by Picton *et al.* (1974) that EPs to clicks during sleep show substantial enhancement of the N_{290} component.

The best-controlled paradigm for obtaining EP indicators of selective attention was used by Hillyard *et al.* (1973). Concurrent sequences of tone pips were presented via earphones, with 800-Hz pips to one ear and 1500-Hz pips to the other. About 10% of the pips were of slightly higher frequencies and the healthy adult subjects were instructed to count these signal tones to one ear at a time. Thus the subjects were in attentive states throughout the session, with attention directed to stimuli in one or the other ear. Comparisons of vertex EPs between stimuli to the two ears showed significantly higher N_{80} amplitudes to stimuli in the attended than in the nonattended ear, with amplitude differences of 20–78% for different subjects. Also, a late positive (P_{300}) component was found only to the higher-pitched signal tones in the attend series, while the amplitudes of other late components were not affected by the experimental variables. These findings were interpreted as cortical reflections of two distinct processes of selective attention that seem to correspond to Broadbent's (1970) distinction between stimulus set and response set. Since the experiment required the subject to attend to the signal pip and also to respond appropriately (count), these attentive sets may be reflected, respectively, by the N_{80} and P_{300} components. This interpretation may also be applied to earlier findings of P_{300} during selective attention (Donchin and Cohen, 1967; Harter and Salmon, 1972; Sutton *et al.*, 1965).

The paradigm of Hillyard *et al.* (1973) has been used in our research with MBD children. In view of the difficulty of the task, in the first study (Zambelli *et al.*, 1977) a group of 14-year-old boys was selected from the files of a children's clinic. Nine boys were chosen who had been diagnosed as MBD, met the HK criteria of pronounced hyperactivity and attentive deficits, and had responded to stimulant medication. Although their behavioral symptoms had subsided and medication had been discontinued, their EPs on the selective attention task differed from those of age-matched controls. Whereas the N_{80} amplitudes for the control group were significantly greater to the stimuli in the attend than in the nonattend channels, with a median difference of 21%, no significant amplitude differences were found for the clinical group (median difference of 5%). Moreover, when the boys were tested for button presses to the signal pips, the clinical group made significantly fewer correct responses than the controls and almost 4 times as many errors of commission. This investigation is currently being continued in a second study (Loiselle *et al.*, 1977) with 12-year-old MBD boys and controls. The results obtained thus far, with 12 HK boys and age-matched controls, are consistent with the earlier findings. The N_{80} amplitude differences between attend and nonattend stimuli are significantly smaller for the HK group than for the control group, with the former also making substantially more button-press errors. Comparisons of the button-press responses between age groups from the two studies indicate fewer errors by the older boys, both clinical and control. These findings provide evidence for dysfunctions in the neural substrates of attentive processes.

This brief review of the EP literature indicates the potential usefulness of this procedure with HK children and points the direction for further research. It is important to conduct well-controlled experiments with normal subjects for identification of specific EP components, such as N_{80} and P_{300}, that reflect distinct attentive processes. The paradigms should then be applied to carefully selected groups of clinical children. The findings of abnormal EP components might be important in the differential diagnosis of MBD subgroups, such as hyper- and hypoactive children. The previous attempts of using EP measures for predictions of drug responses have not been productive. The EP technique should be used only after establishment of objective measures for drug responses and identification of the relevant EP components.

143

MINIMAL BRAIN
DYSFUNCTION:
PSYCHOLOGICAL AND
NEUROPHYSIO-
LOGICAL DISORDERS
IN HYPERKINETIC
CHILDREN

THE HK SYNDROME AND FRONTAL LOBE DYSFUNCTIONS

It has been emphasized that the terms "MBD" and "HK" are symptomatic lables and do not designate any known brain damage or dysfunction. However, the evidence for psychological and neurophysiological aberrations in HK children provides support for inferred brain dysfunctions. An adequate hypothesis should delineate the brain structures involved and specify the modes of neuronal disorders. The constellation of psychological disorders in HK children, namely, inadequate attention, inadequate impulse control, and inadequate planning of response sequences, appears analogous to that found in patients with known damage to the anterior dorsolateral and polar segments of the frontal lobes. The main characteristics of the frontal lobe syndrome have been summarized by Pontius (1973) as the inability to construct a plan of action ahead of the act, to execute this plan, and to reprogram ongoing activity whenever necessary. Experimental evidence for these dysfunctions has been obtained by Milner and her associates from groups of patients who had sustained differing circumscribed cortical resections for the relief of epilepsy. Compared to other surgical groups, patients with dorsolateral frontal resections were specifically impaired on the Wisconsin Card Sorting Test (Milner, 1963) and on visually (Milner, 1965) and tactually (Corkin, 1965) guided maze learning. Their errors on these tasks were the consequence of excessive response perseverations and those of "broken rules"; e.g., when the patients were questioned, they gave correct statements concerning the rules for the task and recognized their error responses. As Milner (1964) concluded, the intellectual ability of the frontal lobe patients was within normal limits on many tasks, but deficiencies occurred in situations which require frequent shifting of response tendencies and inhibitions of perseverative interference from previous sensory input. These findings and conclusions are consistent with those reported by Luria (1973) and Teuber (1964).

The evidence for physiological dysfunctions in frontal lobe patients is unfortunately sparse and has been reported primarily in the Russian literature by Luria and his associates. These investigators have found pronounced irregularities in electrophysiological measures of orienting responses, as indicated by sluggish changes to differing stimuli (Luria, 1973), as well as abnormalities in cortical evoked potentials (Simernitskaya, 1973). EP research with normal subjects has provided indications for frontal lobe involvement in attentive processes. Picton *et al.* (1974) determined scalp distributions of EPs to clicks and found maximum amplitudes for several late components, especially N_{80} and P_{160}, from the fronto-central region.

The findings from several lines of research provide evidence for late developmental processes of the frontal lobes. Myelinization of the neurons in these areas and of thalamofrontal tracts is slow and not completed until the late adolescent years (Yakovlev and Lecours, 1967). Furthermore, systematic investigations of EPs (Beck *et al.*, 1975) have shown age-related changes in latencies and especially in amplitudes of late components. Amplitudes increased substantially from birth to 5–7 years and then declined gradually until they attained stable levels at 15–17 years. Impressive evidence regarding the development of frontal lobe functions has been obtained from tests on the delayed-response task with infant and juvenile monkeys whose dorsolateral prefrontal cortex had been ablated in the neonatal period (Goldman, 1974). These monkeys could perform adequately on the task until the age of about 36 months, while older frontally ablated monkeys were severely impaired. Additional findings with reversible cooling of prefrontal cortex (Goldman and Alexander, 1977) indicate task deficits only for 34- to 36-month-old monkeys, the age that is close to sexual maturity. These findings indicate that the prefrontal areas do not become functional until pubescence and that the task is mediated in younger monkeys by other forebrain structures, probably the caudate nucleus. Recent anatomical studies (Goldman and Nauta, 1977) have shown intact neuronal pathways in infant brains between prefrontal cortex and cortical and subcortical structures. Thus there seems to be a wide age gap between the structural and functional maturation of dorsolateral prefrontal cortex.

Evidence for the implication of forebrain structures in the HK syndrome has been obtained from pharmacological and neurochemical investigations. The excitatory effects of amphetamines in the nervous system are the consequence of their actions on synaptic processes of catecholamines, specifically dopamine and norepinephrine. Amphetamine interferes with the reuptake of these neurotransmitters and can also bring about their release into the synaptic cleft. Other CNS stimulants such as methylphenidate presumably act in similar ways (Snyder and Meyerhoff, 1973). It has also been possible to distinguish between the effects of amphetamine on the dopaminergic and norepinephrinergic transmitter systems. Neurochemical research with the two isomers, *d*-amphetamine and *l*-amphetamine, has found that the former is about 10 times as potent as the latter in affecting norepinephrinergic transmission, whereas both isomers are about equally potent for dopaminergic processes (Snyder and Meyerhoff, 1973). Therefore, the findings of nearly equal effectiveness of both amphetamine isomers on behavior ratings in HK children (Arnold *et al.*, 1972, 1973) have been explained by excitation of the dopaminergic neural system. Distinct neuroanatomical pathways have also been identified for the two transmitter substances. The norepinephrine synapses are widely distributed in subcortical structures, in the limbic system, and over the entire cerebral cortex, while 90% of dopamine transmitters are concentrated in the nigrostriatal system, which terminates in the caudate-putamen structure (Snyder and Meyerhoff, 1973). The caudate nucleus also receives efferents from the cerebral cortex, especially the prefrontal areas. Close functional associations

145

MINIMAL BRAIN
DYSFUNCTION:
PSYCHOLOGICAL AND
NEUROPHYSIO-
LOGICAL DISORDERS
IN HYPERKINETIC
CHILDREN

between prefrontal cortex and caudate have been found with lesion studies in monkeys. The same forms of behavioral impairments have been obtained with discrete lesions in the caudate and with circumscribed resections of prefrontal segments that project to their respective zone in the caudate (Rosvold and Szwarc-bart, 1964).

Physiological experiments have shown that cortex exerts mainly excitatory influences on the caudate and that this structure, in turn, has widespread inhibitory effects over cortical and subcortical structures (Buchwald *et al.,* 1967). These findings provide direct support to the concept of the important role of prefrontal cortex in the execution of behavioral responses. Consequently, it seems possible to postulate a simple model for deficient neuronal processes in HK children that takes into account the two sets of impressive findings, namely, the disorders in attention and impulse control and the improvements in these functions with stimulant medication. Dysfunctions in prefrontal cortex would lead to inadequate excitation of caudate neurons and, consequently, to impairments in inhibitory control of psychological processes and motor responses. Stimulant drugs have the effects of raising the levels of caudate excitation, which would compensate, at least partially, for the deficient frontal lobe excitatory influences. This view is supported by the research findings of autonomic nervous processes in HK children (Zahn *et al.,* 1975).

The concept of putative frontal lobe dysfunctions in HK should, like all hypothetical models, help to delineate the directions for future investigations and aid in the formulation of improved methods of treatment and prognosis. More research is clearly needed for clarification of the HK children's specific difficulties in attentive processes and for obtaining additional electrophysiological measures of these dysfunctions. With regard to diagnosis, we are impressed by Douglas's (1974) conclusion "that it may be worth considering an approach in which the existing diagnostic labels are ignored and subjects are chosen instead on the basis of attentional problems and poor impulse control" (p. 159). She recommends the use of tests that have differentiated between HK and normal children and have also shown signficant changes with stimulant drug treatment. These tests should include the CPT, signaled RT task, MFF, and Porteus Maze. The test scores should be related to the electrophysiological measures of attention. Also, determination of the optimal drug dosage for each HK child should be based on his cognitive task performance rather than on behavioral measures, in view of the findings by Sprague *et al.* (1974).

The pervasiveness of impaired attention and impulse control in HK children indicates the need for determining appropriate training procedures that will remediate these disorders. Unfortunately, none of the techniques used thus far have been found to be effective (Douglas, 1974; Messer, 1976). A review of different procedures for improving performance on the MFF task by normal impulsive children (Messer, 1976) indicated the most promising results with a scanning procedure in which the child recited the instructions aloud. This method is consonant with Luria's (Luria and Luria, 1966) formulation for the development of cognitive functions, namely, that voluntary control over the child's behavior is attained first by verbalization and then by internalization of verbal

JOHN S. STAMM AND
SHARON V. KREDER

commands. The effectiveness of verbal mediation in problem solving was investigated by Palkes *et al.* (1972), who tested 30 HK boys (7–13 years old) by differing procedures on the Porteus Maze (Porteus, 1965) under several conditions. Verbalization resulted in reductions of some types of errors, but did not facilitate maze learning. These findings emphasize the difficulties in developing techniques that will improve attentive processes in HK children.

The evidence for the late maturation of frontal lobe functions stresses the need for investigations of HK children during their adolescent years. There is little evidence concerning the outcome of their neurodevelopmental processes. These may continue until normal maturational levels are attained, or may stabilize at below-normal levels. Both of these outcomes may be expected in different adolescents, in view of the great individual variabilities in dysfunctions of HK children. It seems clear that HK children are not "out of the woods" during their pubescent years, even though their hyperactive symptoms subside. Therefore, substantial research effort is required for assessment of the HK adolescent, and longitudinal studies are needed for obtaining early indicators for the ultimate outcome of this disorder in each child.

REFERENCES

Anderson, R. P., Halcomb, C. G., and Doyle, R. B. The measurement of attentional deficits. *Exceptional Children*, 1973, *39*, 534–539.

Anderson, R. P., Halcomb, C. G., Gordon, W., and Ozolins, D. Measurement of attention/distractibility in LD children. *Academic Therapy*, 1974, *9*, 261–266.

Arnold, L. E., Wender, P. H., McCloskey, K., and Snyder, S. H. Levoamphetamine and dextroamphetamine: Comparative efficacy in the hyperkinetic syndrome. *Archives of General Psychiatry*, 1972, *27*, 816–822.

Arnold, L. E., Kirilkuk, V., Corson, S. A., and Corson, E. O. Levoamphetamine and dextroamphetamine: Differential effect on hyperkinesis in children and dogs. *The American Journal of Psychiatry*, 1973, *130*, 165–169.

Bala, S. P. Eye movements of hyperkinetic children. Doctoral dissertation, City University of New York, 1976.

Beck, E. C., Dustman, R. E., and Schenkenberg, T. Life span changes in the electrical activity of the human brain as reflected in the cerebral evoked response. In J. M. Ordy and K. R. Brizzee (eds.), *Neurobiology of Aging: An Interdisciplinary Life Span Approach*. New York: Plenum, 1975.

Bradley, C. The behavior of children receiving benzedrine. *The American Journal of Psychiatry*, 1937, *94*, 577–585.

Bradley, C. Benzedrine and dexedrine in the treatment of children's behavior disorders. *Pediatrics*, 1950, *5*, 24–37.

Broadbent, D. E. Stimulus set and response set: Two kinds of selective attention. In D. I. Mostovsky (ed.), *Attention: Contemporary Theory and Analysis*. New York: Meredith, 1970.

Buchsbaum, M., and Wender, P. Average evoked responses in normal and minimally brain dysfunctioned children treated with amphetamine. *Archives of General Psychiatry*, 1973, *29*, 764–770.

Buchwald, N. A., Hull, C. D., and Truchtenberg, M. C. Concomitant behavioral and neural inhibition and disinhibition in response to subcortical stimulation. *Experimental Brain Research*, 1967, *4*, 58–72.

Campbell, S. B., Douglas, V. I., and Morgenstern, G. Cognitive styles in hyperactive children and the effect of methylphenidate. *Journal of Child Psychology and Psychiatry*, 1971, *12*, 55–67.

Cantor, H. Role of the neurologist in management of children with learning disabilities. In J. Harstein (ed.), *Current Concepts in Dyslexia*. St. Louis: Mosby, 1971.

Cantwell, D. P. *The Hyperactive Child*. New York: Spectrum, 1975a.

Cantwell, D. P. Epidemiology, clinical picture and classification of the hyperactive child syndrome. In D. P. Cantwell (ed.), *The Hyperactive Child*. New York: Spectrum, 1975b.

Capute, A. J., Niedermeyer, E. F. L., and Richardson, F. The electroencephalogram in children with minimal cerebral dysfunction. *Pediatrics,* 1968, *41*, 1104.

Chapman, R. M., and Bragdon, H. R. Evoked responses to numerical and non-munerical visual stimuli while problem solving. *Nature (London),* 1964, *203*, 1155–1157.

Clements, S. D. Task force one: Minimal brain dysfunction in children. National Institute of Neurological Diseases and Blindness, Monograph No. 3, U.S. Department of Health, Education, and Welfare, 1966.

Cohen, N. J., and Douglas, V. I. Characteristics of the orienting response in hyperactive and normal children. *Psychophysiology,* 1972, *9*, 238–245.

Cohen, N. J., Douglas, V. I., and Morgenstern, G. The effect of methylphenidate on attentive behavior and autonomic activity in hyperactive children. *Psychopharmacologia,* 1971, *22*, 282–294.

Cohen, N. J. Weiss, G., and Minde, K. Cognitive styles in adolescents previously diagnosed as hyperactive. *Journal of Child Psychology and Psychiatry,* 1972, *13*, 203–209.

Connors, C. K. A teacher rating scale for use in drug studies with children. *American Journal of Psychiatry,* 1969, *126*, 152–156.

Connors, C. K. Symptom patterns in hyperkinetic, neurotic, and normal children. *Child Development,* 1970, *41*, 667–682.

Connors, C. K. Pharmacotherapy of psychopathology in children. In H. C. Quay and J. S. Werry (eds.), *Psychopathological Disorders of Childhood.* New York: Wiley, 1972.

Connors, C. K., Rothschild, G. H., Eisenberg, L., Stone, L., and Robinson, E. Dextroamphetamine in children with learning disorders. *Archives of General Psychiatry,* 1969, *21*, 182–190.

Connors, C. K., Taylor, E., Meo, G., Kurtz, M. A., and Fournier, M. Magnesium pemoline and dextroamphetamine: A controlled study in children with minimal brain dysfunction. *Psychopharmacologia,* 1972, *26*, 321–336.

Conrad, W. G., Dworkin, E. S., Shai, A., and Tobiessen, J. E. Effects of amphetamine therapy and prescriptive tutoring on the behavior and achievement of lower class hyperactive children. *Journal of Learning Disabilities,* 1971, *4*, 509–517.

Corkin, S. Tactually guided maze learning in man: Effects of unilateral cortical excisions and bilateral hippocampal lesions. *Neuropsychologia,* 1965, *3*, 339–351.

Czudner, G., and Rourke, B. P. Age difference in visual reaction time of "brain damaged" and normal children under regular and irregular preparatory interval conditions. *Journal of Experimental Child Psychology,* 1972, *13*, 516–526.

Davis, H. Enhancement of evoked cortical potentials in humans related to a task requiring a decision. *Science,* 1964, *145*, 182–183.

Donchin, E., and Cohen, L. Averaged evoked potentials and intramodality selective attention. *Electroencephalography and Clinical Neurophysiology,* 1967, *22*, 537–540.

Douglas, V. I. Stop, look and listen: The problem of sustained attention and impulse control in hyperactive and normal children. *Canadian Journal of Behavioral Science,* 1972, *4*, 259–282.

Douglas, V. I. Sustained attention and impulse control: Implications for the handicapped child. In J. A. Swets and L. L. Elliott (eds.), Psychology and the Handicapped Child. Washington, D.C.: U.S. Department of Health, Education, and Welfare, DHEW Publ. No. (OE) 73-05000, 1974.

Dykman, R. A., Ackerman, P. T., Clements, S. D., and Peters, J. E. Specific learning disabilities: An attentional deficit syndrome. In H. Mykelbust (ed.), *Progress in Learning Disabilities,* Vol. 2. New York: Grune and Stratton, 1971.

Dykman, R. A., Peters, J. E., and Ackerman, P. T. Experimental approaches to the study of minimal brain dysfunction: A follow-up study. *Annals of the New York Academy of Sciences,* 1973, *205*, 93–108.

Eason, R. G., Harter, M. R., and White, C. T. Effects of attention and arousal on visually evoked cortical potentials and reaction time in man. *Physiology and Behavior,* 1969, *4*, 283–289.

Firestone, P., and Douglas, V. The effects of reward and punishment on reaction times and autonomic activity in hyperactive and normal children. *Journal of Abnormal Child Psychology,* 1975, *3*, 201–215.

Garfinkel, B. D., Webster, C. D., and Sloman, L. Methylphenidate and caffeine in the treatment of children with minimal brain dysfunction. *American Journal of Psychiatry,* 1975, *132*, 723–728.

Goldman, P. An alternative to developmental plasticity: Heterology of CNS structures in infants and adults. In D. Stein, J. Rosen, and N. Butters (eds.), *Plasticity and Recovery of Function in the Central Nervous System.* New York: Academic Press, 1974.

Goldman, P. S., and Alexander, G. E. Maturation of prefrontal cortex in the monkey revealed by local reversible cryogenic depression. *Nature (London),* 1977, *267*, 613–615.

147

MINIMAL BRAIN
DYSFUNCTION:
PSYCHOLOGICAL AND
NEUROPHYSIO-
LOGICAL DISORDERS
IN HYPERKINETIC
CHILDREN

Goldman, P. S., and Nauta, J. H. Columnar distribution of corticocortical fibers in the frontal association, limbic and motor cortex of the developing rhesus monkey. *Brain Research,* 1977, *122,* 393–413.

Gross, M. B. Caffeine in the treatment of children with minimal brain dysfunction or hyperkinetic syndrome. *Psychosomatics,* 1975, *16,* 26–27.

Gross, M. B., and Wilson, W. C. *Minimal Brain Dysfunction.* New York: Bruner/Mazel, 1974.

Grünewald-Zuberbier, E., Grünwald, G., and Rasche, A. Hyperactive behavior and EEG arousal reactions in children. *Electroencephalography and Clinical Neurophysiology,* 1975, *38,* 149–159.

Haider, M., Spong, P., and Lindsley, D. B. Attention, vigilance, and cortical evoked potentials in humans. *Science,* 1964, *145,* 180–182.

Hall, R. A., Griffin, R. B., Moyer, D. L., Hopkins, K. H., and Rappaport, M. Evoked potential, stimulus intensity, and drug treatment in hyperkinesis. *Psychophysiology,* 1976, *13,* 405–418.

Halliday, R., Rosenthal, J. H., Naylor, H., and Callaway, E. Averaged evoked potential predictors of clinical improvement in hyperactive children treated with methylphenidate: An initial study and replication. *Psychophysiology,* 1976, *13,* 429–440.

Harter, M. R., and Salmon, L. E. Intra-modality selective attention and evoked potentials to randomly presented patterns. *Electroencephalography and Clinical Neurophysiology,* 1972, *32,* 605–613.

Hillyard, S. A., Hink, R. F., Schwent, V. L. , and Picton, T. W. Electrical signs of selective attention in the human brain. *Science,* 1973, *182,* 177–180.

Hughes, J. R. Electroencephalography and learning disabilities. In H. R. Myklebust (ed.), *Progress in Learning Disabilities,* Vol. 2. New York: Grune and Stratton, 1971.

Kagan, J. Reflection-impulsivity: The generality and dynamics of conceptual tempo. *Journal of Abnormal Psychology,* 1966, *71,* 17–24.

Kagan, J., Rosman, B. L., Day, D., Albert, J., and Phillips, W. Information processing in the child: Significance of analytic and reflective attitudes. *Psychological Monographs,* 1964, 78 (1, Whole No. 578).

Keogh, B. K. Hyperactivity and learning disorders: Review and speculation. *Exceptional Children,* 1971, *38,* 101–109.

Keogh, B. K., and Donlon, G. M. Field dependence, impulsivity, and learning disabilities. *Journal of Learning Disabilities,* 1972, *5,* 331–336.

Kinsbourne, M. Minimal brain dysfunction as a neurodevelopmental lag. *Annals of the New York Academy of Sciences,* 1973, *205,* 268–273.

Knights, R. M., and Hinton, G. The effects of methylphenidate (Ritalin) on the motor skills and behavior of children with learning problems. *Journal of Nervous and Mental Diseases,* 1969, *148,* 643–653.

Laufer, M. W., and Denhoff, E. Hyperkinetic behavior syndrome in children. *Journal of Pediatrics,* 1957, *50,* 463–474.

Loiselle, D. L., Zambelli, A. J., and Stamm, J. S. Auditory evoked potentials as measures of selective attention in older MBD children. Paper presented at International Neuropsychological Society, Santa Fe, New Mexico, 1977.

Luria, A. R. The frontal lobes and the regulation of behavior. In K. H. Pribram and A. R. Luria (eds.), *Psychophysiology of the Frontal Lobes.* New York: Academic Press, 1973.

Luria, A. R., and Luria, F. A. *Speech and the Development of Mental Processes in the Child.* London: Staples, 1966.

Messer, S. B. Reflection-impulsivity: A review. *Psychological Bulletin,* 1976, *83,* 1026–1052.

Millichap, J. G. Drugs in management of minimal brain dysfunction. *Annals of the New York Academy of Sciences,* 1973, *205,* 321–334.

Millichap, J. G., Aymat, F., Sturgis, L. H., Larsen, K. W., and Egan, R. A. Hyperkinetic behavior and learning disorders. III. Battery of neuropsychological tests in controlled trial of methylphenidate. *American Journal of Diseases of Children,* 1968, *116,* 235–244.

Milner, B. Effects of different brain lesions on card sorting: The role of the frontal lobes. *Archives of Neurology,* 1963, *9,* 90–100.

Milner, B. Some effects of frontal lobectomy in man. In J. M. Warren and K. Akert (eds.), *The Frontal Granular Cortex and Behavior.* New York: McGraw-Hill, 1964.

Milner, B. Visually guided maze learning in man: Effects of bilateral hippocampal, bilateral frontal, and unilateral cerebral lesions. *Neuropsychologia,* 1965, *3,* 317–338.

Naatanen, R. Anticipation of relevant stimuli and evoked potentials: A comment of Donchin and Cohen's "Averaged evoked potentials and intramodality selective attention." *Perceptual and Motor Skills,* 1969, *28,* 639–646.

149

MINIMAL BRAIN
DYSFUNCTION:
PSYCHOLOGICAL AND
NEUROPHYSIO-
LOGICAL DISORDERS
IN HYPERKINETIC
CHILDREN

Palkes, H., Stewart, M., and Freedman, J. Improvement in maze performance of hyperactive boys as a function of verbal-training procedures. *The Journal of Special Education,* 1972, *5*, 337–342.

Penfield, W., and Jasper, H. *Epilepsy and the Functional Anatomy of the Human Brain.* Boston: Little, Brown, 1954.

Picton, T. W., Hillyard, S. A., Krausz, H. I., and Galambos, R. Human auditory evoked potentials. I. Evaluation of components. *Electroencephalograpy and Clinical Neurophysiology,* 1974, *36*, 179–190.

Pontius, A., Dysfunction patterns analogous to frontal lobe system and caudate nucleus syndromes in some groups of minimal brain dysfunction. *Journal of the American Medical Women's Association,* 1973, *26*, 285–292.

Porges, S. W., Walter, G. F., Korb, R. J., and Sprague, R. L. The influences of methylphenidate on heart rate and behavioral measures of attention in hyperactive children. *Child Development,* 1975, *46*, 727–733.

Porteus, S. D. *Porteus Maze Tests: Fifty Years Application.* Palo Alto, Calif.: Pacific Books, 1965.

Prichep, L. S., Sutton, S., and Hakerem, G. Evoked potentials in hyperkinetic and normal children under certainty and uncertainty: A placebo and methylphenidate study. *Psychophysiology,* 1976, *13*, 419–428.

Ross, D. M., and Ross, S. A. *Hyperactivity: Research, Theory, and Action.* New York: Wiley, 1976.

Ross, J. J., Childres, D. G., and Perry, N. J., Jr. The natural history and electrophysiological characteristics of familial language development. In P. Satz and J. J. Ross (eds.), *The Disabled Learner.* Rotterdam: Rotterdam University Press, 1973.

Rosvold, H. E., and Szwarcbart, M. K. Neural structures involved in delayed-response performance. In J. M. Warren and K. Akert (eds.), *The Frontal Granular Cortex and Behavior.* New York: McGraw-Hill, 1964.

Rourke, B. P., and Czudner, G. Age differences in auditory reaction time of "brain damaged" and normal children under regular and irregular preparatory interval conditions. *Journal of Experimental Child Psychology,* 1972, *14*, 372–378.

Satterfield, J. H. Evoked cortical response enhancement and attention in man: A study of responses to auditory and shock stimuli. *Electroencephalography and Clinical Neurophysiology,* 1965, *19*, 470–475.

Satterfield, J. H., and Dawson, M. E. Electrodermal correlates of hyperactivity in children. *Psychophysiology,* 1971, *8*, 191–197.

Satterfield, J. H., Cantwell, D. P. Lesser, L. I., and Podosin, R. L. Physiological studies of the hyperkinetic child: I. *The American Journal of Psychiatry,* 1972, *128*, 1418–1424.

Satterfield, J. H., Lesser, L. I., Saul, R. E., and Cantwell, D. P. EEG aspects in the diagnosis and treatment of minimal brain dysfunction. *Annals of the New York Academy of Sciences,* 1973, *205*, 274–282.

Satterfield, J. H. Cantwell, D. P., and Satterfield, B. T. Pathophysiology of the hyperactive child syndrome. *Archives of General Psychiatry,* 1974, *31*, 839–844.

Satz, P., and Van Nostrand, G. K. Developmental dyslexia: An evaluation of a theory. In P. Satz and J. J. Ross (eds.), *The Disabled Child: Early Detection and Intervention.* Rotterdam: Rotterdam University Press, 1973.

Schnackenberg, R. C. Caffeine as a substitute for schedule II stimulants in hyperkinetic children. *American Journal of Psychiatry,* 1973, *130*, 796–798.

Simernitskaya, E. G. Application of the method of evoked potentials to the analysis of activation processes in patients with lesions of the frontal lobes. In K. H. Pribram and A. R. Luria (eds.), *Psychophysiology of the Frontal Lobes.* New York: Academic Press, 1973.

Sleator, E. K., and Sprague, R. L. Dose effects of stimulants in hperkinetic children. *Psychopharmacology Bulletin,* 1974, *10*, 29–33.

Sleator, E. K., von Neumann, A., and Sprague, R. L. Hyperactive children. A continuous long-term placebo-controlled follow-up. *Journal of the American Medical Association,* 1974, *229*, 316–317.

Snyder, S. H., and Meyerhoff, J. H. How amphetamine acts in minimal brain dysfunction. *Annals of the New York Academy of Sciences,* 1973, *205*, 310–320.

Spong, P., Haider, M., and Lindsley, D. B. Selective attentiveness and cortical evoked responses to visual and auditory stimuli. *Science,* 1965, *148*, 395–397.

Sprague, R. L., Barnes, K. R., and Werry, J. S. Methylphenidate and thioridazine: Learning, reaction time, activity, and classroom behavior in disturbed children. *American Journal of Orthopsychiatry,* 1970, *40*, 615–628.

Sprague, R. L., Christensen, D. E., and Werry, J. S. Experimental psychology and stimulant drugs. In C. K. Conners (ed.), *Clinical Use of Stimulant Drugs in Children.* The Hage: Excerpta Medica, 1974, 141–164.

Spring, C., Greenberg, L., Scott, J., and Hopwood, J. Electrodermal activity in hperactive boys who are methylphenidate responders. *Psychophysiology*, 1974, *4*, 436–442.

Sroufe, L. A., Sonies, B. C., West, W. D., and Wright, F. S. Anticipatory heart rate deceleration and reaction time in children with and without referral for learning disability. *Child Development*, 1973, *44*, 267–273.

Stewart, M. A., Pitts, F. N., Craig, A. G., and Dieruf, W. The hyperactive child syndrome. *Amerian Journal of Orthopsychiatry*, 1966, *36*, 861–867.

Sutton, S., Braren, M., Zubin, J., and John, E. R. Evoked potential correlates of stimulus uncertainty. *Science*, 1965, *148*, 395–397.

Sykes, D. H., Douglas, V. I., and Morgenstern, G. Sustained attention in hyperactive children. *Journal of Child Psychology and Psychiatry*, 1973, *14*, 213–220.

Tecce, J. J. Attention and evoked potentials in man. In D. I. Mostovsky (ed.), *Attention: Contemporary Theory and Analysis*. New York: Meredith, 1970.

Teuber, H. L. The riddle of frontal lobe function in man. In J. M. Warren and K. Akert (eds.), *The Frontal Granular Cortex and Behavior*. New York: McGraw-Hill, 1964.

Weiss, G., Minde, K., Douglas, V., Werry, J., and Sykes, D. Studies on the hyperactive child. V. The effects of dextroamphetamine and chlorpromazine on behavior and intellectual functioning. *Journal of Child Psychology and Psychiatry*, 1968, *9*, 145–156.

Weiss, G., Minde, K., Werry, J. S., Douglas, V., and Nemeth, E. Studies on the hyperactive child. VIII. Five-year follow-up. *Archives of General Psychiatry*, 1971, *24*, 409–414.

Wender, P. H. (ed.), *Minimal Brain Dysfunction in Children*. New York: Wiley-Interscience, 1971.

Werry, J. S. Developmental hyperactivity. *Pediatric Clinics of North America*, 1968, *15*, 581–599.

Wilkinson, R. T., and Lee, M. V. Auditory evoked potentials and selective attention. *Electroencephalography and Clinical Neurophysiology*, 1972, *33*, 411–418.

Witkin, H. A., Dyk, R. B., Faterson, H. F., Goodenough, D. R., and Karp, S. A. (eds.), *Psychological Differentiation*. New York: Wiley, 1962.

Worden, F. G. Attention and auditory electrophysiology. In E. Stellar and J. M. Sprague (eds.), *Progress in Physiological Psychology*, Vol. 1. New York: Academic Press, 1966.

Yakovlev, P. I., and Lecours, A. R. The myelogenetic cycles of regional maturation of the brain. In A. Minkowski (ed.), *Regional Development of the Brain in Early Life*. Oxford: Blackwell, 1967.

Zahn, T. P., Abate, F., Little, B. C., and Wender, P. H. Minimal brain dysfunction, stimulant drugs, and autonomic nervous system activity. *Archives of General Psychiatry*, 1975, *32*, 381–387.

Zambelli, A. J., Stamm, J. S., Maitinsky, S., and Loiselle, D. L. Auditory evoked potentials and selective attention in formerly hyperactive adolescents. *The American Journal of Psychiatry*, 1977, *134*, 742–747.

PART IV

Language Mechanisms and Their Disorders

7

Speech Perception and the Biology of Language

SALLY P. SPRINGER

INTRODUCTION

Despite 25 years of intensive research, only very limited progress has been made in the development of machines capable of speech understanding (Lea, 1974; Rubenstein, 1974). The difficulties that have beset efforts to construct such devices are testimony to the complexity of the relationship between sound and meaning present in every natural language.

The nature of speech as an acoustic signal may be appreciated with the aid of a sound spectrograph that displays speech visually as a time-by-frequency plot. Figure 1 presents a spectrogram of the utterance "This is a sound spectrogram." The reader should attempt to segment the display before reading the caption that performs that task for him. This exercise illustrates an important characteristic of speech. Although it is perceived as a series of discrete, nonoverlapping units, the acoustic substrate is intergraded to a large degree. Silent periods in speech do not always occur at word boundaries, and may in fact occur at intuitively unlikely places—in the middle of words themselves. The individual sound units, or phonemes, that compose speech are fused into one another in the acoustic representation. With few exceptions, it is difficult to determine where one phoneme begins and another ends.

Difficulty in segmenting the speech signal is in part responsible for the trouble even highly trained investigators have reading spectrograms (Fant, 1962; Liberman *et al.*, 1967*b*). Further contributing to the problem is a lack of invariance in the acoustic structure of phonetic segments. For example, the acoustic shape of

SALLY P. SPRINGER Department of Psychology, State University of New York, Stony Brook, New York 11794.

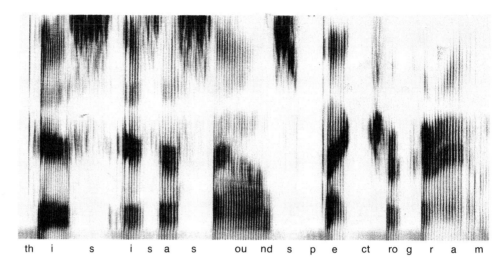

th i   s   i s a s   ou nd s p e   ct ro g   r   a   m

Fig. 1. Wide-band sound spectrograms of the utterance "This is a sound spectrogram." Ordinate displays frequency from 80 Hz to 7 KHz. Courtesy of M. Bischoff and F. Poza, Stanford Research Institute.

/d/ in the English word "deep" is different from its form in "deck," which is in turn different from its acoustic shape in "duke." The listener perceives the initial segments in these three words to be identical, although the physical structure of /d/ is not invariant and depends on the context in which it occurs (Liberman *et al.*, 1954).

Although the intergraded nature of the speech signal and the lack of acoustic invariance pose substantial difficulties for those who wish to read spectrograms or build voice-operated typewriters, speech perception proceeds for most human beings with intact hearing in an entirely effortless fashion. How is this possible? It has been suggested that the ease with which human listeners process spoken language is a consequence of the operation of special mechanisms, intimately related to speech production, that are speech and species specific (Liberman, *et al.*, 1967*a*).

In their now-classic paper, Liberman *et al.* (1967*a*) present the view that speech is a complex code in which a perceived phonetic message does not have a one-to-one relationship with the acoustic signal that conveys it. The sounds of speech are not isolatable units concatenated as the proverbial "beads on a string" of traditional linguistic analysis; rather, at each moment in time in the speech stream, information is transmitted in parallel about one or more adjacent phonetic segments. This complexity is necessary, it is argued, to overcome the limitations set by the resolving power of the ear. Speech can be understood at rates of up to 30 phonetic segments per second, while the auditory system appears capable of resolving only a fraction of that number of discrete units. Parallel transmission of information serves to reduce the number of units to a manageable number at the cost of a complex relationship between acoustic structure and phonetic message— phonemes do not take forms that are context invariant.

Liberman *et al.* (1967*a*) propose that in the absence of acoustic invariance to subserve the perception of the same phoneme in different contexts the listener finds invariance in the motoric commands to the articulatory system. The acoustic signal is processed by reference to the manner in which it is produced. This view, positing that a listener is capable of understanding speech because of his tacit knowledge of the way it is generated, is referred to as the "motor theory" of speech perception. The reader is referred to Liberman *et al.* (1967*a*) and Cooper (1972) for a fuller explication of this and related theories.

The phenomena of categorical perception, selective adaptation, and ear asymmetries in dichotic listening have each been offered in support of the notion that the perception of speech differs from the perception of other sounds and is uniquely human (Liberman, 1970*a,b;* Mattingly and Liberman, 1969; Wood, 1975). The purpose of this chapter is to review these phenomena that characterize the perception of speech, examining the evidence as it bears on the issue of whether special, speech- and species-specific processing mechanisms need be postulated to account for them. This question, of course, is of considerable interest to neurobiology and the efforts to discover the neural substrates of language.

SOME FUNDAMENTALS

Evaluation of the investigations to be discussed in later sections requires an understanding of the acoustic and linguistic properties of the stimuli they employ. This brief digression into the basic principles of speech production and the nature of the cues that have been shown to be important in the perception of certain speech sounds will provide the necessary background for the reader with no previous knowledge in this area. (See Stevens and House, 1972, for additional background.)

The flow of air from the lungs provides the source of acoustic energy for the sounds of speech. This energy is then "filtered" by the supralaryngeal vocal tract, the resonance characteristics of which are a consequence of its cross-sectional area function. The resonances produced, known as formants, are represented as dark bands on a spectrographic display, and are numbered with respect to their position on the frequency scale. The first formant (F1) is the lowest in frequency, the second (F2) the next higher, and so forth. While natural speech may contain upwards of three formants, most of the information in the signal is contained in the lowest two or three formants, and good-quality synthetic speech may be produced in many instances with F1 and F2 alone.

Speech sounds may be grouped according to classification schemes based on similarities in the ways in which the sounds are produced by human talkers. The articulation of consonant sounds may be described in terms of their place of articulation, their manner of articulation, and the presence or absence of vocal fold vibration (voicing). The sounds /b/, /d/, and /g/ share the same manner of articulation; the breath stream is blocked momentarily at the point of articulation, allowing pressure buildup, and is then released in each case. Known as stop consonants because of this manner of production, they differ from each other in place of articulation. Closure occurs at the lips for /b/, the dental ridge for /d/, and

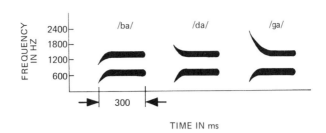

Fig. 2. Schematic spectrograms of two-formant syllables differing in place of articulation. After Delattre *et al.* (1955).

the soft palate for /g/. The places of articulation are referred to as bilabial, alveolar, and velar, respectively.

Figure 2 presents schematic spectrograms of the syllables /ba/, /da/, and /ga/ "(bah," "dah," and "gah"); these spectrograms permit visual inspection of the acoustic consequences of differences in place of articulation. These syllables differ only in the direction and extent of the change taking place in F2 during the first 50 msec of the syllable. This F2 transition, rising to its final value appropriate for the vowel in /ba/, falling in /da/, and falling sharply in /ga/, has been shown to be an important cue for the identification of these sounds (Liberman *et al.*, 1954).

Since vocal fold vibration accompanies the release of the supraglottal closure in /b/, /d/, and g/, these sounds are referred to as voiced. This is in contrast to /p/, /t/, and /k/, also stop consonants with bilabial, alveolar, and velar places of articulation, respectively, where the onset of vocal fold vibration lags release of the sounds. Such phonemes are classified as voiceless. The consonants /b/ and /p/, for example, are said to differ in voice onset time (VOT) (Lisker and Abramson, 1964), with the onset of voicing delayed in /p/ relative to /b/.

Figure 3 presents a spectrographic display of the acoustic manifestation of

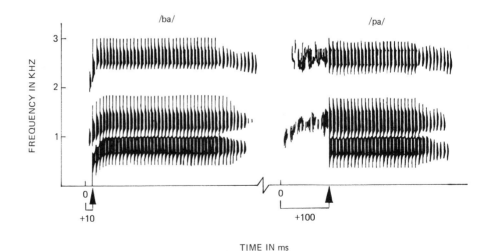

Fig. 3. Spectrograms of syllables differing in voice onset time. After Abramson and Lisker (1973).

VOT. Voice onset time is represented by the delay in onset of F1 relative to F2 and F3. The syllable on the left, heard as /ba/ by speakers of English, has a VOT value

157

SPEECH PERCEPTION
AND THE BIOLOGY OF
LANGUAGE

VOT. Voice onset time is represented by the delay in onset of F1 relative to F2 and F3. The syllable on the left, heard as /ba/ by speakers of English, has a VOT value of 10 msec—the onset of F1 lags the onset of F2 and F3 by 10 msec. A VOT value of 100 msec is illustrated at the right of Fig. 3. Listeners perceive the syllable as /pa/ when the VOT value is 30 msec or greater.

Vowel sounds differ from consonants in that the outgoing breath stream has relatively free movement through the vocal tract; shape and size of the air passages determine their acoustic structure. Spectrographically, isolated vowels appear as a set of steady-state formants. Different vowels may be produced synthetically by varying the relative postion of the formants in terms of frequency.

The development of speech synthesis devices has made it possible to generate speech sounds that vary along place of articulation and VOT dimensions, as well as along other continua. These synthetically produced speech sounds form the basis for much of the research in the discussions that follow.

CATEGORICAL PERCEPTION

Perception is said to be categorical when subjects are able to discriminate among a set of stimuli only to the extent that they can assign different labels to them (Studdert-Kennedy *et al.*, 1970). Categorical perception has been described as a special property of speech sounds that is "unusual, if not unique, since in the perception of nonspeech sounds many more stimuli can be discriminated than can be identified" (Mattingly *et al.*, 1971).

A series of synthetically generated stimuli that differ from each other in equal steps along a particular acoustic continuum form the starting point for demonstrations of the categorical nature of speech perception. Investigators (Liberman *et al.*, 1957; Mattingly *et al.*, 1971; Barclay, 1972; Pisoni, 1973) have varied the direction and extent of the second formant transition to construct such a series, e.g., /b/-/d/-/g/, while others (Liberman *et al.*, 1961; Pisoni and Lazarus, 1974) have employed a continuum of stimuli that differ in linearly equivalent steps along the dimension of VOT, e.g., /d/-/t/.

Typically, the stimuli from the series chosen are randomly ordered and presented repeatedly to subjects for identification, followed by tests that assess the ability of the same individuals to discriminate pairs of stimuli selected from the series. Figure 4 presents idealized data from a hypothetical study employing eight stimuli. The labeling function reveals the existence of a phonetic boundary located at a point along the continuum intermediate between stimuli 4 and 5. Syllables to the left of this boundary are consistently assigned to category A, while to the right of the boundary they are identified as members of category B. When discrimination is tested, stimuli 4 and 5, assigned to different phonetic categories, are readily discriminable, while discrimination of the stimuli selected from within a phonetic category is at chance level. The location of discrimination peaks at phonetic boundaries and discrimination troughs within phonetic categories is predicted by the categorical perception model. While results obtained in actual experiments depart somewhat from this idealized representation, many studies report a good

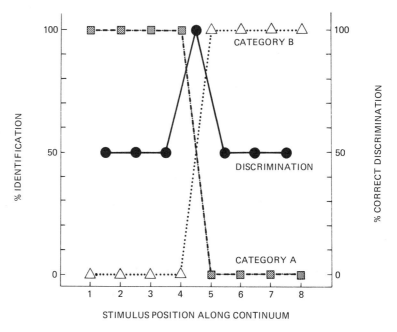

Fig. 4. Idealized identification and discrimination functions reflecting categorical perception of stimuli along a continuum. After Studdert-Kennedy *et al.* (1970).

fit between observed discrimination functions and those predicted from identification data assuming that labeling constrains discrimination.

Similar phenomena are not observed with other acoustic continua such as frequency or intensity. While the listener may be limited to 7 ± 2 categories with which to label stimuli along a frequency continuum, for example, his capacity to discriminate among pairs of pure tones far exceeds what one would predict if discrimination were constrained by labeling (Miller, 1956). Moreover, not all speech sounds that can be ordered along a continuum show categorical perception as defined here. Vowel continua, such as one from /ɪ/ to /ɛ/ to /ae/ (as in "pit," "pet," and "pat"), show less steep labeling functions as well as good within-category discrimination (Eimas, 1963; Fry *et al.*, 1962; Stevens *et al.*, 1969).

Taken as a group, these results have been used to support the notion of a special processor for certain classes of speech sounds that serves to "extract" the phonetic message, subsequently rendering the auditory properties of the acoustic signal unavailable to the listener (Liberman *et al.*, 1972; Pisoni, 1973). The vowel/consonant difference was interpreted as reflecting the lesser degree of context-conditioned variation shown by the vowels; i.e., vowels tend to be acoustically invariant across contexts and hence they would not rely as much on a special processor for the recovery of their phonetic message.

ROLE OF TASK FACTORS

The issue of categorical perception reflecting special, speech-specific processes has been a controversial one (Lane, 1965; Studdert-Kennedy *et al.*, 1970).

One line of research has demonstrated that the extent to which a particular set of speech stimuli will be perceived categorically is a function of the way the stimuli are presented to the subject. Exposure to the entire series of consonant–vowel syllables in an ordered fashion prior to discrimination, for example, considerably improved within-category discrimination along a VOT continuum under certain conditions (Pisoni and Lazarus, 1974). The implication here is that listeners can discriminate subtle, within-category differences if they know in advance what they are listening for.

The role of short-term memory factors in categorical phenomena has also been explored. Pisoni (1973) tested the hypothesis that the differences found between consonants and vowels might be related to differences in the degree to which information about acoustic structure remained in a short-term store. By using a same/different discrimination paradigm and varying the interval between presentation of the members of a stimulus pair, he showed that vowels look more and more categorical as the interval increases.

The phenomenon of categorical perception, then, appears considerably more flexible than original formulations had allowed. However, it is important to make the distinction between what subjects characteristically *do* when listening to the sounds of speech and what they *can do* given appropriate training and/or task manipulations. It is really the former that is of interest to those who would understand speech perception as an integral part of human communication.

Categorical Phenomena with Nonspeech

Bearing more directly on the issue of categorical perception as a speech-specific phenomenon is a second line of investigation demonstrating that categorical-like phenomena, far from being unique to speech, are common in both audition and vision (Cutting and Rosner, 1974; Locke and Kellar, 1973; Miller *et al.*, 1976). Using a Moog synthesizer, Cutting and Rosner (1974) generated a continuum of sawtooth waveforms, approximately 1000 msec in duration, that differed in rise time from 0 to 80 msec in 10-msec steps. When randomly ordered and presented to subjects for labeling as "plucked" or "bowed" sounds, listeners very consistently categorized items with rise times of 30 msec or less as plucked and those with rise times greater than 50 msec as bowed. The identification functions were steep, showing that there was little ambiguity in labeling except for the 40-msec item. Discrimination performance could be predicted quite well on the basis of these identification data. Discrimination between two stimuli was good if they straddled the 40-msec pluck–bow boundary, while the same difference in rise time between stimuli labeled both as "pluck" or "bow" produced significantly poorer discrimination. Thus a series of stimuli not heard as speechlike met the criteria for categorical perception.

A more recent nonspeech investigation by Miller *et al.* (1976) provides some insights into the factors that determine whether or not a set of stimuli will be perceived categorically. Their stimuli consisted of noise–buzz sequences in which the onset of a noise preceded that of 500-msec buzz in 10-msec steps from −10 to +80 msec, with both terminating simultaneously. Identification (as noise or no noise) and discrimination functions were obtained from a group of subjects, with the labeling data used to generate the discrimination functions predicted by the categorical perception model. A comparison of predicted and obtained discrimination data revealed relationships strikingly similar to those found in studies employing synthetic speech stimuli along a VOT continuum; i.e., the locations of discrimination peaks were well predicted, and within-category performance was somewhat underestimated. Control stimuli composed of noises equal in duration to the leading portions of the noise–buzz sequences did not produce comparable results indicative of categorical perception.

In their discussion, Miller *et al.* (1976) state that it is "probably important to note that where categorical perception is demonstrated, it is a single component of a stimulus complex that is the variable. It is likely that the unchanged or constant part of the stimulus complex provides an immediate stimulus context against which the effects of the changed component are judged." Such context is absent, they observe, when subjects make judgments about the frequency or intensity of a series of pure tones, two oft-cited examples of perception that is not categorical, and it is absent in their own control stimuli that show no evidence of categorical perception.

It is of interest to compare the latter observation with the results obtained when nonspeech control stimuli are fashioned from portions of the synthetic speech stimuli on which the categorical perception phenomenon is based. For stimuli varying along place of articulation, for example, F2 transitions alone have been used as controls (Mattingly *et al.*, 1971). These short segments are not perceived as speech but are heard as birdlike chirps. Since the syllables along the place-of-articulation continuum used differed only in the direction and extent of the F2 transitions, failure to observe categorical perception with these contol stimuli has been interpreted in support of the speech-specific processor hypothesis. Acoustic cues must be presented in speech context, in this view, for the phenomenon of categorical perception to occur (Mattingly *et al.*, 1971). However, similar context sensitivity has now been demonstrated for noise–buzz stimuli, suggesting that categorical perception may be viewed in terms of psychophysical boundaries or thresholds that are encountered as one component of a stimulus complex is changed relative to the remainder of the complex. Miller *et al.* (1976) do not provide a way to determine a priori the location of these psychophysical boundaries or the kinds of stimulus continua that will exhibit them; what they do provide are convincing data to demonstrate that all of the criteria of categorical perception may be met by stimuli in no way heard as speechlike.

Developmental and Comparative Investigations

Developmental and comparative approaches to categorical perception have produced data of considerable relevance, if not of unequivocal interpretation, to the issue of the possible uniqueness of speech perception. If the processing of human speech requires special, species-specific mechanisms, infrahuman primates and other organisms should not demonstrate the phenomena that derive from the operation of such mechanisms. To the extent that the capacity shows evolutionary development, however, organisms phylogenetically more related to man may show greater evidence of similar perceptual functioning than more distant evolutionary relatives. The degree to which human infants demonstrate the phenomena characteristic of their species will depend on the role played by experience as well as maturational factors.

STUDIES OF CATEGORICAL PHENOMENA IN INFANTS. A number of studies have explored the ability of infants to discriminate speech sounds along the same continua studied in categorical perception investigations with adults (for reviews, see Eimas, 1975b; Morse, 1978). The logic is similar in each case. If the infants hear speech sounds in the same way as adults, then discrimination of sounds that fall within an adult phonetic boundary should be poor. Discrimination of sounds that straddle the adult phonetic boundary should be good, however, as it is in adults. One of two response measures, high-amplitude sucking (HAS) and heart rate (HR), has generally been employed to tap infant perceptual abilities. (See Morse, 1974, for a discussion and comparison of these paradigms.)

With the HAS procedure, the presentation of a speech stimulus is made contingent on the infant's rate of nonnutritive sucking. Sucking increases over a baseline level following the establishment of the contingency relationship, with the rate decreasing over time as the stimulus presumably loses its reinforcing properties for the infant. An increase in sucking rate following substitution of a new stimulus, relative to the rate when the stimulus is unchanged, is seen as reflecting the infant's capacity to discriminate the two stimuli.

The HR paradigm makes use of the finding that heart rate deceleration typically accompanies the presentation of a new stimulus to the infant, with the degree of deceleration decreasing or habituating over the course of repeated presentations of the same item. Discrimination is said to have occurred when dishabituation, or recovery of heart rate deceleration, occurs on presentation of a new stimulus in comparision to heart rate without stimulus change.

In one of the earliest investigations of infant speech perception, Eimas *et al.* (1971) used a HAS procedure to study the perception of syllables along a /ba/-/pa/ continuum in 1- and 4-month-olds. Between-category-shift infants were initially presented with either a +20-msec or a +40-msec VOT syllable, and then shifted to the other after habituation had taken place. This condition is referred to as "between category" since the /b/-/p/ phonetic boundary in English is approximately +25 msec. The two syllables presented thus belonged to different categories, and the shift following habituation was between phonetic categories. A similar procedure was followed for the within-category infants who were exposed to pairs of stimuli whose members belonged to the same phonetic category, i.e., −20 msec VOT and 0 msec VOT, heard as /ba/, or +60 msec VOT and +80 msec VOT, heard as /pa/. Control infants heard one of the six syllables throughout the study; following attainment of the habituation criterion, the infants continued to hear the same stimulus contingent on sucking.

Subsequent to the change in stimulus, the between-category-shift infants showed a greater rate of responding than did the control group, while the within-category-shift group did not differ significantly from the control level. These results were interpreted in terms of the infant's ability to hear the change in stimulus when it involved a shift to a different adult phonetic category, whereas such a change was not discriminable (at least not to the extent that it affected sucking rate) when the stimulus differed acoustically in a linearly equivalent amount but fell within the same adult phonetic category. Work of this nature has been extended to other speech continua as well, generally mirroring the findings obtained with adults (Eimas, 1974a,b; 1975a).

Role of Linguistic Experience. Recently, investigators have begun to explore the role played by what must be the rather limited linguistic experience of the infant (Lasky *et al.*, 1975; Streeter, 1976). These studies make use of the observation that not all languages partition the VOT continuum in the same fashion as English. Streeter (1976) worked in Kenya with infants whose parents spoke Kikuyu, a Bantu language that has only one bilabial stop, a prevoiced /b/, in which voicing precedes articulatory release by an average of 64 msec. Using a HAS procedure with stimuli similar to those of Eimas *et al.* (1971), she observed that Kikuyu infants discriminated the contrast appropriate for their native language, as well as the contrast found in English but not used in Kikuyu. Morse (1978) notes, however, that there is little evidence in her data to suggest that the discrimination of the English contrast is categorical in nature for these infants. This fits nicely with findings by Eimas (1975b) that suggest that American infants can discriminate a change across the prevoiced–voiced boundary found in Kikuyu, but not categorically as they do the English /b/-/p/ contrast.

The capacity of human infants to discriminate speech sounds in a manner lawfully related to the way in which adults label those sounds is an extremely interesting finding and one which may be added to the ever-growing list of abilities not previously thought to be present in infants. The extent to which these demonstrations bear on innate, speech-specific processing mechanisms, however, depends on additional evidence. It would be of value to know, for example, if infants show signs of categorically perceiving nonspeech stimuli. In a HAS study using sawtooth wave forms varying in rise time (the pluck–bow stimuli), Jusczyk *et al.* (1977) showed that infant discrimination may be predicted from the categorical labeling of adults with these items. Thus the evidence for categorical perception as a general sensory phenomenon has been extended to include infants as well as adults.

Animal Studies. Perhaps the most stringent tests of the hypothesis that many of the perceptual phenomena characteristic of speech require special, speech-specific processing mechanisms will come from investigations with animals. A strong form of the model (Mattingly and Liberman, 1969) posits that the link between speech perception and production precludes the possibility that infrahuman primates process speech in the same way as human adults and infants, since they lack the capacity to produce the relevant sounds (Liberman, 1974). Similarities between the perception of speech by man and monkey could be accommodated, however, by a weaker hypothesis that adopts a general evolutionary view; such a model would predict, though, that the similarities extend to infrahuman primates only.

Several investigators have studied the discrimination of speech sounds by infrahuman primates (Morse and Snowdon, 1975; Sinnott *et al.*, 1976; Waters and

Wilson, 1976). Using a HR paradigm to assess discrimination along a place-of-articulation continuum in rhesus monkeys, Morse and Snowdon (1975) found evidence of both within- and between-category discrimination, with discrimination across a phonetic boundary superior to that obtained when stimuli were selected from within a phonetic category. A comparison of the monkey data with results obtained from 3-month-old human infants in a similar paradigm (Miller and Morse, 1976) revealed that the rhesus monkey is better able to discriminate stimuli within a phonetic category than is the human infant, while both subject populations show better discrimination between than within categories.

A strong form of the special processor model would require that stimuli differing by acoustically equivalent amounts be equally discriminable for the monkey regardless of how they are classified by human listeners . The results obtained by Morse and Snowdon (1975), however, suggest that stimuli that straddle human phonetic boundaries are especially discriminable to the monkey, although the discrimination is less categorical in nature than that observed with human adults or infants. Would exposing these monkeys to an auditory environment similar to that of the human infant serve to reduce the level of within-category discrimination, in the same fashion that discrimination appears to be more categorical in human infants for those phonetic distinctions to which they have had early exposure? This experiment remains to be done.

An investigation of the discrimination of stimuli differing in VOT in chinchillas provides a test of the weaker form of the special processor model (Kuhl and Miller, 1975). The animals were trained to discriminate synthetic 0-msec VOT and +80-msec VOT alveolar stop-vowel syllables in a go–no go avoidance paradigm and then tested for generalization to intermediate stimuli along the continuum. The generalization function obtained showed a sharp boundary at 33.5 msec VOT, strikingly similar to the 35.2 msec VOT phonetic boundary established by human listeners with these stimuli. Since no one is likely to defend the existence of speech-specific, phonetic processing in the chinchilla, Kuhl and Miller (1975) argue that an explanation of these results is best sought in auditory psychophysics and that it is reasonable to consider extending such an explanation to the perception of these sounds by human listeners.

It has been suggested, however, that the correspondence between the human identification boundary and the chinchilla generalization function may be a fortuitous consequence of training the animals on end-point stimuli whose mean VOT value roughly approximates the human phonetic boundary (Morse, 1978; Liberman, 1976). The animals may have bisected the stimulus range in some fashion, producing, by chance, a function similar to the one found with human listeners. Waters and Wilson's (1976) work with a similar paradigm in rhesus monkeys has been offered in support of this argument since the generalization functions obtained in their study did vary with the end-point stimuli used. It should be noted, however, that work with human subjects has recently indicated a relationship between the range of VOT values employed and the location of the phonetic boundary subsequently observed (Brady and Darwin, cited in Darwin, 1976; Studdert-Kennedy, 1976). Moreover, when the chinchilla is tested for discrimination of stimuli along the VOT continuum, discriminability is best at the perceptual boundary defined in the Kuhl and Miller (1975) "labeling" experiments (Kuhl, 1976). These data strongly argue that range effects are not entirely responsible for the similar location of human and chinchilla boundaries.

To conclude this section, it is interesting to note that at least one set of investigators (Snowdon and Pola, 1978) has begun to study the perception of monkey vocalizations by the monkeys themselves, with preliminary evidence suggesting that it takes a categorical form. When these vocalizations are presented to human listeners, categorical-like performance is not obtained. Such investigations meet a longstanding need for a less anthropocentric approach to vocal communication and may prove valuable in understanding human speech in the context of principles that govern vocal communication in general.

Selective Adaptation

Relatively recently, investigators in speech perception have considered the possibility that feature detector mechanisms may contribute to speech processing (Abbs and Sussman, 1971; Studdert-Kennedy, 1974). A feature approach to the analysis of speech sounds is not new; various systems of linguistic features have been proposed to describe the structure of phonemes (e.g., Jakobson *et al.,* 1963; Halle, 1964; Chomsky and Halle, 1968). The notion that these features may have biological reality in the form of neural networks with the specific function of responding to those features is, however, of recent origin. An impressive body of evidence pointing to the existence of property detectors in the human visual system that are involved in the perception of visual displays (e.g., Blakemore and Campbell, 1969; Blakemore and Sutton, 1969; McCollough, 1965) has encouraged the search for similar mechanisms operating in the auditory modality to mediate the perception of speech.

Eimas and Corbit (1973) were the first to test hypotheses derived from a speech feature detector model with human listeners. They postulated that feature detector mechanisms sensitive to VOT were responsible for the perception of voicing contrast, e.g., /b/-/p/ in English. Two sets of detectors, each maximally responsive to a different range of VOT values, were proposed. A phoneme would be heard as voiced when excitation of the short VOT detectors exceeded that of the detectors sensitive to longer VOT values, while the perception of a voiceless consonant would follow from greater activation of the detectors tuned to the long end of the VOT range. The voiced–voiceless boundary would correspond to the point along the VOT continuum that activated the two types of feature analyzers equally.

Data consistent with this model were obtained by Eimas and Corbit (1973) in a series of selective adaptation experiments. Representative of these studies is one that employed stimuli along a /ba/-/pa/ VOT continuum. Modeling their investigations after a paradigm that had proved to be successful in studying feature detectors in vision (Barlow, 1972), Eimas and Corbit (1973) attempted to fatigue one of the two sets of feature detectors they had postulated by repeated presentation to subjects of either a −10-msec VOT stimulus heard as voiced, i.e., /ba/, or a

+60-msec VOT syllable whose consonant was perceived as voiceless, i.e., /pa/. Repetitions of the adapting syllable occurred at the rate of approximately 2/sec in blocks 1 min long. Interspersed between adapting blocks were presentations of the remaining items from the VOT continuum that the subjects were asked to identify as /ba/ or /pa/.

When the identification functions obtained after adaptation were compared with those of the same subjects prior to adaptation, differences were found in the location of the category boundaries. After exposure to the −10-msec VOT stimulus, subjects experienced a boundary shift toward the voiced end of the continuum, i.e., listeners assigned fewer stimuli to the voiced category. Adaptation with the voiceless stop produced the opposite effect—fewer stimuli were heard as voiceless. Adaptation trials, then, served to shift the locus of the phonetic boundary toward the adapting stumulus. This is precisely what would be expected if the outputs of two sets of feature detectors, each tuned to a different range of VOT values, had been differentially affected by adaptation such that the detectors less fatigued contribute relatively more to the resulting percept.

To ensure that the adaptation effect was indeed due to a change in perception and not merely reflective of a bias in labeling sounds as /ba/ or /pa/, pairwise combinations of the items along the VOT continuum were presented for discrimination both before and after the adaptation procedure. Postadaptation discrimination functions mirrored the shifts that had taken place in the phonetic boundary, in good agreement with predictions from a categorical model. This modification of the ability to discriminate sounds as a consequence of adaptation argues strongly for the hypothesis that adaptation served to alter perception. Reliable adaptation effects have subsequently been replicated for stimuli varying in VOT (Eimas *et al.*, 1973; Cooper, 1974*c*) and extended to stimuli varying in place of articulation (Cooper, 1974*b*; Ades, 1974).

FUNCTIONAL LOCUS OF ADAPTATION—SOME CONSIDERATIONS

At this point, it is appropriate to pose the question that was asked of categorical perception: Do these phenomena derive from mechanisms that are specific to speech? Phrased differently, what is the functional locus of the selective adaptation effect? Does it reflect the operation of detectors responsive to properties of speech as an acoustic signal, or, alternatively, does it reflect mechanisms that are speech specific in that they serve to extract phonetic information from incoming stimuli? Investigators seeking to answer these questions have commonly employed one of two research strategies.

The first involves the use of adapting stimuli in which the relevant acoustic cues have been taken out of speech context, e.g., F2 transitions alone. Appropriate boundary shifts induced by the repeated presentation of relevant cues in isolation would be interpreted in terms of an auditory locus for the effect, while failure to find evidence of adaptation would be seen as support for the speech-specific (phonetic) nature of the phenomenon. The second strategy varies acoustic structure of the adapting and test stimuli while retaining the phonetic relationship between them. For example, in studies of adaptation along place of articulation continua, this may be achieved by employing a different vowel in the adapting and test stimuli. Transitional cues important for the identification of stop consonants in syllable initial position, it will be remembered, are markedly different for the same consonant in different vowel contexts. If phonetic information is extracted by the feature detectors, adaptation should be independent of the vowel context of the adapting stimulus. If the feature analyzers are sensitive to particular acoustic parameters of the stimulus, however, variations in vowel context (and hence acoustic structure) should markedly reduce the degree of adaptation.

Experimental Tests

A clear-cut picture of the functional locus of the adaptation phenomenon has not emerged from either strategy. Several investigators have failed to obtain significant adaptation effects with acoustic cues in isolation (Eimas *et al.*, 1973; Diehl, 1975), while others report adaptation effects (Tartter and Eimas, 1975). Similarly, adaptation effects are reduced or absent in some studies if the adaptation stimulus and the continuum tested differ acoustically while sharing a relevant phonetic feature (Cooper, 1974*a,b*), while at the same time there is evidence that the perceived phonetic nature of the stimulus may, under certain conditions, play a more important role than its acoustic structure (Ades, 1974, experiment 2; Diehl, 1975; Cooper and Blumstein, 1974).

An appreciation for the nature of the conflicting data as well as for the ingenuity of researchers in this area may be gained from a brief examination of two recent studies. The acoustic cues for /b/ and /d/ in the syllables /bae/ and /dae/ (as in "bat" and "dab") are roughly mirror images of the cues for the same consonants in the syllables /aeb/ and /aed/. Ades (1974, experiment 1) reasoned that boundary shifts along /bae/-/dae/ and /aeb/-/aed/ place-of-articulation continua should be readily obtained with either set of syllables as adapting stimuli if feature detectors are responsive to linguistic (phonetic) information. Boundary shifts occurred, however, only in those conditions in which the consonant appeared in the same syllable position for both adapting and test stimuli; i.e., /b/ and /d/ in syllable final position did not produce adaptation along a continuum in which they appeared in syllable initial position, and vice versa. This study may be interpreted as supporting the importance of acoustic cues in eliciting the adaptation phenomenon.

In another test of the auditory–phonetic distinction, Cooper (1975) asked subjects to monitor a series of visually presented words containing either voiced or voiceless stop consonants. Viewing either set of words produced boundary shifts along an auditorily presented /ba/-/pa/ continuum in the expected directions. This investigation, of course, did not involve any acoustic input, and hence it is difficult to argue that adaptation of feature detectors sensitive to acoustic parameters of a stimulus had taken place. Cooper interpreted these data in terms of detectors responsive to phonetic features, and concluded that the adaptation literature points to the existence of feature analyzers at both the auditory and phonetic levels.

It is of interest to note that some recent work in human visual perception is at least consistent with the idea that higher-level cognitive processes may serve as inputs to feature detector mechanisms traditionally thought to be tied only to physical aspects of stimulation (Smith and Over, 1975). Smith and Over (1975) have shown that prolonged viewing of figures containing subjective contours in which there are no luminance discontinuities at the location of the perceived borders produces tilt aftereffects similar to those found when observers view actual lines at different orientations. The aftereffect phenomenon is generally interpreted as reflecting the fatigue of orientation-sensitive detectors in the visual system, and hence this investigation implicates the role of these property analyzers in the perception of subjective as well as real contours.

DEVELOPMENTAL AND COMPARATIVE ASPECTS OF ADAPTATION PHENOMENA

Although selective adaptation studies per se have not been conducted with infants or infrahuman mammals, Eimas (1975b) notes important parallels between adaptation studies and the methodology employed in investigations of categorical perception in infants.

Both HR and HAS procedures involve repeated presentations of a stimulus analogous to the repetitions of the adaptor in selective adaptation studies. These repeated presentations could suffice to fatigue one set of detectors, thereby decreasing the novelty of the stimulus. Presentation of an acousticaly different stimulus that excited the same detectors would not be perceived as novel, while a subsequently presented stimulus from a different phonetic category would excite a different set of detectors and show dishabituation in response to it. It is only a small step to extend this type of analysis to the work with infrahuman primates using the HR paradigm (Morse and Snowdon, 1975). Thus it may be the case that the process of selective adaptation underlies the evidence for categorical perception in infants and in some of the studies with infrahuman mammals.

THE RIGHT EAR ADVANTAGE IN DICHOTIC LISTENING

The evidence most directly linking speech perception to specific biological mechanisms comes from studies of hemispheric asymmetry of function. The asymmetry between the hemispheres in the capacity to produce propositional speech is well known from clinical observations; asymmetries in the processes involved in speech perception have been explored primarily in experimental investigations using the dichotic listening paradigm.

"Dichotic" refers to the simultaneous presentation of two different inputs, one to each ear. Kimura (1961a) was the first to report that when subjects listened to three pairs of dichotically presented spoken digits in rapid succession they were better able to identify the digits delivered to the right ear. Subsequent work with patients who had undergone sodium amytal testing to determine the hemisphere housing the centers responsible for expressive language demonstrated a relationship between ear superiority in the dichotic task and the location of the speech center (Kimura, 1961*b*). The ear contralateral to the hemisphere specialized for speech production typically performed at a higher level than the ear ipsilateral to the speech center. To explain the absence of ear asymmetries when stimuli are presented to just one ear at a time, Kimura (1961*a*) cited the work of Rosenzweig (1951) that indicated stronger contralateral ear–cortex representation in cats. In addition, she hypothesized that, under conditions of dichotic presentation, suppression or inhibition of ipsilaterally transmitted information takes place.

A right-handed person shows a right ear advantage, therefore, because stimuli presented to his right ear have a more direct access to the speech hemisphere than do left ear items. Kimura (1961*a*) did not mention the role of interhemispheric connections in her early models, but subsequent investigators suggested that the probable path for the left ear items was first to the right hemisphere, followed by transfer via the cerebral commissures to the left hemisphere (Sparks and Geschwind, 1968). Loss associated with this process was believed responsible for the advantage enjoyed by the right ear.

These observations have important implications for the mechanisms underlying speech perception since they suggest that the processes involved in the perception of speech are lateralized much in the same way as expressive mechanisms. Shankweiler and Studdert-Kennedy (1967) sought to determine whether a lateralized processor existed for speech at a very basic level—the perception of meaningless syllables differing only in their initial consonants. By presenting single, pairwise combinations of the syllables /pa/, /ta/, /ka/, /ba/, /da/, and /ga/ on each trial, Shankweiler and Studdert-Kennedy (1967) were able to eliminate the contribution of short-term memory and meaningfulness as variables operating to affect performance in the dichotic listening task. They observed a significant advantage in favor of the right ear with their task, a result that argued for the existence of lateralized speech-processing mechansims operating at the level of the raw units of speech. Subsequent work has replicated and extended these observations (Studdert-Kennedy and Shankweiler, 1970; Berlin and McNeil, 1976).

The remainder of this section will deal with the question of whether the asymmetries observed in the dichotic listening task can be attributed to lateralized processing and, if so, whether any of that processing is speech specific as opposed to a more general property of the auditory system.

ASYMMETRY OF PROCESSING OR OUTPUT?

Mindful of results with commissurotomy patients that indicated that differences in output capacity between the hemispheres could masquerade as processing differences (Gazzaniga and Sperry, 1967), Springer (1971) noted that dichotic listening studies typically required subjects to verbally report, aloud or in writing, the material presented on a trial. She argued that such a procedure confounds processing and output functions, and hence that the ear asymmetry might merely reflect the well-known asymmetry in expressive language capacity rather than a difference in speech processing as such. Using stimuli similar to those employed by Shankweiler and Studdert-Kennedy (1967), she modified the dichotic task to permit a go–no go manual response that presumably could bypass left hemisphere output centers. Reaction time data obtained with the dichotic detection task showed that right ear target items were responded to 50 msec more quickly than left ear targets, consistent with the interpretation that the ear asymmetry phenomenon is at least in part perceptual in nature.

Darwin (1971) approached the processing/output question somewhat differently. Instead of varying response mode with a fixed set of stimuli, he held the response constant while varying acoustic cues in a set of consonants. Darwin made use of the fact that there are two main types of acoustic cues for fricative consonants such as /f/: frication or noise and formant transitions to the adjacent vowel. He compared the magnitude of the ear difference obtained when fricative initial syllables synthesized with formant transitions in addition to frication were presented dichotically with that found when the fricative initial syllables used were cued by frication alone. He found an advantage in favor of the right ear in the condition in which the stimuli contained formant transitions, while no asymmetry was found with the frication-only items. If ear differences were determined simply by output mechanisms, the two conditions in this study should have produced equivalent asymmetries since each syllable is identified by the same response.

THE CASE FOR TWO LEFT HEMISPHERE MECHANISMS

Several investigators have analytically approached the characteristics of stimuli that appear to engage the hypothesized lateralized processor. Darwin (1971) demonstrated that a right ear advantage could be obtained when synthetic fricative-vowel syllables containing formant transitions were presented dichotically, while similar syllables constructed without transitions failed to produce a right ear advantage. The role of formant transitions was thus implicated by this result, fitting nicely with observations that isolated vowels, which do not contain transitional information, produce smaller right ear advantages than stop-vowel syllables (Shankweiler and Studdert-Kennedy, 1967; Cutting, 1974).

Further support for the view of the left hemisphere as an extractor of information from rapidly changing frequency patterns comes from the work of Halperin *et al.* (1973). These investigators found a shift from a left ear to a right ear advantage as a function of the number of alternations in sequences of dichotically presented tones. Stimuli containing two alternations produced a right ear advantage, while a left ear superiority was observed for stimuli without such changes.

Although a case may be made for a left hemisphere auditory specialization that subserves speech but is more general in nature, it is important to note that not all speech stimuli need possess formant transitions to show a right ear advantage. Weiss and House (1973) demonstrated that a right ear advantage appeared in a task with dichotically presented vowels when the signal-to-noise ratio was unfavorable; a more favorable signal-to-noise ratio did not reveal any asymmetry. The results suggest that asymmetries may be masked if the dichotic task is not sufficiently taxing. In terms of the neural model of dichotic listening presented earlier, asymmetries in processing may not be observed unless the left ear to left hemisphere route results in sufficient degradation of the left ear input to place it at a disadvantage relative to the right ear stimulus. By making the task more difficult, one moves the dichotic "observation window" to a region more sensitive to differences between the ears. This result suggests that the left hemisphere may be specialized to process all speech sounds regardless of the presence of particular acoustic properties.

In an interesting experiment designed to assess the contribution of acoustic as well as these more abstract "phonetic" factors to the ear asymmetry phenomenon, Cutting (1974) employed stimuli with phonetically impossible formant transitions; use of a synthesizer allowed him to create stimuli whose transitions could never be produced by a human vocal tract. Dichotic presentation of these stimuli in a temporal order judgment task produced a right ear advantage identical to that found with stimuli containing phonetically appropriate transitions. An auditory device serving to extract formant transition information was thus implicated by these results. Cutting (1974) interpreted his data as supporting the operation of a lateralized phonetic device as well, however, since sine wave stimuli with transitions but lacking formant structure showed reduced right ear advantages relative to stimuli that are more speechlike.

To summarize, there is evidence to support the idea that important contributors to the left hemisphere's ability to process speech are mechanisms designed to extract patterns of rapidly changing frequency information. That this is not a complete characterization of lateralized left hemisphere mechanisms is suggested by the numerous observations that ear asymmetries may be found for speech stimuli lacking these properties. Data exist, then, to support both an auditory and a speech-specific functional locus for the right ear advantage.

DEVELOPMENTAL AND COMPARATIVE INQUIRIES

The ontogeny and phylogeny of the cerebral asymmetries reflected in the right ear advantage are of considerable interest, both practical and theoretical. While these issues do not bear directly on the general problem of a possible special status for the mechanisms that process speech, they will be briefly discussed here because of their relevance to the biological foundations of language.

Several studies have employed the dichotic listening paradigm to determine the age at which the right ear advantage first manifests itself (Kimura, 1963; Gilbert and Climan, 1974; Nagafuchi, 1970). Recent work has indicated that the right ear advantage is present in children as young as 2 years of age. Until recently, attempts to investigate asymmetries in even younger populations have been thwarted by the limited response repertoires of the subjects. Entus (1975) and Best and Glanville (1976), however, have taken dichotic listening into the crib by employing high-amplitude sucking and heart rate deceleration paradigms, respectively, in lieu of verbal and manual responses employed with older subjects.

Entus delivered consonant-vowel syllable pairs dichotically to 3-week-old infants, contingent on their rate of HAS. After the sucking response had habituated, the stimulus in one ear was changed while the other ear continued to receive the stimulus heard during habituation. Significantly greater recovery of sucking rate occurred when the right ear stimulus was changed compared to the left, while a left ear superiority emerged when notes from different musical instruments were delivered dichotically. Entus's work provides support for the assertion that hemispheric asymmetry of function is present at birth. Best and Glanville (1976) obtained similar results using heart rate as a dependent measure.

Differential processing as a function of hemisphere and type of stimulus in infants has also been demonstrated electrophysiologically by Molfese *et al.,* (1975). Using infants ranging in age from 1 week to 10 months, Molfese *et al.* have shown that the amplitude of the average evoked response to consonant-vowel syllables is greater in the left hemisphere, while the reverse is true when nonspeech stimuli are presented. Both the dichotic paradigm and electrophysiological data, then, support the idea that asymmetries in the processing of speech sounds are functional at or shortly after birth in the human infant.

To this author's knowledge, there have been no attempts to apply dichotic listening methodology to the study of hemispheric asymmetry in infrahuman mammals. Hamilton (1977) has reviewed much of the existing research on hemispheric asymmetry in infrahuman mammals and concludes that there is little evidence for asymmetries on the basis of the tests charateristically employed in unilateral ablation and split-brain studies. He notes, however, that these tests are, for the most part, crude and simplistic, and that future investigations should take into account the type of lateralization found in man as a model for the animal studies. The ability to form intermodal associations has been considered crucial to the development of language, and a recent study by Dewson (1976) has provided some preliminary evidence for left hemisphere specialization in the performance of an intermodal, delayed-response task. Dewson (1976) taught monkeys to push a red light at various delays after hearing a tone and a green light after hearing a noise. Defects following lesions of the superior temporal gyrus depended on the locus of the lesion. The three left hemisphere lesioned animals could no longer perform the task with delays greater than 1 or 2 sec, while the two monkeys with right hemisphere lesions were unaffected by the surgery. This work must be regarded as preliminary, however, and the question of the evolution of hemispheric asymmetry awaits further research.

SUMMARY AND FURTHER QUESTIONS

The preceding pages have asked whether it is necessary to postulate special, speech-specific, species-specific mechanisms to account for the phenomena of categorical perception, selective adaptation, and ear asymmetries in dichotic listening. Much of the literature reviewed suggests that the answer is no. Categorical phenomena are observed with nonspeech stimuli (Miller *et al.,* 1976), and the few investigations employing infrahuman subjects indicate that these animals display categorical-like behavior in response to speech sounds along F2 or VOT continua (Morse and Snowdon, 1975; Kuhl and Miller, 1975). Boundary shifts following selective adaptation appear in many cases to require acoustic as well as phonetic similarities between adapting and test stimuli (Ades, 1974), and appropriate nonspeech segments excised from speech stimuli are often successful as adapting stimuli (Tartter and Eimas, 1975). Research in dichotic listening has indicated that formant transitions may play an important role in engaging the lateralized processor (Darwin, 1971), and that nonspeech stimuli with appropriate properties may engage it as well (Cutting, 1974).

The picture is far from clear-cut, however. The categorical performance evidenced by nonhuman primates differs in important ways from that shown by human listeners (Sinnott *et al.*, 1976; Morse and Snowdon, 1975), and quantitative comparisons of categorical perception with speech and nonspeech stimuli have not been made. Boundary shifts along a VOT continuum may be induced by repeated presentations of a visual stimulus (Cooper, 1975), and right ear advantages are larger when appropriate acoustic cues are embedded in speech context (Cutting, 1974).

It may be the case, however, that categorical perception, selective adaptation, and ear asymmetries in dichotic listening are not the best phenomena with which to test the hypothesis that the perception of speech is unique. They are somewhat contrived, and are much less compelling than the simple observation, made by any human listener, that "deep," "duke," and "deck," while different, share in common their initial segment. Would a monkey be aware of the relationship between these stimuli that is so salient for human listeners? Liberman (1976) suggests that tests be extended further to determine if animals treat as perceptually equivalent the same phonemes cued by very different acoustic cues. Attempts to ask these questions of human infants have just begun (Fodor *et al.*, 1975) and will undoubtedly be extended to infrahuman primates as well.

Without waiting for the answers, however, one can go on to inquire about the role played by phonetic processing in the perception of speech viewed more broadly than it has been considered here. Speech perception does not end when the listener recovers the phonetic structure of a speech signal; it ends when he recovers the meaning conveyed by it. Must phonetic analysis, whether the output of a special processor or not, precede the extraction of meaning from speech? Some recent evidence obtained from so-called split-brain subjects suggests that this is not necessarily the case.

Springer and Gazzaniga (1975) and Zaidel (1978) have studied the capacity of the right cerebral hemisphere in commissurotomized adults to process syllables composed of a stop consonant and vowel. Pairs of syllables were delivered dichotically with the experimental task designed in both studies to optimize processing and output of stimuli presented to the left ear/right hemisphere. Left ear performance, however, was at chance level compared to nearly perfect performance of stimuli routed to the right ear/left hemisphere. The same patients who displayed an inability to process the stop-vowel syllables in the right hemisphere were able to respond to the presentation of spoken words and sentences when response choices were restricted to the right hemisphere (Zaidel, 1978; Gazzaniga and Sperry, 1967). Thus the right hemisphere in these patients proved unable to make certain phonetic distinctions, although it did demonstrate the capacity to deal with words and sentences meaningfully. That phonetic analysis as such is not part of the

repertoire of the right hemisphere is further supported by the inability of that half
brain to rhyme (Levy, 1974).

173

SPEECH PERCEPTION
AND THE BIOLOGY OF
LANGUAGE

Several explanations of these phenomena are possible. For example, phonetic
analysis may occur bilaterally for certain speech sounds, such that the "auditory
comprehension" demonstrated by the right cerebral hemisphere may be a result
of the partial information that it is able to extract from the acoustic signal. The
right hemisphere would be unable to recover the complete phonetic structure of
an utterance, but information sufficient for comprehension would be available.

Alternatively, phonetic analysis may be unnecessary to the process of speech
understanding in some instances. The right hemisphere may demonstrate a mode
of speech perception in which holistic processing plays an important role. The
superiority of the right cerebral hemisphere for holistic processing in the visual
modality has been well documented (for a review, see Levy, 1974), and it is
reasonable to suppose that a similar processing strategy might apply when that
hemisphere is required to process speech.

It has been argued that speech analysis that bypassed recovery of phonetic
segments would be of limited utility given the vast number of possible words and
the difficulties in isolating them from the speech stream (Liberman and Pisonl,
1978). However, enough evidence exists in support of a mode of speech processing that bypasses phonetic analysis under certain conditions that it is worthy of
further investigation to determine these limitations. It is possible that, although
the processes underlying the recovery of phonetic segments from the speech
stream are speech and species specific, auditory comprehension may proceed
without them.

REFERENCES

Abbs, J. H., and Sussman, H. M. Neurophysiological feature detectors and speech perception: A
discussion of theoretical implications. *Journal of Speech and Hearing Research,* 1971, *14*, 23–36.
Abramson, A. S., and L. Lisker. Voice timing perception in Spanish word-initial stops. *Journal of
Phonetics,* 1973, *1*, 1–8.
Ades, A. E. How phonetic is selective adaptation? Experiments on syllabic position and vowel environ-
ment. *Perception and Psychophysics,* 1974, *16*, 61–66.
Barclay, R. Noncategorical perception of a voiced stop. *Perception and Psychophysics,* 1972, *11*, 269–274.
Barlow, H. Single units and sensation: A neuron doctrine for perceptual psychology? *Perception,* 1972,
1, 371–394.
Berlin, C., and McNeil, M. Dichotic Listening. In N. Lass (ed.), *Contemporary Issues in Experimental
Phonetics.* Springfield, Ill.: Thomas, 1976.
Best, C., and Glanville, B. A cardiac measure of cerebral asymmetries in infant auditory perception.
Paper presented at 48th annual meeting of the Midwestern Psychological Association, Chicago,
1976.
Blakemore, C., and Campbell, F. W. On the existence of neurons in the human visual system selectively
sensitive to the orientation and size of retinal images. *Journal of Physiology,* 1969, *203*, 237–260.
Blakemore, C., and Sutton, P. Size adaptation: A new aftereffect. *Science,* 1969, *166*, 245–247.
Chomsky, N., and Halle, M. *The Sound Pattern of English.* New York: Harper and Row, 1968.
Cooper, F. S. How is language conveyed by speech? In J. Kavanagh and I. Mattingly (eds.), *Language by
Eye and by Ear—The Relationships between Speech and Reading.* Cambridge, Mass.: MIT Press, 1972.
Cooper, W. E. Contingent feature analysis in speech perception. *Perception and Psychophysics,* 1974*a*, *16*,
201–204.
Cooper, W. E. Adaptation of phonetic feature analyzers for place of articulation. *Journal of the Acoustical
Society of America,* 1974*b*, *56*, 617–627.

Cooper, W. E. Selective adaptation for acoustic cues of voicing in initial stops. *Journal of Phonetics,* 1974c, *2,* 303–313.

Cooper, W. E. Selective adaptation to speech. In F. Restle, R. Shiffrin, N. Castellan, H. Lindman, and D. Pisoni (eds.), *Cognitive Theory,* Vol. 1. New York: Wiley, 1975.

Cooper, W. E., and Blumstein, S. E. A "labial" feature analyzer in speech perception. *Perception and Psychophysics,* 1974, *15,* 591–600.

Cutting, J. E. Two left hemisphere mechanisms in speech perception. *Perception and Psychophysics,* 1974, *16,* 601–612.

Cutting, J. E., and Eimas, P. Phonetic feature analyzers and the processing of speech in infants. In J. Kavanagh and J. Cutting (eds.), *The Role of Speech in Language.* Cambridge, Mass.: MIT Press, 1975.

Cutting, J. E., and Rosner, B. S. Categories and boundaries in speech and music. *Perception and Psychophysics,* 1974, *16,* 564–571.

Darwin, C. The perception of speech. In E. Carterette and M. Friedman (eds.), *Handbook of Perception,* Vol. VII. New York: Academic Press, 1976.

Darwin, C. J. Ear differences in the recall of fricatives and vowels. *Quarterly Journal of Experimental Psychology,* 1971, *23,* 46–62.

Delattre, P., Liberman, A., and Cooper, F. Acoustic loci and transitional cues for consonants. *Journal of the Acoustical Society of America,* 1955, *27,* 769–773.

Dewson, J. H.,III. Preliminary evidence of hemispheric asymmetry of auditory function in monkeys. In S. Harnad (ed.), *Lateralization in the Nervous System.* New York: Academic Press, 1976.

Diehl, R. The effect of selective adaptation on the identification of speech sounds. *Perception and Psychophysics,* 1975, *17,* 48–52.

Eimas, P. The relationship between identification and discrimination along speech and nonspeech continua. *Language and Speech,* 1963, *6,* 206–217.

Eimas, P. Lingusitic processing of speech by young infants. In R. Schiefelbusch and L. Lloyd (eds.), *Language Perspectives—Acquisition, Retardation, and Intervention.* Baltimore: University Park Press, 1974a.

Eimas, P. Auditory and linguistic processing of cues for place of articulation by infants. *Perception and Psychophysics,* 1974b, *16,* 513–521.

Eimas, P. Auditory and phonetic coding of the cues for speech: Discrimination of the r-l distinction by young infants. *Perception and Psychophysics,* 1975a, *18,* 341–347.

Eimas, P. Developmental studies of speech perception. In L. B. Cohen and P. Salapatek (eds.), *Infant Perception.* New York: Academic Press, 1975b.

Eimas, P., and Corbit, J. D. Selective adaptation of linguistic feature detectors. *Cognitive Psychology,* 1973, *4,* 99–109.

Eimas, P., Siqueland, E., Juszyck, P., and Vigorito, J. Speech perception in infants. *Science,* 1971, *171,* 303–306.

Eimas, P., Cooper, W. E., and Corbit, J. D. Some properties of linguistic feature detectors. *Perception and Psychophysics,* 1973, *13,* 247–252.

Entus, A. K. Hemispheric asymmetry in processing of dichotically presented speech and nonspeech sounds by infants. Paper presented at the Society for Research in Child Development, 1975, Denver.

Fant, C. G. M. Descriptive analysis of the acoustic aspects of speech. *Logos,* 1962, *5,* 3–17.

Fodor, J., Garrett, M., and Brill, S. Pi Ka Pu: The perception of speech sounds by prelinguistic infants. *Perception and Psychophysics,* 1975, *18,* 74–78.

Fry, D. B., Abramson, A. S., Eimas, P., and Liberman, A. M. Identification and discrimination of synethetic vowels. *Language and Speech,* 1962, *5,* 171–189.

Gazzaniga, M. S., and Sperry, R. W. Language after section of the cerebral commissures. *Brain,* 1967, *90,* 131–148.

Gilbert, J. H. V., and Climan, I. Dichotic studies in 2–3 year olds: A preliminary report. Speech Communication Seminar, Stockholm, 1974.

Halle, M. On the basis of phonology. In J. A. Fodor and J. J. Katz (eds.), *The Structure of Language.* Englewood Cliffs, N.J.: Prentice-Hall, 1964.

Halperin, Y., Nachshon, I., and Carmon, A. Shift of ear superiority in dichotic listening to temporally patterned verbal stimuli. *Journal of the Acoustical Society of America,* 1973, *53,* 46–50.

Hamilton, C. R. An assessment of hemispheric specialization in monkeys. In S. Dimond (ed.), *Evolution and Lateralization of the Brain,* New York: The New York Academy of Sciences, 1977.

Jakobson, R., Fant, G., and Halle, M. *Preliminaries to Speech Analysis: The Distinctive Features and their Correlates.* Cambridge, Mass.: MIT Press, 1963.

Jusczyk, P., Rosner, B., Cutting, J., Foard, C., and Smith, L. Perception of nonspeech by infants. *Perception and Psychophysics,* 1977, *21,* 50–54.

Kimura, D. Some effects of temporal lobe damage on auditory perception. *Canadian Journal of Psychology,* 1961*a, 15,* 156–165.

Kimura, D. Cerebral dominance and the perception of verbal stimuli. *Canadian Journal of Psychology,* 1961*b, 15,* 166–171.

Kimura, D. Speech lateralization in young children as determined by an auditory test. *Journal of Comparative and Physiological Psychology,* 1963, *56,* 899–902.

Kimura, D. Functional asymmetry of the brain in dichotic listening. *Cortex,* 1967, *3,* 163–178.

Kuhl, P. Speech perception by the chinchilla: Categorical perception of synthetic alveolar plosive consonants. Paper presented at the 92nd meeting of the Acoustical Society of America, 1976, San Diego.

Kuhl, P., and Miller, J. Speech perception by the chinchilla: Voiced-voiceless distinction in alveolar plosive consonants. *Science,* 1975, *190,* 69–72.

Lane, H. The motor theory of speech perception: A critical review. *Psychological Review,* 1965, *72,* 275–309.

Lasky, R., Syrdal-Lasky , A., and Klein, D. VOT discrimination by four to six month old infants from Spanish environments. *Journal of Experimental Child Psychology,* 1975, *20,* 215–225.

Lea, W. Computer recognition of speech. In T. A. Sebeok (ed.), *Current Trends in Linguistics,* Vol. 12. The Hague: Mouton, 1974.

Levy, J. Psychobiological implications of bilateral asymmetry. In S. J. Dimond and J. G. Beaumont (eds.), *Hemisphere Function in the Human Brain.* London: Paul Elek, 1974.

Liberman, A. M. Some characteristics of perception in the speech mode. In D. A. Hamburg (ed.), *Perception and its Disorders—Proceedings of ARNMD,* Vol. 12. Baltimore: Williams and Wilkins, 1970*a.*

Liberman, A. The grammars of speech and language. *Cognitive Psychology,* 1970*b, 1,* 301–323.

Liberman, A. Discussion paper. In S. R. Harnad, H. D. Steklis, and J. Lancaster (eds.), *Origins and Evolution of Language and Speech,* New York: The New York Academy of Sciences, 1976.

Liberman, A. M., and Pisoni, D. B. Evidence for a special speech perception subsystem in the human. In T. H. Bullock (ed.), *Recognition of Complex Acoustic Signals.* Berlin: Dahlem Konferenzen, 1978.

Liberman, A. M., Delattre, P. C., Cooper, F. S., and Gerstman, L. J. The role of consonant-vowel transitions in the perception of the stop and nasal consonants. *Psychological Monographs,* 1954, *68,* (Whole No. 379).

Liberman, A. M., Harris , K. S., Hoffman, H. S., and Griffith, B. C. The discrimination of speech sounds within and across phoneme boundaries. *Journal of Experimental Psychology,* 1957, *54,* 358–368.

Liberman, A. M., Harris , K. S., Kinney, J. A., and Lane, H. The discrimination of relative onset-time of the components of certain speech and nonspeech patterns. *Journal of Experimental Psychology,* 1961, *61,* 379–388.

Liberman, A. M., Cooper, F. S., Shankweiler, D. P., and Studdert-Kennedy, M. Perception of the speech code. *Psychological Review,* 1967*a, 74,* 431–461.

Liberman, A. M., Cooper, F. S., and Studdert-Kennedy, M. Why are spectrograms hard to read? *Annals of the Deaf,* 1967*b, 113,* 127.

Liberman, A. M., Mattingly, I., and Turvey, M. Language codes and memory codes. In A. W. Melton and E. Martin (eds.), *Coding Processes in Human Memory.* New York: Wiley, 1972.

Lieberman, P. On the evolution of language: A unified view. *Cognition,* 1974, *2(1),* 59–94.

Lisker, L., and Abramson, A. S. A cross language study of voicing in initial stops: Acoustical measurements. *Word,* 1964, *20,* 384–422.

Locke, S., and Kellar, L. Categorical perception in a nonlinguistic mode. *Cortex,* 1973, *9,* 355–369.

Mattingly, I., and Liberman, A. M. The speech code and the physiology of language. In K. N. Liebovic (ed.), *Information Processing in the Nervous System,* New York: Springer-Verlag, 1969.

Mattingly, I., Liberman, A. M., Syradal, A. K., and Halwes, T. Discrimination in speech and nonspeech modes. *Cognitive Psychology,* 1971, *2,* 131–157.

McCollough, C. Color adaptation of edge detectors in the human visual system. *Science,* 1965, *149,* 1115–1116.

Miller, C. L., and Morse, P. A. The heart of categorical speech discrimination in young infants. *Journal of Speech and Hearing Research,* 1976, *19,* 578–589.

Miller, G. A. The magical number seven plus or minus two, or, some limits on our capacity for processing information. *Psychological Review,* 1956, *63,* 81–96.

Miller, J. D., Wier, C. C., Pastore, R. E., Kelly, W. M., and Dooling, R. M. Discrimination and labeling of noise–buzz sequences with varying noise-lead times: An example of categorical perception. *Journal of the Acoustical Society of America,* 1976, *60,* 410–417.

Molfese, D. L., Freeman, R. B., Jr., and Palermo, D. S. The ontogeny of brain lateralization for speech and nonspeech sounds. *Brain and Language,* 1975, *2,* 356–368.

Morse, P. A. Infant speech perception: A preliminary model and review of the literature. In R. Schiefelbusch and L. Lloyd (eds.), *Language Perspectives—Acquisition, Retardation, and Intervention.* Baltimore: University Park Press, 1974.

Morse, P. A. Infant speech perception: Origins, processes, and alpha centauri. In Proceedings of the NICHD Conference on "Early Behavioral Assessment of the Communicative and Cognitive Abilities of the Developmentally Disabled", in press.

Morse, P., and Snowdon, C. An investigation of categorical speech discrimination by rhesus monkeys. *Perception and Psychophysics,* 1975, *17,* 9–16.

Nagafuchi, M. Development of dichotic and monaural hearing abilities in young children. *Acta Otolaryngologica,* 1970, *69,* 409–415.

Pisoni, D. B. Auditory and phonetic memory codes in the discrimination of consonants and vowels. *Perception and Psychophysics,* 1973, *13,* 253–260.

Pisoni, D. B., and Lazarus, J. H. Categorical and noncategorical modes of speech perception along the voicing continuum. *Journal of the Acoustical Society of America,* 1974, *55,* 328–335.

Pisoni, D. B., and Task, J. Reaction times to comparisons within and across phonetic categories. *Perception and Psychophysics,* 1974, *15,* 285–290.

Rosenzweig, M. R. Representations of the two ears at the auditory cortex. *American Journal of Physiology,* 1951, *167,* 147–158.

Rubenstein, H. Computer applications: An overview. In T. A. Seabeok (ed.), *Current Trends in Linguistics,* Vol. 12. The Hague: Mouton, 1974.

Shankweiler, D., and Studdert-Kennedy, M. Identification of consonants and vowels presented to left and right ears. *Quarterly Journal of Experimental Psychology,* 1967, *19,* 59–63.

Sinnott, J. M., Beecher, M. D., Moody, D. B., and Stebbins, W. C. Speech sound discrimination by monkeys and humans. *Journal of the Acoustical Society of America,* 1976, *60,* 687–695.

Smith, A., and Over, R. Tilt aftereffects with subjective contours. *Nature (London),* 1975, *257,* 581–582.

Snowdon, C. T., and Pola, Y. V. Intraspecific and interspecific responses to synthesized pygmy marmoset vocalications. *Animal Behavior,* 1978, *1,* 192–206.

Sparks, R., and Geschwind, N. Dichotic listening in man after section of neocortical commissures. *Cortex,* 1968, *4,* 3–16.

Springer, S. P. Ear asymmetry in a dichotic listening task. *Perception and Psychophysics,* 1971, *10,* 239–241.

Springer, S. P., and Gazzaniga, M. S. Dichotic listening in partial and complete split brain subjects. *Neuropsychologia,* 1975, *13,* 341–346.

Stevens, K. N., and House, A. S. Speech perception. In J. V. Tobias (ed.), *Foundations of Modern Auditory Theory,* Vol. 2. New York: Academic Press, 1972.

Stevens, K. N., Liberman, A. M., Ohman, S. E. G., and Studdert-Kennedy, M. Cross-language study of vowel discrimination. *Language and Speech,* 1969, *12,* 1–23.

Streeter, L. Language perception of two month old infants shows effects of both innate mechanisms and experience. *Nature (London),* 1976, *259,* 39–41.

Studdert-Kennedy, M. The perception of speech. In T. A. Seabeok (ed.), *Current Trends in Linguistics,* Vol. 12. The Hague: Mouton, 1974.

Studdert-Kennedy, M. Stimulus range as a determinant of phoneme boundaries along synthetic consonant continua. Paper presented at the 92nd meeting of the Acoustical Society of America, 1976, San Diego.

Studdert-Kennedy, M., and Shankweiler, D. Hemispheric specialization for speech perception. *Journal of the Acoustical Society of America,* 1970, *48,* 579–594.

Studdert-Kennedy, M., Liberman, A. M., Harris, K. S., and Cooper, F. S. Motor theory of speech perception: A reply to Lane's critical review. *Psychological Review,* 1970, 234–249.

Tartter, V., and Eimas, P. The role of auditory feature detectors in the perception of speech. *Perception and Psychophysics,* 1975, *18,* 293–298.

Waters, R., and Wilson, W. Speech perception by rhesus monkeys: The voicing distinction in synthesized labial and velar stop consonants. *Perception and Psychophysics,* 1976, *19,* 285–289.

Weiss, M. S., and House, A. S. Perception of dichotically presented vowels. *Journal of the Acoutical Society of America,* 1973, *53,* 51–58.

Wood, C. Auditory and phonetic levels of processing in speech perception. *Journal of Experimental Psychology—Human Perception and Performance,* 1975, *104*, 3–20.

Zaidel, E. Auditory language comprehension in the right hemisphere following cerebral commissurotomy and hemispherectomy: A comparison with child language and aphasia. In E. Zurif and A. Caramazza (eds.), *The Acquisition and Breakdown of Language: Parallels and Divergencies.* Baltimore: Johns Hopkins University Press, 1978.

8

Origins and Distribution of Language

OSCAR S. M. MARIN, MYRNA F. SCHWARTZ, AND
ELEANOR M. SAFFRAN

INTRODUCTION

Implicit in the title of this chapter is the promise that we will try to relate the evolutionary history of language to the current distribution of language function in the brain. Unfortunately, this is a promise we are unable to fulfill. At present there are simply too few points of contact between these two areas of limited knowledge for one to inform the other.

Some readers may take issue with this contention, noting quite rightly that neurological evidence has already been used to frame or support arguments about the origins of language. Before we spell out what we take to be the limitations of this theorizing, we will review some of the neurological data, and the arguments that derive from them.

1. The language apparatus is located in the midst of the cortical sensorimotor system, and includes an area of association cortex that is in close proximity to receptive areas concerned with vision and somesthesis, as well as with audition. This area, sometimes defined as the inferior parietal lobule, is a rather recent phylogenetic development and increases significantly in size from ape to man (Geschwind, 1965).

Geschwind (1964, 1965) has speculated that it is the emergence of the parietal association area that first allows for the development of cross-modality associations

OSCAR S. M. MARIN, MYRNA F. SCHWARTZ, AND ELEANOR M. SAFFRAN   Department of Neurology, Baltimore City Hospitals, and The Johns Hopkins University School of Medicine, Baltimore, Maryland 21224.

OSCAR S. M. MARIN,
MYRNA F. SCHWARTZ,
AND ELEANOR M.
SAFFRAN

that, while possible in other primates (e.g., Davenport, 1976), achieve great functional significance only in man. Among the relationships made possible by the convergence of input in this parietal association area are the sound-meaning associations necessary for language (Geschwind, 1965).

2. It is possible to recognize in the language area a receptor-effector polarity which, in accordance with the principle of organization of other subsystems, extends from posterior, post-Rolandic receptive areas to more anterior Rolandic and pre-Rolandic motor areas of the cerebral cortex. There is a network of fibers (the arcuate fasciculus) that connnects the auditory area with frontal and prefrontal motor areas in man, and probably to some extent in other primates as well (Geschwind, 1965).

Geschwind (1965, 1970) has argued that the arcuate connection between the auditory and motor areas accounts for man's ability to imitate auditory stimuli and that it is therefore critical for the vocal learning that is essential to human language. This speculation follows from the belief that lesions in the arcuate fasciculus specifically interfere with vocal imitation in man (Geschwind, 1965, 1970; but see Rasmussen and Milner, 1975, for conflicting observations).

3. Language functions are strongly lateralized in the left hemisphere, in most instances in concordant relation to the side of handedness.

The fact that language and the dominant hand are controlled by the same hemisphere has led to a number of speculations. In particular, this relationship is often cited in support of a gestural origins theory—that symbolic communication began, among our hominid ancestors, in the gestural mode (e.g., Hewes, 1973; Steklis and Harnad, 1976). If speech was indeed preceded by a gestural language, it is likely that the machinery for acoustic-vocal communication would have developed in the hemisphere that controlled the dominant, gesturing hand. The fact that the cortical areas controlling hand and mouth are in close proximity has also been used to support the gestural origins theory (e.g., Holloway, 1976; Jaynes, 1976; Steklis and Harnad, 1976); the notion is that the kind of neuronal organization that evolved to support manual communication eventually spilled over into neighboring areas of the brain.

4. While human language is predominantly if not exclusively a neocortical function, primate vocalization seems to be organized at a subcortical level.

On the basis of this observation, it is argued that speech did not evolve out of the vocalization behavior of subhuman primates (Myers, 1976; Robinson, 1976). The discontinuity argument is then used to support the theory that language had its origins in the gestural mode (e.g., Steklis and Harnad, 1976).

This is about as far as the neurological data will take us in the attempt to trace the origins of human language. It is obviously a fragmentary account; it tells us little about the origins of speech, little about its semantic structure, nothing at all about the evolution of phonology or syntax. If we want to ask about the emergence of these functions, we will not be helped by the neurological literature, because in truth there is nothing known about the brain mechanisms which underlie them, or indeed any other psychological function which cannot be described in associationistic terms.

Beyond the level of gross anatomical correlation, we actually know very little about the functional organization of the nervous system (e.g., Maturana, 1970; Pribram, 1971; Lenneberg, 1975; Marin, 1976). With regard to the brain-language relationship, we are restricted to explanations based almost entirely on the connections between functionally distinct neuronal populations, whose internal operations are not yet understood. This level of explanation works for certain aspects of language—it has been very profitably applied to concrete naming, for example (Geschwind and Kaplan, 1962; Geschwind and Fusillo, 1966)—but its power is definitely limited.

Before we can extrapolate from the brain to the various nonassociative dimensions in language, we will have to understand how it is that neuronal aggregates with similar connectivity patterns behave in rather different ways—how it is, for example, that similar brain structures subserve language function on one side of the brain and not the other. At our present level of description, we cannot even account for the fact that certain language functions (syntax and phonology) are spared the ravages of diffuse cortical degeneration, while others (lexical and semantic functions) are profoundly impaired (Whitaker, 1976; Schwartz, *et al.,* in press). The explanation for such differences will probably be found at a physiological level, but the necessary principles of physiological microorganization still elude us.

Comparative anatomy will not provide much help either until we have a better functional description for the anatomy. How are we, for example, to explain the fact that other primates show anatomical asymmetries (Yeni-Komshian and Benson, 1976) of the sort that are thought to reflect the lateralization of language function when observed in man (Geschwind and Levitsky, 1968; Witelson and Pallie, 1973; Wada *et al.,* 1975)? At present, anatomical comparisons rest almost entirely on size differences, and, as Holloway (1976) and others have pointed out, it is unlikely that human language can be accounted for solely in terms of "extra neurons"; rather, there must have been some reorganization in the function of existing brain tissue which we are not yet in a position to understand.

Thus we will not frame our discussion of the origins of language in terms of our current understanding of the brain. Instead, we will consider the two issues separately. First, we discuss the evolution of language from a purely functional perspective: What were the cognitive developments that eventuated in language? How can we explain the emergence of the acoustic-vocal mode? What were the origins of lexical processes and of syntax? Then we turn to the question of how language is presently distributed in the brain.

EVOLUTION OF LANGUAGE

COGNITIVE PREREQUISITES

Language is a good deal more than speech, and in accounting for the evolution of language we have to account for more than the form which the language code has taken. When humans cannot hear or speak, they develop alternate forms of communication; and, when investigators have taken care to

OSCAR S. M. MARIN,
MYRNA F. SCHWARTZ,
AND ELEANOR M.
SAFFRAN

cast the symbols in an appropriate mode, other primates have also shown some capacity for symbolic communication. Speech burgeoned in our hominid ancestors only because there was a cognitive apparatus to take advantage of it.

What are the roots of this cognitive capacity? We can look at the evolution of cognition as a progressive change in sensibility that defines, at each phylogenetic level, the scope of the organism's interaction with the environment. At the earliest stage, the organism's relationship to the external world is limited to a chemical exchange with the immediate milieu. Later, with the development of exteroception, the organism begins to orient itself in space, localizing stimulus events with respect to its body surface and reacting to them by modifying its shape or changing its location. The interaction at this stage is entirely autoreferential; sensibility is limited to stimuli impinging directly on the body surface and the organism itself is the reference point for all events. The organism's reaction to sensory stimuli is immediate.

At the next stage, the organism expands its purview with respect to space and also with respect to time. With the development of telereceptors, it becomes possible to appreciate relationships among objects in the external world. The organism may operate autoreferentially for the purpose of orientation, but it also begins to have the capacity to observe external events as they relate to one another.* To operate within this expanded space, it is necessary to expand the temporal properties of behavior. The response to the environment is no longer always immediate; behavior is integrated over longer temporal intervals. Temporal integration, in turn, implies memory: the organism's response to the proximal stimulus is determined, in part, by the record of what came before. It also follows that behavior is no longer completely under genetic control but is shaped to an increasing degree by the organism's interaction with the environment. Concomitant with this capacity to objectify the external world and to withhold immediate response to external events is the progressive detachment of perception from emotion: we have an organism that is capable not only of feeling but also of knowing.

Another significant change is the shift from feature detection to figural synthesis. In the case of the lower vertebrates, perception is largely restricted to a set of features that are determined genetically and that have clear significance for survival. Behavior depends on the detection of single features irrespective, for the most part, of their context. For higher mammals, and certainly for primates, there is much greater variety to perceptual experience. While the sensory analyzers remain capable of detecting isolated features, behavior is rarely based on them. Instead, the features are integrated into complex configurations, some of which depend on the record of previous experience ("analysis by synthesis") and not on sensory data alone. The set of possible percepts thus undergoes tremendous expansion.

This expanded perceptual capacity allows the organism to take advantage of a wider range of environmental stimuli. Given that an object or event is perceived,

---

*It is interesting, in this respect, that the visual system appears to have evolved two separate mechanisms, a neocortical system concerned with object perception—an alloreferential spatial system—and an older tectal system concerned with ocular movements and immediate adjustments to the environment—an autoreferential mechanism, in the terms we are using here (Schneider, 1969).

its survival value can be tested. The organism is thus equipped to deal with external variability, whether self-imposed, as in the case of migratory species, or induced by climactic change. But there are some problems with perceptual expansion. The perceptual world is now in constant flux, particularly for organisms that follow a migratory existence, as do many higher primates and as, apparently, did early man. The memory load would become intolerable if not for another phylogenetic trend—the increasing ability to categorize events, to encode experience at more abstract levels of representation. For while it is advantageous to be able to perceive novel configurations that may prove to have adaptive significance, it is not clear that the organism needs to keep a veridical record of its vast perceptual experience. In order for the foraging primate, for example, to determine that the leaves of a particular bush are edible, the bush need not be an exact replica of bushes feasted on before; the animal only needs to perceive a few distinguishing features to recognize that this bush is an instance of a type of vegetation that has proved to be edible in the past. Abstraction and categorization therefore complement perceptual variability, allowing efficient use of the wide range of perceptual experience to which the organism is now open.

The potentialities for categorization increase still further if information can be integrated across sensory modalities. As Laughlin and d'Aquili (1974) have put it,

> two visual percepts may generate more different visual associations than similar ones. If we use only visual associations, these percepts might not be classified together. But if we take into consideration all the possible associations in all sense modalities, it is probable that similarities frequently override dissimilarities, allowing large groups of objects to be classified together. In other words, cross-modal transfer permits the construction of classes of objects where formerly insufficient information was available in any one sensory storage system to serve as the basis for that classification. We now have an adaptive mechanism that is capable of generating classes of objects, or, in more traditional language *concepts*. (p. 53)

In addition to creating categories that might not otherwise have been possible, intermodal association provides the basis for a more abstract mode of representation; it allows an item to "be represented in memory in a unified way despite the different modalities in which the species may have experienced the item" (Premack, 1976*a*, p. 559). Contrary to what was previously thought (e.g., Geschwind, 1965), nonhuman primates are capable of forming intermodal associations (e.g., Davenport, 1976; Premack, 1976*a*), although their abilities in this respect are clearly limited when compared with those of man.

Thus we have brought the organism to the point where, given the pressure to communicate and the availability of a suitable modality, it might invent a language. It appears to have, at the least, the conceptual foundations for a lexicon*; what it

---

*This account resembles, in some respects, the one provided by Geschwind (1964, 1965). He has argued, from a neuroanatomical perspective, that the development of "nonlimbic" (i.e., cross-modal) associations led, eventually, to the capacity for naming. The dichotomy that we have termed autoreferential and alloreferential is paralleled, in his discussion, by "sensory-limbic" and "nonlimbic" associations. Geschwind attributes the appearance of cross-modal integration to the increased development of the inferior parietal cortex. We have taken a more functional approach because we do not believe that the anatomical argument, as presently formulated, particularly elucidates the language origins question.

OSCAR S. M. MARIN,
MYRNA F. SCHWARTZ,
AND ELEANOR M.
SAFFRAN

needs is a symbol system with which to represent these concepts. Presumably, this was the cognitive status in which Washoe (Gardner and Gardner, 1969), Sara (Premack, 1971), and Lana (Rumbaugh and Gill, 1976) awaited their mentors, who supplied the symbol system, together with pressures that the animals might not have met with in their natural state. The nature of this prelinguistic conceptual system is currently being illuminated by these attempts to teach language to chimpanzees. It appears to be rather an impressive system; as Premack (1971, 1976*b*) has shown, these animals not only are capable of making reference based on rich mnestic representations; they also can recognize cause-effect and second-order relations (that, for example, the relation color-of, as it applies to apple and red, is the same as the relation between banana and yellow). Their capacity to symbolize, however, is latent, expressed, as far as we know, only under these unusual experimental conditions. This is only one of several as yet unexplained gaps between other intelligent species and linguistically endowed man.

ORIGINS OF SPEECH

The foundations for symbolic communication were laid in this perceptual/cognitive domain. The next step is to determine how the symbols were first represented—whether language began in the gestural mode (Hewes, 1973; Steklis and Harnad, 1976) or took on its acoustic-vocal shape from the very beginning. Perhaps the best argument for the gestural hypothesis is that it provides natural precursors for arbitrary symbols in object pointing and iconic symbolization; in the case of vocal communication, precursors have been more difficult to find. But even if language began with gesture, we must still explain its evolution in the acoustic-vocal mode.

Most nonhuman primates do possess a repertoire of sounds which they utilize in communicating. But their vocalizations rarely constitute a complete message. More typically, they form only one part of a complex behavioral display that also involves gestures, postures, and facial expressions. The relative unimportance of the vocal component is testified to by the assertion of at least one primatologist that, in contrast to a blind animal, the ape or monkey deprived of hearing would probably function quite normally in its social interactions (Lancaster, 1968).

It is generally agreed that the nonhuman primate does not use the auditory medium to communicate whatever conceptual knowledge it possesses. The vocal repertoire appears to relate to affective rather than cognitive dimensions, the nature of the signal reflecting the emotional disposition of the caller (Green, 1975; Itani, 1963; Rowell and Hinde, 1962). If primates do communicate at all about the environment (see Menzel, 1974), it is probably through the totality of their gestures, rather than by means of meaning-laden vocalization.

We can say with some certainty that the communication system of the nonhuman primate does not exploit the auditory-vocal medium for purposes of symbolic expression. Yet somewhere in the evolution of the hominid line, speech did emerge as the dominant vehicle for semantically based language. How this development came about and why are the central questions in the search for speech origins.

WHY A VOCAL LANGUAGE? A FUNCTIONAL LOOK AT SPEECH. Audition provides an excellent medium for symbolic communication. Relative to the visual system, it stands isolated from the organism's representation of reality—a secluded channel through which the distinction between symbol and referent is assured (Marin, 1976). There are other advantages to an auditory-based language. The acoustic signal is effective in darkness, over long distances, and across barriers; since it does not occur against a background of ongoing stimulation, its onset is particularly distinctive and salient; in order to process the signal, the listener need not be oriented toward its source; and, finally, its production need not interrupt ongoing activity.

All these are advantages inherent in the use of ear and mouth for purposes of communication. But these alone do not capture what it is about human speech and speech perception that makes this transmission mode so well suited to the demands for rapid and efficient exchange of semantically rich messages. The key to its effectiveness lies not in its general properties but rather in those aspects of its structure which appear, at this stage of our knowledge, to be specific to speech.

Phonetic Structure of Speech. Let us consider, for example, how it is possible to communicate through the auditory mode the enormous range of lexical distinctions which the perceptual/cognitive apparatus we described earlier is capable of making. It is inconceivable that the vocal tract as we know it could generate enough differentiable contrasts to map sound onto this profusion of meanings in a one-to-one fashion. The solution to this problem is to use a restricted set of sound contrasts and to convey information by means of their sequential configuration. This is precisely what we have in the phonetic structure of speech. The sequencing of phonemes is limited only by the constraints of the articulators, leaving the system open to a potential infinitude of new combinations, and hence new meanings.

Syntax. If we question how it is that speech reflects the *quality* of the semantic message—its complexities and abstractions—we find the answer in yet another aspect of its structure which has no clear parallel in animal communication (Marler, 1975; Nottebohm, 1975; but see Beer, 1976). Syntax is the critical property: the system of rules which governs the juxtaposition of lexical items and in so doing adds new information of a particular kind. It is through the syntactic structure of our utterances that we *comment on* the lexical items—specifying their relation to one another and to the dimensions of time and space. Thus it is syntax which allows us, through language, to go beyond naming.

Nowhere is this fact more evident than in the speech of aphasic patients who have lost the ability to utilize syntax but who nevertheless retain a sizable lexical vocabulary. In any attempt at narrative, we see that their output is primarily holophrastic and concrete, biased toward specific reference and the naming of people, objects, and situations known to the listener. In this way, the aphasic manages to communicate who and what are the subjects of the discourse, but not who-did-what-to-whom, or for what reason. (For further consideration of this lexical-syntactic dissociation in aphasia, the reader is referred to Goodglass and Geschwind, 1976; Jakobson, 1971; Luria, 1975; Marin *et al.*, 1976.)

The Speech Code. How do we account for the speed and efficiency of spoken language? We know that there are limitations in the rate at which discrete acoustic

OSCAR S. M. MARIN,
MYRNA F. SCHWARTZ,
AND ELEANOR M.
SAFFRAN

events can be perceived. Does the capacity to process speech sounds reflect this limiting factor? The answer seems to be no; there is something special about auditory processing in the speech mode.

We have already said that speech is composed of articulated sounds organized temporally into meaningful patterns. In point of fact, these patterns are generally produced with an amazing rapidity, made possible by the capacity for independent movement of the various articulators in rapid and automatic sequences. This capacity is seen in no other species (Lieberman, 1968).

Indeed, so rapid is this temporal neuromuscular patterning of speech sounds that successive articulatory movements overlap one another. As a result, the distinctiveness of constituent phonemes is generally lost in the acoustic signal; any clearly defined auditory segment provides information, in parallel, about two or more successive phonemes. In reality, then, the phonemic elements of a spoken message do not constitute a string of discrete acoustic events; they are rather restructured or "encoded" at the level of the articulators (Liberman *et al.,* 1967; Studdert-Kennedy, 1974).

How, then, does the listener recover the phonemic structure, as he must do if he is to comprehend the message? One widely held view is that he utilizes perceptual capacities specific to the task of speech processing.

In the last decade, a very strong argument has been made for the existence of a neural mechanism specialized to decode the speech cues on the basis of quite abstract phonetic information (e.g., Cooper, 1974; Eimas and Corbit, 1973). Its operation is characterized by the *categorical* perception of acoustic properties; either acoustic variation within phonemic categories is not perceptible at all, or else the distinguishing auditory information is not held on to long enough to be useful in performing the standard discrimination tasks. Dichotic listening experiments and clinical studies have tended to localize this specialized speech decoder in the left hemisphere. Infant conditioning work has shown that it is functional soon after birth (Eimas, 1974; Eimas *et al.,* 1971; Miller and Morse, 1976).

We can conclude that the key to the efficiency of speech lies here, in the speech-processing apparatus. The average listener can comprehend speech spoken at the rate of up to 30 phonemes per second; yet discrete nonspeech sounds are incomprehensible at this rate (Liberman *et al.,* 1967). It appears that through the specialized encoding and decoding mechanisms of speech the limitations of temporal resolution in the mammalian auditory system have been overcome.

In summary, human speech reveals a structure which is elegantly tailored to the demands for expressing rapidly and efficiently a virtually limitless set of semantic categories. We do not see, nor should we expect to see, these same structural properties in the vocal communication of other primates.

But does this mean that speech did not evolve out of those more primitive systems? Several investigators have attempted to argue precisely this. They claim that it is only man's *paralinguistic* vocal repertoire of cries, moans, laughter, etc., which is functionally homologous with the vocalizations of apes and monkeys. Speech, they argue, arose *de novo* in the hominid line in response to unique pressures for rapid and intelligent communication (Dingwall, 1975; Lancaster, 1968; Myers, 1976; Robinson, 1967; 1976).

We are not entirely comfortable with this assertion. It rests heavily on anatomical evidence which is less than compelling. In addition, we have seen that related anthropocentric claims have failed to withstand close empirical scrutiny. Consider, for example, that only a few years ago one was on firm ground with the argument that man alone possessed the cognitive structures to support language. Since we now know that apes can learn to communicate by means of linguistically based symbol systems, we are forced to consider the possibility that man is not unique in his capacity to abstract and represent the semantic categories which underlie human language.

Another example comes out of recent developments in the speech perception literature, where, under the impetus of the theory of the specialized speech decoder, a few investigators have begun to look at "speech perception" in nonhuman species. Their findings have been startling. Kuhl and Miller (1975), for example, reported that chinchillas trained to respond differentially to speech sounds differing in a single phonetic feature not only generalized to novel instances produced by new speakers but also differentiated these stimuli at the same "phonetic boundaries" as human subjects. Evidence for enhanced discrimination across "phonetic boundaries" has also been reported for rhesus monkeys (Morse and Snowdon, 1975).

These data compel us to ask whether, or more realistically in what way, the perceptual mechanisms used for processing speech reflect prelinguistic capacities shared with other species (Warren, 1976). At the very least, they point out that the development of speech probably proceeded along lines which emphasized certain perceptual contrasts already built into the mammalian auditory system. Other evidence suggests that at least the first stages of speech perception involve the operation of auditory feature analyzers—specialized receptors for transient acoustic events which are probably not unique to man but rather are represented in a wide range of mammalian species (Morse, 1976; Tartter and Eimas, 1975).

In general, the lesson seems to be that language does indeed have a biological history, of which we now know only bits and pieces. The last few years have taught us the value of comparative studies which pose specific questions derived from theories of language. When this approach is coupled with a sensitivity to ethological considerations, the results can be particularly enlightening. We see this in the work of a few zoologists who, working from the premise of biological continuity, utilize the methodological and conceptual advances in speech research to uncover possible precursors of speech in the vocal repertoire of nonhuman primates.

VOCALIZATIONS IN THE NONHUMAN PRIMATE. As in the case of speech, the vocalizations of apes and monkeys are produced by bursts of acoustic energy that are modified by the resonances of the supralaryngeal vocal tract. In both cases, the character of the acoustic signal is determined by the energy source and by the momentary size and shape of the supralaryngeal vocal tract. What sets speech apart is the *variety* of configurations which the supralaryngeal vocal tract can assume, and this, it would appear, is a result of man's unique capacity to manipulate, in a fluid and coordinate manner, his several articulators, most importantly the tongue. In contrast, nonhuman primates make little use of the articulators in their cries. Lieberman (1968) reports that the tongue is not utilized at all, and cites vocal tract anatomy as a limiting condition.

Nevertheless, it is a fact that even with these anatomical limitations a large

OSCAR S. M. MARIN,
MYRNA F. SCHWARTZ,
AND ELEANOR M.
SAFFRAN

number of the sound contrasts utilized in human speech are possible, and indeed have been observed in a subset of the vocalizations of modern primates (Lieberman, 1973). Can we identify in the calls of apes and monkeys the precursors of human speech? Some recent studies provide an interesting functional perspective.

Andrew (1976), for example, has observed that primate calls which are speechlike in their tonal structure and resonances are not likely to be recorded in distress or distant-contact calls. He studied the nature and distribution of one class of speechlike calls, the "humanoid grunt," and found it present in the close contact communications of some primate species which form strong affectional bonds (e.g., baboon, *Papio hamadryas*). Andrew notes that the acoustic properties of these speechlike calls convey information about the size and proportion of the vocal tract. As such, they are particularly well suited to the task of individuating the caller and may serve an important role in the formation and maintenance of social bonds.

A similar conclusion was reached by Green (1975) in his study of vocal communication in the Japanese monkey *(Macaca fuscata)*. Green noted that the class of articulated calls, the "girneys," was the only class of calls exchanged *between* animals, and was usually done in a tête-à-tête fashion. These calls, he claims, "seem to aid in welding a social bond, particularly among unrelated individuals" (p. 97).

Both Andrew and Green suggest that these articulated close-contact calls, with their potential significance for social stability, may represent the precursors of human speech sounds.* It is interesting to note that both the girneys and the humanoid grunts feature prominent tongue and lip movements in addition to voiced elements. As such, they contradict Lieberman's (1968) assertion of minimal involvement of the articulators in the vocalizations of nonhuman primates. It may be that once we know what to look for, and where to look, the body of evidence for speechlike utterances in our primate ancestors may become more impressive.

Marler (1975), noting that human speech sounds are not discrete but rather intergrade into one another, suggests that we pay special attention to those classes of primate vocalizations which are similarly organized. He has linked the occurrence of such graded repertoires to primate species (like the chimpanzee) whose ecology and social structure are similar to what has been postulated for early man, i.e., those characterized by large, nonterrestrial, multimale social orders in which most communication is within rather than between troops. Presumably, such a graded system, amplified and sharpened by simultaneous visual contextual information, allows for the exchange of more subtle messages than is possible within a system of nonoverlapping signals (see Green, 1975, for confirmation).

If we can extrapolate from modern primates to our ape and early humanoid ancestors, we can propose, as Mattingly (1972) has done, that the latter probably possessed a vocal repertoire with a limited phonetic structure, lacking in syntactic organization and functionally restricted to a social/affective role. Mattingly gives

*Green (1975) provides additional evidence for this speculation by noting that the "girneys" are structurally labile in situations where there are no obvious changes in the comportment of the vocalizing monkey. Thus it differs from other, nonarticulated calls where the structural grading correlates quite closely with variations in demeanor, arousal, etc., of the caller. The occurrence of girneys may therefore be less tightly constrained by emotional factors.

an ethological account of the eventual expansion and differentiation of the phonetic repertoire within the human species. He proposes that at this prelinguistic stage of its evolutionary history, speech served man as a social releaser—a means of eliciting appropriate behavioral responses from conspecifics in a wide variety of circumstances. In that role, speech was probably subject to pressures for greater species differentiation through progressive elaboration of its phonetic structure. The anatomical evolution of the human vocal apparatus apparently reflects these pressures. From an early apelike form, limited in the range of possible phonetic contrasts, it has undergone modifications which have made it a more effective vehicle for the production of speech sounds, at the cost of less efficiency in its primary functions of breathing, swallowing, etc. (Lieberman, 1973).

Mattingly (1972) also goes on to discuss the changes in speech structure, particularly the development of syntax, which became necessary when speech came to serve meaning rather than affect. But when in man's evolutionary history that critical change came about, and under what conditions, are questions left unanswered, not just by Mattingly, but in all current theories of language.

This is an additional but directly related gap in our understanding of language origins. The proposed expansion of the vocal repertoire which we have postulated, and which is a precondition for a semantically based vocal language, would certainly have necessitated a major shift in the ontogenetic development of vocalization. Genetic preprogramming would not suffice; a greatly expanded repertoire implies a capacity for vocal learning.

ORIGINS OF VOCAL LEARNING. At what point in human evolution did this proposed shift from genetic control to vocal learning occur? Can we identify nonhuman primates which acquire a vocal repertoire by reference to auditory models? We do not yet know. In studies of bird song development, the role of auditory feedback has been evaluated with great effectiveness by the combined techniques of early deafening, auditory isolation, and foster rearing by parents of different species (see reviews by Konishi and Nottebohm, 1969; Marler, 1976). No comparable studies have been performed with primates.* Yet these data are of enormous potential value, for one might reasonably speculate, as Nottebohm (1975) has done, that the introduction of an auditory-based vocal ontogeny was a critical step in the evolution of language—one which set the stage for additional modifications in the structure and function of the vocal repertoire.

We conceive of this critical step as mediated by the progressive encephalization of vocal motor control. According to this notion, the requirement for auditorily guided vocalization furthered the incorporation of existing efferent mechanisms into the evolving cortical motor system, specialized for precisely such sensory-guided movements (Denny-Brown, 1966; Luria, 1966). Once this level of control was established, other advantages of a cortical motor representation would

---

*There are other lines of evidence which speak to the capacity of vocal learning in nonhuman primates. One of these is the possible existence of regional dialects in the vocal repertoire. Premack (1976a, p. 555) cites a study by Green demonstrating the existence of such dialects in the Japanese monkey and pointing to the role of learning in their acquisition. Experimental evidence for vocal learning in traditional conditioning paradigms has been more difficult to find (see Myers, 1976).

OSCAR S. M. MARIN,
MYRNA F. SCHWARTZ,
AND ELEANOR M.
SAFFRAN

have ensued: among them, the development of flexible and open motor programs such as operate in the production of phonetic strings (Luria, 1966), fluid and automatic execution of these motor programs (Lieberman, 1973; Moscovitch, this volume), and the capacity for voluntary initiation of these motor programs (Jackson, 1884).

All these are general properties of a cortical motor representation; parallel developments can be pointed to in the area of forelimb dexterity (Noback and Moskowitz, 1973; Steklis and Harnad, 1976). Applied to the vocal repertoire, these modifications would have made possible many of the characteristics of speech which we enumerated earlier.

Anatomical Distribution of Vocal Motor Control in Nonhuman Primates. The conclusion from most studies of neural correlates is that only in man is there a cortical locus for vocal motor control. Present-day primates, it is held, do not have their vocal motor programs represented in neocortical areas, but rather in subcortical and predominantly limbic structures. This is important because it is primarily on the basis of this assertion that some investigators have argued for the discontinuity between speech and the vocalizations of nonhuman primates. We quote Bryan Robinson:

> It appears that human speech and primate vocalization depend on two different neural systems. This one is neocortical; the other, limbic. This suggests that human speech did not develop "out of" primate vocalization, but arose from new tissue which permitted it the necessary detachment from immediate, emotional situations. The neurological evidence suggests that human language arose in parallel with primate vocalization. (Robinson, 1967, p. 353)

Before considering the evidence for this assertion, let us take care to state the question clearly. We want to know the nature of the distribution of vocal motor programs in the primate brain. The analogous interest, with regard to human speech, concerns the efferent systems responsible for the successive and simultaneous coordination of the articulators and of the laryngeal/respiratory apparatus for purposes of speech production. Evidence from studies of brain-damaged individuals strongly implicates the posterior frontal region of the left hemisphere. However, if we were to broaden our interests even slightly, this claim to anatomical discreteness would no longer hold. For example, if we inquire about lesions which alter the probability of initiation of the speech act, the rate of speech, or its appropriateness, we see implicated a wide range of neural structures, both cortical and subcortical. These distinctions have generally been overlooked in attempts to localize primate vocalization.

What do we know about the anatomical distribution of vocal motor mechanisms in the brain of nonhuman primates? Not very much. Most of the evidence comes from brain stimulation studies. Experimenters have probed for positive sites in the brains of rhesus monkeys *(Macaca mulatta)* (Kaada, 1951; Robinson, 1967; Smith, 1945), squirrel monkeys (Jurgens *et al.*, 1967; Jurgens, 1969), and gibbons (Apfelbach, cited in Nottebohm, 1975). The results have been quite uniform; natural, identifiable vocalizations are elicited most readily from subcortical, particularly limbic, structures. The anterior cingulate region, amygdala, septum, stria terminalis, preoptic area, and hypothalamus are most frequently implicated. There is, furthermore, a systematic organization such that specific vocalizations tend to occur in certain loci and not in others (Robinson, 1967; Jurgens *et al.*, 1967). Neocortical stimulation sites, on the other hand, are generally silent (but see Dusser de Barenne *et al.*,1941), although stimulation in the inferior motor strip and surrounding tissue does result in observable movements of the mouth, tongue, lips, and larynx (Sugar *et al.*, 1948).

While these stimulation studies are widely cited in support of a limbic substrate for vocal responses (e.g., Robinson, 1976), they may in fact be saying little about the distribution of motor programs. The subcortical sites from which vocalizations can be elicited are known to be critically involved in the creation and alteration of motivational and emotional states. It is likely that they achieve their effect on behavior by exerting an inhibitory or excitatory influence on efferent systems located elsewhere in the nervous system (Milner, 1970). Thus stimulation of these brain sites may elicit vocalizations only indirectly, e.g., by creating the affective state in which the call is typically manifested. This interpretation is consistent with the following observations: (1) that the elicited vocalizations appear natural both to the human observer (Kaada, 1951; Robinson, 1967; Smith, 1945) and to spectographic analysis (Jurgens *et al.*, 1967) and (2) that they are frequently embedded in complex behavioral sequences involving autonomic and somatic components (e.g., Smith, 1945).

If we are correct in this interpretation, then the positive findings from stimulation studies have little to tell us about the organization of vocal motor mechanisms in the primate brain. On the other hand, they do show that these vocalizations are components of behavioral repertoires under the influence of emotional and motivational states. As such, these findings reinforce the functional distinction between speech and the primate vocal repertoire alluded to earlier.

The stimulation technique is notoriously "unphysiological." In some cases, its effect is to disrupt rather than to stimulate. Thus, when the human brain is stimulated in its anterior, neocortical "speech area," the result is never natural speech, but rather the *interruption* of ongoing speech in the awake and conversing patient (Penfield and Roberts, 1959). Does stimulation of the analogous areas in the primate brain similarly disrupt ongoing vocalizations? The relevant studies have yet to be performed (see Nottebohm, 1975, for methodological suggestions).

Most of our knowledge about anatomical correlates of human language comes from the study of brain-damaged individuals. It is well known, for example, that people who suffer lesions in and around the inferior sensorimotor regions of the dominant hemisphere are unable to produce normally structured speech. If neocortical sensorimotor regions played a similarly critical role in the vocal production of nonhuman primates, then experimentally induced lesions made in these areas should certainly impair their vocal behavior. So far this has not proved to be the case. Kaada (1951), in an early study with macaque and cercopithecus monkeys, reported that bilateral ablation of the lower precentral region on the lateral surface of the frontal lobes, together with the rest of the motor areas, was without any effect on stimulation-elicited vocalizations. Sutton *et al.* (1974), using rhesus monkeys, found no disruption of a learned phonatory cry after extensive neocortical lesions. They did observe, however, that these cries were weaker and a good deal less frequent after ablations involving the cingulate and subcallosal gyri. Finally, Myers and co-workers found in rhesus monkeys that bilateral neocortical lesions which were restricted to the homologues of the human "speech areas" were without substantial effect on vocal responses. In contrast, lesions outside these "speech areas," in neocortical regions known to regulate social behavior, produced dramatic decreases in vocalization, in some cases verging on muteness (Myers, 1976).

The results of these several studies are certainly suggestive, but they must be interpreted with caution. For one thing, decisions about where to make the lesions were dictated by a model of language organization in the human brain (Geschwind, 1970), which is in several respects inadequate. In addition, these studies were performed without benefit of recent advances in classification of the primate vocal repertoire. Thus "it is as if investigators trying to plot speech areas in the human brain were unable to tell normal language apart from all its possible distortions and from nonspeech utterances" (Nottebohm, 1975, p. 87). These lesion studies fail to assess the effect of neocortical ablation on the structural integrity or functional appropriateness of vocalizations as they occur in the natural setting; the dependent variable is rather the frequency or probability of responding. This is an important point because, in fact, it is the case with humans also that the most dramatic alterations in speech *dynamics* (in the extreme case, mutism) occur with lesions *outside* the boundaries of the speech area (Luria, 1966).

As we stressed earlier, recent field and laboratory studies are providing valuable clues about where in the primate vocal repertoire we might profitably look for the precursors of speech. A program of neurobiological research which utilized that information would address the following issues: Within a particular primate group, are the graded elements of the vocal repertoire more vulnerable to neocortical lesions than the discrete calls? Are articulated calls more vulnerable than nonarticulated calls? Can we see evidence for progressive encephalization of vocal motor control as we ascend the phylogenetic scale of primates (as suggested by Sutton *et al.*, 1974, on the basis of neurophysiological studies)? In particular, does there tend to be more neocortical involvement in those great apes which utilize part of their vocal repertoire for social-affective exchanges, much as early man probably did?

If these questions are to be properly addressed in the future, there will have to develop a closer interaction than has heretofore existed between those researchers who refine the functional descriptions and those who search for anatomical correlates (cf. Nottebohm, 1975).

DISTRIBUTION OF LANGUAGE FUNCTIONS IN THE BRAIN

INTRODUCTION

We turn now to the question of the neural substrate for language: how are language functions distributed in the human brain? In answering this question, we will, of necessity, draw most of our evidence from ablation studies—studies of patients with losses of brain tissue resulting from disease processes or surgical intervention. The logic of this approach is, of course, that if damage to a particular area of the brain affects language function, then that area must have contributed to language function in the normal state. However, lesions in many parts of the brain affect language in a rather general way by altering the rate, frequency, or efficiency of language production. Frontal lobe lesions, for example, can result in mutism, not because the patient is incapable of speech, but because the lesion compromises voluntary behavior in general (Luria, 1966). Thus we will attribute language function only to those regions where damage or stimulation of brain tissue alters the structure of the language process rather than the efficiency of its use.

Two generalizations can safely be made with respect to the anatomical distribution of language: (1) the special machinery for language is primarily neocortical, and (2) it is localized, for the most part, in the left cerebral hemisphere. Possible qualifications of the first assertion will be discussed at the end of this section. We will begin with the evidence for hemispheric specialization and go on to discuss the intrahemispheric distribution of language function. We will also touch on the problem of changes in language distribution during ontogeny.

HEMISPHERIC SPECIALIZATION FOR LANGUAGE

There is, by now, a large body of evidence to support a left hemisphere localization for language, at least in most adults of the species. But while it might have been concluded, just a few years ago, that the right hemisphere was completely devoid of linguistic ability, it is now apparent that this view requires some modification. We will summarize, first, the evidence that supports a left hemisphere localization for language and go on to discuss the possibility of right hemisphere language function.

EVIDENCE FOR LEFT HEMISPHERE LANGUAGE. The evidence for left hemisphere specialization for language dates back at least a century (see Penfield and Roberts, 1959, for a historical summary) and comes principally from the following sources:

Brain Lesions. The incidence of language deficits with damage to the left cerebral hemisphere is about 70% in the general population; with right hemisphere lesions, the incidence drops to 1 or 2% (Penfield and Roberts, 1959; Russell and Espir, 1961).

Wada Test. It is possible to anesthetize the hemispheres independently by injecting sodium amytal into the ipsilateral carotid artery (Wada, 1949). During the few minutes that one hemisphere is deactivated, the other can be tested for language function. Left carotid injection disrupts speech in 90% of the right-handers tested, while the comparable figure for right-sided injection is only about 10% (Branch *et al.*, 1964).*

---

*This figure is somewhat higher than would be predicted from the incidence of language impairment with right hemisphere lesions. The disparity is probably explained by the fact that the Wada Test—a difficult procedure that is used primarily to establish language localization prior to surgery—was not performed on a normal population. The patients used in the Branch *et al.* (1964) study were epileptics, some of whom may have had early left hemisphere lesions which led to transfer of language functions to the right. Although some attempt was made to eliminate such patients from the data analysis, it is possible that some of them had been asymptomatic in childhood and could not, therefore, be identified as having had early lesions.

OSCAR S. M. MARIN,
MYRNA F. SCHWARTZ,
AND ELEANOR M.
SAFFRAN

Commissurotomy and Hemispherectomy. Each hemisphere can be studied more adequately when it is isolated from the other. This is possible in the split-brain patient, where the connections between the hemispheres have been severed, or in hemispherectomy cases, where one hemisphere has been removed entirely. The isolated left hemisphere proves to be normal or near normal in language function (Gazzaniga, 1970; Smith, 1974), while the right demonstrates only the limited linguistic abilities that we will describe in some detail below.

Electrical Activity. Language-related asymmetries have been observed in the electrical activity of the brain. Verbal activity tends to suppress the α rhythm over the left hemisphere more than it does on the right (Butler and Glass, 1976), and auditory evoked potentials recorded from the left hemisphere are more sensitive to the linguistic properties of the acoustic stimulus than evoked potentials recorded from the right (e.g., Morrell and Salamy, 1971; Wood, 1975; Molfese *et al.*, 1975).

Interference with Motor Activity. If language is well lateralized, verbal operations might be expected to interfere with the ability to carry out other lateralized functions such as fine motor control of the hand. Several investigators have found that concurrent verbal activity interferes more with right than with left hand performance on finger-tapping and dowel-balancing tasks (e.g., Kinsbourne and Cook, 1971; Lomas and Kimura, 1976).

Dichotic and Split-Field Studies in Normals. It is possible to get some measure of hemispheric specialization in normal subjects by addressing competing stimuli to the two ears. The right ear typically shows an advantage in dichotic listening tasks when verbal stimuli, such as words and stop consonants, are used (e.g., Kimura, 1967; Studdert-Kennedy and Shankweiler, 1970; Studdert-Kennedy *et al.*, 1972). Ear differences under dichotic stimulation are thought to reflect inequalities in the pathways from the two ears such that, while each hemisphere receives input from both ears, the contralateral pathway is more effective (Kimura, 1967; Sparks and Geschwind, 1968).* The implication of the right ear advantage for most speech sounds is therefore that phonetic processing mechanisms are lateralized in the left hemisphere.

In the visual modality, input can be addressed separately to the two hemispheres by means of the split-field technique. The method involves presenting parafoveal stimuli tachistoscopically, at exposures too brief to permit lateral eye movements. It is typically found that the left hemisphere is superior to the right in the recognition of letters and words (e.g., McKeever and Huling, 1971; Moscovitch, 1973, 1976*a*).

LEFT-HANDERS. The general picture thus far is of complete left hemisphere control of language function, at least in righthanders. The situation differs somewhat in the left-handed population, where evidence from brain lesions (e.g., Gloning *et al.*, 1969; Hécaen and Sauget, 1971), amytal tests (Branch *et al.*, 1964; Milner, 1974), and dichotic and split-field studies (e.g., Zurif and Bryden, 1969; McKeever *et al.*, 1975) indicates that language is less well lateralized, at least in familial left-handers. The distribution of language function between the hemispheres in left-handers will be considered below.

---

*But see Kinsbourne (1974) for an alternate view.

EVIDENCE FOR RIGHT HEMISPHERE LANGUAGE. But even in right-handers, the restriction of language ability to the left hemisphere seems to be less complete than had previously been thought. What is most intriguing about this evidence is that the right hemisphere seems more capable of supporting some aspects of language function than others. The apparent restrictions on right hemisphere language representation should help to elucidate what it is that the more linguistic left hemisphere is specialized for.

Most of the evidence comes from studies of split-brain and commissurotomy patients, where right hemisphere language processes can be studied without interference from the left. This evidence should be interpreted cautiously, however, since (1) it is based, thus far, on very few cases; (2) in most of these patients, it is possible that early damage to the left hemisphere caused some transfer of language function to the right, and therefore that the level of right hemisphere language function is not representative of the normal state; and (3) the tasks employed to test right hemisphere language function are not always adequate measures of the linguistic abilities ostensibly under investigation. It is therefore important to seek confirming evidence from patients with right hemisphere lesions and from experiments with normals. We will consider various aspects of language, as follows:

Oral Language. The right hemisphere of the split-brain patient appears totally mute. When there is a verbal response to a stimulus perceived only by the right hemisphere, it is usually inappropriate—quite clearly a confabulation produced by the left (Gazzaniga, 1970; Levy *et al.,* 1971). Some verbal output is possible, however, in left hemispherectomy cases, where there is no competition for control of the vocal apparatus. When the left hemisphere is removed early in life, speech, along with most other language functions, transfers readily to the remaining hemisphere. Postpubertal cases, which would provide a better indication of right hemisphere language representation in the normal adult brain, are rare, but the available data do suggest that such patients are capable of some verbal output (see Moscovitch, 1973, 1976b, for a compilation of these cases). The most detailed reports (of the same patient) by Gott (1973) and Zaidel (1978) indicate that the speech production of the isolated right hemisphere is, at best, nonfluent, largely holophrastic, agrammatic, and dysarthric; that its expressive vocabulary is limited; and that it is prone to semantic errors in naming tasks. In contrast to this picture of effortful and impoverished speech, these patients are apparently able to sing, often with complete lyrics and with good articulation (Smith, 1966; Gott, 1973).

Receptive Language: Lexical Abilities. The receptive language functions of the isolated right hemisphere are, in general, better developed than its expressive functions. The right hemisphere in both split-brain and hemispherectomy patients does fairly well in vocabulary tests that involve matching a spoken word to a pictorial representation of its meaning. Age-level scores of 11 and 16 years were achieved by two split-brain patients (Zaidel, 1976); two left hemispherectomy patients scored somewhat lower, at about the 8-year level (Smith, 1966; Gott, 1973).

Some evidence of right hemisphere involvement in lexical functions is also found in patients with right hemisphere lesions, who are impaired relative to

OSCAR S. M. MARIN,
MYRNA F. SCHWARTZ,
AND ELEANOR M.
SAFFRAN

normals in vocabulary tests but not in comparable tests of phonological and syntactic function (Lesser, 1974). Recent data from split-field studies of normal subjects also suggest that the right hemisphere has some form of lexical representation (see below).

Receptive Language: Phonetic Abilities. While the right hemisphere appears to have some ability to understand spoken words, at least in the context of the multiple choice picture vocabulary test (Zaidel, 1976), it is not clear that it does so by analyzing the auditory stimulus phonetically. It is in this area that the investigation of the language capacities of the isolated right hemisphere has been least satisfactory. This is unfortunate, particularly in light of the contention, based on normal dichotic listening studies (Studdert-Kennedy and Shankweiler, 1970; Studdert-Kennedy *et al.*, 1972) and evidence from brain-damaged patients (Oscar-Berman *et al.*, 1975; Saffran *et al.*, 1976), that the phonetic apparatus is strongly lateralized on the left.

Zaidel (1978) has made some attempt to look at right hemisphere phonetic processing abilities in two commissurotomy patients and in one patient with a left hemispherectomy. He found that the right hemisphere was fairly good at discriminating between phonemically similar words, but it is difficult to determine from his data whether this performance was based on an analysis of phonetic features or possibly on auditory characteristics alone (for a discussion of the auditory-phonetic distinction, see Studdert-Kennedy, 1976). Zaidel (1978) also reports that the right hemisphere performed at chance level on a stop-consonant identification task and concludes that it is unable to analyze the speech signal phonetically. However, the identification task, which requires the subject to match the auditory signal (e.g., "da") with a printed letter (e.g., "D"), may be difficult for the right hemisphere for reasons having nothing to do with phonetic analysis; as will be seen below, the direct association of grapheme with phoneme is another task that the right hemisphere is probably unable to do.

Receptive Language: Syntactic Abilities. Early studies of right hemisphere language in split-brain patients suggested that comprehension was limited to simple nouns and adjectives; verbs were not understood at all (Gazzaniga, 1970; Gazzaniga and Hillyard, 1971). More recent studies by Zaidel (1978) suggest greater syntactic competence than had previously been suspected, with average right hemisphere performance (of the two split-brain patients and one left hemispherectomy patient) at the 4- to 6-year-old level. The syntactic comprehension tasks were, however, heavily weighted toward grammatical morphemes (functors, such as pronouns and prepositions, and affixes, such as tense and number markers and comparative endings), and did not adequately assess the right hemisphere's understanding of intermorphemic relationships such as clause structure and word order. It is this structural aspect of syntax that proves difficult for aphasics with otherwise good comprehension (Caramazza and Zurif, 1976; Scholes, 1978; Schwartz *et al.*, 1978), and it is also at the structural level that the performance of patients whose left hemispheres were removed in infancy begins to break down (Dennis and Kohn, 1975; Dennis and Whitaker, 1976). It is evident even from these possibly inflated estimates, however, that the syntactic competence of the isolated right hemisphere lags significantly behind its lexical development.

Reading and Writing. When we turn to written language, the right hemisphere's abilities seem, in general, less impressive than its ability to deal with speech. In the split-brain patient, the right hemisphere is able to match printed words with their meanings, but only if the stimuli are simple adjectives or concrete nouns (Gazzaniga, 1970; Gazzaniga and Hillyard, 1971); its ability to write is minimal, again limited mostly to nouns (Levy *et al.*, 1971). There is evidence of limited reading ability in at least one left hemispherectomy patient, whose capacity to encode the meanings of printed words exceeded her ability to read them aloud (Gott, 1973). There is no evidence of writing ability in the hemispherectomy cases reported thus far.

Several recent studies in normal subjects also suggest a right hemisphere capacity for reading. While the conclusion of a host of split-field studies has been that there is a left hemisphere *superiority* for the recognition of verbal stimuli (e.g., Moscovitch, 1976*a*), these studies do not provide an absolute measure of right hemisphere performance. Some indication that the right hemisphere is actually processing the graphemic stimuli as words, rather than simply transferring them to the left for linguistic analysis, comes from studies of word recognition across word classes. In comparing the effects of presenting abstract and concrete words to the two visual fields, it is found that the right visual field advantage is greater for abstract than for concrete words (Ellis and Shepherd, 1974; Day, 1976; Hines, 1976, 1977). The word class experiments force the conclusion that the normal right hemisphere has some capacity for word recognition, albeit limited. The ability to read concrete words accords well with other evidence of right hemisphere lexical representation.

Nature of Right Hemisphere Language. Two additional pieces of evidence may provide further insights into the nature of language representation in the minor hemisphere. The first comes from an examination, again by Zaidel (1977), of right hemisphere performance on the Token Test, a task that places heavy demands on auditory short-term memory.* Despite its ability to comprehend the lexical items themselves, and some evidence that it retains a good deal of the lexical information in the stimulus sentences, the right hemisphere of split-brain and hemispherectomy patients does rather poorly on this test.

Zaidel (1977) attributes this problem to an inability to preserve the sequential information in the stimulus sentence (e.g., asked to "Pick up the yellow circle and the red rectangle," the patient might retrieve the yellow rectangle and the red circle), and characterizes it as a short-term memory defect.† This kind of short-term memory impairment, with loss of sequential information but relative preservation of the items themselves, is characteristic of aphasics with articulatory disorders and nonfluent speech and has been attributed to the inability to rehearse material at a subvocal level (Saffran *et al.*, 1977). Given that the right hemisphere is severely limited in verbal output, it may be limited as well in the ability to encode

---

*The subject has to respond to a set of increasingly complex nonredundant commands, e.g., "Pick up the small white circle and the large yellow rectangle."

†An alternative explanation is a syntactic one—that the patient fails to appreciate the modifier-noun relationship that is signaled by word order. However, Zaidel (1978) reports that the right hemisphere also performs poorly on sequential pointing span tasks.

OSCAR S. M. MARIN,
MYRNA F. SCHWARTZ,
AND ELEANOR M.
SAFFRAN

information in a form suitable for rehearsal. Some evidence from split-brain patients suggests that this is indeed the case. Levy and Trevarthen (cited in Levy, 1974) found that while the right hemisphere may be able to go from sound *to* meaning, as shown by its performance on vocabulary tests, it is unable to generate phonology *from* meaning, as shown by its inability to match objects according to the acoustic similarity of their names (e.g., "bee" with "key").* Thus the right hemisphere short-term memory deficit may reflect a more basic deficit in phonological encoding.

It is likely, therefore, that right hemisphere language representation is normally limited to a rather impoverished lexicon consisting principally of concrete words. This lexicon is capable of relating sounds and graphemes to meaning, but it does not seem to operate in the reverse direction; it cannot generate phonology from meaning. There is also reason to believe that the right hemisphere has only limited syntactic competence. As we will see below, syntax may very well depend on the same kind of brain organization that subserves motor speech.

DISTRIBUTION OF LANGUAGE FUNCTIONS IN LEFT-HANDERS. As we have noted above, left-handers show less hemispheric asymmetry with respect to language function than is typically found in the right-handed population. We may ask, then, whether *all* aspects of language are uniformly distributed between the hemispheres in left-handers, or whether some functions show more of a bilateral distribution than others.

The data, while not plentiful, are at least suggestive. One source of information is the Wada Test, where language lateralization is indicated by mutism or dysphasic speech production during the period of hemispheric deactivation by sodium amytal (Branch *et al.*, 1964). In a group of 74 left-handers with no clinical evidence of early left hemisphere injury, 23 (32%) showed disruption of speech production with right-sided injection; of these, almost half also became dysphasic with left-sided injection (Milner, 1974). Expressive language function therefore appears to be represented in the right hemisphere in a minority of left-handed individuals. If we look now at the incidence of different types of language dysfunction in left-handers with right or left hemisphere lesions, we find the following pattern (based on data from Hécaen and Sauget, 1971): there is a tendency, as the sodium amytal data would suggest, toward a higher incidence of expressive disturbances with left than with right hemisphere lesions; comprehension disturbances, however, occur with about equal frequency in the right and left lesion groups. This suggests a more symmetrical distribution of receptive than expressive language functions in left-handers. A comparison with right-handers further supports the idea that receptive language functions are bilaterally distributed in left handers. If we compare left- and right-handers with left hemisphere lesions, we find that while the incidence of expressive disturbances is approximately equal in the two groups, comprehension disorders are about 3 times more frequent in the right-handers (Hécaen and Sauget, 1971); The bilateral representation of comprehension mechanisms presumably protects against receptive impairment in left-handers.

*To perform this task, it is not necessary to be able to articulate the rhyming words. Patients who are unable to express the stimulus words, because of either articulatory impairment (Nebes, 1975) or anomic disturbance (Marin *et al.*, 1976), have been able to perform the rhyming task.

It is likely that the degree of bilaterality of language representation varies considerably in the left-handed population even within the group of familial left-handers. This is a problem that is only now being addressed (e.g., Lishman and McMeekan, 1977). The major purpose of earlier studies was to demonstrate differences in brain organization between right- and left-handers, and the data (ear differences, for example, in dichotic listening tasks) were therefore expressed as differences between group means (e.g., Zurif and Bryden, 1969). What is needed now to assess interhemispheric language distribution in left-handers is to examine difference scores within individuals—differences between the ears, between the two visual fields, and, in brain-damaged patients, between scores on different types of language tasks. What seems already clear, however, is that the distribution of language functions in the brains of left-handed individuals is more variable and probably more diffusely organized than it is in right-handers (Hécaen and Sauget, 1971; Brown and Hécaen, 1976).*

Changes in Language Distribution during Ontogeny

Although there is already evidence of left hemisphere specialization for language in the neonate (Molfese *et al.*, 1975), the right hemisphere is able to assume control of language function if the left is damaged early in life—at least up to age 5 (Krashen, 1973) and possibly until puberty (Lenneberg, 1967). This raises the question of whether language develops for a time in both hemispheres, or whether the right acquires language de novo when the need arises. The strongest evidence for early right hemisphere involvement in language function is the much higher incidence of language deficits with right-sided lesions in children than in adults—about 30% as compared with 4% (Witelson, 1976). This difference is the more impressive if one considers, as Witelson (1976) has done, that these reports of childhood aphasia are based primarily on clinical impressions of language output, and that verbal output appears to be the most left lateralized of all language functions in the adult.

But in evaluating this evidence it must be remembered that the functional consequences of brain damage are generally less specific in children than adults. The childhood aphasias produced by left hemisphere lesions, whatever their location, always involve restricted verbal output; fluent, Wernicke-type aphasias of the adult type are not seen in children (Brown and Hécaen, 1976). Whether the differences between children and adults reflect maturational changes in brain function that allow specific subsystems to operate more independently or whether actual shifts in functional localization occur is not yet clear. It is possible, as Brown and Hécaen (1976) have suggested, that the more symmetrical distribution of language functions between the hemispheres and the apparent lack of intrahemispheric specialization in children both reflect a tendency toward diffuse organization of language functions in the immature brain. With maturation, language would become progressively left lateralized, and its functions better differentiated

---

*Evidence from dichotic listening experiments suggests that there is variability in the degree of lateralization of language functions in the right-handed population as well (Shankweiler and Studdert-Kennedy, 1975). However, variability seems to be more common and more extreme in the left-handers.

OSCAR S. M. MARIN,
MYRNA F. SCHWARTZ,
AND ELEANOR M.
SAFFRAN

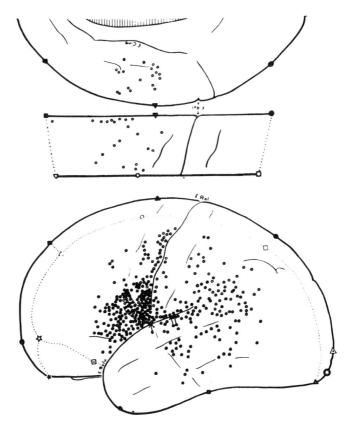

Fig. 1. Left hemisphere loci where electrical stimulation resulted in interference with speech production. The types of interference included total speech arrest, hesitation, slurring, repetition of words and syllables, word substitutions, and inability to name. The stimulation points in the upper portion of the figure lie within the supplementary motor area. From Penfield and Roberts (1959).

within the left hemisphere itself. Brown and Hécaen further suggest that bilateral language representation in left-handers be viewed as an arrest in this process; language bilaterality in left-handers would then be explained as incomplete left lateralization rather than as anomalous migration of language to the right.

DISTRIBUTION OF LANGUAGE IN THE LEFT HEMISPHERE

From brain lesion and stimulation data, it is possible to identify an area of the left hemisphere that plays a special role in language. Stimulation within this area momentarily disrupts speech production (Penfield and Roberts, 1959), and lesions within its boundaries produce at least a temporary but often a permanent impairment of language function (e.g., Conrad, 1954; Russell and Espir, 1961). It will be seen from Figs. 1 and 2 that this area is primarily confined to the lateral surface of the left hemisphere,* and that it includes and surrounds the auditory receptive

*The stimulation studies of Penfield and Roberts (1959) suggest that the more dorsal supplementary motor area (Fig. 1) is also involved, but language disturbances have rarely been reported with lesions in this area.

area in the temporal lobe and the inferior Rolandic motor area that controls the face and tongue. There is some evidence from studies based on well-circumscribed surgical excisions that the area just in front and just behind the Rolandic fissure may not be essential for language function (Rasmussen and Milner, 1975), in which case the language cortex would take on a more bifurcated appearance. In any event, lesions outside this general area do not seem to result in language impairment (Fig. 2).

The task of localizing particular aspects of language function *within* the left hemisphere language cortex is more difficult and much more controversial. There is a wide range of opinion, from the views of extreme localizationists who have proposed specific centers for writing and the like (e.g., Exner, 1881; Henschen, 1920) to antilocalizationists who maintain that the language area functions as a whole (e.g., Jackson, 1932; Marie, 1926). In the middle ground, there has been fairly widespread acceptance of a neuroanatomical model first proposed by Wernicke (1874) and recently revived by Geschwind (1970). The model (Fig. 3) postulates two language centers, a speech reception center in the left temporal lobe (Wernicke's area) and an expressive component located more anteriorly in the frontal lobe (Broca's area); a fiber tract that connects these two areas (the arcuate fasciculus) permits imitation of speech sounds and facilitates vocal learning.

The model is simple, and in its translation of linguistic associations into connections in the brain is intuitively appealing. But it is limited in the kinds of functions it attempts to explain—syntactic and semantic processes, for example, are excluded—and will not, therefore, serve the purposes of the linguist or psychologist who is interested in how language, as he defines it, is organized in the

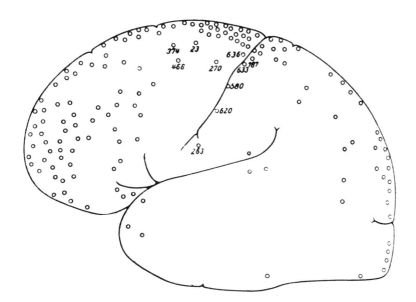

Fig. 2. Sites where damage to the left hemisphere did not give rise to language disturbances. The circles correspond to the approximate centers of the lesions as indicated by skull defects. The numbered circles indicate cases that were regarded as anomalous. From Conrad (1954).

OSCAR S. M. MARIN,
MYRNA F. SCHWARTZ,
AND ELEANOR M.
SAFFRAN

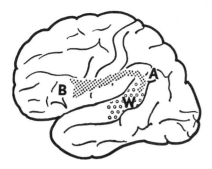

Fig. 3. Location of Broca's (B) and Wernicke's (W) areas and the arcuate fasciculus (A) connecting them. From Geschwind (1970).

brain. Taken even on its own terms, the model is not firmly supported by the available data. Mohr (1976) has shown, contrary to widespread belief, that Broca's area (the foot of the third frontal convolution (see Fig. 3) is not essential to language production; speech is no more than transiently affected unless the lesion extends beyond Broca's area. This conclusion has been reached by other investigators as well (e.g., Conrad, 1954; Penfield and Roberts, 1959). With respect to the posterior speech zone, there is no doubt that the area around the temporoparietal junction is critically involved in language comprehension; but the location of Wernicke's area, operationally defined as the region which, when damaged, gives rise to Wernicke's aphasia (see Goodglass and Kaplan, this volume, for a description of this syndrome), is not at all clear (Bogen and Bogen, 1976). The role of the arcuate pathway in relating the functions of the anterior and posterior speech zones has also been questioned (Rasmussen and Milner, 1975).

In fact, if we adhere closely to the data, we find that we can say little about the neuroanatomical distribution of language beyond the fact that there seem to be two poles of activity within the language area, that these two poles are in the proximity of cortical mechanisms for motor control and for auditory reception, and that these areas differ somewhat in function.

Lesions in the anterior, Rolandic portion of the language area tend to result in disturbances that are predominantly, but not exclusively, of an expressive nature (Figs. 4 and 5). Some of these disturbances are purely articulatory (Fig. 4), while in other cases more central aspects of the language processes are involved as well (Fig. 5). The data in Figs. 4 and 5 are taken from a study by Conrad (1954), who does not provide a detailed description of these more linguistic impairments; however, since he refers to the cases in Fig. 5 as "Broca's aphasias," we can assume that they correspond to a disorder characterized by nonfluent,* poorly articulated, agrammatic speech production with generally well-preserved comprehension (see Goodglass and Kaplan, this volume, for further description).

More posterior lesions, in the region of the temporoparietal junction, affect both receptive and expressive language functions (Fig. 6). The receptive symptomology runs the gamut from isolated disorders of phoneme perception (e.g., Saffran *et al.*, 1976) to generalized comprehension disturbances that may not involve phonetic impairment (Blumstein, 1978). The expressive component of

*It has been held that decreased fluency is diagnostic of a pre-Rolandic lesion (Benson, 1967). However, recent data indicate that fluency may be compromised by posterior lesions as well (Karis and Horenstein, 1976).

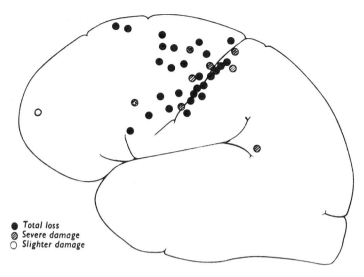

Fig. 4. Sites where lesions produced only articulatory disturbances, other language functions remaining intact. As in Fig. 2, each circle indicates the midpoint of the skull defect, not the actual extent of the lesion. From Conrad (1954).

these posterior aphasias seems primarily to involve lexical and phonemic selection, as opposed to syntactic structure and phonemic articulation (e.g., Jakobson, 1971; Luria, 1975; Marin *et al.,* 1976). Disturbances of lexical function alone can occur with lesions over a wide area of the left hemisphere (Fig. 6), a fact that is consistent with the obvious complexity of the naming process, which involves mechanisms ranging from perceptual operations to articulation (e.g., Geschwind, 1967). One further generalization that can be made with a fair degree of certainty is that posterior lesions, extending from the posterior temporoparietal area into the

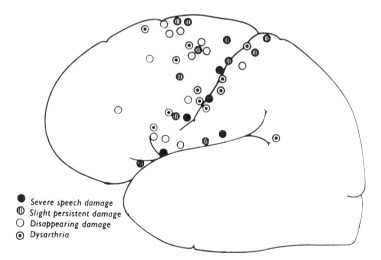

Fig. 5. Sites where lesions resulted in Broca's aphasias. As in preceding figures, circles are central points of skull defects. From Conrad (1954).

OSCAR S. M. MARIN,
MYRNA F. SCHWARTZ,
AND ELEANOR M.
SAFFRAN

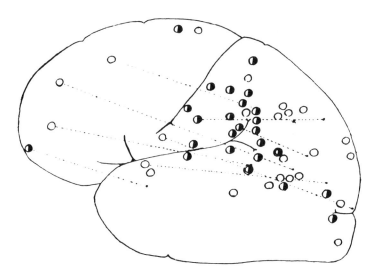

Fig. 6. Sites where the lesion resulted in word-finding deficits (○) and word-finding deficits combined with receptive disturbances (◐). Again, the circles correspond to the midpoints of skull defects. From Conrad (1954).

occipital lobe, can specifically disrupt reading (e.g., Russell and Espir, 1961; Hécaen and de Angelergues, 1964).

While the localization picture as presented in Figs. 4–6 would probably be acceptable to most aphasiologists, it should be cautioned that the actual data are a good deal less precise than the maps would seem to indicate. Each point in these figures represents the center of a trephine hole or a skull fracture, not a well-circumscribed, punctate lesion. The Conrad (1954) study from which these figures are drawn is not atypical in this respect; most large-scale attempts to localize language function have been based on skull data (e.g., Russell and Espir, 1961; Luria, 1970) rather than on the more accurate but less readily obtainable information provided by histological examination or surgical excision. The lesion data that comprise the bulk of the evidence for language localization are, therefore, fairly gross, and other methods that might be used for this purpose, such as brain stimulation and recording, have not yet proved to be discriminative enough to localize particular aspects of language function. Fortunately, there is hope for the future in new computerized radiographic techniques that can localize brain lesions fairly easily and precisely. But even if the localization problem can be solved, there remain some difficulties in the design and interpretation of lesion studies, and it may be worthwhile to discuss them here.

The lesion method has inherent limitations; as Jackson (1884) pointed out long ago, localizing a symptom is not necessarily the same as localizing a function, and we are not always careful about making this distinction. In the case of language, it is conceivable that the pattern of deficit seen in some patients with left hemisphere lesions represents the expression of right hemisphere language capacity rather than residual left hemisphere function. We might, for example, observe relative sparing of lexical compared with syntactic function in some patients, not because the lesion differentially affects syntax, but because the right hemisphere is able to support one of these functions more adequately than it can the other. It has in fact been shown that deactivation of the right hemisphere by intracarotid amytal injection suppresses residual language function in some aphasic patients (Kinsbourne, 1971, 1975). There is need to devise some less stressful means of evaluating right hemisphere contributions to language behavior and to incorporate this test into future studies of language localization.

Of more difficulty is the nature of the lesion itself. The brain insult—usually a biological accident, uncontrollable in location or extent—would seem an inappropriate tool with which to probe so complex a functional system. We have been encouraged to find, however, that in at least some proportion of cases the lesion rather specifically disrupts a particular aspect of language function (Marin *et al.*, 1976). The challenge for neuropsychology is how best to make use of this information. As we have pointed out before (Marin *et al.*, 1976), the selection of the independent variable is a critical question in this research: do we ask what changes in language behavior result from damage to a particular part of the brain, or do we begin with a particular kind of language deficit and *then* determine the site of the responsible lesion? Were we dealing with controlled, delimited lesions, this decision might not appreciably affect the outcome of our study (although it is certainly conceivable that various linguistic subsystems so overlap in their anatomical distribution that small differences in the lesion might result in large differences in behavior). But in the case of aphasia we clearly are not; the lesions are often fairly large, almost always irregular, and rarely reproducible. From the standpoint of experimental design, it makes more sense for the experimenter to designate as the independent variable the parameter over which he has most control. In this case, the linguistic parameter can be carefully specified, using the appropriate language tasks, while there is no comparable control over the anatomical variable; to designate the lesion as the fixed parameter is therefore to introduce unnecessary variation. The linguistic variable would also seem to have a logical priority in this research; if we are interested in delineating functional systems in the brain, we should frame the inquiry in terms of the functional units we wish to uncover. We would argue, therefore, that the first consideration in aphasia research should be the specification of the language variable. Cases must be selected on a linguistic basis and the lesion data organized with respect to linguistic criteria.

Given that we do not yet have such data, what can we say about the localization of particular aspects of language function within the brain? The speculations that follow are based on observed patterns of association and dissociation of symptoms in aphasia (see also Marin *et al.*, 1976; Goodglass and Geschwind, 1976).

While there is little direct evidence to link syntactic function, per se, with particular brain structures, there is a strong association, in aphasia, between syntactic impairment and disturbances of articulation; it is possible to find articulatory deficits without loss of syntax, but cases of agrammatism rarely, if ever, occur without concomitant articulatory impairment. There is some evidence that patients with agrammatic speech production (for a description, see Goodglass and Geschwind, 1976; Goodglass and Kaplan, this volume) also have specific deficits in

OSCAR S. M. MARIN,
MYRNA F. SCHWARTZ,
AND ELEANOR M.
SAFFRAN

syntactic comprehension, other aspects of language comprehension remaining intact (Caramazza and Zurif, 1976; Scholes, 1978; Schwartz *et al.*, 1978). The deficit therefore appears to be truly a syntactic one, and the association with articulatory impairment clearly implicates structures in the anterior part of the language area (Fig. 5), where the final organization of the instructions to the vocal apparatus is likely to take place. The association between articulatory and syntactic deficit has been pointed out before, and, as Jakobson (1971) has argued, there are some similarities between these processes; both involve the combination and sequencing of elements—phonemes in the one case, lexemes and morphemes in the other—and both may therefore depend on the same basic type of neuronal organization.

The fact that lexical processes can be disrupted independently of syntactic operations, both as a result of focal brain injury (Marin *et al.*, 1976) and in cases of diffuse cortical degeneration (Whitaker, 1976; Schwartz *et al.*, in press), suggests that lexical functions depend on a different kind of neuronal organization. Lexical operations are probably more diffusely organized than syntactic functions; they may even extend into the right hemisphere where, as we have seen above, there are some indications of lexical representation. There is also some evidence that lexical processes, particularly referential processes, tend to be localized more posteriorly in the brain (Fig. 6), in closer proximity to the perceptual systems that provide the sense data for reference.

With respect to phonological operations, the data present a confusing picture. Evidence from patients with unilateral lesions (Oscar-Berman *et al.*, 1975; Saffran *et al.*, 1976) certainly points to a left hemisphere locus for phonetic processing, but the split-brain and hemispherectomy data are ambiguous on this point. Within the left hemisphere, the auditory association area of the temporal lobe seems a likely locus, but recent studies of speech perception in aphasic patients indicate that phonetic deficits are not reliably associated with particular aphasic syndromes and hence, one might conclude, with particular anatomical loci (Blumstein, 1978; Blumstein *et al.*, 1977). It has been claimed, in fact, that deficits in phonetic perception occur more frequently in patients with articulatory disorders than in patients with posterior aphasic syndromes (Basso *et al.*, 1977), an association that would seem to provide support for a motor theory of speech perception (Liberman *et al.*, 1967). It is possible, however, that patients with anterior lesions have particular difficulty with the kinds of tasks used to study phonetic analysis rather than with phonemic perception per se.

On the production side, phonological errors are found in patients with both anterior and posterior lesions (e.g., Blumstein, 1973). This is consistent with a model of language organization in which instructions for lexical items originate in posterior brain mechanisms but are sent forward to anterior motor speech mechanisms for final assembly and output.

SUBCORTICAL STRUCTURES AND LANGUAGE

Interest in the possible role of subcortical structures in language has centered on certain thalamic nuclei, principally the ventrolateral nucleus and the pulvinar and, to a lesser extent, the globus pallidus. Both lesions and stimulation in these areas cause some disruption of language behavior, particularly when the affected structure is on the left (e.g., Fedio and Van Buren, 1975; Riklan and Cooper, 1975; Ojemann, 1976). Insofar as it has been tested, language comprehension does not appear to be affected; the deficits are most evident in tests of verbal memory function and in certain aspects of speech production. Word-finding difficulty has been reported with both thalamic and pallidal lesions, and anomic responses, including paraphasia and perseveration, have been observed with stimulation of the ventrolateral nucleus and portions of the pulvinar (Ojemann, 1976). Others have described effects on the timing, accuracy, completeness, and fluency of oral expression (Darley *et al.*, 1975; Riklan and Cooper, 1975).

Rather than inferring from this evidence that these subcortical structures are specifically involved in particular aspects of the language process, we can explain the effects in terms of changes in the activation or tone of the speech cortex. Similar effects on naming and on verbal memory, and on parameters such as the rate and flow of speech, are observed in fatigue and in various toxic and drug states and are best interpreted as signs of cortical inefficiency rather than as indices of specific functional involvement. The effects appear to have some specificity because some stages of language processing may be more dependent on high levels of cerebral activation (Riklan and Cooper, 1975). Whether the lateralized nature of these thalamic and pallidal influences reflects only the predominance of ipsilateral connections from these subcortical areas to the speech cortex, or whether there is something intrinsically linguistic about these influences (they might, for example, form part of a specific attentional mechanism for language), is not yet clear.*

SOME IMPLICATIONS FOR LANGUAGE ORIGINS

Thus while other neural systems may play a supportive role in language behavior, the language apparatus itself seems fairly well restricted to the area of the left hemisphere delineated earlier in this chapter, with perhaps some limited representation in the right hemisphere as well. As we suggested, the differences between left and right hemispheric language functions may give us some further clues to the nature and perhaps to the origins of left hemisphere specialization for language.

Current evidence suggests that vocal output is the most completely lateralized aspect of language function, while lexical processes appear to have the most bilateral distribution. We know less about the extent to which the right hemisphere shares in syntactic and phonological functions, but the available data suggest that its abilities in these areas are less well developed than its capacity for lexical representation.

How can we account for what appears to be strongly left-lateralized control over the vocal apparatus? As Marin (1976) has commented, the vocal organ is unusual among structures under voluntary control in that it is unitary. Paired

*For a more extensive review of this problem, we refer the reader to Ojemann (1976) and to *Brain and Language,* Vol. 2, No. 1, 1975, an entire issue devoted to this subject.

OSCAR S. M. MARIN,
MYRNA F. SCHWARTZ,
AND ELEANOR M.
SAFFRAN

structures, like the forelimbs, are each represented on different sides of the brain, but the vocal apparatus is innervated by both hemispheres. Thus it might be open to conflicting articulatory instructions if both hemispheres were capable of providing them. It may be for this reason that *functional* control over the vocal apparatus is well lateralized, which appears to be the case for other complex behaviors like bird song (Nottebohm and Nottebohm, 1976) as well as for language in man.

The choice of the left over the right hemisphere as the locus for motor speech organization almost certainly had to do with an earlier established right-hand preference in the hominid line (Dart, 1949). Vocal sequencing and manual sequencing may depend on the same basic type of neural organization, a possibility that receives some support from the association between linguistic and apraxic disturbances with posterior left hemisphere lesions (Kimura, 1976). Given that motor control for language had become established in the left hemisphere, there might then have been a tendency for other language functions to organize themselves in proximity to the motor speech cortex; thus the left hemisphere would have been the locus for the increasing specialization of auditory mechanisms that would provide the perceptual basis for vocal learning, as well as for the development of syntactic mechanisms involved in the higher-order programming of motor speech output. Aspects of lexical representation might develop, to some extent, in both hemispheres, because of their relationship to perceptual function.

A rather similar argument has recently been made by Premack (1976a). Commenting on the evidence that other species have shown some capacity to perceive acoustic stimuli categorically, Premack goes on to say:

> The neuroanatomical properties underlying categorical perception, be it of speech or non-speech sounds, may be quite primitive. Consider that monkeys have relatively little voluntary control of vocalization and yet discriminate speech sounds categorically. Speech-sound discrimination may thus depend on properties of the auditory system laid down before brain lateralization and even before encephalization of the auditory-vocal system. This could suggest that the productive and receptive structures for speech had separate evolutionary histories, the receptive occurring well before the productive. From this one might infer that lateralization had more to do with the production than with the comprehension of speech sounds. (Premack, 1976*a*, p. 558)

We should add, with Premack (1976*a*), that "all of this is recognizably speculative."

REFERENCES

Andrew, R. J. Use of formants in the grunts of baboons and other nonhuman primates. *Annals of the New York Academy of Sciences,* 1976, *280*, 673–693.

Basso, A., Casati, G., and Vignolo, L. A. Phonemic identification defect in aphasia. *Cortex,* 1977, *13*, 84–95.

Beer, C. Some complexities in the communication behavior of gulls. *Annals of the New York Academy of Sciences,* 1976, *280*, 413–432.

Benson, D. F. Fluency in aphasia: Correlation with radioactive scan localization. *Cortex,* 1967, *3*, 373–394.

Blumstein, S. E. *A Phonological Investigation of Aphasic Speech.* The Hague: Mouton, 1973.

Blumstein, S. E. The perception of speech in pathology and ontogeny. In A. Caramazza and E. B. Zurif (eds.). *The Acquisition and Breakdown of Language: Parallels and Divergencies.* Baltimore: Johns Hopkins University Press, 1978.

Blumstein, S. E., Baker, E., and Goodglass, H. Phonological factors in auditory comprehension in aphasia. *Neuropsychologia,* 1977, *15,* 19–30.

Bogen, J. E., and Bogen, G. M. Wernicke's region—Where is it? *Annals of the New York Academy of Sciences,* 1976, *280,* 834–843.

Branch, C., Milner, B., and Rasmussen, T. Intracarotid sodium amytal for the lateralization of cerebral speech dominance: Observations in 123 patients. *Journal of Neurosurgery.* 1964, *21,* 399–405.

Brown, J. W., and Hécaen, H. Lateralization and language representation. *Neurology,* 1976, *26,* 183–189.

Butler, S. R., and Glass, A. EEG correlates of cerebral dominance. In A. H. Riesen and R. F. Thompson (eds.), *Advances in Psychobiology,* Vol. 3. New York: Wiley, 1976.

Caramazza, A., and Zurif, E. B. Dissociation of algorithmic and heuristic processes in language comprehension: Evidence from aphasia. *Brain and Language,* 1976, *3,* 572–582.

Conrad, K. New problems of aphasia. *Brain,* 1954, *77,* 491–509.

Cooper, W. E. Adaptation of phonetic feature analyzers for place of articulation. *Journal of the Acoustical Society of America,* 1974, *56,* 617–628.

Darley, F. L., Brown, J. R., and Swenson, W. M. Language changes after neurosurgery for Parkinsonism. *Brain and Language,* 1975, *2,* 65–69.

Dart, R. A. The predatory implemental technique of *Australopithecus. American Journal of Physical Anthropology,* 1949, *7,* 1–38.

Davenport, R. K. Cross-modal perception in apes. *Annals of the New York Academy of Sciences,* 1976, *280,* 143–149.

Day, J. The right hemisphere knows concrete words but not abstract ones. Paper presented to the Eastern Psychological Association, New York, April 1976.

Dennis, M., and Kohn, B. Comprehension of syntax in infantile hemiplegics after cerebral hemidecortication: Left-hemisphere superiority. *Brain and Language,* 1975, *2,* 472–482.

Dennis, M. and Whitaker, H. A. Language acquisition following hemidecortication. *Brain and Language,* 1976, *3,* 404–433.

Denny-Brown, D. *The Cerebral Control of Movement.* Springfield, Ill.: Thomas, 1966.

Dingwall, W. O. The species-specificity of speech. *Georgetown University Round Table on Language and Linguistics.* Washington, D.C.: Georgetown University Press, 1975, 17–62.

Dusser de Barenne, J. G., Carol, H. W., and McCulloch, W. S. The "motor" cortex of the chimpanzee. *Journal of Neurophysiology,* 1941, *4,* 287–303.

Eimas, P. D. Auditory and linguistic processing of cues for place of articulation by infants. *Perception and Psychophysics,* 1974, *16,* 513–521.

Eimas, P. D., and Corbit, J. D. Selective adaptation of linguistic feature detectors. *Cognitive Psychology,* 1973, *4,* 99–109.

Eimas, P. D., Siqueland, E. R., Jusczyk, P., and Vigorito, J. Speech perception in infants. *Science,* 1971, *171,* 303–306.

Ellis, H. D., and Shepherd, J. W. Recognition of abstract and concrete words presented in the left and right visual fields. *Journal of Experimental Psychology,* 1974, *103,* 1035–1036.

Exner, S. *Untersuchungen über die Lokalisation der Funktionen in der Grosshirnrinde des Menschen.* Vienna: W. Braumuller, 1881.

Fedio, P., and Van Buren, J. M. Memory and perceptual deficits during electrical stimulation in the left and right thalamus and parietal subcortex. *Brain and Language,* 1975, *2,* 78–100.

Gardner, R., and Gardner, B. Teaching sign language to a chimpanzee. *Science,* 1969, *165,* 664–672.

Gazzaniga, M. S. *The Bisected Brain.* New York: Appleton-Century-Crofts, 1970.

Gazzaniga, M. S., and Hillyard, S. A. Language and speech capacity of the right hemisphere. *Neuropsychologia,* 1971, *9,* 273–280.

Geschwind, N. The development of the brain and the origin of language. *Monograph Series on Language and Linguistics,* No. 17. Washington, D.C.: Georgetown Universtiy Press, 1964.

Geschwind, N. Disconnexion syndromes in animals and man: Parts I and II. *Brain,* 1965, *88,* 237–294; 585–644.

Geschwind, N. The varieties of naming errors. *Cortex,* 1967, *3,* 97–112.

Geschwind, N. The organization of language and the brain. *Science,* 1970, *170,* 940–944.

Geschwind, N., and Fusillo, M. Color-naming defects in association with alexia. *Archives of Neurology,* 1966, *15,* 137–146.

Geschwind, N., and Kaplan, E. A human cerebral deconnection syndrome. *Neurology,* 1962, *12,* 675–685.

Geschwind, N., and Levitsky, W. Human brain: Left-right asymmetries in temporal speech region. *Science*, 1968, *161*, 186.

Gloning, I., Gloning, K., Haub, G., and Quatember, R. Comparison of verbal behavior in right-handed and non right-handed patients with anatomically verified lesion of one hemisphere. *Cortex*, 1969, *5*, 43–52.

Goodglass, H., and Geschwind, N. Language disorders (aphasia). In E. C. Carterette and M. Friedman (eds.), *Handbook of Perception*, Vol. VII. New York: Academic Press, 1976.

Gott, P. Language following dominant hemispherectomy. *Journal of Neurology, Neurosurgery and Psychiatry*, 1973, *36*, 1082–1088.

Green, S. Variation of vocal pattern with social situation in the Japanese monkey (*Macaca fuscata*): A field study. In L. A. Rosenblum (ed.), *Primate Behavior*, Vol. 4. New York: Academic Press, 1975.

Hécaen, H. and de Angelergues, R. Localization of symptoms in aphasia. In A. V. S. de Reuck and M. O'Connor (eds.), *Disorders of Language*. London: Churchill, 1964.

Hécaen, H., and Sauget, J. Cerebral dominance in left-handed subjects. *Cortex*, 1971, *7*, 19–48.

Henschen, S. E. *Klinische und Anatomische Beitrage zur Pathologie des Gehirns*, Vols. 5, 6, and 7. Stockholm: Nordiska Bokhandeln, 1920–1922.

Hewes, G. W. Primate communication and the gestural origin of language. *Current Anthropology*, 1973, *14*, 5–12.

Hines, D. Recognition of verbs, abstract nouns and concrete nouns from the left and right visual half-fields. *Neuropsychologia*, 1976, *14*, 211–216.

Hines, D. Differences in tachistoscopic recognition between abstract and concrete words as a function of visual half-field and frequency. *Cortex*, 1977, *13*, 66–73.

Holloway, R. L. Paleoneurological evidence for language origins. *Annals of the New York Academy of Sciences*, 1976, *280*, 900–912.

Itani, J. Vocal communication of the wild Japanese monkey. *Primates*, 1963, *4*, 11–66.

Jackson, J. H. The evolution and dissolution of the nervous system. *British Medical Journal*, 1884, *1*, 591, 660, 703.

Jackson, J. H. *Selected Writings of J. Hughlings-Jackson*. J. Taylor (ed.). London: Hodder and Stoughton, 1932.

Jakobson, R. Linguistic types of aphasia. In *Roman Jakobson, Selected Writings II*. The Hague: Mouton, 1971.

Jaynes, J. The evolution of language in the late Pleistocene. *Annals of the New York Academy of Sciences*, 1976, *280*, 312–325.

Jurgens, U. Correlation between brain structure and vocalization type elicited in the squirrel monkey. *Proceedings of the Second International Congress of Primatology* (Atlanta, Ga.), 1969, *3*, 28–33.

Jurgens, U., Maurus, M., Ploog, D., and Winter, P. Vocalization in the squirrel monkey (*Saimiri sciureus*) elicited by brain stimulation. *Experimental Brain Research*, 1967, *4*, 114–117.

Kaada, B. R. Somato-motor, autonomic, and electrocorticographic responses to electrical stimulation of "rhinencephalic" and other structures in primates, cat and dog. *Acta Physiologica Scandinavica*, 1951, *24* (Suppl. No. 83).

Karis, R., and Horenstein, S. Localization of speech parameters by brain scan. *Neurology*, 1976, *26*, 226–230.

Kimura, D. Functional asymmetry of the brain in dichotic listening. *Cortex*, 1967, *3*, 163–178.

Kimura, D. The neural basis of language qua gesture. In H. Whitaker and H. A. Whitaker (eds.), *Studies in Neurolinguistics*, Vol. 2. New York: Academic Press, 1976.

Kinsbourne, M. The minor cerebral hemisphere as a source of aphasic speech. *Archives of Neurology*, 1971, *25*, 302–306.

Kinsbourne, M. Mechanisms of hemispheric interaction in man. In M. Kinsbourne and W. L. Smith (eds.), *Hemispheric Deconnection and Cerebral Function*. Springfield, Ill.: Thomas, 1974.

Kinsbourne, M. Minor hemisphere language and cerebral maturation. In E. H. Lenneberg and E. Lenneberg (eds.), *Foundations of Language Development: A Multidisciplinary Approach*, Vol. 2. New York: Academic Press, 1975.

Kinsbourne, M., and Cook, J. Generalized and lateralized effects of concurrent verbalization on a unimanual skill. *Quarterly Journal of Experimental Psychology*, 1971, *23*, 341–345.

Konishi, M., and Nottebohm, F. Experimental studies in the ontogeny of avian vocalizations. In R. A. Hinde (ed.), *Bird Vocalizations*. Cambridge: Cambridge University Press, 1969, pp. 29–48.

Krashen, S. Lateralization, language learning, and the critical period: Some new evidence. *Language Learning*, 1973, *23*, 63–74.

Kuhl, P. K., and Miller, J. D. Speech perception by the chinchilla: Voiced-voiceless distinction in alveolar plosive consonants. *Science*, 1975, *190*, 69–72.

Lancaster, J. B. Primate communication systems and the emergence of human language. In P. C. Jay (ed.), *Primates*. New York: Holt, 1968.

Laughlin, C. D., and d'Aquili, E. G. *Biogenetic Structuralism*. New York: Columbia University Press, 1974.

Lenneberg, E. H. *Biological Foundations of Language*. New York: Wiley, 1967.

Lenneberg, E. H. In search of a dynamic theory of aphasia. In E. H. Lenneberg and E. Lenneberg (eds.), *Foundations of Language Development: A Multidisciplinary Approach*, Vol. 2. New York: Academic Press, 1975.

Lesser, R. Verbal comprehension in aphasia: An English version of three Italian tests. *Cortex*, 1974, *10*, 247–263.

Levy, J. Psychological implications of bilateral asymmetry. In S. J. Diamond and J. G. Beaumont (eds.), *Hemisphere Function in the Human Brain*. New York: Wiley, 1974.

Levy, J., Nebes, R. D., and Sperry, R. W. Expressive language in the surgically separated minor hemisphere. *Cortex*, 1971, *7*, 49–58.

Liberman, A. M., Cooper, F. S., Shankweiler, D., and Studdert-Kennedy, M. Perception of the speech code. *Psychological Review*, 1967, *74*, 431–461.

Lieberman, P. Primate vocalizations and human linguistic ability. *Journal of the Acoustical Society of America*, 1968, *44*, 1574–1584.

Lieberman, P. On the evolution of language: A unified view. *Cognition*, 1973, *2*, 59–94.

Lishman, W. A., and McMeekan, E. R. L. Handedness in relation to direction and degree of cerebral dominance for language. *Cortex*, 1977, *13*, 30–43.

Lomas, J., and Kimura, D. Interhemispheric interaction between speaking and sequential manual activity. *Neuropsychologia*, 1976, *14*, 23–33.

Luria, A. R. *Higher Cortical Functions in Man*. New York: Basic Books, 1966.

Luria, A. R. *Traumatic Aphasia*. The Hague: Mouton, 1970.

Luria, A. R. Basic problems of language in the light of psychology and neurolinguistics. In E. H. Lenneberg and E. Lenneberg (eds.), *Foundations of Language Development: A Multidisciplinary Approach*, Vol. 2. New York: Academic Press, 1975.

Marie, P. *Travaux et Mémoires*, Vol. 1. Paris: Masson, 1926.

Marin, O. S. M. Neurobiology of language: An overview. *Annals of the New York Academy of Sciences*, 1976, *280*, 900–912.

Marin, O. S. M., Saffran, E. M., and Schwartz, M. F. Dissociations of language in aphasia: Implications for normal function. *Annals of the New York Academy of Sciences*, 1976, *280*, 868–884.

Marler, P. On the origin of speech from animal sounds. In J. F. Kavanagh and J. E. Cutting (eds.), *The Role of Speech in Language*. Cambridge, Mass.: MIT Press, 1975.

Marler, P. An ethological theory of the origin of vocal learning. *Annals of the New York Academy of Sciences*, 1976, *280*, 386–395.

Mattingly, I. G. Speech cues and sign stimuli. *American Scientist*, 1972, *60*, 327–337.

Maturana, H. R. *Biology of Cognition*. Biological Computer Laboratory, Report 9.0. Urbana, Ill.: Department of Electrical Engineering, University of Illinois, 1970.

McGlone, J., and Davidson, W. The relation between cerebral speech laterality and spatial ability with special reference to sex and handedness. *Neuropsychologia*, 1973, *11*, 108–113.

McKeever, W., and Huling, M. Lateral dominance in tachistoscopic word recognition performances obtained with simultaneous bilateral input. *Neuropsychologia*, 1971, *9*, 15–20.

McKeever, W. F., Gill, K. M., and Van Deventer, A. D. Letter versus dot stimuli as tools for "splitting the normal brain with reaction time." *Quarterly Journal of Experimental Psychology*, 1975, *27*, 363–373.

Menzel, E. W. A group of young chimpanzees in a one-acre field. In A. M. Schrier and F. Stollnitz (eds.), *Behavior of Nonhuman Primates*, Vol. 5. New York: Academic Press, 1974.

Miller, C. L., and Morse, P. A. The "heart" of categorical speech discrimination in young infants. *Journal of Speech and Hearing Research*, 1976, *19*, 578–589.

Milner, B. Hemispheric specialization: Scope and limits. In F. O. Schmitt and F. G. Worden (eds.), *The Neurosciences: Third Study Program*. Cambridge, Mass.: MIT Press, 1974.

Milner, P. M. *Physiological Psychology*. New York: Holt, Rinehart and Winston, 1970.

Mohr, J. P. Broca's area and Broca's aphasia. In H. Whitaker and H. A. Whitaker (eds.), *Studies in Neurolinguistics*, Vol. 1. New York: Academic Press, 1976.

Molfese, D. L., Freeman, R. B., and Palermo, D. S. The ontogeny of brain lateralization for speech and non-speech stimuli. *Brain and Language*, 1975, *2*, 356–368.

Morrell, L. K., and Salamy, J. G. Hemispheric asymmetry of electrocortical responses to speech stimuli. *Science*, 1971, *174*, 164–166.

OSCAR S. M. MARIN,
MYRNA F. SCHWARTZ,
AND ELEANOR M.
SAFFRAN
Morse, P. A. Speech perception in the human infant and rhesus monkey. *Annals of the New York Academy of Sciences,* 1976, *280*, 694–707.

Morse, P. A., and Snowdon, C. T. An investigation of categorical speech discrimination by rhesus monkeys. *Perception and Psychophysics,* 1975, *17*, 9–16.

Moscovitch, M. Language and the cerebral hemispheres: Reaction time studies and their implications for models of cerebral dominance. In P. Pliner, L. Krames, and T. Alloway (eds.), *Communication and Affect: Language and Thought.* New York: Academic Press, 1973.

Moscovitch, M. On the representation of language in the right hemisphere of right-handed people. *Brain and Language,* 1976a, *3*, 47–71.

Moscovitch, M. On interpreting data regarding the linguistic competence and performance of the right hemisphere: A reply to Selnes. *Brain and Language,* 1976b, *3*, 590–599.

Myers, R. E. Comparative neurology of vocalization and speech: Proof of a dichotomy. *Annals of the New York Academy of Sciences,* 1976, *280*, 745–757.

Nebes, R. D. The nature of internal speech in a patient with aphemia. *Brain and Language,* 1975, *2*, 489–497.

Noback, C. R., and Moskowitz, N. The primate nervous system: Functional and structural aspects in phylogeny. In J. Buettner-Janusch (ed.), *Evolutionary and Genetic Biology of Primates,* Vol. I. New York: Academic Press, 1973.

Nottebohm, F. A zoologist's view of some language phenomena with particular emphasis on vocal learning. In E. H. Lenneberg and E. Lenneberg (eds.), *Foundations of Language Development,* Vol. 1. New York: Academic Press, 1975.

Nottebohm, F., and Nottebohm, M. E. Left hypoglossal dominance in the control of canary and white-crowned sparrow song. *Journal of Comparative Physiology,* Series A, 1976, *108*, 171–192.

Ojemann, G. A. Subcortical language mechanisms. In H. Whitaker and H. A. Whitaker (eds.), *Studies in Neurolinguistics,* Vol. 1. New York: Academic Press, 1976.

Oscar-Berman, M., Zurif, E. B., and Blumstein, S. E. Effects of unilateral brain damage on the processing of speech sounds. *Brain and Language,* 1975, *2*, 345–354.

Penfield, W., and Roberts, L. *Speech and Brain Mechanisms.* Princeton, N.J.: Princeton University Press, 1959.

Premack, D. Language in chimpanzee? *Science,* 1971, *172*, 808–822.

Premack, D. Mechanisms of intelligence: Preconditions for language. *Annals of the New York Academy of Sciences,* 1976a, *280*, 544–561.

Premack, D. *Intelligence in Ape and Man.* New York: Halsted Press, 1976b.

Pribram, K. *Languages of the Brain: Experimental Paradoxes and Principles in Neuropsychology.* Englewood Cliffs, N.J.: Prentice-Hall, 1971.

Rasmussen, T., and Milner, B. Clinical and surgical studies of the cerebral speech areas in man. In K. J. Zulch, O. Creutzfeldt, and G. C. Galbraith (eds.), *Cerebral Localization.* New York: Springer-Verlag, 1975.

Riklan, M., and Cooper, I. S. Psychometric studies of verbal functions following thalamic lesions in humans. *Brain and Language,* 1975, *2*, 45–64.

Robinson, B. W. Vocalization evoked from forebrain in *Macaca mulatta. Physiology and Behavior,* 1967, *2*, 345–354.

Robinson, B. W. Limbic influences on human speech. *Annals of the New York Academy of Sciences,* 1976, *280*, 761–77.

Rowell, T. E., and Hinde, R. A. Vocal communication by the rhesus monkey *(Macaca mulatta). Proceedings of the Zoological Society, London,* 1962, *138*, 279–294.

Rumbaugh, D. M., and Gill, T. V. The mastery of language-type skills by the chimpanzee *(Pan). Annals of the New York Academy of Sciences,* 1976, *280*, 562–578.

Russell, W. R., and Espir, M. L. E. *Traumatic Aphasia.* London: Oxford University Press, 1961.

Saffran, E. M., Marin, O. S. M., and Yeni-Komshian, G. H. An analysis of speech perception in word deafness. *Brain and Language,* 1976, *3*, 209–228.

Saffran, E. M., Marin, O. S. M., Schwartz, M. F., and Rubman, A. C. Two mechanisms of auditory verbal STM impairment in aphasia. Paper presented at the Fifth Annual Meeting of the International Neuropsychology Society, Sante Fe, New Mexico, February 1977.

Schneider, G. E. Two visual systems. *Science,* 1969, *163*, 895–902.

Scholes, R. Syntactic and lexical components of sentence comprehension. In A. Caramazza and E. B. Zurif (eds.), *The Acquisition and Breakdown of Language: Parallels and Divergencies.* Baltimore: Johns Hopkins Press, 1977.

Schwartz, M. F., Marin, O. S. M., and Saffran, E. S. Dissociations of language function in dementia: A case study. *Brain and Language,* in press.

Schwartz, M. F., Saffran, E. M., and Marin, O. S. M. Syntactic comprehension in agrammatic aphasics.

Paper presented to the Sixth Annual Meeting of the International Neuropsychology Society, Minneapolis, February 1978.

Shankweiler, D., and Studdert-Kennedy, M. A continuum of lateralization for speech perception? *Brain and Language,* 1975, *2,* 212–225.

Smith, A. Speech and other functions after left (dominant) hemispherectomy. *Journal of Neurology, Neurosurgery and Psychiatry,* 1966, *29,* 467.

Smith, A. Dominant and nondominant hemispherectomy. In M. Kinsbourne and W. L. Smith (eds.). *Hemispheric Deconnection and Cerebral Function.* Springfield, Ill.: Thomas, 1974.

Smith, W. K. The functional significance of the rostral cingular cortex as revealed by its responses to electrical excitation. *Journal of Neurophysiology,* 1945, *8,* 241–255.

Sparks, R., and Geschwind, N. Dichotic listening in man after section of neocortical commissures. *Cortex,* 1968, *4,* 3–16.

Steklis, H. D., and Harnad, S. R. From hand to mouth: Some critical stages in the evolution of language. *Annals of the New York Academy of Sciences,* 1976, *280,* 445–455.

Studdert-Kennedy, M. The perception of speech. In T. A. Sebeok (ed.), *Current Trends in Linguistics,* Vol. XII. The Hague: Mouton, 1974.

Studdert-Kennedy, M. Speech perception. In N. J. Lass (ed.), *Contemporary Issues in Experimental Phonetics.* Springfield, Ill.: Thomas, 1976.

Studdert-Kennedy, M., and Shankweiler, D. Hemispheric specialization for speech perception. *Journal of the Acoustical Society of America,* 1970, *48,* 579–594.

Studdert-Kennedy, M., Shankweiler, D., and Pisoni, D. Auditory and phonetic processes in speech perception: Evidence from a dichotic study. *Cognitive Psychology,* 1972, *3,* 455–466.

Sugar, O., Chusid, J. G., and French, J. D. A second motor cortex in the monkey *(Macaca mulatta). Journal of Neuropathology and Experimental Neurology,* 1948, *7,* 182–189.

Sutton, D., Larson, C., and Lindeman, R. R. Neocortical and limbic lesion effects on primate phonation. *Brain Research,* 1974, *71,* 61–75.

Tartter, V. C., and Eimas, P. D. The role of auditory feature detectors in the perception of speech. *Perception and Psychophysics,* 1975, *18,* 293–298.

Wada, J. A new method for the determination of the side of cerebral speech dominance: A preliminary report on the intra-carotid injection of sodium amytal in man. *Medical Biology,* 1949, *14,* 221.

Wada, J. A., Clarke, R., and Hamm, A. Cerebral hemispheric asymmetry in humans. *Archives of Neurology,* 1975, *32,* 239–246.

Warren, R. M. Auditory perception and speech evolution. *Annals of the New York Academy of Sciences,* 1976, *280,* 708–717.

Washburn, S. L., and Strum, S. C. Concluding comments. In S. L. Washburn and P. Dolhinow (eds.), *Perspectives on Human Evolution,* Vol. 2. New York: Holt, Rinehart and Winston, 1972, pp. 469–489.

Wernicke, C. The symptom complex of aphasia. Translation of 1874 paper in R. S. Cohen and M. W. Wartofsky (eds.), *Boston Studies in the Philosophy of Science,* Vol. 4. Dordrecht, The Netherlands: Reidel, 1969.

Whitaker, H. A case of the isolation of the language function. In H. Whitaker and H. A. Whitaker (eds.), *Studies in Neurolinguistics,* Vol. 2. New York: Academic Press, 1976.

Witelson, S. F. Early hemisphere specialization and interhemisphere plasticity: An empirical and theoretical review. In S. Segalowitz and F. Gruber (eds.), *Language Development and Neurological Theory.* New York: Academic Press, 1976.

Witelson, S. F., and Pallie, W. Left hemisphere specialization for language in the newborn: Neuroanatomical evidence of asymmetry. *Brain,* 1973, *96,* 641–646.

Wood, C. C. Auditory and phonetic levels of processing in speech perception: Neurophysiological and information processing analyses. *Journal of Experimental Psychology: Human Perception and Performance,* 1975, *104,* 3–20.

Yeni-Komshian, G. H., and Benson, D. A. Anatomical study of cerebral asymmetry in temporal lobe of humans, chimpanzees and rhesus monkeys. *Science,* 1976, *192,* 387–389.

Zaidel, E. Auditory vocabulary in the right hemisphere following brain bisection and hemidecortication. *Cortex,* 1976, *12,* 191–211.

Zaidel, E. Unilateral auditory language comprehension on the Token Test following cerebral commissurotomy and hemispherectomy. *Neuropsychologia,* 1977, *15,* 1–18.

Zaidel, E. Auditory language comprehension in the right hemisphere: A comparison with child language and aphasia. In A. Caramazza and E. B. Zurif (eds.). *The Acquisition and Breakdown of Language: Parallels and Divergencies.* Baltimore: Johns Hopkins University Press, 1978.

Zurif, E. B., and Bryden, M. F. Familial handedness and left-right differences in auditory and visual perception. *Neuropsychologia,* 1969, *7,* 179–187.

9

Thalamic Mechanisms in Language

Jason W. Brown

Introduction

Although there are reports in the early literature of lesions of the thalamus in association with disorders of perception, for example, de Morsier's (1938) case of pulvinar lesion with "peduncular hallucinosis," as well as with disorders of cognition, such as Grunthal's (1942) case of "thalamic dementia," it was not until the monograph by Penfield and Roberts (1959) that attention was focused on the thalamus in relation to language organization. In this monograph, it was proposed that the thalamus, specifically the nucleus pulvinaris, was a way station in language processing between the anterior and posterior speech zones. While no persuasive evidence was presented in support of this hypothesis, it was at least consistent with the enormous expansion of pulvinar over the mammalian series leading to man, as well as with the presence of major fiber pathways between pulvinar and the posterior temporoparietal cortex.

Subsequently, the development of stereotactic surgery for the treatment of movement disorders, particularly for Parkinson's disease and dystonia, led to the investigation of psychological function following surgical lesion in various thalamic sites. In spite of the obvious importance of and interest in this region, it is striking how little we still know of the behavioral consequences of thalamic lesions in man. Unlike other areas, the thalamus is not often preferentially involved in neurological disease, nor is it commonly the site of localized vascular lesion. Surgical ablation has been carried out only in a few nuclear groups and only in subjects with

Jason W. Brown   Department of Neurology, New York University Medical Center, Goldwater Memorial Hospital, Roosevelt Island, New York 10044.

preexisting neurological disorders, so that even there we see the effects on an ongoing pathological state rather than in a normal brain.

Nonetheless, over the last 20 years renewed interest in the role of the thalamus in language and cognition has given rise to new observations and experimental studies. It is the purpose of this chapter to review some of this material in relation to present concepts of language-brain relationships (see Fig. 1).

In man, the pertinent observations can be grouped into the following categories: lesions which result from (1) degenerative, (2) vascular, or (3) neoplastic involvement of the thalamus, or (4) surgical thalamotomy.

DEGENERATIVE LESIONS

Several patients have been described with progressive symmetrical bilateral degeneration of the thalamus. The first case was reported by Stern (1939) in a 41-year-old man with a dementia progressing rapidly over a 1-year period. The

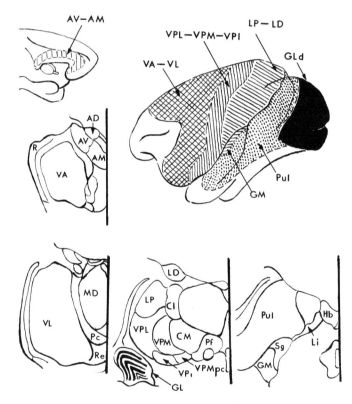

Fig. 1. Thalamic nuclei and cortical projections. VA, n. ventralis anterior; AM, n. anteromedialis; AV, n. anteroventralis; AD, n. anterodorsalis; R, n. reticularis; VL, n. ventralis lateralis; MD, n. medialis dorsalis; PC, n. paracentralis; VPM, n. ventralis posteromedialis; VPL, n. ventralis posterolateralis; Pf, n. parafascicularis; VPi, n. ventralis posteroinferior; PUL, pulvinar; Re, n. reuniens; LD, n. lateralis dorsalis; LP, n. lateralis posterior; CL, n. centralis lateralis; CM, n. centrum medianum; GM, medial geniculate; GL, lateral geniculate; Li, n. limitans; Hb, n. habenularis; Sg, n. suprageniculatus. Modified from Eyzaguirre and Fidone (1975).

principal features were severe impairment of memory, orientation, and attention, with perseveration, confabulation, drowsiness, inertia, and lack of initiative; peculiar mannerisms, sucking of the lips, and extreme restlessness were also described. The patient was uncommunicative and showed little attention to questions or commands, but did not use wrong words. There was no difficulty in expression; the patient simply spoke less and less. Understanding became impaired and he was eventually unable to read or write. There was also a tendency to repeat actions and words (echopraxia, echolalia), and "the whole mental atmosphere was weird, uncanny and crafty." Aphasia, apraxia, and agnosia were said to be absent. Neurological findings were limited to mild left lower facial weakness, loss of the pupillary and convergence reflex, and bilateral grasping and sucking reflexes. The autopsy revealed no evidence of gross cortical atrophy, but on microscopic examination there was severe bilateral symmetrical degeneration of the thalamus, primarily involving the anterior, medial, and lateral nuclei and centromedian. Posterior ventral, reticular, and midline nuclei and geniculate bodies were spared. The cerebral cortex showed some lipoid neuronal atrophy and recent gliosis, with dense subcortical gliosis considered to be senile changes. There was some bilateral atrophy of the medial sector of dorsal and ventral inferior olivary laminae and gliosis of the superior colliculi. Stern (1939) commented that this was a system degeneration in the thalamus, sparing the phylogenetically older nuclear groups (e.g., midline nuclei, ventral nucleus, and geniculate bodies), possibly an atypical form of Creutzfeldt-Jakob disease.

A few years later, Grunthal (1942) reported another case, unsatisfactory for the reason of mental deficiency prior to the development of dementia and a course of 26 years. Grunthal considered a vascular pathology in the thalamus, but subsequent authors have argued that atrophic dementia was present. These cases are both discussed in a paper by Schulman (1957) in which a further case is described, a 50-year-old man with a rapidly progressive dementia leading to death in 7 months. The picture was characterized by recent memory impairment, reduced digit span, difficulty with simple arithmetic, and hesitancy or blocking in speech, although neither dysarthria nor aphasia was present. The patient showed no concern about his illness, and was facetious, with frequent smiling and laughing. Moderate ataxia was present in all limbs, with choreoathetosis and increased deep reflexes on the right side. The patient's behavior gradually became more bizarre, with episodes fluctuating between quiet stupor and sudden crying, shouting, and violent laughter. Speech was ultimately reduced to a state of virtual muteness. On postmortem study, serial sections of the thalamus demonstrated severe degeneration in n. dorsomedialis, n. ventralis, posterolateralis, dorsolateralis, reticularis, and anterior pulvinar. Moderate degeneration was found in n. anterodorsalis and ventralis anterior, and mild changes were found in the centromedian. No changes were noted in intralaminar and midline nuclei, geniculate bodies, or posterior pulvinar, and the remainder of the brain was essentially normal except for mild gliosis in the rostrodorsal periphery of the red nucleus and in the bilateral rubrothalamic radiations. Following Stern, Schulman noted the preferential involvement of the neothalamus, but he also mentioned certain inconsistencies such as the severe involvement of the reticular nucleus and the sparing of the posterior pulvinar. He did not emphasize a relation to Creutzfeldt-Jakob disease, although, according to Garcin *et al.* (1963), when this case was presented to the American Association of Neuropathology in December 1955, this possibility was specifically mentioned by Adams in the ensuing discussion.

Garcin *et al.* (1963) subsequently reported a further case and concluded that the disorder was a localized form of Creutzfeldt-Jakob disease. Their patient, a 56-year-old man, developed apathy, memory difficulty, dysarthria, and choreoathetosis leading to coma and death in 9 months. Pathological findings were mainly in the thalamus, with bilateral symmetrical neuronal loss and gliosis especially affecting n. dorsomedialis, ventralis lateralis, and pulvinar. Minor lesions in F_3, insula, and inferior olives were present. The striatum was normal, with no senile or inflammatory changes.

Subsequent papers dealing with this subject include those of Nayrac *et al.* (1965), Castaigne *et al.* (1966), and Martin (1966). A report by Daniels (1969) described a 55-year-old man with personality change, irritability, and impairment of recent memory which rapidly progressed to confusion, global dementia, and death over a 5-month period. This patient also had a syndrome of inappropriate antidiuretic hormone secretion in association with bronchogenic carcinoma. Pathological examination disclosed symmetrical bilateral degeneration of the thalamus, with neuronal loss and gliosis most severely affecting n. dorsomedialis. Moderate involvement of the anterior group, centromedian, n. ventralis lateralis, posteromedialis, and pulvinar was present. The disorder was considered a remote effect of the carcinoma.

Reyes *et al.* (1976) reported a 38-year-old woman with Hodgkin's disease who developed an impairment in recent and remote memory and diminished attention span. The patient showed "withdrawn behavior," continued to deteriorate, and died several weeks later. Postmortem examination disclosed a neuroaxonal dystrophy involving primarily the thalamus symmetrically, and presumed to be a secondary effect of the Hodgkin's disease.

In sum, although there are few reported instances of degenerative change limited to the thalamus, it is nevertheless possible to delineate some general features of the resultant dementia. The onset is characterized by apathy and indifference, with gradual uninterest and slowing of activity. Speech also becomes slowed, although dysarthria is not apparently a prominent feature. There is loss of recent memory, and the patient does not have full insight into the nature of his condition. Although the mental state is characterized by a progressive retardation of all functions, restlessness, bizarre behavior, inappropriate laughing, and echo reactions may also occur. It is evident that while the tendency toward a catatonic state may be punctuated by psychotic episodes the overall course is rapid and generally leads to coma and death within a year. Pathological changes tend to be limited to the thalamus, with symmetrical bilateral degeneration affecting principally, although not exclusively, the neothalamic groups, n. dorsomedialis, anterior nucleus, centromedian, and pulvinar. A relation to Creutzfeldt-Jakob disease has been stressed in a few reports, and in two cases the syndrome has been considered a remote effect of cancer. It appears likely that the principal nuclei involved in the dementia of thalamic degeneration are n. dorsomedialis, pulvinar, and/or anterior nucleus. The recent correlation by Victor *et al.* (1971) of Korsakoff amnesia with lesions in n. dorsomedialis and perhaps pulvinar is consistent with this conclusion. There are also important negative cases, such as the patient of Adams and Malamud (1971) with bilateral symmetrical degeneration of centrum medianum without language disorder or dementia.

Vascular Lesions

Another line of evidence pointing to the possible role of the thalamus in cognition and language function concerns those patients with documented unilateral and/or bilateral thalamic vascular lesions. This material can be discussed under two major categories, patients with bilateral thalamic encephalomalacia and patients with unilateral hemorrhagic or ischemic damage to the thalamus.

Unilateral Cases

It is generally considered that thalamic infarction may be accompanied by some language disturbance, although few pertinent cases are available. Most of the early work developed out of the description by Dejerine and Roussy (1906) of a thalamic syndrome, and the occurrence in some cases of defects in speech. Perhaps the first case to be studied from this point of view was the report by Walther (1945) of a 54-year-old right-handed man with two apoplectic attacks leading ultimately to a syndrome characterized by dullness, apathy, confusion, and difficulty in formulating thought and finding words.

Certainly, the most publicized case of unilateral thalamic lesion is that of Penfield and Roberts (1959). Their patient, said to be aphasic, was diagnosed as having a small hemorrhage in the pulvinar on the basis of clinical studies. However, the brevity of the clinical description and the lack of postmortem verification leave both the diagnosis and localization in some doubt. About the same time, Fisher (1959) noted the occurrence of dysphasia as a cardinal feature of thalamic hemorrhage.

Two cases of unilateral thalamic lesion were described by Sager *et al.* (1965, in Botez and Barbeau, 1971). Both patients were said to show "receptive dysphasia" following cerebrovascular accidents of 7 and 14 days' duration. Postmortem examination disclosed hemorrhagic softening in the left posterior thalamus without cortical involvement.

Subsequently, Ciemins (1970) described two patients with aphasia and left thalamic hemorrhage. The first case was of a 53-year-old man with incomplete and fragmentary sentences. There was little spontaneous speech and the patient responded only to questions. Repetition was normal, simple objects could be named, and simple commands could be carried out. A large hemorrhagic lesion was found in the left thalamus. In this case, the description suggests as much an aspontaneity of speech as a true aphasia. Moreover, the course was rapid, only 22 days, and the patient was somnolent, with bilateral Babinski responses suggesting bilateral involvement. The second case was of a 61-year-old woman with some speech disturbance, e.g., speech was "feeble" for several years prior to death; a thalamic infarct was found at necropsy.

Mohr *et al.* (1975) reported two cases of hemorrhage involving, but not confined to, the left thalamus (localization by CT scan). Both patients showed paraphasic speech and good (echolalic) repetition, but in the context of obvious somnolence or disorientation. While the authors make a claim for a specific language disorder associated with a left thalamic lesion, it is not unlikely that the language disorder was part of a general confusional state related to the acute mass lesion rather than to a lesion specifically in the thalamus. Certainly, the intermittent nature of the language disorder seems to argue against an effect of a fixed lesion.

Luria (1976) has observed two cases in which a left thalamic lesion was inferred from the clinical picture, with paraphasic impairments in speech and repetition. These "quasiaphasic" symptoms are presumed secondary to a defect in stimulus filtration rather than to a primary disruption of language.

Recently, Rubens and Johnson (1976) have described another case, with CT scan demonstration of a left thalamic hemorrhage. This patient had "bursts of almost entirely unintelligible logorrheic speech with frequent phonemic paraphasia often resulting in neologisms." In contrast to Luria's case, but similar to those of Mohr, repetition was correct but echolalic. Also, as with Mohr's cases, the intermittent nature of the symptoms could reflect pressure or other effects from an acute mass lesion, i.e., acute confusion, rather than an aphasia of thalamic origin. This is further suggested by the fact that the patient improved into a more typical confusional state.

It would appear that at least two different "syndromes" can occur with an acute left vascular lesion of the thalamus, either a state of mutism, which may or may not be aphasic in nature, or a picture of intermittent logorrheic jargon with or without echolalia, which may or may not be a confusional state. The following personal cases are examples of each of these types.

CASE REPORT. A 68-year-old hypertensive right-handed woman had a sudden collapse in December 1970, with flaccid right hemiparesis, right visual field defect, and diminished sensation on the right side. Initially, she was mute and unable to follow commands. Repeated lumbar punctures revealed elevated opening pressure and bloody fluid; EEG showed left hemispheric slowing. Over the subsequent weeks, there was no change in her status. On repeat examination 8 weeks later, she was alert but inattentive to the right side. There was still a flaccid right hemiplegia, absent response to pain on the right side, and loss of response to visual threat in the right visual field. Deep reflexes were brisk on the right, with bilateral Babinski responses.

The patient was aphonic, with no attempt at vocalization. There was no response to repetition, naming, or verbal or written commands. She was unable to write or draw, and made no response to whole-body commands or tests utilizing imitation. The family was questioned and confirmed the total lack of speech and speech comprehension. There was no change in her condition until death 2 months after admission.

Pathological examination revealed a brain weight of 1300 g; macroscopic sections showed possible slight thinning of the cortical mantle. There was a hemorrhagic lesion restricted largely to the region of the left thalamus (Fig. 2). The lesion extended posteriorly to a thin ribbon involving the tapetum and optic radiations, and anteriorly up to, although sparing, the anterior nucleus of the thalamus. Major thalamic groups involved were pulvinar, ventralis posterior, and lateralis, and the posterolateral portion of n. dorsalis medialis and centrum medianum. As noted in Fig. 2, the posterior limb of the internal capsule and part

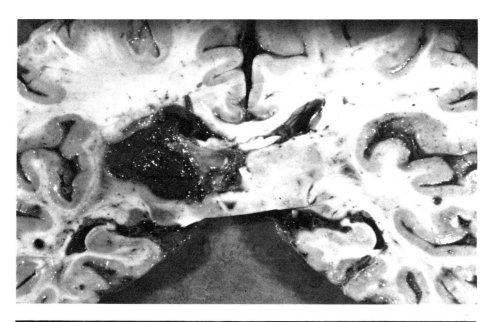

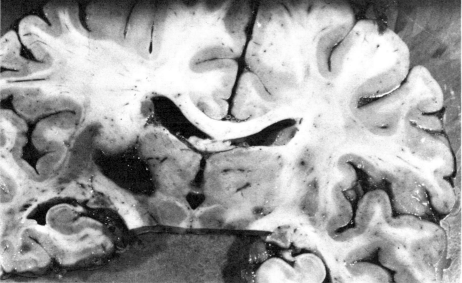

Fig. 2. Hemorrhage in left thalamus. (Reprinted with permission from Brown, 1974.)

of the putamen and left hippocampal commissure were involved. A small area (4 mm) of cystic encephalomalacia was present in the right internal capsule. The midbrain, pons, and medulla were normal except for a slight decrease in size of the left corticospinal tract. The cerebellum was normal. Microscopic examination of the left temporoparietal cortex was negative. Basal ganglia and the thalamus showed accumulation of gitter cells, with fragmentation of myelin and areas of necrosis. There were large amounts of hemosiderin deposit present at the periphery of the infarct and left lateral ventricle. Some vacuolation and decrease of myelin were noted in the left corticospinal tract.

CASE REPORT. A 76-year-old man developed an acute intracerebral hemorrhage, with mild right hemiparesis, no sensory impairment, and difficulty with speech. The patient was not personally examined, but was described as "speaking in an unknown language or in gibberish." It was said that he "made no sense in English." Some observers thought he may have been trying to speak in German, but there is no indication of prior facility with this language. Repetition was not described, but he was reported to have followed verbal commands well. A CT scan showed a left thalamic hemorrhage (Fig. 3). Over the next few days, the aphasia resolved to a state of confusion and disorientation. Six days later, he developed a recurrent left thalamic hemorrhage, again confirmed by CT scan. At this time, he was said to have an "expressive aphasia." One day later, he was noted to be

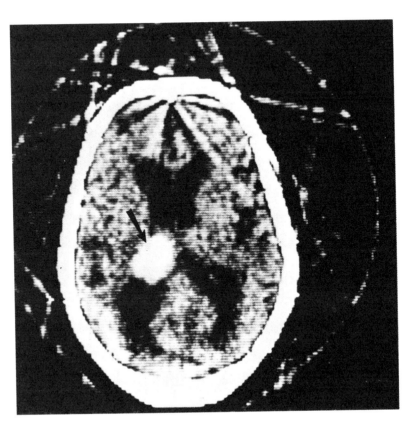

Fig. 3. CT scan showing hemorrhage in left thalamus.

dysarthric and "not clear mentally." Another observer stated that he was able to speak and complained of weakness in his limbs. The following day he was "talking more clearly," and the next was "conversing in English," although it would seem that complete recovery from the aphasia had not yet occurred. Shortly after, the patient went into coma and expired.

On postmortem examination (Dr. G. Budzilovich), the brain weight was 1300 g, and the external appearance was unremarkable. Coronal sections confirmed the presence of a hemorrhage in the left thalamus extending into the left lateral ventricle. Moderate generalized ventricular dilatation was noted. The overlying cortex was grossly normal, although full histological study was not carried out.

DISCUSSION. Of these two cases, the first is more characteristic of unilateral thalamic vascular lesion, with a picture of mutism and failure to respond to comprehension testing. In this respect, such cases are comparable to those of thalamic degeneration or tumor (see below), where apathy, disorientation and confusion, word-finding difficulty, and aspontaneity of speech lead to an end state of (akinetic) mutism. The picture may be difficult, if not impossible, to distinguish from a global aphasia, especially in view of the apparent relationship to left-sided vascular lesions. It would be important to study recovery in patients of this type, to determine if the evolution is through an aphasic stage. If it should prove that such patients are truly mute rather than aphasic, the predilection for left thalamic lesions could be explained through the tendency for acute involvements of the dominant hemisphere to produce bilateral manifestations, while the effects of acute right hemispheric pathology tend to be limited to that hemisphere.

In the second case, the description of "gibberish" speech suggests a possible correspondence to cases with logorrheic jargon. In this case, as in the others described, the thalamic lesion has generally been hemorrhagic in nature. In such cases, symptoms fluctuate due to pressure shifts. Logorrheic jargon is well known in patients with marked confusion; neologisms and paraphasias may also occur. In the second patient, the aphasia resolved into a confusional state after several days, suggesting that the initial language disorder was a manifestation of the more profound degree of confusion.

BILATERAL CASES

Bilateral cases are among the earliest reports of vascular involvement of the thalamus giving rise to language disorder and are generally included as instances of the so-called arteriopathic thalamic dementia, with descriptions of thalamic degeneration. Even the original case of Grunthal (1942) has been classified with both the vascular and the atrophic dementias. The initial description was Schuster's (1936, 1937) case (No. 11) of a 49-year-old woman with a sudden onset of coma resolving into a state of aspontaneity, apathy, indifference, and memory disorder. There was no evidence of aphasia, but speech was described as atonal, poorly articulated, and similar to parkinsonian speech. The author suggested a comparison with akinetic mutism. Postmortem findings were of bilateral necrosis involving the paraventricular region, the internal nuclei, the medial portion of the lateral nucleus, and the centrum medianum.

According to Botez and Barbeau (1971), the only two cases on record of bilateral thalamic softening with impaired speech fluency are those of Marinesco *et al.* (1935) and Kreindler *et al.* (1962). The patients in these studies were not thought to represent instances of pure aphasia but rather of speech aspontaneity and/or mutism.

In an excellent review, Castaigne *et al.* (1966) described two patients, the first a 76-year-old woman with left hemiparesis, inattention, and a dementia characterized by aspontaneity of movement and speech with severe memory disturbance. Speech consisted of incessant mumbling, which was stereotyped in a weak voice without intonation. Repetition of words and short phrases was possible, naming was good for objects, and there was no disturbance of comprehension at a simple level, both for written and for spoken language. It was specifically mentioned that aphasic disturbances were absent. Postmortem findings were of bilateral thalamic softening restricted to the retromammillary peduncle and intralaminar formation, affecting the left ventralis anterior and part of the dorsolateral and paracentral nuclei. Their second case was of a 67-year-old woman with the sudden onset of a vascular accident and coma which evolved into dementia persisting over 3 years until death. There was marked disturbance of attention and memory; WAIS IQ was 70; there was no evidence of aphasia. Postmortem examination showed bilateral softening in the thalamus involving on the left especially the paracentral group and the inferior part of n. dorsomedialis and ventralis anterior, and on the right n. parafascicularis and dorsomedialis.

Recently, Delay and Brion (1962) described a case of true aphasia with thalamic lesion. This 48-year-old woman had a rapid onset of delirium and depression leading to dementia with paranoia, auditory hallucinations, intellectual reduction, and impaired memory. Paramnesia was present, and there was only partial awareness of the disorder. There were no neurological signs. The authors noted that a Wernicke's aphasia was present, although details were not given. The patient showed progressive deterioration, and terminated in a state of epileptic seizures with a right hemiparesis. Postmortem findings were of diffuse arteriosclerosis, but the cortex was intact. There were a small area of old encephalomalacia in the white matter of T_4 on the left, vascular lesions in the left amygdaloid region, and lacunae in the putamen and cerebellum. The major lesions involved the thalamus in a bilateral and symmetrical fashion, with old areas of softening in the left and right n. dorsomedialis and right pulvinar and an organized thrombus in the right lateral nuclear group. In view of the finding of Wernicke's aphasia, it is regrettable that the pathological picture was so diffuse.

Apart from these cases, there are only anecdotal references to thalamic dementia on an arteriopathic basis. Nielson (1965) commented on the occurrence of defects in attention with bilateral thalamic degeneration, and there are scattered cases of stupor, apathy, and/or indifference with similar pathology. In a related study, Segarra (1970) discussed akinetic mutism as a manifestation of small lesions in the midbrain and the thalamus. Particularly important are the midline nuclei, both of his cases having lesions of n. dorsomedialis and centrum medianum. This is further evidence for the essential similarity of thalamic apathy and the akinetic mute state.

There are numerous cases in the literature of unilateral and bilateral thalamic neoplasms in which dementia was a prominent symptom. Smyth and Stern (1938) reported two cases of small intrinsic thalamic tumor without somnolence in which dementia was the presenting complaint. The dementia was characterized by inattention, forgetfulness, and disorientation, and the pathology concerned the medial portion of the thalamus, possibly n. dorsomedialis. Cheek and Taveras (1966) agreed with this conclusion and insisted that dementia could occur with thalamic tumor without hydrocephalus or massive white matter involvement. Delay and Brion (1962) concluded that bithalamic tumor can present with early dementia as a specific sign prior to increased intracranial pressure. Other references are Cremieux *et al.* (1959), Nayrac *et al.* (1965), and McEntee *et al.* (1976).

The picture that emerges is of a generally bilateral but occasionally unilateral thalamic glioma, usually in the region of the third ventricle, presenting with early mental change. The dementia is characterized by slowness of activity and ideation, apathy, aspontaneity, and moderate to marked impairment of memory. Catatonic or delirious episodes or even frank psychosis may occur. Attention is certainly reduced, and in many cases it is unclear whether a confusional state or a true dementia is present. In cases where the tumor originates extrinsic to the thalamus, there is gradual encroachment on the lateral nuclei. Here, dementia is apparently a part of late confusion, somnolence, or obtundation. However, with intrinsic tumor, especially if the tumor originates medially, the dementia may be the earliest sign and will be apparent well before there is demonstrable ventricular enlargement or elevated intracranial pressure.

In sum, there is little to distinguish the dementia of thalamic glioma from the vascular or degenerative states which have been discussed. Diagnosis depends on the history and on the ancillary findings of hydrocephalus and elevated intracranial pressure.

Surgical Lesions

Various thalamic nuclei have been explored surgically for the treatment of psychiatric disease, pain states, seizures, and movement disorders. Regarding lesions of n. ventralis lateralis, a large literature has accumulated (e.g., Bell, 1968; Riklan and Levita, 1969) and will not be discussed at length in this chapter. Most authors have demonstrated mild general decrement on intellectual testing following bilateral lesions, with some evidence (Riklan and Levita, 1969; Ojemann and Ward, 1971) that lesions in the speech-dominant hemisphere entail further deficit in verbal memory and in verbal IQ. In various series (e.g., Waltz *et al.,* 1966; Allen *et al.,* 1966; Hermann *et al.,* 1966), aphasia has been reported as a sequel in anywhere from 2% to 10% of cases, and relates especially to procedures in the dominant hemisphere. However, careful studies of post-thalamotomy "dysphasia" have not been carried out, and it is not clear whether they simply represent speech reduction and/or dysarthria. When present, aphasia usually lasts only a week or two following surgery, rarely persisting beyond the third or fourth week. Since testing has usually been carried out several days after surgery without immediate postoperative observation, it has not been possible to eliminate general factors such as edema, subsequent hemorrhage into a lesion, and general effects of ventriculography. Moreover, most reports concern parkinsonian patients, many no doubt with preexisting mild dementia in association with diffuse brain pathology, and comparisons are lacking with thalamotomy effects in subjects without such preexisting problems.

In other studies, Spiegel *et al.* (1955) have reported a variety of changes following bilateral surgical lesions of n. dorsomedialis. Disturbances of memory and orientation have been described, as well as a disorder in the "time sense," chronotaraxis. Mark *et al.* (1963) have described relief of pain without apparent change in mentation following surgical lesions in the parafascicular and intralaminar nuclei; lesions in the anterior nucleus produced euphoria with some change in affect and pain relief. Alterations in mentation were not described. Sugishita *et al.* (1973) described a 62-year-old man who developed a "pure agraphia" which persisted for 6 weeks following left CM-thalamotomy for intractable facial pain. Mild constructional disability was present, but no disorder of language was observed. In contrast, Jurko and Andy (1973) noted few cognitive changes following surgical lesion of the centrum medianum. These authors did note varying degrees of impairment on cognitive tests with lesions in other thalamic sites. Of interest was their finding of greater impairment on the Bender-Gestalt Test after right thalamic lesion.

PULVINECTOMY

Surgical interest in the pulvinar developed largely out of the theory of Penfield and Roberts (1959) that the speech functions of the various cortical language areas are coordinated by way of reciprocal projections to the pulvinar (Fig. 4). This hypothesis led to studies by Ojemann *et al.* (1968), who described "dysnomia" on stimulation in three subcortical sites in right-handed (mainly parkinsonian) subjects, the left pulvinar and deep parietal white matter of both hemispheres. However, stimulation in parietal white matter produced a more densely anomic state (omissions) than stimulation in pulvinar (misnaming), and white matter stimulation also had the more severe effect on verbal memory, findings which might have suggested the dysnomia to be a cortical rather than subcortical effect. The recent demonstration by Ojemann (personal communication, 1976) of similar effects on direct cortical stimultion is consistent with this interpretation.

There is also evidence (Ojemann, 1976) that stimulation in the dominant thalamus enhances later retrieval of material presented during the stimulation period, an effect which has apparently not been duplicated by neocortical stimulation. Whether this also represents a distant effect—in this case on limbic structures—or is attributable to thalamic mechanisms concerned directly with memory or with attentional processes has not yet been determined.

In a more recent paper, Van Buren and Borke (1969) studied serial sections of thalamus in several patients with cerebral lesions and aphasia. Marked degener-

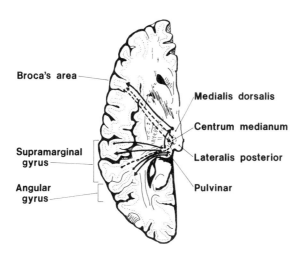

227

THALAMIC
MECHANISMS IN
LANGUAGE

Fig. 4. Thalamocortical systems in relation to language zones. (Modified from Penfield and Roberts, 1959.)

ation of the pulvinar was found in a case of global aphasia and moderate degeneration in another case. On the basis of these findings, the authors argued that the anterior superior pulvinar was important in language function. Subsequently, Ojemann and Ward (1971) concluded from stimulation studies that the anatomical substrate for speech includes the pulvinar and *en passage* fibers related to the centrum medianum and n. dorsomedialis (for comment on these studies, see Brown, 1973).

We have had the opportunity to study over 30 patients with cryogenic surgical lesion in the pulvinar (Brown, 1972, 1973). This procedure was initially carried out in the hope of benefit for severe permanent aphasia, but was extended to incapacitated dystonic patients when some favorable effect on motor tone was observed.

Unilateral. Most of the 30 patients in the unilateral group were right-handed. There were also several instances of structural brain damage (vascular, traumatic) and cerebral palsy. It was found that subjects with normal preoperative language and cognitive function, and without structural brain damage, showed no evidence of aphasia or dementia following cryopulvinectomy in the presumed speech-dominant hemisphere. Moreover, there was no evidence of spatioconstructional disturbance in patients undergoing surgery in the presumed nondominant hemisphere (Fig. 5). Some patients showed immediate postoperative decrement in verbal learning on supraspan word recall and paired associates, but there was no indication that verbal material learned prior to surgery was affected by the operation. This alteration was not absolutely related to dominant-side surgery, although statistical analysis of side preference was not carried out. Mild reduction in digit span was also noted. In a few patients with preexisting structural lesion and with borderline language or cognitive function, cryopulvinectomy in the dominant hemisphere did induce further deterioration. In one such patient with head trauma and bilateral brain damage, right hemiparesis, mild dementia, and some word-finding difficulty, a marked dysnomic state at times approximating

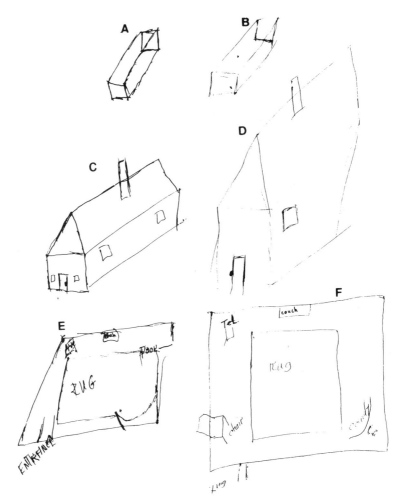

Fig. 5. Performance before (A,C,E) and after (B,D,F) right pulvinectomy on copying a cube, drawing a house, and drawing a map of patient's living room. (Reprinted with permission from Brown, 1974.)

semantic jargon followed left cryopulvinectomy. There was gradual improvement over a 4- to 6-week period to the preoperative level. A second patient with longstanding hemispheric atrophy and right hemiparesis but without preoperative language defect developed dysnomia following pulvinectomy in the atrophic hemisphere. This patient also showed resolution over a period of a few weeks. A third patient with a cerebrovascular accident, right hemiparesis, and resolved anterior aphasia had transient postoperative hesitation on naming and mild vocabulary impairment, particularly noticeable on tests utilizing low-frequency words. However, in the more optimal surgical group, the dystonics, the majority of whom had normal or above-average IQ and intact preoperative language function, no deterioration in language was observed. Some degree of aspontaneity and mild inconstant mood changes were also noted.

BILATERAL. In three cases studies with extensive pre- and postoperative language testing, there was no evidence of an aphasic impairment following bilateral cryopulvinectomy. In two patients, the presence of severe limb dystonia prevented thorough evaluation of writing and spatioconstructional ability, although no postoperative change was judged to be present. This was corroborated in a third case where more extensive evaluation was possible. Moreover, there was no right-left disorientation, misidentification of fingers, alexia, or dyscalculia; visual imagery was unchanged, and there was no hallucinatory or psychotic behavior. In two patients, IQ testing showed a slight decrement. In a third case, marked decrement occurred in the period following left pulvinectomy and prior to right pulvinectomy, a time during which no surgery occurred. Subsequent repeat testing demonstrated moderate return. The principal findings, as in the unilateral cases, were of some impairment on tests of verbal learning, e.g., supraspan word recall and paired associates, and reduced digit span (see Brown, 1974). An example of writing and drawing prior to initial surgery and following bilateral pulvinar lesions in one of these cases is illustrated in Fig. 6.

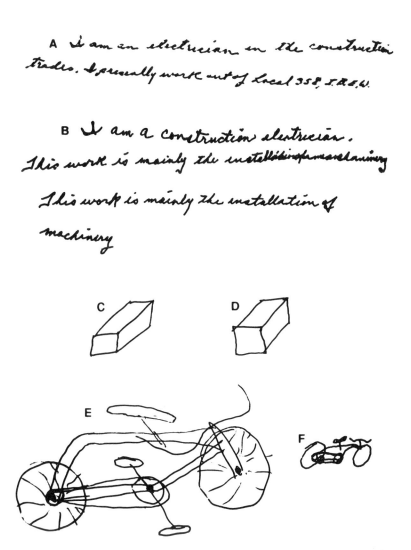

Fig. 6. Performance before surgery (A,C,E) and following bilateral pulvinectomy (B,D,F) on spontaneous writing, copying a cube, and drawing a bicycle. (Reprinted with permission from Brown, 1974.)

The study of these cases has demonstrated relatively minor changes in language function following unilateral or bilateral pulvinectomy. This finding has been confirmed in a recent paper by Vilkki and Laitinen (1976). The principal postoperative changes were restricted to a slight reduction in digit span, mild aspontaneity, and some impairment on tests of verbal learning. Some patients gave the impression of mild dullness, expressed in slowness of response, hesitation, or in the general appearance and manner of the patient, but this could not be specified on psychological testing. A comparison of the subtest scores for pulvinectomy and routine thalamotomy (Riklan and Cooper, 1975) did not show an appreciable difference in the pattern of impairment. Spatioconstructional ability, imagery, praxis, and calculations were judged to be essentially unchanged. In one patient, macrographic drawing was noted after right cryopulvinectomy, and, in another patient, micrography was found following the second side of a bilateral procedure. These alterations are discussed by Mendilaharsu *et al.* (1968) in relation to parietal lobe involvement. Some tendency toward simplification of drawing was occasionally found in the absence of other signs of constructional disability.

Apart from the above, postoperative changes in affect were not observed. However, the procedure was carried out in only a few subjects with preexisting emotional disorder. In two patients with a left hemispheric lesion, pulvinectomy in the damaged hemisphere accentuated preexisting aggressive behavior. In two other patients with pathological lability, there was mitigation of the emotionality following right pulvinectomy. These patients all had preexisting structural brain damage.

In general, the findings in these cases, impairment of verbal memory and a suggestion of mental dulling and aspontaneity, correspond quite well with the symptoms of nonsurgical lesion in other neothalamic groups, Review of our pathological material (Fig. 7) indicates that ordinarily only about 20% of the pulvinar was involved by the cryogenic lesion. This might account for the relative lack of major deficit following surgery.

The possible importance of lesion size is illustrated by the following unique case in which pulvinectomy was done together with ablation in other thalamic sites.

CASE REPORT

Preoperative Evaluation (July 20, 1971). The patient was a 45-year-old man with longstanding dystonia; he had an eighth-grade education, could read and write, and was strongly right-handed with no family history of left-handedness. Conversational speech and comprehension were relatively normal, although the patient appeared somewhat dull. Proverbs were done concretely, there was difficulty with dates, and he could not remember the names of many previous presidents. Given three words and tested 5 min. later for recall, he produced all three correctly. On a test of supraspan recall with ten items, scores were 4, 5, 6, 7, and 8 over five trials. The impression was of some memory impairment with either mental retardation or mild dementia.

Operation (July 21, 1971). The patient underwent stereotaxic surgery with the placement of extensive cryogenic lesions in the ventralis lateralis, ventralis posterolateralis, centrum medianum, and pulvinar on the left side.

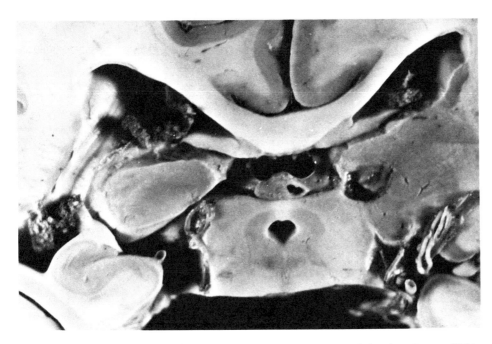

Fig. 7. Cryogenic surgical lesion in the pulvinar. (Reprinted with permission from Brown, 1974.)

Postoperative Evaluation (July 28, 1971). At this time, speech appeared greatly reduced in quantity and articulation was slightly more impaired than prior to surgery but dysarthria was not clearly present. Utterances consisted for the most part of one- or two-word phrases, generally monotonous, grammatically correct, and with perseveration. Asked how he was feeling, he replied, "Okay" or "Better"; when asked about his work, he said, "My work has got better." Asked to describe the job of a policeman, he said, "A policeman has got a better job than the average guy." Many questions were not answered at all, and all responses showed an extremely long latency. Motor series were done slowly but correctly. He followed a conversation but failed on many tests of speech comprehension. For example, asked to point to the door, he sat blankly without a response. Asked to point to each of three objects on command, he correctly pointed to only two, and could not point to objects on a functional description.

Repetition was excellent. He named about 80% of objects and showed excellent phonemic cueing to objects not named spontaneously. Occasionally, there was complete blocking without response. There did not appear to be a difference in performance on visual or tactile naming. However, there was some difficulty in object identification beyond a naming disorder. For example, he was able to correctly identify a spoon, a lock, a football, a comb, and a battery, respectively, but when shown a toothbrush he stated that he did not know what it was, could not describe it or demonstrate its use, was unable to select the correct name from a group of names offered, and, when finally given the correct name, rejected it. When he was then asked to demonstrate how a toothbrush should be used, he did so correctly, and finally agreed that the object might be a toothbrush. No paraphasias were heard, either the object being named correctly or the patient saying, "I don't know."

On tests of color naming, substitution of color names was noted. The patient could not point correctly to colors on command. Naming of body parts was similarly impaired. He was able to read simple words but could not indicate objects whose names he had just read. When shown an object and given a choice of four written names, he was unable to select the correct name. Constructional ability was extremely poor. He was unable to write his first name with his left hand (severe dystonia on the right side). Simple commands were done well, such as making a fist or saluting, but inappropriate movements were noted. Facial praxis could not be evaluated because of dystonic grimacing.

Visual fields appeared intact, but there was difficulty with voluntary gaze to the right. The patient did not attend well to objects on the right side. There was a tendency for head turning to the right but a deviation of the eyes to the left. He was able to reach out and touch objects presented in the left visual field better than objects presented on the right side. Spontaneous and following eye movements were normal. There was difficulty when asked to look to the right, the left, or up and down. Finally, there was definite blunting of affect with little insight into the disorder and extreme inattentiveness.

Second Postoperative Evaluation (August 5, 1971). Two weeks following surgery, little change was noted, the patient still showing marked lack of spontaneity in speech and behavior, prolonged latency for response, and frequently no response at all. On comprehension testing, he pointed to objects with greater success, repetition was still excellent, and naming was slightly improved, although he was still at times unable to identify common objects.

In summary, this 45-year-old man with some preoperative impairments showed considerable deterioration following an extensive surgical lesion in the left thalamus. The postoperative state was characterized by marked retardation in speech and behavior, inattentiveness, impaired object recognition and reaching in the visual field. Conversational speech consisted of one or two words or, less commonly, longer phrases, generally grammatically intact, the most striking feature being that of slowness and occasional perseveration. Repetition was excellent while comprehension was impaired. Most objects were named correctly, with failures suggesting an agnosic deficit. Substitutions were noted on color naming, but otherwise no phonemic or verbal paraphasias occurred. Responses were characterized by marked slowness, often without a response at all. There was also an impression of some memory loss and dementia.

Medial Geniculotomy

This procedure was carried out in one patient with jargon aphasia in an attempt to mitigate the speech disorder. The case is described in full as a unique instance of a stereotaxic lesion in the medial geniculate body of the dominant hemisphere. The rationale for this operation has been previously discussed (Brown, 1975).

Case Report. A 64-year-old woman had a stable jargonaphasia for 18 months following a stroke. Neurological findings consisted of right hemiparesis with minimal right facial weakness, marked weakness in the right arm with flexion rigidity, and moderate weakness and rigidity of the right lower extremity. Response to pain was symmetrical. Deep reflexes were increased on the right side, Babinski reflexes were absent, and there was no visual field defect. Speech consisted of fluent, voluble neologistic jargon. There was active gesture and euphoria, with no evidence of speech awareness. Comprehension was nil, with no response to verbal commands, object pointing, yes/no questions, or whole-body commands. The only sign of comprehension was eye closure to command, response to her name, and puzzlement when addressed by the examiner in jargon. Repetition and naming were severely jargonized without recognizable links to test items. Reading, writing, and constructional ability were nil. Psychological testing was not possible. An EEG and previous brain scan disclosed a left posterior temporal abnormality. The patient was observed for several months prior to surgery without change in these findings.

Intracarotid Amytal Test. Bilateral intracarotid amytal testing was carried out on separate days. Left-sided injection produced loss of speech save for a "bu, bu, bu" stereotypy. The patient remained able to close her eyes to command. On right injection, jargon persisted, with loss of eye closure. This suggested that the neologistic jargon and eye closure were left and right hemisphere dependent phenomena, respectively.

Surgery and Postoperative Evaluation. In October 1972, a cryogenic lesion was made in the left medial geniculate body, with freezing down to $-90°C$ for 2 min at a point 1 mm below and behind the posterior commissure and 15 mm from the midline. Postoperatively, there was no attempt to speak until the sixth day, when whispered jargon similar to that on preoperative testing appeared. Speech volume gradually increased over the next 2 or 3 days up to the normal level. The patient responded to her name, and, with eyes closed, stopped talking to a whispered "shh" sound.

Neurological examination was unchanged and, although testing was difficult, there was no evidence of auditory or vestibular dysfunction. Bedside ice water calorics elicited symmetrical nystagmus on stimulation of either ear. There was no behavioral evidence of auditory hallucinations. Hearing seemed intact bilaterally, with rapid orientation to whisper or other sounds on either side and with either ear occluded. When approached from behind and her name whispered, the patient promptly turned toward the sound source. Requests for eye closure in a barely audible whisper elicited immediate correct responses. She could be aroused from sleep by noise, and there was no evidence of auditory neglect or inattention. Audiometric testing disclosed ability to turn in the direction of speech sounds in various positions of the acoustic field.

Repeat language testing over a 6-week period did not disclose a change in the fluent neologistic jargon. Other parameters of language testing remained unchanged. There was a suggestion of slightly improved speech intelligibility on conversational material.

The failure to initiate speech in the immediate postoperative period occurred with otherwise good gesture and attention. Speech returned as a whisper, with gradually increasing volume. Preoperative audiometric testing indicated that speech volume could be controlled by input volume; i.e., the patient spoke with normal volume to an input of 65 dB and whispered when the input dropped to 45 dB. This suggests that the postoperative speechlessness and whispering may have been acoustically determined.

DISCUSSION

This review of the thalamus and disorders of language and cognition has centered chiefly on the complex of symptoms associated with different types of thalamic pathology. While it would have been preferable to consider such symptoms in relation to specific thalamic groups, this has not been possible because of the scarcity of pathological cases with restricted vascular lesions. Regarding the surgical material, only a few nuclei have been explored, and in such cases one cannot ignore the fact that the preexisting neurological deficit has an influence on the postoperative behavior.

There is some evidence to suggest that lesion of the nucleus ventralis lateralis produces mild intellectual changes similar to those following lesion of the pulvinar (Riklan and Cooper, 1975). Stereotaxic lesion of the nucleus dorsomedialis has produced memory impairment (Spiegel et al., 1955), but such cases, few in number, have not been carefully studied. Natural lesions of the anterior nucleus may also lead to memory impairment, as in the Korsakoff syndrome, although Victor et al. (1971) have attributed this to pathology in the dorsomedialis. In view of the evident difficulty in establishing correlations between lesion and symptom—no less at the thalamic than the cortical level—caution should be exercised in assigning functions to specific nuclear groups. This is even more true for stimulation studies where distant effects are always a possibility. In this regard, claims for a localization of language in anterior superior pulvinar appear to go well beyond the experimental evidence.

The effort to establish such correlations comes from the view of the thalamus as a collection of separate nuclei connected to different areas and subserving different functions. However, it can also be argued that the thalamus is a hierarchically organized structure in which levels (nuclear groups) have evolved in company with the cortical zones to which these levels project. The concept of successive levels of functional thalamic organization laid down in the course of evolution has been discussed by Ris et al. (1972). These authors have delineated six stages in the phylogenesis of the thalamus: a *spinal* or *reflex* level in relation to certain nuclei of the ventral basal complex; a *reticular* level in relation to nonspecific thalamic nuclei; a *cerebellar* level in relation to the ventral anteroventrolateral complex; a *midbrain tectal* level in relation to the primate pulvinar inferior or the lateralis posterior of other mammals; a *limbic* level in relation to the anterior nuclei and medial parts of the medial-dorsal nucleus; and a *neocortical* level in relation to the pulvinar and lateral portions of the medial dorsal nucleus.

Sanides (1970) has argued that stages in thalamic differentiation can be viewed as emergent zones which differentiate together with their cortical projection areas. Both the thalamic nucleus and its cortical projection zone can be viewed as part of the same level in brain evolution. In this way, the nuclei of the thalamus come to be understood not as control centers facilitating, inhibiting, or otherwise influencing some extrinsic area but rather as components of more widely distributed anatomical levels. The thalamic nucleus participates with its "projection" zone in the mediation of cognitive events specific to that structural level of which it is but one component.

Since thalamic differentiation follows an evolutionary course parallel to that of the neocortex, the symptomology of thalamic lesions should occur as a destructuring of this phylogenetic organization. In other words, thalamic pathology should show a level-by-level correspondence with pathology of the cortex. Symptoms of a lesion in a particular thalamic nucleus should resemble those of a lesion in the cortical zone related to that nucleus. Thus the picture of a lesion of the pulvinar should be of the same general type as that of a temporoparietal lesion, the picture of a lesion in the limbic thalamus should resemble that of the limbic cortex, and so on. With regard to language pathology, there is some preliminary evidence that this may be the case.

Thus there are two "aphasic" syndromes which have been related to thalamic lesions: one is characterized by mutism, the other by fluent jargon. Both occur with acute left thalamic lesion, but only mutism has been described in progressive bilateral cases. While it is yet unclear whether these disorders reflect the disruption of intrathalamic mechanisms, or are referred effects on overlying cortex, and if the former what mechanisms (nuclei) are involved, the approach to thalamus described above permits another interpretation of these symptoms.

Studies in primate have demonstrated prominent connections between the inferior parietal lobule and the pulvinar (Walker, 1938). Using the HRP technique, Kasdon and Jacobson (1978) have shown a more heterogeneous input to this area in monkey but have confirmed the presence of major projections to the inferior parietal lobule from the pulvinar. This arrangement is similar to that in man, where strong connections have been shown to exist between the pulvinar and the inferior parietal and posterior temporal region (Van Buren and Borke, 1969). In contrast, the anterior speech area receives the major projection from the dorsomedial nucleus. This has been demonstrated in monkey by Tobias (1975), and appears also to be the case in man. In sum, the pulvinar is in relation to the generalized neocortex of the posterior sector, and the dorsomedial nucleus is in relation to the generalized neocortex of the anterior sector.

Accordingly, the fluent-nonfluent distinction that seems to prevail in the differentiation of posterior and anterior aphasias at the "cortical" level would be expected also to prevail at the thalamic level. The aphasic jargon which is associated with a (?) pulvinar lesion, and the dysnomia which occurs on pulvinar stimulation, would correspond to the semantic jargon and verbal paraphasia, and anomia, which result from lesions of posterior (transitional and generalized) neocortex. On the other hand, the mutism that occurs with a lesion of (?) dorsomedial nucleus would correspond to the mutism that occurs as a symptom of anterior (transitional and generalized) neocortical lesion. The lack of phonological or articulatory deficit in both the fluent and nonfluent thalamic syndromes would indicate that these nuclei are in functional relationship to the generalized neocortex surrounding the Broca and Wernicke areas, *sensu stricto*, since lesions of these latter areas produce impairment at the phonological stage in language processing (Brown, 1977). Naturally, it is emphasized that this interpretation is quite speculative, and that further study is needed before it can be accepted. This is an important task for the future.

Acknowledgment

The author is most grateful to the editor and publisher of *Confinia Neurologica* for permission to use material and figures from his article that appeared earlier in their publication.

REFERENCES

Adams, J., and Malamud, N. Severe chorea with degeneration of the nucleus centrum medianum. *Archives of Neurology (Chicago* 1971, *24*, 101–105.

Allen, C., Turner, J., and Gadea-Ciria, M. Investigations into speech disturbances following stereotactic surgery for Parkinsonism. *British Journal of Disorders of Communication*, 1966, *1*, 55–59.

Bell, D. Speech functions of the thalamus inferred from the effects of thalamotomy. *Brain*, 1968, *91*, 619–638.

Botez, M., and Barbeau, A. Role of subcortical structures, and particularly of the thalamus in the mechanism of speech and language. *International Journal of Neurology*, 1971, *8*, 300–320.

Brown, J. *Mind, Brain and Consciousness: The Neuropsychology of Cognition*. New York: Academic Press, 1977.

Brown, J. *Aphasia, Apraxia and Agnosia: Clinical and Theoretical Aspects*. Springfield, Ill.: Thomas, 1972.

Brown, J. Observations on cryopulvinectomy. In Cooper, Riklan, and Rakic (eds.), *The Pulvinar-LP Complex*. Springfield, Ill.: Thomas, 1973

Brown, J. Language, cognition and the thalamus. *Confinia Neurologica*, 1974, *36*, 33–60.

Brown, J. The neural organization of language: Thalamic and cortical relationships. *Brain and Language*, 1975, *2*, 18–30.

Brown, J., Riklan, M., Waltz, J., Jackson, S., and Cooper, I. Preliminary studies of language and cognition following surgical lesions of the pulvinar in man (cryopulvinectomy). *International Journal of Neurology* 1971, *8*, 276–299.

Castaigne, P., Buge, A., Cambier, J., Escourolle, R., Brunet, P., and Degos, J. Démence thalamique d'origine vasculaire par ramollissement bilatéral. *Revue Neurologique*, 1966, *114*, 89–107.

Cheek, W., and Taveras, J. Thalamic tumors. *Journal of Neurosurgery*, 1966, *24*, 505–513.

Ciemins, V. Localized thalamic hemorrhage. *Neurology*, 1970, *20*, 776–782.

Cremieux, A., Alliez, J., Toga, M., and Bruno, M. Tumeur thalamique à évolution démentielle rapide. *Annales Medico-Psychologiques*, 1959, *117*, 508–517.

Daniels, A. Thalamic degeneration, dementia and seizures. *Archives of Neurology (Chicago)*, 1969, *21*, 15–24.

Dejerine, J., and Roussy, G. Le syndrome thalamique. *Revue Neurologique*, 1906, *12*, 521–532.

Delay, J., and Brion, S. *Les Démences Tardives* Paris: Masson, 1962.

de Morsier, G. Les hallucinations. *Revue d'Oto-Neuro-Ophthalmologie*, 1938, *6*, 244–352.

Eyzaguirre, C., and Fidone, S. *Physiology of the Nervous System*. Chicago: Year Book Medical Publishers, 1975.

Fisher, C. The pathologic and clinical aspects of thalamic hemorrhage. *Transactions of the American Neurological Association*, 1959, *84*, 56.

Garcin, R., Brion, S., and Khochneviss, A. Le syndrome de Creutzfeldt-Jakob et les syndromes cortico-striés du presenium. *Revue Neurologique*, 1963, *109*, 419–441.

Goldstein, K. *Language and Language Disturbances*. New York: Grune and Stratton, 1948.

Goodglass, H., and Kaplan, E. *Assessment of Aphasia and Related Disorders*. Philadelphia: Davis, 1972.

Grunthal, E. Ueber thalamische Dememz. *Monatsschrift für Psychiatrie und Neurologie*, 1942, *106*, 114–128.

Hermann, K., Turner, J., Gillingham, F., and Gaze, R. The effects of destructive lesions and stimulation of the basal ganglia on speech mechanisms. *Confinia Neurologia*, 1966, *28*, 197–207.

Jurko, M., and Andy, O., Psychological changes correlated with thalamotomy site. *Journal of Neurology Neurosurgery and Psychiatry*, 1973, *36*, 846–852.

Kasdon, D. and Jacobson, S. The thalamic afferents to the inferior parietal lobule of the rhesus monkey. *Journal of Comparative Neurology*, 1978, *177*, 685–705.

Kreindler, A., Nereantiu, F., and Botez, M. Tulburari de constiinta intr-un caz de ramolisment thalamic bilateral. *Neurologia (Bucuresti,* 1962, *7*, 121–129.

Luria, A. Personal communication, 1976.

Marinesco, G., Nicolesco, J., and Nicolesco, M. Lésions bilatérales du thalamus. *Encéphale*, 1935, *30*, 153–170.

Mark, V, Ervin, F., and Yakovlev, P. Stereotactic thalamotomy. *Archives of Neurology (Chicago)*, 1963, *8*, 528–538.

Martin, J. Troubles psychiques dans une atrophie primitive des noyaux thalamiques dorso-medians. *Revue Neurologique*, 1966, *114*, 215–219.

McEntee, W., Biber, M., Perl, D., and Benson, F. Diencephalic amnesia: A reappraisal. *Journal of Neurology, Neurosurgery and Psychiatry*, 1976, *39*, 436–441.

Mendilaharsu, C., Milglionico, A., Mendilaharsu, S., Budelli, R., and Souto, H. A propos d'une épreuve d'étude de l'apraxie constructive. *Acta Neurologica Latinoamericana*, 1968, *14*, 138.

Mohr, J., Watters, W., and Duncan, G. Thalamic hemorrhage and aphasia. *Brain and Language*, 1975, *2*, 3–17.

Nayrac, P., Arnott, G., and Warot, P. Lesions thalamiques et troubles mentaux. *Lille Médical*, 1965, *10*, 692–698.

Nielson. *Agnosia, Apraxia, Aphasia*. New York: Hafner, 1965.

Ojemann, G. Subcortical language mechanisms. In H. Whitaker (ed.), *Neurolinguistics*, Vol. 1. New York: Academic Press, 1976, pp. 103–138.

Ojemann, G., and Ward, A. Speech representation in ventrolateral thalamus. *Brain*, 1971, *94*, 669–680.

Ojemann, G., Fedio, P., and Van Buren, J. Anomia from pulvinar and subcortical parietal stimulation. *Brain,* 1968, *91*, 99–116.

Penfield, W., and Roberts, L. *Speech and Brain Mechanisms*. Princeton, N.J.: Princeton University Press, 1959.

Reyes, M., Chokroverty, S., and Masdeu, J. Thalamic neuroaxonal dystrophy and dementia in Hodgkin's disease. *Neurology*, 1976, *26*, 251–253.

Riklan, M., and Cooper, I. Psychometric studies of verbal functions following thalamic lesions in humans. *Brain and Language*, 1975, *2*, 45–64.

Riklan, M., and Levita, E. *Subcortical Correlates of Human Behavior*. Baltimore: Williams and Wilkins, 1969.

Riss, W., Pederson, R., Jakway, J. and Ware, C. Levels of function and their representation; in the vertebrate thalamus. *Brain Behavior and Evolution*, 1972, *6*, 26–41.

Rubens, A., and Johnson, M. Aphasia with thalamic hemorrhage. Presentation at Academy of Aphasia, Miami, 1976.

Sager, O., Mares, A., and Nestianu, V. *Formatia Reticulata*. Bucharest: Ed. Acad. RSR, 1965.

Sanides, F., Functional architecture of motor and sensory cortices in primates in the light of a new concept of neocortex evolution. In C. R. Noback and W. Montagna (eds.), *The Primate Brain*. New York: Appleton-Century-Crofts, 1970.

Schulman, S. Bilateral symmetrical degeneration of the thalamus. *Journal of Neuropathology and Experimental Neurology*, 1957, *16*, 446–470.

Schuster, P. Beitrage zur Pathologie des Thalamus opticus. *Archiv für Psychiatrie und Nervenkrankheiten*, 1936, *105*, 358–432, 550–622, 1937, *106*, 13–53, 201–233.

Segarra, J. Cerebral vascular disease and behavior. *Archives of Neurology (Chicago)*, 1970, *22*, 408–418.

Smyth, G., and Stern, K. Tumours of the thalamus—a clinico-pathological study. *Brain*, 1938, *61*, 339–374.

Spiegel, R., Wycis, H., Orchinik, C., and Freed, H. Thalamic chronotaraxis. *Archives of Neurology and Psychiatry*, 1955, *73*, 469–471.

Stern, K. Severe dementia associated with bilateral symmetrical degeneration of the thalamus. *Brain*, 1939, *62*, 157–171.

Sugishita, M., Ishijima, B., Hori, T., Fukushima, T., and Iwata, M. "Pure" agraphia after left CM-thalamotomy (Japanese). *Clinical Neurology*, 1973, *13*, 568–574.

Tobias, T., Afferents to prefrontal cortex from the thalamus mediodorsalis nucleus in the rhesus monkey. *Brain Research*, 1975, *83*, 191–212.

Van Buren, J., and Borke, R. Alterations in speech and the pulvinar. *Brain,* 1969, *92*, 255.

Victor, M., Adams, R., and Collins, G. *The Wernicke-Korsakoff Syndrome.* Philadelphia: Davis, 1971.

Vilkki, J., and Laitinen, L. Effects of pulvinotomy and ventrolateral thalamotomy on some cognitive functions. *Neuropsychologia,* 1976, *14*, 67–78.

Walker, A. E., *The Primate Thalamus.* University of Chicago Press, Chicago, 1938.

Walther, H. Uber einen Dammerzustand mit triebhafter Erregung nach Thalamusschadigung. *Monatsschrift für Psychiatrie und Neurologie,* 1945, *3*, 1–16.

Waltz, J., Riklan, M., Stellar, S., and Cooper, I. Cryothalamotomy for Parkinson's disease. *Neurology,* 1966, *16*, 994.

Weinstein, E., and Kahn, R. Nonaphasic misnaming (paraphasia) in organic brain disease. *Archives of Neurology and Psychiatry,* 1952, *67*, 72–80.

10

Aphasias

HENRY HÉCAEN

INTRODUCTION

By "aphasia" is meant disturbances in verbal communication due to circumscribed cerebral lesions. Such a definition is not particularly satisfactory, since the language disorder is defined by the focal lesion giving rise to it rather than by any special feature of the disorder itself.

The complex organization of language, of course, can be disordered at various levels of integration. So we must first specify which disturbances of verbal expression or reception we include in the term "aphasia." Although a clinician has no trouble in distinguishing a motor aphasia from a subcortical dysarthria, or a sensory aphasia from the verbal performance of an incoherent schizophrenic patient, the theoretical basis of such distinctions is often unclear. Very frequently, criteria independent of the linguistic disturbance—for example, associated symptoms and cortical lesions—are taken into consideration in deciding whether and how to separate these disorders. A classic example of such a decision concerns the relation between intellectual disorders and sensory aphasia.

Linguistic methods and concepts seem useful in providing criteria for distinguishing between so-called aphasias and other disorders of language or speech. Aphasias thus may be considered as impairments of the formal language code at different levels of verbal performance. On the one hand, disturbances of the phonological system with the phonetic aspect preserved and, on the other hand, disturbances of the use of syntactic rules can distinguish the expressive aphasias from paretic or ataxic disorders of speech and from demential semantic incoherency, respectively. In the field of receptive disorders, we must distinguish between failures of phonemic discrimination (as in word deafness) and mere lowering of

HENRY HÉCAEN   Unité des Récherches Neuropsychologiques et Neurolinguistiques, Ecole des Hautes Etudes en Sciences Sociales, Paris 75014, France.

auditory acuity that may lead to poor detection of some of the sounds of language. At another level, failure to understand verbal commands must be distinguished from the incomprehension of dementia, which is not limited to the verbal code.

Delusional and schizophrenic patients' language, despite its neologisms, its agrammaticism, and its semantic anomalies, which resemble the jargon of Wernicke's aphasia, indicates not a disorganization of the code itself but rather the use of a neocode whose rules depend on the underlying psychological disorder.

This categorization of language pathology in aphasia must permit a better integration between descriptions from linguistic methods and descriptions relating to clinical-anatomical findings, even going so far as the inclusion of anatomical-physiological models to help elucidate the mechanisms of the disorganizations.

History

Aphasia, as a problem of language articulation caused by cerebral lesion, was not studied until the second half of the nineteenth century.

Despite interesting remarks and pertinent observations (see Benton and Joynt, 1960), despite publications by Gall (1811–1819), and despite the profound impact of phrenological theories, in particular their influence on the conceptions of localization of Bouillaud (1825), it was not until April 18, 1861, that actual investigation of aphasia began. On that day, Broca presented to the Société d'Anthropologie de Paris the case of a subject who could not speak and for whom postmortem examination revealed specifically the part of the frontal lobe that must have been the site for the faculty of articulated language. Four years later, Broca also established the principle of left hemispheric dominance for this same faculty.

Another major moment in the history of aphasia was in 1874, when Wernicke showed that lesioning of another part of cortex, the first temporal convolution, caused a loss of memory for auditory images of words. The symptoms which result from this lesion are primarily an abundance of mispronounced words and a deficit in verbal comprehension. Wernicke also introduced a model for the functioning of language which takes into account both clinical and anatomical data; the associationist model which Bastian had proposed in 1869 had been a first approximation. Word deafness consequent to destruction of the verbal auditory center is the essential characteristic of receptive or sensory aphasia; absence of auditory control over his own production of language provokes an incoherence of expression in the patient. Inversely, motor aphasia is an expressive aphasia determined by the destruction of the center which commands the movements of organs of speech. From this model, Wernicke deduced that there must exist a third aphasia corresponding to the destruction of pathways which connect one center to another: the patient should understand verbal signs, since the auditory verbal center is intact, but he would lose control over his verbal utterances. The passage from reception to expression is altered, and the aphasic cannot repeat what one says to him, even though it is comprehended. Derived from a theoretical scheme, this aphasia that Wernicke called "conduction aphasia" was later established as a clinical reality.

Endowing neurologists with an associationist model, Wernicke opened a particularly fertile line of research, allowing the establishment of particular forms of aphasic disorders based on topography of lesion sites. Correlations between lesion sites and particular forms of aphasia were successfully confirmed by research and were synthesized by Dejerine (1914) at the end of the period of investigation. Nevertheless, the success of this method caused researchers to interpret clinical-anatomical data in light of their theoretical deductions, thereby multiplying the hypothetical centers and pathways needed to explain cerebral mechanisms of language.

The second historical period consisted of a reaction against the excessive and abusive interpretations of associationists. Some individuals had already expressed their reservations—indeed, had expressed their opposition—to the accepted conception, among them was Jackson, whose influence was not felt until much later. A strong but warranted attack by Marie (1926) advocated a unitary conception of aphasias (excluding Broca's region of the language zone), and recalled the critical methodology of von Monakow (1914), the observations of Head (1926), and, above all, the gestalt theories of Gelb and Goldstein (1920), such that not only were the theoretical conceptions elaborated since Wernicke overturned, but also a large portion of the clinical-anatomical relationships suggested by these theories were discarded.

Gelb and Goldstein emphasized the difference, within the language, between the sensorimotor processes which constitute the instrumentalities and the psychological processes evaluated in terms of a thought-language dialectical relationship; language is an integral part of the human organism in general, and, consequently, aphasia cannot be seen as a specific deficit but rather as a general defense process whereby the organism responds to a particular distress. If the perturbations of instrumentalities depend on localized lesions, the perturbation of the function of language cannot be attributed to a specific lesion. It is the product of the alteration of a dynamic, functional ensemble, and results from a dedifferentiation of the figure-ground relation. What unifies the various aphasic symptoms is the loss of a categorizing attitude, that is, the capacity to comprehend reality as a symbol of something and for that something to be susceptible to representing diverse realities. The patient no longer imagines relationships that exist between an item and the things that it symbolizes; he can no longer establish an attitude of classification toward it. From abstract language, the aphasic regresses to a simple automatic verbal knowledge, toward a more concrete level of realized language.

The holistic conceptions of cerebral functioning dominated the entire interwar period. Furthermore, these globalist theories received support from the experimental findings of Lashley (1923), who affirmed principles of cerebral equipotentiality and of mass action.

It would be unjust not to underline the work of certain authors, independent of any theory, who attempted either to specify clinical-anatomical correlations (Foix, 1928) or to proceed with descriptive analysis of language disorders with more objective techniques (Weisenburg and McBride, 1935).

The last historical period began with a renewed interest in localization. Studies on the aphasic sequelae of warwounded patients allowed confirmation of relationships between the lesion site and aspects of disorders. But aphasiology is currently distinguished essentially by two lines of research, one represented by a revival of the connectionist model, the other by the introduction of linguistic methods and psycholinguistics into the study of language disorders.

The reenlivened connectionist model is a result of clinical-anatomical studies by Geschwind (1965) and investigations of split-brain patients. The accent is placed on the destruction of pathways, and no longer on destructions of centers. Such an approach demands that the observer demonstrate normal performances in the tasks that do not require passage of information through the pathways affected by the lesion. This model requires a suite of new modes of exploring behavior.

Not until Roman Jakobson in 1956 did a true line of research in neurolinguistics begin. Clearly, in 1941, Jakobson had already suggested the problem himself while researching analogies between the stages of development of language and of states of pathological disorganization. Also, in 1947, Luria had presented an analysis of different types of posttraumatic aphasia, taking account of linguistic principles as well as of different levels of language structure. Most dramatic however, was the publication of *Fundamentals of Language* by Jakobson and Halle (1956), which marks the debut of real neurolinguistics. A theoretical analysis of aphasic disorders was presented. Admitting a bipolar structure of normal language, these authors presented a classification based on a dichotomy of these disorders and, on the basis of two methods of structuring of linguistic signs, paradigmatic and syntagmatic, postulated that the language of aphasics no longer translates the structural bipolarity of normal language but rather that a single scheme of connections is used to the exclusion of the other.

In the two decades that followed this theoretical analysis, neurolinguistic studies attracted more and more attention from aphasiologists. The application of linguistic models and methods, of psycholinguistic techniques, and of experimental phonetics improved the conceptions to permit better descriptions of various disorders of verbal behavior caused by cerebral lesions and to establish thereby a more precise typology of aphasias.

It is with these facts in mind that we shall discuss the aspects of disorders of verbal behavior and their relation to different lesion sites.

Neurolinguistic Classification and Description of Aphasias

Any description of aphasia syndromes naturally implies a classification which is itself founded on implicit or explicit physiopathological presuppositions and on the arbitrary application of the theoretical model accepted. The proposed classifications have been numerous, but in their diversity one easily sees in them two fundamentally different tendencies which have opposed each other through the history of the conceptions of aphasia, and which still oppose each other. The first, with a description of the diverse modalities of aphasia, on theoretical as well as clinical bases suggests a classification in which specific forms are in some ways fixed in the type of distinct disorganization that differentiates them; the second, after eliminating isolated disorders of expression or of reception, sees a unique phenomenon in aphasia.

The problem of the typology of aphasia does not necessarily present itself for those who support the second hypothesis. However, the most extreme partisans of a unitary aphasia themselves proposed a typology, but emphasizing that certain of these forms did not pertain to the aphasia framework (anarthria, pure alexia, etc.) or that the diverse aspects of real aphasic disorders were due only to added pathological phenomena, nonlinguistic ones included.

The physiopathological interpretation underlay the classification of the period of the associationist schemas. The opposition between Dejerine and Marie (1908) ended this period and opened the following period. Dejerine admitted the distinction of Broca's aphasia and sensory aphasia without overlooking their possible addition toward a global aphasia, and he recognized pure forms of aphasia. For Marie, the problem of classification did not suggest itself, sensory aphasia being the only aphasia. He was ultimately forced to admit diverse clinical aspects and to recognize that they result from different lesion substrates.

We find this disagreement in the principal classification proposed by clinicians, whatever their suggested criteria.

Neurolinguists allow more coherent descriptions. It is therefore necessary to define the sense of this neurolinguistic approach, making precise its goals and methods. Description of various disorders of verbal performance resulting from focal cortical lesions; recognition of similarities and differences in verbal performances with respect to them, according to lesion topography; research on intervening factors in these perturbations and in their pattern of interaction depending on the task and the sensory channel—these steps appear to be the necessary stages in neurolinguistic research, stages corresponding more to aspects of the same research than to different chronological stages of analysis.

Associations between neurolinguistic syndromes, thusly isolated, and other neuropsychological defects should naturally be kept in mind: the relationship to various apraxias and agnosias, to intellectual deterioration, to disorders of memory, etc.

Finally, anatomical-pathological conditions (mass and nature of the lesion) must not be neglected, nor should the age, the sociocultural level, or the polyglottism of the subject himself. Ultimately, comparisons of peculiarities of pathological verbal behavior in subjects speaking different languages (tonal languages, languages with two systems of writing) or using systems of signs (deafmutes) should furnish very interesting information on the nature of the linguistic disorder.

The topology that we have suggested is hardly definitive, but it seems useful to present it as consistent with results already obtained. This classification harmonizes with established classical clinical-anatomical facts. Even though it may be only an artifact of the investigative method, this harmony justifies the effort to synthetize.

Conscious of the risk that our approach involves, we nevertheless feel that the methods used will ultimately justify its legitimacy, correct its excesses, and reduce its limitations, if it is possible for us, over a large series of collected observations, without preselection, to find groupings and after testing to establish correlations between the results of examination of cognitive abilities and neurological findings. The anatomical criteria should finally permit appreciation of whether or not neurolinguistic and neuropsychological groupings reflect different nervous mechanisms.

Then, and only then, will it be possible to understand the interference of different factors in a mixed syndrome where the ensemble of disorders certainly is not manifest as a simple addition but rather as an interaction of deficits and a reorganization of remaining functional possibilities to overcome the resulting perturbations.

DISORDERS OF ORAL LANGUAGE

EXPRESSIVE APHASIAS. Expressive aphasias must be divided into three subgroups: the first two varieties are very close to one another, and the third diverges notably from the others while conserving the essential negative characteristics of expressive aphasia, disorders of reception and of verbal comprehension being either absent or relatively secondary.

In this ensemble it might be necessary to include another variety: transcortical motor aphasia described by Wernicke (1903) as a result of a rupture between Broca's center and the superior center for concepts. According to him, its characteristics are a dearth of spontaneous language, the presence of automatic language and repetition, and conservation of verbal comprehension. This form, accepted by Goldstein (1948) as language akinesia, corresponds to the dynamic aphasia of Luria (1969). In fact, it may not be a real aphasia, but more a phenomenon of lack as described by Kleist (1933) in cases of anterior or medial (supplementary motor area) frontal lesions.

Aphasia of Phonemic Production. Aphasia of phonemic production corresponds to "motor aphasia" of the classical literature, to the "anarthria" of Marie (1926), to the "verbal aphasia" of Head (1926), and to the "syndrome of phonetic disintegration" of Alajouanine *et al.* (1939). The writing disorders are quasiconstant, wherein, most frequently, the character and intensity do not parallel those of perturbations in speech, to such a point that, classically, a pure motor aphasia might be considered present where graphic disorders were absent.

Dejerine (1914), while he accepted the existence of the syndrome, denied that it had a single anatomical correlate, since the syndrome could be found following cortical (foot of F_3) and subcortical lesions. Hécaen and Consoli (1973) studied 19 subjects with anatomically verified lesions limited to Broca's area. Within this group of 19 subjects, a subgroup with lesions restricted to the cortical surface had a cluster of signs which corresponded to pure motor aphasia: decreased verbal fluency and dysprosody (slowness, dysrhythmia, and syllabation), even in the absence of dysarthric deformations. Reading, writing, and auditory comprehension were within normal limits, although spelling was impaired.

Most usually, however, since lesions do not limit themselves to the surface of Broca's area, the disorders of language also influence written expression, and even verbal comprehension, realizing Broca's picture of aphasia as understood by Dejerine.

The emission of language can, in the most aggravated form of motor aphasia, be totally blocked. From the first question posed, the patient, who cannot respond, resorts to an intense gesticulation to indicate the impossibility of expressing himself. He finally can emit several inarticulate groans. Often the patient is limited to a single syllable or to several syllables of greater or lesser complexity, and empty of meaning. Thus Broca's patient pronounced only "tan tan tan."

At a less severe level, the patient uses a reduced verbal stock wherein units suffer multiple deformations (literal paraphasias) which correspond to disorders in the phonic constitution of the item.

In general, the prosody of language, i.e., the expressive intonation, the rhythm, and the intonation, is only slightly or not at all altered in motor aphasics. However, Monrad-Krohn (1947) insisted on dysprosody as a possible concomitant of motor aphasia, or as a simple sequela. This perturbation of the prosodic qualities of speech can give a foreign-sounding accent to a language. Or the dysprosody can simply consist of a decrease of flow with syllabic scansion where each utterance is pronounced syllable by syllable, each of the syllables consisting of an autonomous articulation. Spectrographic analysis of speech in such cases reveals only the decrease of flow, while the formant structure and consonant transitions are normal.

Naming naturally cannot be explored if disorders of expression are too great; when a certain degree of expression is possible, most generally the patient can name objects presented, but arthric deformations are manifest in his responses.

Disorders of auditory verbal comprehension or of written material are present in the initial period, but they attenuate quickly. Recently, however, a new analysis of our observations dealing with only verified posterior frontal or anterior Rolandic lesions has forced us to admit that they can persist in a relatively severe form in a certain number of cases, especially if the lesion is extensive in depth.

As a general rule, writing disorders are present except in pure motor aphasia, and their main characteristic is literal paragraphia; the grapheme generally can be executed, but at the word level there are omissions, distortions, additions, and substitutions of graphemes. The sentence level hardly ever is attained. Spelling, moreover, shows grave disorders. This agraphia of expressive aphasia is marked by three dissociations: the disorder affects only writing to dictation and spontaneous writing, while copying is unimpaired; the writing of dictated words is much better than that of nonsense syllables; and figures and numbers are generally well written.

The possibility of singing is usually preserved: melody is hummed without words, and song can often favor verbal expression.

Associated disorders are acalculia (written or mental); buccolingual-facial apraxia, especially when the speech disorder is acute; and sometimes left ideomotor apraxia. There is either a right hemiplegia or a brachiofacial or brachial monoplegia, at least initially; sensory disturbances are likewise found almost invariably.

Neurolinguistic studies (Cohen *et al.*, 1963; Shankweiler and Harris, 1966; Johns and Darley, 1970; S. Blumstein, 1973) allowed classification of disorders of oral expression at a phonetic level and specification of the character of "arthric" difficulties: permanence of the vocalizing system, more marked deficit of fricatives and liquids than of stop consonants, reductions of consonant groups, phenomena of vowel or consonant anticipation, even syllabic, and phenomena of perseveration. The variability of responses includes, in addition, the conservation of the phonological system, wherein only zones of deficient distribution are observed.

Shankweiler and Harris insist on the variability of substitutions and on the absence of systematization of errors according to place of articulation, and underline that the origin of the disorder need not depend on a paretic or spastic state of articulatory muscles; rather, one must envisage a disorganization of the process by which phonological units are encoded.

Johns and Darley (1970) insisted on the difference between articulatory disorders due to motor aphasia and those based on defective neuromotor projection systems (dysarthria) and those due to sensory or perceptual impairment. These authors called the defect "apraxia of speech" and underlined the distinctive characteristics of this syndrome: the presence of alterations of volitional articulation manifested by variability of phoneme production; anticipatory errors; unrelated and additive substitutions, repetitions, and blocks; "conduites d'approche" and dysprosody.

Phonetic research was undertaken with regard to verbal utterances of expressive aphasias. In the case of articulation disorders of aphasic type, if the spectrogram shows no new precision, the electromyogram of the buccophonatory muscles reflects a production or an impossibility of independent movements of articulatory muscles (Shankweiler *et al.*, 1968).

Agrammatic Aphasia or Disorder of Syntactic Production. Agrammatic aphasia is more a variant of the previous form than it is a distinct form. Here expression is characterized by a discourse of isolated words, substantives, and verbs in nominal form with reduction of grammatical words, even when well pronounced.

Linguistic analysis of agrammatism was first undertaken by Pick (1913) and by Isserlin (1922); it has been done more systematically these past few years.

According to Cohen and Hécaen (1965), the deficit in agrammatism is disorganization of the structure of the immediate constituents of the sentence or those of relation between the immediate constituents. Contrasts between syntactic variants are suppressed. Agrammatism is different from motor aphasia, where the deficit relates to the program of phonetic production, since the constituent morphemes are spoken without error in spontaneous speech and the phonic deficit appears only at the level of repetition of words and nonsense syllables. The specific distribution of errors does not necessarily appear initially, but certainly ultimately; conservation of prosody of the pronounced elements confers them with a sentence value. The deficit thus has two aspects: reduction of syntactic patterns and conservation of lexemes with concurrent inpoverishment of lexical stock. The explicit references to the situation are replaced by implicit references, such that as a result of the reduction of syntactic patterns, functional-grammatical words are less often spoken than others.

In a completely different perspective, Goodglass (1968) defines motor agrammatism as a disorder of language at a much simpler level than that of syntax:

inhibition of initiation and flux of speech. Agrammatism would essentially be noted by an association between the difficult production of small groups of words and the omission of initial, unstressed functors, these same words being capable of pronunciation in a statement if they are placed after a fully stressed word. Essentially this agrammatism would depend on the necessity for the patient to make a first utterance, to find a salient word, usually a significant noun or verb. This character of salience is defined as a result of the combined effect of (1) the intonational stress, (2) the phonological prominence, and (3) the informational load. Functional words usually possess only a weak degree of these three aspects and so disappear from the aphasic statement.

According to Goodglass, the absence of rhythm and intonation would result from this limitation to salient words; the agrammatic patient guards only "a residual knowledge of the manner by which certain words can be placed to make certain sentences." A primitive rule therefore persists, substituting for other rules no longer known.

This interpretation counters certain objections such as the conservation of intonation contours of emitted word-sentences and the persistence of agrammatism in writing. Goodglass admits another agrammatism of a so-called conceptual type, not so specific as Broca's aphasia. It would be characterized by a confusion between prepositions of time and space, the gender of pronouns, and the time of verbs, and would also reflect as much on comprehension as on expression of grammatical discriminations.

Ultimately, in a series of psycholinguistic studies on the grammar of aphasics, Goodglass (1976) observed a similarity of aphasic performance irrespective of clinical type. He suggested that the hierarchy of agrammatical errors revealed with structured psycholinguistic testing of aphasics may not reflect a purely linguistic disturbance. Performance factors such as sentence length, word frequency, and especially stress were found to contribute significantly to the patient's apparent grammatical defect. Goodglass concluded that linguistic impairments in aphasia cannot be explained exclusively by reference to linguistic theories of derivational or transformational complexity but must be considered in terms of a performance model.

From a linguistic analysis of the performances of agrammatic patients, Tissot *et al.* (1973) objected to previous interpretations of the syndrome of agrammatism. While underlining the uniqueness of the syndrome, they define it as a difficulty of mastering the grammar. This "syndrome of disintegration of grammar" is therefore opposed to the syndrome of phonetic disintegration of motor aphasics. In the group thus defined, the performances of subjects on linguistic tests allowed the authors to define three subgroups.

1. Agrammatisms with a morphological predominance. Deficits of production of morphological opposites, of morphological derivatives, and of articles and difficulties in the correction of morphological marks are very notable. On the other hand, the word order of a statement is conserved.

2. Agrammatisms without major morphological disorders, with predominant syntactic disorder. The structure of statements is very different. Conventional

word order is no longer respected, and there are major difficulties in putting missing lexemes in sentences left for completion. But, contrarily, the patients of this group easily find morphological opposites.

3. Pseudoagrammatism with dysprosody (Goodglass).

The authors conclude that the two real forms of agrammatism that they have isolated represent two poles of agrammatism, indicative of a certain degree of independence of syntactic (and morphological) mechanisms. In the agrammatism without major morphological disorder, syntactic perturbations relating to deep structure of the language dominate. In the first variety, what is deficient is the technique of transformation, especially morphological, relating to surface structure of the language.

Even though verbal comprehension seems intact in agrammatism, more precise tests may reveal that the deficit is not limited to expression. There may well be a selective deficit of a level of language. Zurif *et al.* (1972) asked patients for a judgment of syntactic proximity between words (presented in triads) within a sentence; they found that the deficit was qualitatively identical between the reception and the production of the sentence; hence a simple procedure of economy could not be offered as explanation.

In fact, agrammatics base their judgments according to a hierarchical scheme which excludes nonessential elements (grammatical words), while normal subjects take advantage of the surface syntactic structure of the sentence.

Conduction Aphasia or Phrastic Programming Aphasia. The reality of conduction aphasia, first postulated theoretically by Wernicke (1874), was subsequently confirmed by a number of observations. For some, however, it did not correspond to more than a fortuitous association of symptoms or a regressive stage of sensory aphasia.

Construction aphasia is defined by the presence of paraphasias in spontaneous language and by disorders of repetition, occasionally of writing, and furthermore is contrasted by an absence of real disorders of comprehension. Paraphasias based on telescoping of words or on confusion of words phonetically close occasionally render communication difficult, so much so that the patient who is conscious of his deficit tries to correct them by successive approximations (conduites d'approches). Sentences are limited to attempts or to simple clauses not related to one another, with stops and intercalation of adverbs such as "then" and "later;" with each change of enunciation, fluency of speech is lessened. On the other hand, automatic series are better expressed.

In repetition, errors are manifest, even for monosyllables, and they multiply with the number of syllables equally well for repetition of words or nonsense syllables, these become considerable during the repeating of sentences. The lesser errors can be corrected secondarily. Even when the patient is particularly vigilant, he repeats in a hesitating fashion and stresses each syllable.

Naming of objects is often very disturbed; either the patient can find no nouns, even approximately, or the attempts give rise to paraphasias (substitution, phonic errors of which the patient is aware and which he attempts to correct. Following the investigation of Yamadori and Ikumura (1975) of a case of conduction aphasia in a Japanese, it is known that the anomia cannot be merely a simple association but is an integral part of this kind of aphasia.

Verbal comprehension appears, however, to be little altered. The patients recognize the grammatical or agrammatical character of sentences presented to them. They are also capable of performing grammatical transformations. Comprehension of written orders is generally good; on the other hand, reading aloud is slow and difficult and paralexias are considerable.

Writing disorders are consistently found. Graphic production shows autocontrol with frequent crossing out, overwriting, and stopping. The graphemes are correctly formed, but there are disturbances of the structure of words similar to the literal paragraphia in motor aphasia but with some telescoping or even substitutions or omissions of lexemes. The writing of dictated single words is better than that of nonsense syllables. At the sentence level there is usually some impairment; subordinate and coordinate clauses may be formed, but at the same time function words are left out and there also are slight syntactic deficiencies. Copying remains unimpaired, and figures and numbers are correctly written, but spelling is always faulty.

Conduction aphasia is associated with acalculia and disturbance of reproduction of rhythmical structures and frequently, despite some exceptions, with bilateral somatognosic and ideomotor or constructive apraxic disorders. There are no motor defects, sensory disorders are slight, and the visual field is generally unimpaired.

The accepted name for this variety of aphasia reveals the interpretation given of it as a result of the theoretical model of Wernicke: the lesion which causes it ruptures the connections between the zones of reception and expression of language, and so prohibits the repetition and the control of Wernicke's area over expression. After a long period of discredit, this connectionist interpretation was brillantly restored to value by Geschwind (1965). Konorski (1961) and Benson *et al.* (1973) also support this interpretation. However, other authors did not want to see in this more than a fortuitous conjunction of symptoms or an aspect of regression of a sensory aphasia (e.g., Kleist, 1933). For Goldstein (1948), on the other hand, conduction aphasia—a well-defined syndrome—constitutes a prelinguistic deficit. This disorder interdicts the process which goes from thought to language, hence the name he uses, "central aphasia." It represents a disorder of inner speech. In the conduction aphasic there exists a loss of voluntary attitude which normally permits structuring of verbal knowledge into verbal formulas; while the verbal sounds can be recognized, the subject becomes incapable of realizing a simultaneous synthesis of words to be emitted.

Linguistic analysis of these aphasics has permitted new interpretations. Hence in 1964, Dubois *et al.*, from a study of six very pure cases of this aphasia, concluded that conduction aphasia depends on a disorder of phrastic programming.

Conduction aphasia is characterized first by a twofold integrity: (1) integrity of reception of verbal messages and (2) integrity of the relation of the subject to the utterance he makes, to the significance he gives to it, and to the situations in which he is placed. The patient controls his emissions, as is shown by his frequent self-correction. The intonation conserves all its wealth of expressiveness except for abnormal pauses.

Conduction aphasia appears to be an alteration of the capacity for "phrasic programming." Even though the possibility to produce utterances and to handle the grammatical code persists, the concatenations of realized elements are profoundly disturbed as is made evident by tests of repetition and of simulated generation of sentences. The deficit in the tests of repetition (words, nonsense syllables, sentences) increases on the one hand as a function of the number of syllables or of words in the sentence, and on the other hand as a function of the number of transformations that the sentence contains, i.e., a function of length and complexity.

The difficulty a patient encounters in producing a sentence on the presentation of several isolated words is of the same order. These difficulties have the following aspects: neglect of one or several proposed words, simple juxtaposition of one of the words after the others have been integrated into the sentence, considerable difficulty in initiating sentences even though they are correctly produced, and abnormally long pauses between syntagmatic groups. The phonic difficulties are manifest at the level of selectional paradigmatic units and at the level of phrastic concatenation.

These phonic difficulties are qualitatively similar to the phonemic difficulties of motor aphasics. Nevertheless, they have certain features that are different—for example, their appearance in the middle of a word and not at the beginning, the frequency of syllable iteration, and less difficulty with words of few syllables than with nonsense words of the same length.

Yamadori and Ikumura (1975) also propose that the deficit involves a disorder of motor encoding with difficulty of establishing the syllabic sequence of the target word. The deficit is as often encountered during repetition as during reading aloud, naming, or writing to dictation. The isolated syllable is produced, but not the syllabic sequence. Yamadori and Ikumura underline that the best performance of the patient in writing *kanji* rather than *kana* corresponds to the interpretation, because in *kanji* writing an exact syllabic sequence is not absolutely necessary.

A completely different interpretation is proposed by Warrington and his colleagues (Warrington and Shallice, 1969; Shallice and Warrington, 1970, 1974). These authors insist on the presence, in aphasia very close or identical to recognized conduction aphasia, i.e., originating from a lesion in the same place, of a selective disorder of auditory verbal short-term memory, whereas short-term visual memory or short-term retention of significant nonverbal sounds is much less disturbed and long-term memory and verbal auditory learning are not disturbed. Their experiments show that the disorder of repetition of a series cannot be uniquely attributed to an expressive deficit since the immediate designation of elements of the series by nonverbal means is as distrubed as by verbal repetition.

Safran and Marin (1975) also found this selective impairment of auditory short-term verbal memory in a case of conduction aphasia. The abnormal performance of their patient during immediate repetitions presents clear characteristics of the delayed recall: the existence of a primacy effect but absence of recency effect (found, however, if the material is presented visually) and an influence of factors such as the meaningfulness or familiarity of the items. In the repetition of sentences the richness of paraphrases shows that the patient is mastering the semantic contents, as long as the syntactic complexity is not too great.

Other research has confirmed that this failure of short-term verbal memory occurs in the auditory more than in the visual modality.

However, it seems to consist more of a quantitative than a qualitative difference, as even the results of Warrington and colleagues show. Tzortzis and Albert (1974) explored short-term memory in the auditory and verbal modality in three patients for verbal and nonverbal material with either verbal or manual responses. In fact, deficits were present in all these tests, but the items were frequently reproduced and the patients failed only to recall the correct order of the items. There did not seem to be a deficit of reproduction since the performance of these patients was as deficient compared to that of normal controls or aphasics of other varieties as it was in matching tasks for sequences.

Strub and Gardner (1974) also admit without totally rejecting the mnemonic factor that the disorder essentially consists of a deficit of selection and arrangement of phonemes in correct sequence.

The difficulty of sequencing or more exactly of memory of sequences could thus be one of the factors responsible for the deficit of linguistic performance recognized as a problem of phrastic programming (Dubois *et al.*, 1964) and of phonemic combination (Strub and Gardner, 1974).

In fact, it is quite possible that the discrepancy of various results just cited is due to the existence of diverse varieties of the syndrome of conduction aphasia. Certain anatomical indications permit consideration of this possibility (Benson *et al.*, 1973).

AMNESIC APHASIAS: DISORDERS OF MORPHEME SELECTION. *Non-Modality-Specific Forms.* Probably all aphasics have a reduced stock of words available for speech, or a reduced access to a preserved stock, thus a naming deficit or word-finding disturbance is a regular feature of the aphasic syndromes; and various theories have been proposed to account for the several different varieties of naming disorders observed clinically.

However, one group of aphasic subjects seems to be isolable from other groups by manifesting a selective loss of lexical items in the presence of fluent articulation, preserved grammar, and intact comprehension. This selective impairment is called "anomia," and the syndrome within which this impairment is found is called "anomic aphasia" or "amnesic aphasia."

Pitres first proposed clinical autonomy for this syndrome in 1898, claiming the basic defect to be a simple forgetting of words. Dejerine (1914), while accepting the existence of word-finding difficulty, felt that an isolated anomic syndrome was quite rate. Marie (1926) recognized the syndrome only as a residual defect of Wernicke's aphasia.

Clinically, one sees rambling but uninformative and circumlocutory speech. Discourse, while essentially fluent, may be punctuated by pauses during which the patient attempts to find the correct word. Indefinite nouns and verbs take the place of the precisely correct lexical item desired, and may be used repetitively. Periphrases, descriptions of a word rather than the word itself, and even explanatory gestures substitute for the target word. Tests of naming demonstrate a hierarchy of difficulty, with nouns being most severely impaired, and verbs and adjectives next.

An essential question to be resolved is whether the deficit in morpheme selection is a single neuropsychological deficit, regardless of the clinical context in which it appears, or if it represents different defects with a common clinical manifestation. For Goldstein (1948), true amnesic aphasia results from an underlying defect in abstract attitude, and this syndrome should be distinguished from other disorders in which a word-finding defect is present. As causes for these other disorders of word-finding ability one would find either a deficit of the instrumentalities of language or a general disorder of memory. True amnesic aphasia, on the other hand, is the expression of a basic loss of orientation to words as symbols which stand for concepts. These patients have an associated difficulty in understanding abstract concepts and fail on tasks which require sorting by category.

Neurolinguistic studies are beginning to clarify the naming disorders. Oldfield (1966) demonstrated that word frequency is a significant variable. This result was similar to that of Wepman *et al.* (1956), who had earlier found an overuse of high-frequency words, regardless of grammatical class, in the speech of aphasics.

Ramier (1972) studied naming with an extensive battery of tests in 83 subjects with left hemispheric lesions. She was able to demonstrate the existence of a true, pure syndrome of amnesic aphasia. The syndrome was rare (three cases out of 83) and was characterized by a unity or similarity of defective naming performances, regardless of the type of stimulus material or the modality of presentation, while all other aspects of verbal behavior were entirely normal. The types of errors were for the most part either failures to respond or claims of not knowing or forms of verbal predication. When verbal substitutions were made, they were always semantically close to the target. Phonological cueing facilitated response. Word-finding deficits in spontaneous speech were not necessarily linked to the naming disorder. Recovery in these pure forms of amnesic aphasia was always rapid. Lesions were located in the temporal lobe in all three patients.

Other studies have provided evidence that word-finding ability may be a function of the semantic category of the word involved (Yamadori and Albert, 1973).

Also to be considered in the process of naming is the amount of information available in the sensory input. For the visual modality (Bisiach, 1966) reduction of total information available reduced the ability of aphasics to name the objects, even though recognition by multiple choice was intact.

Modality-Specific Forms. Naming difficulty may be limited to stimuli presented in a single sensory modality while being preserved for stimuli presented in other modalities. Thus Freund (1888) described a case of optic aphasia in which the naming disorder appeared with stimuli in the visual modality, but not with stimuli in the auditory modality. Geschwind and Kaplan (1962) demonstrated modality-specific tactile aphasia in the left hand of a patient with callosal transection. After studying the dissociation of visual and tactile naming in a group of aphasics, Spreen *et al.* (1966) concluded that although word-finding difficulty is ordinarily not modality specific, some aphasic patients have a clear dissociation of naming ability depending on the modality of stimulus presentation.

Explanation of the syndrome of optic aphasia has been based on two anatomical lesions: one being a left occipital lesion producing a right homonymous hemianopia, the other a lesion of the splenium of the corpus callosum. The naming disorder would result from a disconnection of the right occipital lobe— the only region capable of receiving visual inputs—from the language centers in the left hemisphere (Geschwind, 1965). As with optic aphasia, tactile aphasia represents a callosal disconnection syndrome. A highly demonstrative case of optic aphasia was reported more recently by Lhermitte and Beauvois (1973). Naming disorders were limited to stimuli presented in the visual modality. Evocation of names (word finding) in response to oral description of an item was preserved. This subject had a coexistent agnosic alexia and an agnosia for colors. The authors believed that the term "visuoverbal disconnection" both described the syndrome and provided an adequate explanation for its cause.

Not all authors have accepted the explanation of visuoverbal disconnection to account for optic aphasia. Occasional observations of modality-specific aphasias associated with temporal lobe lesions permit one to conclude that callosal lesion cannot be the only explanation for all cases of this syndrome.

THE GROUP OF SENSORY APHASIAS. *General Clinical Features.* Sensory aphasia (also called "syntactic aphasia" by Head, 1926; "receptive aphasia" by Weisenburg and McBride, 1935; "acoustic aphasia" by Luria, 1969; and Wernicke's aphasia) is characterized primarily by a disorder in verbal reception and comprehension, although other associated defects are the rule. Since the original descriptions by Bastian (1869) and Wernicke (1874), the clinical features have been frequently commented on. Spontaneous speech output is fluent, or indeed hyperfluent, with an increased rate of words per minute and an inability to bring a sentence to a close ("press of speech"). Intonation pattern and facial and gestural expression remain normal, even while the content of the utterance is incomprehensible. This incomprehensibility of verbal output is not due to a deformation of the word in its motor production (as in motor aphasia), but rather is due to substitution of an incorrect lexical item for a correct one (paraphasia), without the patient himself being aware of this substitution. Multiple paraphasias added to the circumlocutory speech due to word-finding difficulties result in a verbal output, called "jargonaphasia," which permits of virtually no meaningful communication. Repetition is impaired, but to varying degrees depending on the type of sensory aphasia. Naming and word finding are defective.

Comprehension defect, the hallmark of the syndrome, may vary from mild to total, and is seen for both spoken and written language. Evaluation of auditory comprehension in terms of the linguistic level at which the comprehension defect occurs—phonemic, semantic, syntactic—has allowed a more refined delineation of separable syndromes within the general category of the sensory aphasias.

Reading aloud, by contrast with reading comprehension, is sometimes possible, although paralexias may be frequent. Writing of name, address, and some words or short phrases may be adequate: however, paragraphic errors are abundant. Longer phrases and sentences cannot be written. The writing disorder, in fact, seems to us to reflect precisely the character and intensity of the oral language disorder. Copying ability, on the other hand, may be reasonably well preserved. Spelling is impaired.

Associated nonlinguistic defects may often include ideomotor, ideational, and constructional apraxias, acalculia, visual recognition defects, and finger agnosia. These defects are not constant, however. General neurological examination may show nothing more than a right hemianopia or quadrantanopia.

If this is the clinical schematic aspect of sensory aphasia, the complexity of this symptomatology and also its variability from one case to another or from one group of cases to another should be underlined, because they are what makes intervention of different factors in different proportions probable.

It has been known for a long time that a selective disorder of verbal reception could be found, the exception being the pure state, and more often clearly predominant over other disorders of verbal performance.

Pure Word Deafness. For word deafness to be called pure, the disorder must be strictly limited to the recognition of sounds of language, at least after the initial phase. In the chronic stage, the patient does not understand anything spoken to him aloud, cannot capture words, and cannot write to dictation, but spontaneous writing is intact.

The syndrome is thus constituted only by the loss of comprehension and repetition of speech and by the impossibility of writing to dictation. Words are perceived by the patient as either an indistinct murmur or as sounds in a foreign language. Occasionally these patients seize certain words in the interior of a sentence and attempt to interpret the context from this reception of varied quality. Theoretically, spontaneous language should be normal in cases of pure word deafness; more often, in the spontaneous language of these patients paraphasias can be observed and several words are missing. Verbal naming and reading are often good. Spelling is only rarely intact. Copied writing is perfect in the majority of cases; in spontaneous writing, it is common to note several forgotten letters or syllables or missed words.

The symptomatology is limited to the domain of language, and most often no praxic or gnosic phenomena appear.

In several observations, it has been noted that the patient is only slightly aware of his problem. This anosognosia seems more often to affect paraphasias in tests of repetition or particularly in spontaneous language, and rarely verbal incomprehension.

By definition, this syndrome does not include an auditory deficit, at least one important enough to compromise the reception of the sounds of language. This indispensable point has often been difficult to make clear, and certainly was before the introduction of audiometric methods. If the existence of severe deficits of auditory perception in cases of word deafness is established, then it seems difficult to admit that these deficits are sufficient to explain verbal agnosia.

Detailed psychoacoustic studies of Jerger *et al.* (1969) and of Chocholle *et al.*

(1975) confirmed this, citing results sufficiently supportive but not identical. It must be stressed that Jerger's patients had a disorder of temporal sequencing of two sounds (Efron, 1963) and that this deficit did not exist in Chocholle's patient. Other authors equally did not find this in patients with severe disorders of reception of verbal material. This disorder of temporal auditory acuity cannot therefore be considered as a necessary condition for word deafness.

Inattention to auditory stimuli with indifference to speech is signaled in a number of observations. But this auditory inattention can itself dissipate while word deafness persists unchanged.

The association of word deafness with nonrecognition of melodies and of meaningful sounds is frequent but not constant. Certain patients are always capable of perceiving vowels, of recognizing characteristics of individual voices, and even of identifying a particular accent, while they fail totally in tests of phonemic discrimination (see particularly Denes and Semenza, 1975). The inverse dissociation has also been observed (Albert *et al.*, 1972). It seems difficult to envisage pure word deafness as only a "fragment of cortical deafness" (Goldstein *et al.*, 1975). Safran *et al.* (1976) showed in a subject affected with a quasi-pure word deafness that comprehension of words was improved when they were presented in context. From such evidence it became accepted that such subjects have a disorder at the phonetic level which can be partially surmounted by recourse to semantic or prosodic indices. The disorder can even not involve auditory reception exclusively, as in the "verbally deaf" patient of Denes and Semenza (1975), who, although capable of matching meaningful sounds with the image of the object that produced it, could not name the object after its sound.

Sensory Aphasias. Adjacent to this selective disturbance in the recognition of the auditory signs of language known as word deafness, there are cases called "sensory aphasia" wherein the inverse is true: words and nonsense syllables can be recognized and repeated, while complex orders presented orally or in writing give rise to failures. These cases speak in favor of the intervention of diverse factors in the most complex cases of sensory aphasia (Hécaen *et al.*, 1968; Hécaen, 1972). Two of these factors seem to be particularly dissociable, one corresponding to the aspect of word deafness and the other to that of disordered comprehension. Finally, there appears to be a third factor, a nonlinguistic one which affects verbal performance, conferring on it a particular character. We have qualified it provisionally as an attentional disorganization.

A quantitative analysis of a series of observations of sensory aphasia (Hécaen, 1969) permitted us to find in two-thirds of these cases self-distinguishing aspects of different profiles in verbal performance (thematic coherence of spontaneous speech, word–nonsense syllables discrimination, verbal comprehension, repetition of words and of nonsense syllables, comprehension of written orders, naming).

1. Sensory Aphasia with Predominance of Word Deafness: Word deafness is marked in spontaneous language as well as in tests of repetition and in writing and reading by a certain number of characteristics which clearly specify it.

Spontaneous Language: logorrhea with paraphasias is common to all varieties, the discourse maintains a unique theme, and the transmitted information constitutes a coherent ensemble despite the anomaly of the sentences. The paraphasias, relatively small in number, are usually in close relation with the context; they are especially of the telescopic type, or phonic approximations.

Repetition: Patients do not treat words and nonsense syllables differently. The quantity of errors is considerable since no item is repeated correctly. The performance is very distant from the model. It must be noted that the response always uses the phonemic stock of the language and that each phoneme of an auditory sequence is isolatedly recognizable and transcribable. Isolated syntagms are repeated as unique items, without dissociation of sound flow; repetition of simple sentences considerably accentuates this trait.

Oral verbal comprehension is null as a result of a disorder of verbal reception.

The discordance is clear between spontaneous writing and writing to dictation, with copied writing being well realized. In essence, spontaneous writing although always disturbed remains possible, thematic coherence is relatively conserved, and paragraphias are relatively less abundant.

Decoding of the written message is always superior to that of spoken messages; the visual channel can remain the only means of entry to communicate with the patient. Naturally, paralexias increase according to the complexity of the text being read.

2. Sensory Aphasia with Predominance of Verbal Comprehension Disorder. The pattern is very different here from the preceding pattern, reception of verbal signs being relatively conserved. By schematizing and taking extreme forms which exist for word deafness, but which are only theoretical for this variety, one could find a point-by-point opposition of each possible performance.

Spontaneous verbal expression: This is extremely diffluent and characterized by a continuous nonachievement and an unfinished embedding of successive sequences. Paraphasias can be numerous, often in the form of substitutions leading to shifts in meaning. The speech is also characterized by ungrammaticalities, and at the same time, even more than in the previous type, is interspersed with stereotyped sentences. Anosognosia seems particularly frequent.

Repetition: The performances vary with the linguistic nature of the item to be repeated: they are better on meaningful words than on nonsense syllables. For words, length is a facilitating factor (less difficulties on longer words), whereas the converse holds for nonsense syllables (the number of errors increases with the number of syllables). The erroneous repeated word here has a close connection with the stimulus; errors illustrate all types of phonemic permutations, but in all cases the structural pattern of the French syllable is preserved. Within this pattern, the errors seem to be purely random (e.g., one type of consonant does not lead to one type of substitution).

Unlike in word deafness, the repetition of sentences remains possible, at least elementary ones. Disturbances manifest themselves with an increase of syntagmatic combination. The disorganizations which appear are essentially reinterpretations of the proposed sentence, from isolated semantic and phonic elements which have been retained.

The comprehension of orders given in writing as well as orally is very disturbed, while phonemic discrimination is altered relatively little.

The important findings of Blumstein *et al.* (1977) must be mentioned here concerning the relative conservation of the capacity for phonemic discrimination in words or in nonsense syllables, or in syllabic structures, and conservation of the discrimination of the order of phonemes in subjects with Wernicke's aphasia having severe comprehension deficits. These discriminations were much more disturbed in Broca's aphasia with disorder of comprehension. The authors themselves note that it is nevertheless in the group of Wernicke's aphasics that a certain relation existed between the comprehension disorder and the degree of phonemic discrimination. So it seems that this relation may not be uniform in Wernicke's aphasics.

The dissociation in writing, is the inverse of that described for the preceding form. Dictation of words gives satisfactory results, but for nonsense syllables errors are frequent, with graphemic substitutions. Spontaneous writing, on the other hand, gives rise to considerable paragraphias.

This description effectively corresponds to that for transcortical sensory aphasia, first postulated by Lichteim (1885) and subsequently described by Wernicke (1903). Goldstein (1948) accepted the reality of this form of aphasia, but rejected the associationist explanation provided by Lichteim and Wernicke, according to which the center for auditory memory images was disconnected from the center for concepts. The causes of the defect were a diminution of attention and acoustic memory and a mild disturbance in the relationship between instrumentalities of language and nonverbal performance; word concept formation depended on this relationship.

Attentional Disorganization. By "attentional disorganization" we mean (Hécaen *et al.,* 1967) to designate a factor which particularly bears on linguistic performances, although it belongs to a much more general disorder, as is shown by disturbances in other aspects of behavior.

As long as there is no serious comprehension deficit or verbal deafness, which is often the case, the repetition of words, nonsense syllables, and sentences presents no difficulty.

The impairment manifests itself clearly in spontaneous speech and in the tasks of sentence production and transformation. Distractibility and perseveration result fundamentally in utterances characterized by an asemanticism which contrasts with their general conformity to the grammatical patterns of the language.

This form of sensory aphasia is probably rare as an isolated or lasting type. But this attention factor can often be found within more complex forms of sensory aphasia.

Distractibility is shown in spontaneous speech by diffluency; the patient is unable to finish the sentence he has begun. His utterance is made of a series of embedded clauses which start but are not completed; the beginning of a complement or embedding is followed by the beginning of another, and another, in a centrifugal manner, each opening giving rise to another. The result of this endless embedding is a general semantic shift of the utterance.

This distractibility factor thus explains the asemantic character of the utterances, as compared with their relative grammatical correctness—although the grammaticalness mainly holds at the level of basic constitution and phrase structure; beyond that, grammatical mistakes can be found, such as errors in agreement or construction, when sequential constraints are not so powerful. And ungrammaticalness becomes much more marked at the interclausal level, with choice of pronouns, number, etc., not adequate for the phrases they refer to in a preceding clause.

The asemanticism of the utterances can be ascribed to breaking of selectional constraints; sometimes adjectives are selected because they have frequent cooccurrence with the noun, despite the fact that they are inappropriate in the particular situation; but, above all, selectional constraints are violated between the subject noun-phrase and the verb, between a noun and its expansion, etc., with mistakes involving subcategorization such as the animate/inanimate distinction.

The same semantic anomaly, with correct surface structure, is found in the sentences that the patient has to make up with words given to him. In this task too, the breaking of selectional constraints leading to asemantic productions is associated with diffluency (Gosnave, 1977).

Perseveration is manifested by severe echolalia—at least at the onset of illness. It also accounts for the very special character of the spontaneous speech, as the paraphasias arise from the interaction of this perseveration and the substitution phenomena. The utterances are thus marked by numerous iterations and repetitions of sentence patterns.

As for naming, there are on the one hand answers with words having only a very loose semantic relationship to the expected item and on the other hand perseverations.

Finally, writing under dictation and copying are good, apart from a few slips and iterations, but in spontaneous writing there again are found the same features of asemanticism through diffluency and of extraneous additions and complementations.

DISORDERS OF WRITTEN LANGUAGE

As we have seen, disorders in written language, at least when they concern encoding, are almost invariably associated with oral language disorders. However, the two are frequently of different sort and intensity. The features peculiar to the written as compared to the spoken code (perceptual and motor features, conditions of acquisition, and structural differences between the two codes) account for the partial autonomy of the former. Pathological investigation has revealed certain discrepancies between disturbances in written and in oral language. These disorders may even be completely separated; indeed, it is possible to find a dissociation between disorders in the reception and the production of written language.

AGRAPHIAS. In dealing with the graphic or written expression of language and its disorders, one must take into account the distinction between the elementary ability to write, which involves primary motor and perceptual functions, and the symbolic content and linguistic characteristics of the material to be expressed. The graphic code cannot be considered as a simple transcription of the oral code. Graphic expression provides a system of symbols in the spatial sphere, derived from a distinct set of linguistic rules. These rules condition the production of graphemes and their linkage in manuscript writing so as to preserve the individuality of graphemic signs within a broad range of idiolectic variants. At the level of syntax, these rules provide the structure within which graphic output can indicate segmentation, thus avoiding the loss of information which in oral expression may be transmitted by nonsegmental elements, such as intonation, facial and manual gestures, and situational context. These conditions both allow and require a high degree of redundancy for the transmission of grammatical and semantic information.

Graphic activity represents an autonomous model of linguistic performance, closely linked nonetheless to the performance model of oral expression. The relationship between these two performance models may be seen at different stages of writing. For example, aside from their independent significance, graphemic signs have specific articulatory referents with respect to the phonological system of the language under consideration. In addition, written sentences may have a deep structure identical to that of spoken sentences despite different sets of performance rules.

From the foregoing considerations it may be concluded that separable varieties of agraphia may occur, each resulting from breakdown at a different level within one of the several neuropsychological systems on which graphic symbolic expression depends—motor, perceptual, linguistic, etc. Disorders of written expression may be categorized into clinical subgroups: pure agraphia, apraxic agraphia, and aphasic agraphia. In this section we shall consider the first two varieties, aphasic agraphia having been discussed in the appropriate sections dealing with aphasia.

Apraxic Agraphia. Disturbance of gestural capacity has long been recognized as a causative factor in many cases of agraphia. These agraphias have been linked primarily to parietal apraxia, and numerous authors have studied both the motor and the kinesthetic limbs of this practic activity (Ogle, 1867; Kussmaül, 1884; Henschen, 1922; Kleist, 1933; Goldstein, 1948).

Apraxia produces agraphia by impairing the ability to form normal graphemes, with inversions and distortions appearing in their stems. The disorder is seen in all modalities of writing (spontaneous, to dictation, and by copying), although infrequently the ability to spell or compose words with alphabet blocks is retained.

In certain cases, although exceptional, the writing disorder is essentially a praxic disorder, which is also manifest in drawing or constructives, but spelling and the composition of words with alphabet blocks remain intact (Pitres, 1884).

In another type of apraxic agraphia without oral language disorder, the graphic disorder affects mainly the production of graphemes and the praxic disorder is limited to a left unilateral ideomotor apraxia (Hécaen and de Angelergues, 1966). The latter would seem to depend on psychomotor reactions of the grasp reflex or avoidance reactions. This disorder cannot be merely apraxic, since spelling and writing with alphabet blocks are also impaired. The causative lesion may be found in the left medial frontal region. The disorder of writing movements appears to correspond to the tonic disorder, even though the two deficits do not occur in the same hand. Heilman *et al.* (1973) studied agraphia and apraxia in a left-handed patient and suggested that dominance for language and dominance for handedness could be represented separately in the two hemispheres in some individuals, language in the left and handedness in the right. If this is correct, disorders of praxis and disorders of graphic linguistic expression could be found in separate hands.

Apraxic and Alexic Agraphia. The more common variety of apraxic agraphia represents a combination of elements of the syndrome of parietal apraxia and that of alexia with agraphia, and is sometimes called "parietal agraphia." A disturbance in both encoding and decoding of written language is found, although the severity of the defect is not necessarily parallel in the two. Frequently associated with this syndrome are disorders of spoken language, especially amnesic aphasia and mild comprehension difficulty.

The characteristics of this agraphia reflect the apraxic influence; distortions and inversions of graphemes are prominent. The relative conservation of the syntactic structure of a sentence and the conjoint impairment of all modes of writing (spontaneous, to dictation, by copying) also are characteristics of the agraphia. The use of alphabet blocks often improves the situation, but never completely. Spelling errors are numerous, with abundant iterations.

Even though the alexia represents an association that, if not constant, is very frequent, it should be recalled that the severity of the defect is not necessarily parallel in the two disorders.

We consider this variety of agraphia to be distinctive and not a part of aphasia-linked agraphia. Nor can apraxia alone entirely explain the findings. This syndrome represents a basic disorder of written language, to which have been added elements of disordered gestural behavior. The essential defect is in the programming of the graphic message, both at the level of gestural performance and at the level of the organization of linguistic symbolic structures. The defect manifests itself primarily in the graphic production of morphemes, the correspondence between phonic and graphic structures being disrupted.

Pure Agraphia. By "pure agraphia" is meant disordered written language expression in the absence of disorders of oral language, reading, or praxis. In 1965, Benedikt suggested that the parts of the brain controlling written and spoken language may have separate anatomical locations. In 1881, Exner presented evidence in favor of the existence of an independent graphic center at the foot of the second frontal gyrus, separate from Broca's area. Henschen (1922) suggested that there was a motor graphic center located in Exner's area and a sensory graphic center in the angular gyrus. In fact, only Gordinier (1899) and Penfield and Roberts (1959) have obtained precise anatomical data.

Few detailed reports of the clinical and neurolinguistic aspects of isolated disorders of writing have been published (Hécaen *et al.*, 1963; Dubois *et al.*, 1969; Assal *et al.*, 1970; Chedru and Geschwind, 1972). Dubois *et al.* (1969) studied six patients with this syndrome. They found no disorder of oral language or of constructional ability. All of their patients had acalculia and four had general intellectual deterioration. Analysis of graphic output revealed the following features. Although misspelling the words in written expression, the patients were able to spell the same words correctly aloud. No significant differences in total errors were noted between single digits and letters or multidigit numbers and words. Ability to copy was essentially intact, although errors crept in when a patient had to change from one expressive code (e.g., cursive script) to another (e.g., block print). Morphographemic rules of expression were normally maintained, and the correspondence of letter to sound (morphographemic-to-morphophonological relationship) was preserved. Perseverative errors were found in only one patient.

Writing in script by hand and writing by the use of anagram letters were compared. In half the group, writing in manuscript was worse; in two patients, errors were equivalent with either method. Spelling errors were further analyzed. Error types, aside from the perseverative errors of one patient, were errors of combination and of selection, with the central portion of the item accounting for the most errors.

From these observations, the authors concluded that pure agraphia consisted of two main forms of graphic defect: one was a spatiotemporal disorganization specific to graphic activity, isolated from constructional apraxia; the other was a disorder of grapheme selection, even in the absence of impaired ability to name letters.

Also, our observations combined with those of Gordinier and of Penfield and Roberts seem to prove the reality of a pure agraphia dissociated from disorders of oral language. But the observations of Gordinier (1833) and Penfield and Roberts (1959) differ notably from ours. With one exception, our observations can be regrouped into a homogeneous unit. Their observations reveal writing disorders similar to those in expressive aphasias. There are even cases where the agraphia reveals the same aspects, although some disorder of oral expression remains. The discrepancy between the severity of graphic disorders and that of oral language disorders suggests that they are intermediates between pure agraphia and agraphia accompanying expressive aphasia.

A novel form of agraphia, selective for written spelling, was described by Kinsbourne and Rosenfield (1974). The patient had impaired ability to spell by writing and manual sorting, but his ability to spell orally was relatively spared. The authors postulated that the programs which translate letter choice into visual terms for purposes of written (as distinct from oral) spelling may be related to a specific cerebral location (left posterior parasagittal parietal area).

Besides the anatomical factor, other factors are very likely to interfere: degree of mastering the written language in the premorbid state, difference of cerebral functional organization in relation to manual preference, and general intellectual impairment. Chedru and Geschwind (1972) particularly noted that this last factor casts doubt on the role of focal lesions in isolated disorders of writing.

ALEXIAS. The suggestion that disorders of reading are associated with disorders of spoken language is very old. Early authors also posited that difficulties of reading could be manifested independently of disorders of oral expression, and even independently of disorders of writing (Gendrin, 1838, cited by Charcot, 1890). Trousseau (1877), Broadbent (1872), Wernicke (1903), and Kussmaül (1884) described such cases in more and more precise fashion, but Charcot's report in 1890 presented the first really typical case.

However, it was Dejerine who provided the impetus for further study of the syndrome by his publications in 1891 and 1892 of two clearly defined case reports including postmortem findings. For Dejerine, alexia in its pure form was a specialized variety of aphasia.

Since the early period, numerous studies have been devoted to the topic of alexia (see the reviews by Hécaen, 1967; Benson and Geschwind, 1969; Dubois-Charlier, 1971; Hécaen and Kremin, 1976). Despite theoretical and nosological dispute, most authors agree that the alexias may be subdivided on an anatomoclinical basis into three major groups: (1) alexia associated with sensory aphasia, due to lesions of the dominant posterior temporal lobe; (2) alexia with agraphia, due to lesions of the angular gyrus; (3) alexia without agraphia (also called "pure alexia" and, by some, "agnosic alexia").

Alexia with Agraphia. To separate alexia with agraphia clinically from the combination of alexia and agraphia associated with sensory aphasia, one must find impaired ability to read and write in relative isolation from disorders of oral language and calculation (e.g., Dejerine, 1891; Nielsen, 1947; Alajouanine *et al.*, 1960). A lesion of the angular gyrus in the language-dominant hemisphere is generally accepted as the anatomical locus underlying this syndrome, and this syndrome is even called "parietal alexia" by some (Quensel, 1931; Pötzl, 1928; Hoff *et al.*, 1954).

Recognition of letters is generally better preserved than that of words, while context often facilitates the understanding of a sentence. Nonetheless, with longer or more complex sentences, comprehension fails. The way words are read seems to show that the normal perceptual strategy used in reading is lost (Haslerud and Clark, 1957). Disorders of graphic expression of language, while present, may not parallel the severity of the alexia. Kinesthetic feedback does not benefit these patients. Associated disorders include, almost invariably, a mild to moderate anomia. Often, but not always, one may see elements of the Gertsmann syndrome, finger agnosia, dyscalculia, dysgraphia, right-left spatial disorientation, and impairment in the ability to recognize or identify fingers. Hemianopia is not necessarily present.

Pure Alexia. The existence of pure alexia is generally accepted; however, some writers think that it should be separated from language disorders and considered as a special optic agnosia or as the result of a more basic disorder (loss of the ability to structure gestalten).

Pure alexia differs from other reading disorders of cortical origin in that it is accompanied by no language disorder (fluency of speech and understanding are unimpaired), except for verbal recall; there are no spelling disorders and no impairment of the perceptual strategies used in reading; writing is normal, or, at least, the degrees of disturbance in reading and in dictation or spontaneous writing are quite different. Copying, on the other hand, is always impaired. Acalculia is frequent but usually slight; visual agnosia (colors and pictures) is variable. Homonymous right lateral hemianopia is always present.

Evaluation of the reading disorder has revealed different subsets within the main syndrome; however, these varieties of alexia have often been considered to be variations in intensity of the basic disorder. Hécaen (1967), Dubois-Charlier (1971), and Hécaen and Kremin (1976) have conducted neurolinguistic analyses of pure alexia, determining the structural basis of the several varieties: literal, verbal, sentence, and global. By this means they have determined that the different varieties of alexia represent distinctive, although overlapping, disorders.

1. Verbal Alexia: The patients are capable of recognizing most letters or, at least, make only a few errors in their identification. By slowly reading letter by letter the patient is often able to read several words by successive spelling, but the difficulties are manifest if the length of the word is increased. The perceptive strategy appears to be conserved.

Nonsense syllables are also well read. When the disorder is relatively slight and there is hence a possibility that all words can be read, simple orders can sometimes be read and executed.

If digits and isolated numbers containing up to three digits are always well read, errors are noted for large numbers. Several difficulties are found in arithmetic operations, but understanding of the principles most often remains intact.

Copying is almost always disturbed, and sometimes markedly, but transformation from capital to cursive is habitual, and paragraphias are rare.

Writing to dictation and spontaneously shows only minimal dysorthographic errors. The writing of digits and numbers is always well executed.

Visual agnosias (pictures, colors) are often found, but in general they are of a slight degree; right homonymous hemianopia is constant.

2. Literal Alexia: In the identification of letters, which is rarely lost completely, errors are much more numerous than in identification of words. Lexemes are much more well read than functional words and nonsense syllables.

Paralexias are frequent in the reading of words, approximately according to their graphic form and especially for word endings. Paralexias are also produced in the semantic sphere (Beringer and Stein, 1930), the patient occasionally producing the semantic category of the word to be read, but secondarily, with a differentiation; sometimes the word read has only a very uncertain semantic rapport with the item.

In this type of alexia, simple orders are generally read with approximations. Complex orders give rise to a partial apprehension with uncertainty. Reading of a text gives rise to either a complete failure or considerable paralexias.

Reading of digits and numbers appears more disturbed in this group than in the previous one.

Copying is severely impaired in these patients, often taking the form of a slavish reproduction of apparently meaningless forms. In writing spontaneously or to dictation, clear deficits are frequently observed, while writing of isolated words to dictation remains relatively good. Only the writing of isolated digits is possible.

Disordered recognition of pictures and of colors is as frequent as in the previous variety. Several praxic difficulties and several somatognosic difficulties can appear, although they may be slight. Right homonymous hemianopia is frequent but not constant.

What essentially characterizes this form is the impossibility of reading by spelling. A certain number of words are read, but in a paralexic manner; either the word once its start is identified is completed by approximation or invention, or the general meaning of the word is captured ("hospital":"doctor, patient . . . "), or a related graphic form is recognized in the presented word ("hôpital":"habitat").

Goldstein (1948), Faust (1955), and Marshall and Newcombe (1966) noted paralexic aspects very much related to those found during literal alexia despite the presence of several disorders of oral language in these observations. Marshall and Newcombe (1966) analyzed these paralexias quantitatively and qualitatively. The errors are grouped in a selective way as a function of the grammatical class of words presented, total failure being much more frequent for adjectives and verbs than for nouns; and grammatical morphemes are read only exceptionally. Paralexic responses of a semantic type clearly predominate for nouns, while "visual responses" ("next," for "exit") and visual completion ("gentlemen" for "gentle") are relatively predominant for nouns and verbs. In addition, in erroneous responses, whatever the paradigmatic class or the paralexic type, a strong tendency to respond with nouns is noted. Semantic errors go "from almost pure synonymity to cases where the stimulus word and the response error had only one or two semantic markers in common (sick read for ill; historic for ancient; town for city, etc. . . .)."

3. Sentence Alexia: This additional variety of alexia has been proposed as a separate category (Dubois-Charlier, 1971; Hécaen and Kremin, 1976). The ability to read letters and words is largely preserved, along with the ability to read single- and multiple-digit numbers. Errors become numerous, however, with the reading (and comprehension) of simple commands. As the commands or sentences to be read for meaning become longer and more complex, the deficit becomes exaggerated.

4. Global Alexia: This is the inability to read either letters or words, despite the relatively normal ability to read single- and multiple-digit numbers. In this variety of alexia the patient can compensate by kinesthetic feedback. Thus, as noted in the earliest reports (Charcot, 1890; Dejerine, 1892), these subjects can "read" letters and even words by actively tracing the letters with their fingers or by having the examiner move their arms in the air in the pattern of the letter. Spontaneous writing and writing to dictation remain normal. Associated disorders have been variously reported. These may include difficulties with arithmetic operations and with recognition of musical notation (Dejerine, 1892; Hécaen, 1972) and agnosia for colors (Pötzl, 1928). Right homonymous hemianopia is a constant finding.

Neurolinguistic Analyses of Pure Alexias. Hécaen and Kremin (1976) analyzed new cases of pure alexia in the same manner as Dubois-Charlier. This classification of alexias according to the different levels of the graphematic units which reflect the disturbances can be maintained as a result of their findings. But it is also suggested in this report that this classification must be made precise while taking into account three contrasts that stem from the implicated cognitive processes or from the character of the material presented: recognition vs. reading of items, meaningfulness vs. nonmeaningfulness of the items, and combination vs. global comprehension of the material.

The different aspects of reading are certainly not affected in isolation, and there can be no hope of finding the alexic forms that would reveal their isolated involvement. It is more a question of assessing their combination and interaction in the different pathological aspects of reading, which as an initial approximation were described according to the linguistic level (letters, words, sentences) at which the disturbance was predominantly found.

Despite all the reservations that can and should be made with regard to this classification, the fact remains that it does correspond to a certain clinical reality. It seems necessary, however, to reconsider these forms, specifying for each the similarities and differences with regard to the three contrasts described.

1. Verbal Alexia: At the level of graphemes, this type of alexia is characterized by a good ability to read and good recognition of individual letters. There appears, however, to be a deficit in categorization which manifests itself when the patient has to recognize the same letter in different graphic shapes. At the level of words, reading difficulties caused by combination difficulties are observed. These are more or less independent of the factor of "meaningfulness." The recognition of words seems to depend on the nature of the task. Presentation of pictures in a multiple-choice task and presentation of words in a foreign language facilitate the recognition, whereas presentation of part of the letters which make up a word in a task of recognition of mutilated words does not facilitate the recognition. The strategy of reading used is deciphering by successive spelling. An overall (global) understanding of a word is totally impossible.

2. Literal Alexia: Individual letters may be recognized but not read. There is no deficit in categorization. Words (even mutilated words) and nonsense syllables are easily recognized. The ability to read is, however, impaired. Nonsense syllables cannot be read at all, and the responses have no resemblance to the stimulus. The reading strategy used is "global," which produces visual and semantic paralexias.

3. Sentence Alexia: Individual letters are well read, but a deficit in categorization is also found in this form. Recognition of nonsense syllables and words is good. Words may be relatively well read, but nonsense syllables create serious problems. The major impairment is found at the level of written text and sentences, for which both reading and recognition are very deficient. Reading is accomplished on the basis of an overall comprehension of the word. Combination difficulties are found, but at a higher level. They appear to be characterized by the loss of principles of sequence, choice, or coordination of the morphemic items of a sentence or a text. Sentence alexia is thus characterized by the same deficit in categorization as verbal alexia. Combination difficulties also seem to be a common feature of these two types of alexia, but are found at different linguistic levels. At the same time, sentence alexia also has features in common with literal alexia, e.g., the global comprehension strategy used for words and the influence of the factor of meaningfulness on the performance.

ANATOMICAL BASIS OF LANGUAGE

If the first concept of localization of disorders of language appeared with the work of Gall and Bouillaud, it was Broca (1861) who first demonstrated localization of the faculty of articulated language, at the level of the posterior part of third frontal gyrus. In 1874, Wernicke showed the role of a second cortical zone, the first temporal convolution, where a lesion caused another type of aphasia; Dejerine in 1891 recognized the role of lesions of the angular gyrus in disorders of reading, and Exner (1881) hypothesized the existence of a center for writing situated in the posterior part of F_2. On this anatomical base was built the schema which presides over the associationist schemas of aphasia.

Dejerine (1914), like Wernicke denying the autonomy of Exner's center, describes three primary regions within the "zone of language" (Fig. 1): (1) An anterior portion, Broca's area, consisting of the posterior portion of the foot of the third frontal convolution, the frontal operculum, and the immediately adjacent cortical zone (tip of F_3 and foot of F_2) not including the Rolandic operculum; this region extends as far as the anterior portion of the insula: (2) An inferior or temporal portion, Wernicke's area, consisting of the posterior portion of the first and second temporal gyri; this region represents the center for verbal auditory images: (3) A posterior portion corresponding to the angular gyrus; this region represents the center for verbal visual images.

Marie (1926) denied the conceptions of the localizationists and associationists, and specifically concluded that "the foot of the third frontal convolution played no role in aphasia." For Marie, there was only one aphasia, and this always corresponded to a lesion of Wernicke's area, even if the symptoms were variable. Broca's aphasia was conceived of as a combination of Wernicke's aphasia plus anarthria. This anarthria, which was not a part of the true aphasia, resulted from a lesion somewhere within the confines of a subcortical quadrilateral zone. He emphasized that this zone was always involved and that the foot of the third

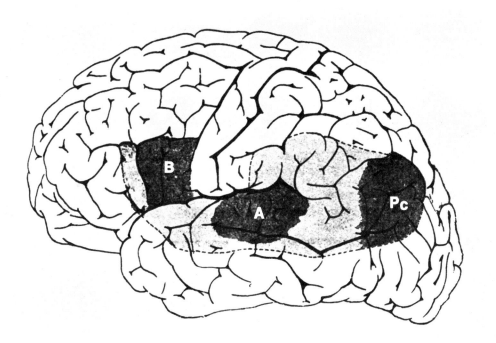

Fig. 1. Zone of language (Dejerine, 1914). B, Broca's area; A, Wernicke's area; Pc, angular gyrus.

frontal convolution was frequently uninvolved in the presence of motor disturbances of language.

Each localizationist who followed presented his own anatomical refinement to the argument (e.g., Henschen, 1922; Kleist, 1933; Nielsen, 1947).

Even Goldstein (1948), the best known of the globalists, after first asserting the impossibility of localizing the functions of language, finally admitted its possibility. He described the existence of disorders of the instrumentalities of language, with specific defects of auditory, visual, and motor "gestalten." These defects corresponded anatomically to the different cortical foci. Nonetheless, Goldstein affirmed that the capacity for inner speech, closely tied to the faculty for abstraction, remained dependent on "the central regions of the cortex."

In the mid-1960s, Geschwind (1965), reviving and reinforcing the anatomical conceptions of Wernicke and Dejerine, provided a compelling theoretical argument concerning the region of the angular gyrus as a critical anatomical development in the evolution of language. By means of its crucial location, abutting the association cortices of three sensory regions (auditory, visual, and somesthetic) and by virtue of its dense polysynaptic connections, the angular gyrus region was able to foster the formation of corticocortical, nonlimbic, cross-modal associations neccessary for certain aspects of human language.

The study of patients with vascular lesions has played a major role in the elaboration of classical aphasiological doctrine. The work of Dejerine and his school was based primarily on the anatomical study of vascular lesions. Special mention, in this regard, should be given to Foix (1928), whose systematic study of the different vascular territories of the brain led to the establishment of a map of the vascular territories of aphasia and the clinical syndromes which depend on the destruction of these vascular territories.

Head injuries from war wounds and accidents have provided large numbers of patients for neuropsychological study. Although the anatomical localization of the lesions in these cases could only be approximate, their great and ever-increasing number and ready availability have prompted many large-scale statistical studies.

All the studies of gunshot wounds of the brain undertaken after World War II (Schiller, 1947; Conrad, 1954; Bay, 1960; Alajouanine *et al.,* 1957; Russel and Espir, 1961) schematically confirm the accepted zones, with a double motor and sensory polarity, while at the same time they show how intricate are the aspects involved. These studies also show the importance of the amount of tissue destroyed in determining the intensity, the persistence, and the global character of language defects. Finally, these authors are in agreement in not recognizing any particular localization value in amnesic aphasia.

Luria based his anatomolinguistic classification of 1947 on studies of aphasics with war-induced head injuries. He divided subjects into the following groups: aphasia with phonemic disintegration due to lesions in the posterior portion of the temporal lobe, aphasia with deficits in the ability to communicate relations (space, time, logicogrammatical forms) due to parietooccipital lesions, aphasia with loss of capacity to synthesize successive elements in a continuous series due to frontotemporal lesions, and dynamic aphasia due to frontal lesions.

Brain tumors producing language defects have also been a source of patient material for neuropsychological study. In such studies most authors have made allowance for the lack of precision of lesion boundaries as well as for the behavioral defect due to increased intracranial pressure which may be added to the focal symptomatology. Of particular interest regarding the relationship of brain tumors to language pathology has been the commonly made observation that word-finding difficulty is frequently the predominant symptom regardless of the localization of the tumor; and this difficulty may remain in isolated fashion for a considerable period of time.

Hécaen and Angelergues (1964) presented a quantitative analysis of the correlations between signs of aphasia and lesion localization in 214 right-handed patients with left hemispheric lesions of diverse etiologies, principally tumors or trauma. An initial observation was that the volume of the lesion, as well as the location, played a major role in producing aphasic symptoms; the greater the lesion volume, the more severe the symptoms. The several symptom patterns of language disorganization varied according to lesion localization. No purely motor aphasic syndromes were found, although Rolandic lesions seemed particularly responsible for articulatory disorders. Lesions affecting the temporal or parietal lobes caused various symptom clusters within the general category of sensory aphasia. The relative degree of severity of agraphia or alexia varied with lesion localization: in temporooccipital lesions, alexia predominated; in parietooccipital lesions, agraphia was more marked than alexia. As for naming defects, these were present regardless of lesion localization. Intensity of naming defect was increased if the lesion was large or if the lesion involved the temporal lobe.

The electrocortical stimulation studies of Penfield and Roberts (1959) have provided additional information concerning language disorders. By stimulating different cortical regions in awake subjects, these authors could provoke disturbances of vocalization, speech arrest, and even aphasiclike symptoms. The speech disturbances were caused by stimulation of either hemisphere; the aphasiclike symptoms (e.g., word-finding difficulty) were found only following simulations in the dominant hemisphere. Three specific cortical regions were associated with speech and language: (1) the inferior frontal region corresponding to Broca's area, (2) the temporoparietal region, and (3) the supplementary motor area.

Fedio and van Buren (1974) produced only responses of aphasic type with stimulation of the left hemisphere, principally of the posterior parietotemporal region. As for the anterior part of the temporal lobe, they obtained only disorders of verbal memory.

CLINICAL-ANATOMICAL ASPECTS. The contribution of these diverse global studies to the knowledge about the location of lesions in the major forms of aphasia permits consideration of not only clinical aspects but also clinical-anatomical aspects. Before schematizing these results, the frequency of mixed forms should be emphasized, but the frequent difficulty of separating, in a radical way, the diverse clinical aspects should also be stressed.

Expression Aphasia. Expression aphasias correspond to anterior lesions involving Broca's region as well as the inferior part of the Rolandic convolutions.

According to Hécaen and Consoli (1973), should a superficial lesion of Broca's area produce only articulatory and/or prosodic disorders, with slight impairment of writing and spelling, then lesions of this same area, but more deep, can cause not only very severe disorders of expression but also disorders of verbal comprehension.

Conduction Aphasia. Wernicke (1874) postulated that a lesion of the insula should produce conduction aphasias. However, most of the later anatomical observations implicated the posterior temporal region, particularly the angular gyrus and the supramarginal gyrus.

Perhaps, then, it is necessary to accept the conclusions of Benson *et al.* (1973) from a review of literature and from their cases that conduction aphasia can be produced by two different lesion sites: one suprasylvian, and in this case apraxic phenomena would appear, and the other temporal, since a few cases were observed without damage of the two gyri, supramarginalis and angularis. In consideration of the disconnectionist interpretation, the role of a lesion in the arcuate fasciculus was largely supported. Indeed, all deep lesions of white matter subjacent to the angular gyrus and supramarginalis would have to destroy the origins of these fibers.

Sensory Aphasia. Sensory aphasias correspond to lesions of Wernicke's area. With posterior damage to this area, toward the angular gyrus, the intensity of disorders of writing and reading increases. As a result of an absence of sufficient anatomical evidence, only a tentative localization for the three aspects of this syndrome can be suggested. If the aspect of word deafness predominates, lesions are located at the level of the first temporal convolution, surrounding Heschl's gyri. When the aspect of disordered comprehension predominates, the lesions will be found in the region of the inferoposterior temporal lobe. Finally, the aspect of attentional disorganization seems, to us, to correspond to lesions of the temporal tip.

Amnesic Aphasia. Amnesic aphasia, in a very general fashion, seems to be determined by lesions at different locations. However, it is particularly frequent and intense with temporal lesions. When the anomic disorder is quasi-isolated, posterior temporal lesions are most frequently if not exclusively encountered.

LESION SITES IN PURE APHASIAS AND ROLES OF SUBCORTICAL STRUCTURES. Two problems also merit consideration here: the lesion sites in pure aphasias, and the role of lesions and stimulation of subcortical structures in disorders of language.

"Pure" Aphasia. 1. Pure Motor Aphasia: Dejerine (1914) and Pelissier (1912) refused to grant anatomical autonomy to pure motor aphasia; cortical lesions (foot of F_3) as well as subcortical lesions could provoke it. Conrad (1954) and Russel and Espir (1961) thought that these exceptional cases could result from partial damage to the Rolandic operculum. In a case of pure phonetic disintegration presented by Alajouanine *et al.* (1949), anatomical examination revealed a softening of three-fifths of the left inferior pre-Rolandic convolution, preserving Broca's area (Lecours and Lhermitte, 1976). According to Mohr (1976), lesions strictly limited to Broca's area determine only arthric and prosodic disorders (apraxia of speech), after the acute phase.

2. Pure Word Deafness: Considered anatomically, the rare observations of pure word deafness can be divided into two groups: bilateral temporal lesions and unilateral left temporal lesions. The question of cortical or subcortical origins for this disorder has been much debated. According to Wernicke, the lesion had to be subcortical, interrupting subcortical auditory fibers in their trajectory toward the center of verbal images.

3. Pure Agraphia: In 1881 Exner and then Henschen posited the existence of a center for writing in area F_2. The cases of pure agraphia on which their opinions were based are not satisfactory, with the exception of the case of Gordinier (1899). Penfield and Roberts (1959) observed transitory agraphia after an excision in areas F_2 and F_3. In the six cases of pure agraphia of Dubois *et al.* (1969), four were due to frontal lesions, although a more precise intrafrontal focus could not be adduced.

Also, several observations of Russel and Espir (1961), one of our cases elsewhere with a particular character (iteration), and an observation of Kinsbourne and Rosenfield (1974) prove the possibility of isolated agraphia due to a posterior parietal lesion.

4. Pure Alexia: In 1892, Dejerine attributed the origin of pure word blindness to an interruption of connections between the calcarine fissure and the angular cyrus caused by a lesion of white matter in the lingual lobe. This lesion site was admitted by many authors, but the role of the callosal lesion in the genesis of alexia already supported by Wernicke (1903) has always had its supporters. Many researchers, however, acknowledge that two lesions are necessary to produce alexia, one being in the white matter of the left lingual and fusiform gyri and the other in the splenium of the corpus callosum. In 1925, Foix and Hillemand, on the basis of anatomoclinical arguments, emphasized the importance of the lesion of the splenium in alexia. Vincent *et al.* (1930) described a neurosurgical case of removal of an occipital tumor, during which part of the splenium was probably damaged. Alexia, which was not present before the operation, appeared postoperatively, but a considerable recovery was evident shortly afterward.

In 1937, Tresher and Ford confirmed that, after a posterior callosal section, one patient was unable to recognize objects and letters in the left visual hemifield or by palpation with the left hand. This was subsequently confirmed by Maspes in 1948 in two patients after a section of the splenium.

The negative findings of Akelaïtis (1943), who studied epileptic patients on whom van Wagenen had performed callosal section, cast some doubt on the role of the callosal lesion in the genesis of alexia. Geschwind (1965, 1966) has provided a new stimulus to the connectionist model, according to which a lesion of the splenium prevents visual input—which does not go farther than the right occipital lobe as a result of the right hemianopsia—from reaching the language areas. This theory has subsequently been widely accepted, particularly because the work of Sperry and Gazzaniga (1967) on patients who had undergone commissurotomy did not confirm any of the negative findings by Akelaïtis.

However, it should be noted that pure alexia can be found in the absence of hemianopia. It is also necessary to explain satisfactorily why the deficit of verbalization does not consistently extend to objects and colors.

Finally, having considered different aspects of pure alexia according to linguistic levels, one should examine to see if different lesion locations can explain the disturbances. Hécaen and Kremin (1976) propose the following tentative systematization: global alexia relates to a double lesion (occipital and callosal); verbal alexia relates to a lesion of the fusiform and lingual gyri; and literal and sentence alexias relate to occipital lesions extending either to the temporal lobe or to the parietal lobe.

Effects of Subcortical Stimulations and Destructions on Language. The surgical procedure of deep subcortical (usually thalamic) destruction of tissue as a treatment for Parkinson's disease has led to an analysis of speech and language defects due to such lesions. Guiot *et al.* (1961) and van Buren (1963) have observed arrest or acceleration of speech and confusion associated with thalamic, caudate, or pallidal stimulation. These speech disorders have not involved phonemic organization, however, but have been disruptions of the rhythm or spontaneous initiation of verbal emission. More convincing has been the work of Ojemann *et al.* (1971) and Fedio and van Buren (1971, 1974), who found anomia, paraphasia, and verbal memory disturbance following stimulation of the left pulvinar and posterocentromedian portion of the ventrolateral nucleus. No such defects were found with stimulation of the right pulvinar or other portions of the thalamus.

These results raise the index of suspicion concerning the possibility that subcortical stimulation or damage can cause aphasic symptomatology. Whether true permanent aphasic syndromes result from purely subcortical lesions is a subject of controversy. On the one hand are the studies against the possibility. For example, Dubois *et al.* (1966) in a neurolinguistic analysis of the language of 20 parkinsonians before and after stereotaxic surgery found no disruption of the linguistic code. Van Buren (1975) reviewed the anatomoclinical evidence regarding the thalamic role in speech and language, and advised caution in assigning to the dominant thalamus more than a minor role in the total speech mechanism.

On the other hand are the case reports and statistical studies in favor of the possibility. For example, Mohr *et al.* (1975) described the behavioral effects of left thalamic hemorrhage in a total of six cases and concluded that a peculiar state of logorrheic paraphasia resembling delirium was sufficiently distinctive to warrant isolation as a language disorder separate from traditional aphasic syndromes. Psychometric studies of patients with surgically induced thalamic lesions have indicated that thalamic nuclei, especially VL and pulvinar, may play a role in verbal functions (e.g., Riklan and Levita, 1969; Riklan and Cooper, 1975; Vilkki and Laitinen, 1974).

In Summary. The wide variety of clinical, anatomopathological, and electrophysiological studies of the past 60 years seems to confirm, with certain exceptions and qualifications, the earlier work of Dejerine. It is reasonable to talk about a "zone of language" present in the dominant hemisphere, situated in the perisylvian region, excluding the frontal and occipital poles and the superior and inferior regions of the hemisphere, and to which must be added the supplementary motor area. However, rather than referring to the limited and rigid concept of a cortical "center" for behavioral function, one should consider the concept of functional zones. A central zone, the classical Wernicke's area, may be essential to all modalities of language. Related to this central zone, a certain number of functional poles may be defined: an anterior motor pole, situated in the classical Broca's region, but perhaps extending to the pre- and postcentral Rolandic region as well; a posterior parietooccipital pole concerned with reading and writing; and a superior pole (parietal) concerned with gestural activity.

Both lesion volume and lesion localization influence language. In addition, inherent in the concept of functional zones is the belief that a supple and dynamic organization of activity underlies the language function for which each zone is preferentially responsible, thus allowing for the often considerable recovery of function seen following aphasia-producing lesions.

HEMISPHERIC REPRESENTATION OF LANGUAGE

After Broca had established, in 1865, that the left hemisphere was dominant for spoken language, that this hemisphere should be dominant for all language functions in right-handers readily became the widespread belief. And in spite of efforts on the part of Jackson (1931)—who held firmly that the right hemisphere played a role in this function, being "the one for the most automatic use of words"—and on the part of other authors such as Pierre Marie (1926), Niessl von Mayendorff (1911), and Liepmann and Pappenheim (1914)—who recognized its participation in certain types of verbal performance,—the right hemisphere was considered merely substitute tissue, at best capable of rough approximation of the function.

The dominance of the left hemisphere remains undisputed. Nevertheless, in the light of recent pathological as well as experimental data from normal subjects, there is a trend toward reexamination of the role of the right hemisphere in right-handers for certain verbal performances.

It is necessary to stress the importance of the role of the right hemisphere in language functions, because of its possible participation in recovery from aphasia or its participation during ontogenesis in normal or neonatally lesioned children. This problem must be investigated while taking into consideration an assortment of data of various value. These concern pathological studies as well as experimental research in normal subjects. Also, the problem must be examined in its relationship to manual preference and, finally, appreciated as a function of the degree of cerebral maturation.

NEUROPSYCHOLOGICAL EVIDENCE SUPPORTING THE NOTION OF RIGHT HEMISPHERE PARTICIPATION IN THE LANGUAGE FUNCTION

CROSSED APHASIA IN RIGHT-HANDERS. In order to account for the exceptions to the rule propounded by Broca according to which right-handers "speak" with their left hemispheres and left-handers with their right hemispheres, the notion of crossed aphasia was set forth. If such crossing is of frequent occurrence in left-handers, aphasia in right-handers resulting from right hemisphere damage remains exceptional, provided that determination is made on the following bases: damage limited to the right hemisphere, no damage incurred during childhood, no left-handers in the family. Following these criteria, Zangwill (1967) evaluated the frequency to be 1.8%, Gloning *et al.* (1969) 1.0%, and Brown and Hécaen (1976) 0.38%. From a recent review of the literature (Brown and Hécaen, 1976), it seems that only nine cases can be maintained with certainty.

RESULTS OF THE WADA SODIUM AMYTAL TEST. By temporarily disturbing the functioning of one hemisphere through the injection of sodium amytal in the carotid artery on that side, Rasmussen and Milner (1977) observed unilateral right hemisphere speech representation in six out of 140 subjects (4%) without evidence of early brain lesion. In the case of subjects who had suffered brain damage during childhood, the percentage rose to 19.

LEFT HEMISPHERECTOMY IN RIGHT-HANDED ADULTS. Experience with left hemispherectomy in right-handed adults is, needless to say, very limited and the documents are not of uniform value. Zollinger (1935) and Crockett and Estridge (1951) described patients whose survival following operation was of relatively short duration. Language behavior in these patients was markedly restricted. All that remained of expressive capacities were "automatic" speech, expletives, and words of overlearned songs. The case reported by Hillier (1954) was that of a 14-year-old child; thus comments regarding language performance would be of uncertain value. Of the patients with left hemispherectomy described by French *et al.* (1955), one, who had been aphasic for 12 years previously when he had undergone an operation for brain tumor, was able to ask simple questions and had a good degree of comprehension. But the patient described by Smith (1966), unlike the other reported patients, had a significant return of language function. Six months after the operation he could produce well-constructed, if short, sentences, and verbal comprehension was fairly good. Writing remained quite poor.

A recent observation by Rössing (1975) also deserves mention. Two years after a left hemispherectomy, speech was fluent and nondysarthric; a corpus of 1600 words consisted mainly of a few functional words that were always the same. Lexemes were virtually absent. Communication was reportedly good.

Despite the undoubted interest of these cases, it would be difficult from so few to draw general conclusions about the language capacity of the right hemisphere.

EFFECTS OF RIGHT HEMISPHERIC LESIONS ON VERBAL PERFORMANCES. Few neuropsychological studies have been devoted to language performances following right hemisphere lesion in right-handers. No obvious aphasic signs have been found.

Nevertheless, Eisenson (1961), Critchley (1962), and Weinstein and Keller (1963) have tried to describe certain language characteristics peculiar to patients with damage to the minor hemisphere. Marcie *et al.* (1965) observed in right anterior lesions disorders of articulation or dysprosody in spontaneous expression and repetition. A recent review of our cases reveals that permanent but minor articulatory disorders occurred in 4% of the 242 and almost always occurred when a contralateral motor deficit was involved. When transitory disorders of expression are taken into account, the percentage increases to 6%.

Disorders of syntactic transformation and vocabulary selection were associated with parietal or parietooccipital lesions. These defects seemed to be perseverative in origin.

Disorders on a test of sentence production, using words provided by the examiner, were also present with temporal lobe lesions, especially those of temporal tip. However, a new analysis of the generated sentences from item words reveals a significant increase in the length of sentences made by right-lesioned subjects (even in the absence of confusion) as compared with the sentences produced by control subjects. But the difference was not significant between the group with temporal damage and that with nontemporal damage. Neither was the difference significant within the temporal lobe group for patients with damage in the anterior region and those without this damage (Gosnave, 1977).

Lastly, mention should be made at least of the disorders of reading and writing and calculation resulting from right hemisphere lesions. In these instances, the disturbance is not related to the faculty of encoding and decoding written entities but rather to the ability for dealing with the spatial factors involved in these skills or with perseveration. It represents one of the several features of the minor hemisphere syndrome (Hécaen *et al.*, 1956), and usually results from a lesion involving the right parietotemporooccipital region.

1. Dyslexia of Spatial Type: Errors are most manifest at the level of textual reading, and rarely at the level of the individual word. The disorder seems to reveal two types of disturbances, often associated: impossibility of fixation of gaze on the word or text with skipping of lines and neglect of the left side of the text.

2. Dyscalculia of Spatial Type: The principles of arithmetical operations are conserved here, but the errors stem from faulty placing of the digits with respect to each other or from neglect of the digits situated on the left.

3. Dysgraphia of Spatial Type: Characteristic features clearly distinguish this type of agraphia from those types related to dominant hemispheric pathology. Graphemes are well formed, and morphosyntactic components of written expression are preserved. Four major features define this clinical syndrome. (a) Some graphemes are produced frequently with one, two, or even more extra strokes, the letters "m," "n," and "u" being especially duplicated. (b) The lines of writing are not horizontal, but slant at variable angles of inclination to the top or bottom of the page. (c) The writing occupies only the right-hand part of the piece of paper. (d) Blanks are inserted between the graphemes which make up the word, which disorganizes the word and destroys its unity.

In a quantitative study of the graphic performances of 82 right-handed patients with unilateral cerebral lesions, Hécaen and Marcie (1974) made the following observations. Only the iteration of strokes and letters and enlargement of the left-hand margin are associated significantly with right hemisphere lesions. On the other hand, the loss of continuity in the writing of words is related to left hemisphere lesions. The spatial origin of enlargement of the left hand margin seems clear and directly related to the presence of unilateral spatial neglect, and the repetition of both pothooks and letters is considered to be a perseverative phenomenon which is evident specifically in the spatial aspects of writing.

SPLIT-BRAIN STUDIES. Tresher and Ford (1937) and Maspes (1948) had observed alexia in the left visual field of patients who had been operated on for sectioning of the splenium. But it is mainly from the results obtained with subjects having total commissurotomies—the now classical split-brain patients—that the participation of the right hemisphere in the language functions was demonstrated. Sperry and Gazzaniga (1967) have effectively proved that if this hemisphere cannot express itself orally or in writing, it is capable of comprehending verbal material.

Auditory comprehension was demonstrated by the capacity of the subjects to retrieve with the left hand an object named aloud by the examiner and hidden among a group of test objects. In this manner, nouns and a few adjectival forms (e.g., geometric shapes) could be understood by the right hemisphere. This was true not only when the object was named directly but also when the object was described by definition.

Visual verbal comprehension in the right hemisphere was demonstrated by flashing a printed word to the left visual hemifield and asking the split-brain patient to retrieve the corresponding object with his left hand from a group of hidden objects. In converse technique, after a hidden test object had first been palpated by the left hand, the patient could successfully indicate the correct name of the test object from a list of printed names or a series of printed names flashed successively to the left hemifield.

However, note must be made of Iwata *et al.'s* (1974) patients whose splenium had been sectioned for the removal of pineal tumors. Two of the three patients evinced no comprehension of words presented to the left visual field and the third showed partial comprehension. The difference between these data and those obtained from patients callotomized for epilepsy must be emphasized, for in contrast to these patients Iwata's patients had not sustained any brain damage during childhood. This would preclude the possibility of any reorganization prior to operation.

In commissurotomized patients studied by Sperry and Gazzaniga (1967) right hemisphere comprehension was best demonstrated for nouns and with nonverbal responses. When a subject was asked to mimic or carry out simple acts, the performance of the right hemisphere was less satisfactory. In testing syntactic capabilities of the right hemisphere, Gazzaniga and Hillyard (1971) concluded that while a moderated semantic capability exists in the right hemisphere of the right-handed split-brain patient, little or no syntactic capability is present.

Using special contact lenses which allowed free eye movement but excluded a desired portion of the visual field, Zaidel (1977a,b) was able to examine under near-normal conditions the language capacity of the right hemisphere of commissurotomized patients. The auditory vocabulary of the disconnected right hemisphere seemed equivalent to that of normal subjects between the ages of 8:1 and 16:3, averaging 11:7.

In the auditory comprehension of language, as evaluated by the Token Test, the right hemisphere proved deficient, its level being comparable to that of a 4-year-old child.

A close look at the errors prevented equating the language competence of the right hemisphere and that of aphasics. The right hemisphere proved more sensitive to perceptual and memory factors and to have a poor short-term verbal auditory memory; aphasics seemed more sensitive to linguistic variables.

Levy and Trevarthen (1973) and Levy (1974) have shown that on presentation of chimerical stimuli composed of two parts of words, the right hemisphere was superior at recognizing the word: split-brain patients would point to the word whose letters had been presented to the left visual field. However, when the subject had to select an image corresponding to the letters presented, the predominance of the left hemisphere was almost total, even though the right hemisphere was always capable of matching a picture with a word when that word was presented in its entirety in the left half-field. The left hemisphere is therefore dominant for semantic decoding, although the right hemisphere is capable of performing such a task.

When the task required breaking down the word into its phonetic constituents rather than grasping the word in its entirety, the right hemisphere failed totally.

Other experiments using tachistoscopic vision (Levy and Trevarthen, 1973) and dichotic listening (Zaidel, 1974) on split-brain subjects further demonstrated that the right hemisphere is incapable of any phonetic matching.

Finally, research on normal subjects with methods of dichotic listening or of tachistoscopic vision has permitted explication of those characteristics of the material or the tasks which for a given subject and under given circumstances maximize the participation of the right hemisphere in verbal functions.

Thus it seems impossible to subscribe to the notion of the absolute dominance of the left hemisphere as far as language is concerned. It may be that the sequential analytical mode of processing that it imposes on input as well as output accounts for the left hemisphere's preeminence in the processing of verbal material. It would thus impose its dominance over material which has to be broken down sequentially into its components or over activities organized in a sequential mode.

The right hemisphere is not deprived of verbal capabilities, and these capabilities do not emerge as the attenuated mirror image of the left hemisphere. They can be defined in negative as well as positive terms. In negative terms, we might say: (1) the right hemisphere lacks or has limited expression potential; (2) it cannot break down a phonological whole into its phonetic components; (3) its short-term auditory verbal memory is severely limited. In positive terms, the right hemisphere allows a global grasp of verbal items—visual or auditory.

Compensatory Role of the Right Hemisphere in Aphasia

The different arguments just discussed force us to envisage a participation of the right hemisphere in the return of language functions after left hemispheric lesions. This compensatory role of the right hemisphere has been supported for a long while, by Niessl von Mayendorff (1911), Nielsen (1947), and Kleist (1933, 1962), functional recuperation being attributed to the functioning of the intact symmetrical area. Goldstein (1948), on the other hand, proved much more skeptical concerning the role the minor hemisphere assumes during restoration of the functions. Luria (1963) emphasized that restoration of function by the other hemisphere occurs much less frequently than it is generally presumed. This type of restoration occurs only in subjects with partial hemispheric dominance in whom both hemispheres actually take part in the language function.

The evidence obtained with several cases of left hemispherectomy and particularly the results with split-brain subjects seem to refute these negative opinions.

Other arguments, somewhat indirect, have also been advanced in support of the right hemisphere's role in language. Kinsbourne (1971), using the Wada test with aphasics, observed no aggravation of the preexisting aphasic syndromes after injection of anytal into the left carotid artery, while injection into the right artery caused complete abolition of speech in two of these subjects.

Likewise, Czopf (1972) performed the anytal test on a number of aphasic subjects. In a first group of old and severe cases of aphasia, injection into the right artery made it totally impossible for the subjects to express themselves whereas injection into the left side in two of these subjects caused much less aggravation of the speech disorders. In other groups of mild and recent cases, worsening of aphasia after right injection was only slight. Czopf deduced from these results that the relationship between the hemispheres is not fixed once and for all but that with time the nondominant hemisphere can assume the functions of the dominant one.

Using dichotic or tachistocopic tasks, Moore and Weidner (1974, 1975) also found better performance in aphasics by the left visual field and left ear for verbal material, which is the inverse of that found in normal subjects. Dichotic listening experiments performed by Schuloff and Goodglass (1969) on subjects with brain damage on one side had already shown a possible, if slight, displacement of dominance for verbal material from the left to the right hemisphere. But the most conclusive finding of this study was the observation of a definite bilateral lowering of performance on material for which the lesioned hemisphere was dominant.

Finally, the compensatory role of the right hemisphere must be invoked in the quasitotal regression of alexias occurring after left occipital lobectomy, as we observed in seven subjects who had undergone this operation, three of whom had a long follow-up (Hécaen *et al.,* 1952). Alexia had been total after intervention. A return to reading, although slow and hesitant, with comprehension of meaning appeared 6 weeks later. However, the patients never totally recovered their preoperative reading speed. This recovery of reading skill after removal of the left occipital lobe contrasted sharply with the usual persistence of alexia due to softening of the territory of the posterior cerebral artery. In this case maybe we should invoke the part played by inhibitory influences emanating from the damaged lobe and preventing the intact right lobe from taking over.

It hence seems impossible now to reject the idea of intervention by the minor hemisphere during the return of certain language functions after left lesions. However, the verbal capacities of the right hemisphere are, as we saw, so different from those of the left hemisphere that major recuperation cannot be attributed to it without discussion. It had appeared generally more plausible to postulate a role for remaining, neighboring tissue in the same hemisphere, whether a result of vicarious functions of these adjacent regions or of a redundancy effect in the interior of the language zone.

Only after massive lesions of the dominant hemisphere do certain verbal abilities reappear, although at a relatively low level, such that intervention of the minor hemisphere should be considered.

APHASIA IN LEFT-HANDERS

At the same time that Broca (1865) was establishing the theory of cerebral dominance which stated that the left hemisphere is dominant for language in right-handed individuals, he was also proposing the converse doctrine that the right hemisphere is dominant for language in left-handers. Cases of crossed aphasia in left-handers reported during and shortly after the studies of Broca were in contradiction to his doctrine. Nonetheless, the cases in spite of their relative frequency were considered to be merely rare exceptions to the basic rule. Finally, in 1936, Chescher proposed that these cases were not simple exceptions; rather, he asserted that cerebral representation for language is basically different for left-handers and right-handers.

This early work was followed by several large-scale, systematic studies of language function in left-handed subjects with unilateral cerebral lesions (Conrad, 1949; Humphrey and Zangwill, 1952; Goodglass and Quadfasel, 1954; Penfield and Roberts, 1959; Russel and Espir, 1961; Hoff, 1961; Hécaen and de Ajuriaguerra, 1956, 1963). These studies demonstrated that cortical organization is different for left- and right-handers. The conclusions of Goodglass and Quadfasel (1954) effectively summarized the various reports: it is not correct to establish a direct and necessary correlation between handedness and cerebral lateralization for language functions; left cerebral dominance for language is more frequent than right-handedness, and right cerebral dominance for language is much less frequent than left-handedness. A résumé of most series reveals that 20–30% of left-handed aphasics have right hemispheric lesions.

Additional studies (Subirana, 1952, 1956; Hécaen and Angelergues, 1962), together with previous reports, repeatedly suggested that aphasia was milder, although more frequent, in left-handers than in right-handers, regardless of the hemisphere damaged. Also, left-handers recovered more quickly and more thoroughly from aphasia than did right-handers.

The study of paroxysmal dysphasias also reveals differences between right- and left-handed subjects. Hécaen and Piercy (1956), studying 126 cases of paroxysmal dysphasia with clearly lateralized epileptogenic foci, concluded that paroxysmal dysphasia of an expressive type was significantly more frequent in left-handers than in right-handers, regardless of the hemisphere damaged.

In left-handers, increased frequency of bilateral representation of language, compared to right-handers, can be observed by utilizing the Wada test. Rasmussen and Milner (1977) ascertained that 15% of 122 left-handers had bilateral representation of language and that another 15% had right hemispheric representation. Taking into account the age at onset of an epileptogenic lesion, in left-handers with early brain damage only 30% had language represented on the left, 51% had language represented on the right, and 19% had cerebral ambilaterality.

In addition, Milner *et al.* (1966) noted that 17 left-handed subjects with bilateral representation of language had a mild disorder following injection of sodium amytal into one side or the other. Finally, in nine of these cases there was a dissociation between the defect in naming and the defect in repetition on command of a spoken series.

These various observations are consistent with the hypothesis that left-handers have a cerebral ambilaterality for language representation.

We have made several analyses of our observations of left-handed subjects with right or left unilateral hemispheric lesions (1956, 1962, 1963, 1971). Both qualitative and quantitative analyses were carried out, with the following main conclusions. The left hemispheric syndrome in left-handers maintains many of the features of the left hemispheric syndrome in right-handers. However, disorders of auditory comprehension, of writing, and of spelling are significantly less frequent in left-handers than in right-handers, while alexia and spatial dyslexia are more frequent. The disorganizations of linguistic, practic, and gnostic behavior found in left-handers with left hemispheric lesions are in the main similar to those found in right-handers with left hemispheric lesions. However, some of the neurobehavioral abnormalities (apraxia for dressing, unilateral spatial agnosia, hemiasomatognosia) found with right hemispheric lesions in right-handers are also seen in left-handers with left hemispheric lesions.

The right hemispheric syndrome in left-handers is characterized by a significantly increased frequency of disorders of spoken and written language expression by comparison to those abnormalities in right-handers with right hemispheric lesions. Left-handers also have an increased frequency of alexia and spatial dyslexia.

Comparison of right and left hemispheric syndromes in left-handers shows fewer differences than does comparison of similar syndromes in right-handers. The main differences are nonlinguistic and lie in the realm of visuospatial perception and constructional abilities. The results are consistent with the hypothesis that left-handers have less hemispheric specialization or more cerebral ambilaterality than do right-handers.

However, observations made in large series of subjects with unilateral hemispheric lesions indicate that left-handers do not form a homogeneous group regarding functional hemispheric asymmetry, as do right-handers. The relationship of a familial history of left-handedness to cerebral organization for language was first invoked by Kennedy (1916), who pointed out that right-handers who developed aphasia after a right cerebral lesion were likely to be members of a left-handed family.

The results of dichotic test of left-handed subjects show a diminution of perceptual asymmetry by comparison with right-handed subjects. (Bryden, 1965; Curry and Rutherford, 1967; Satz *et al.*, 1967). When statistical analyses take into account the presence or absence of a familial history of left-handedness, this diminution in perceptual asymmetry is primarily found in left-handers with a family history of left-handedness (Zurif and Bryden, 1969).

Hécaen and Sauguet (1971) reexamined these issues in 49 brain-damaged left-handers, taking into account the presence or absence of a family history of left-handedness. In the "familial" group of left-handers comparison of performance scores of subjects subdivided into those with left and those with right hemispheric lesions showed no significant differences. By contrast, significant differences were found for the group with "nonfamilial" left-handedness depending on which hemisphere was damaged. This group corresponded more closely in performance to right-handers, since there were virtually no language deficits following right brain damage.

CHILDHOOD APHASIA

A distinction should be drawn between developmental (congenital) aphasia in children and acquired aphasia in children. In the latter, which we shall discuss in this section, language disorders develop after the child has already achieved the capacity for language comprehension and verbal expression.

The clinical pattern of acquired aphasia of childhood has several essential differences from that of adults (Bernhardt, 1885; Guttmann, 1942; Basser, 1962; Lenneberg, 1967; Hécaen, 1976). As early as 1885, Bernhardt observed that acquired aphasia in childhood was relatively frequent, transient, and predominantly of an expressive nature. Freud (1897) clearly distinguished acquired aphasia from developmental language retardation, emphasizing that it occurred with much greater frequency after right hemispheric lesions than did acquired aphasia in adults. In 1942, Guttmann presented the first detailed and systematic analysis of childhood aphasia, describing 16 of his own cases. Most subsequent authors, with occasional exceptions, have tended to agree on the main clinical features. Regardless of lesion localization, the spontaneous speech is nonfluent. Mutism is common initially. Subsequently, there are reduced initiatives for speech, hesitations, dysarthria, and an impoverishment of language with reduced lexical stock. Disturbances of writing are constant. The reported frequency and severity of comprehension defects vary with the study. According to Guttmann (1942) and Branco-Lefevre (1950), disorders of comprehension are rare; according to Alajouanine and Lhermitte (1965) and Collignon et al. (1968), they can be found in one-third of cases of childhood aphasia and may be quite severe.

Hécaen (1976) has recently reviewed his observations on 26 children, aged 3½–15, with cortical lesions. Language disorders were present in 19 of these 26 children. For those with unilateral lesions, a disorder of language was found in 15 of 17 with left hemispheric lesion (one of the two exceptions was left-handed). Thus the frequency of acquired aphasia in the Hécaen series (88% with left-sided lesion, 33% with right-sided lesion) corresponds to that found by Basser (1962) in an earlier study (86% and 46% respectively).

Clinically, two essential characteristics emerged from the Hécaen (1976) study: a positive feature, the frequency of mutism, i.e., loss of ability to initiate speech and, more generally, loss of ability to communicate; and a negative feature, the fact that paraphasias were rare and logorrhea was nonexistent. Articulatory disorders were the rule; and disorders of auditory comprehension occurred in more than one-third of the cases. The finding of poor auditory comprehension was similar to that of Alajouanine and Lhermitte (1965), but in contradiction to the observations of Guttmann (1942) and Branco-Lefèvre (1950), who stressed the rarity of this defect. In those studies in which auditory comprehension was impaired, the comprehension defect often cleared up rapidly after the acute stage. Problems with naming were more frequent and more persistent, however. Disorders of writing appeared to be the most frequent and longest lasting of all language defects. Among the associated neuropsychological symptoms, acalculia was the most common.

Recovery from aphasia also presents characteristics special to the developing brain. Motor aphasia, the usual variety, may have a good prognosis, recuperation often being complete in 4 weeks (Guttmann, 1942). The prognosis in mixed motor and sensory aphasia remains more guarded, however.

In his studies of cerebral dominance for language in the child, Lenneberg (1967) attempted to define a critical period for the acquisition of language, a period corresponding to the development of cerebral dominance. Age at onset of cerebral injury was used as a guide. If aphasia was acquired prior to age 3, recovery was rapid and complete. Before 10 years of age, a true aphasia would develop, but slow recovery was the rule. If the child was between 11 and 14 when brain damage occurred, recovery was less likely. Lenneberg concluded that a period roughly between 2–3 years of age and puberty is a critical period. During this time a state of cerebral plasticity exists; following this period, the hemispheres have achieved their final specialization.

Recently, the conclusions of Lenneberg have been disputed by Krashen (1973), who lowered the end of the period during which transfer between the hemispheres is still possible to 5 years of age. He pointed out that in the series of Basser (1962) there were no instances of aphasia with a right-sided lesion occurring after age 5.

Krashen (1973) compared the frequency of right-sided lesions in several series of childhood aphasias where the lesion occurred before or after 5 years with the frequency of right-sided lesions producing aphasia in adults. He noted that in the older children the percentage of right-sided lesions producing aphasia was similar to that observed in adults. Analyses of the Hécaen (1976) series tend to support this argument. Krashen finds support for this argument as well in the results of studies of dichotic listening, particularly those of Kimura (1963) and Knox and Kimura (1970). The superiority of the right ear, that is, the dominance of the left hemisphere in the reception of verbal material (digits), appears around the age of 6, and that of the left ear (right hemisphere) for familiar sounds around age 5. Since this work, Nagafuchi (1974) and Ingram (1975) have found a right ear superiority for verbal sounds (words) as early as 3 years of age.

Findings from studies of aphasia in childhood thus support the notion that very young children have hemispheric equipotentiality for language and that cerebral dominance is established in the course of maturation.

Thanks in particular to data from Basser (1962), we know also that hemispherectomies performed on either the right side or the left produce similar effects. Permanent dysphasia has never been observed after left hemispherectomy performed for damage having occurred before the acquisition of language.

Finally, we have already discussed the results of the Wada test; lesions of early onset are found to displace the representation of language from the left to the right hemisphere, even in right-handers (Milner, 1974a).

There does appear to be a critical period during which each hemisphere may support verbal activity, but this critical period may be of shorter duration than had been suggested by Lenneberg (1967).

On the other hand, the two other lines of argument plead for hemispheric specialization established much earlier in life or even innate.

First, psychological examination of subjects having had early unilateral hemispheric damage reveals a type of deficit in accordance with the lesioned hemisphere similar to that encountered in adults, i.e., deficits in verbal tasks for left damage, deficits in nonverbal tasks, in particular spatial tasks, for right lesions (McFie, 1961; Fedio and Mirsky, 1969; Woods and Teuber, 1973; Rudel *et al.*, 1974).

A second set of arguments in favor of early specialization derives from anatomical research on the structural asymmetry of the hemispheres in the region of the planum temporale, an asymmetry demonstrated in adults by Geschwind and Levitsky (1968) and in the fetus and newborn by Teszner *et al.* (1972), by Witelson and Pallie (1973), and, above all, by Wada *et al.* (1975). These last authors examined 100 fetal and newborn brains and compared them to 100 adult brains. In newborns as in adults, the planum temporale is larger on the left than on the right in approximately 90% of cases. We hold with these authors that this difference is more marked in adults than in newborns, and that there is very likely a further development of the left planum during maturation.

The existence of this structural difference in embryonic life appears particularly likely if we consider in relation to these observations the behavioral studies, such as those of Eimas *et al.* (1971), which show that infants as early as the first month perceive phonemes in the same categorical fashion as adults.

It appears, then, that we now have evidence, both behavioral and anatomical, for an extremely early—indeed, even innate—lateralization of functional representation. On the other hand, we have also mentioned those findings in favor either of initial hemispheric equipotentiality or of the possibility of functional displacement from one hemisphere to the other.

Against these contradictory findings, it should be noted that a precise study of the verbal capacities of patients subjected to hemispherectomy very early revealed differences depending on the hemisphere affected (Dennis and Whitaker, 1976). In cases when the right hemisphere remains, the deficit is certainly not more or less like an aphasia but rather is a deficit of syntactic abilities in comprehension and in production and manipulation of syntactic relationships; phonemic and semantic abilities develop normally.

It is also important to emphasize that language representation can well be in the left hemisphere, in spite of an early and significant lesion of that side. Using the Wada test, Milner (1974a) demonstrated that language could be represented in the left hemisphere even with considerable involvement of that hemisphere, on the condition that the posterior temporoparietal region was not destroyed. Besides the factor of age, the site of the lesions therefore appears of equal importance in the displacement of functional representation.

The relationship of these various findings on the effects of early hemispheric lesions and on the manner of subsequent language recovery is still not sufficient to construct a precise systematization of the ontogeny of cerebral dominance. While there is no doubt that factors of time and site of lesion are important, the role of experience ought not to be neglected. The concept of a critical period for language acquisition should also be reformulated, as in the work of Fromkin *et al.* (1974) based on observation in a young girl deprived of all verbal stimulation from the age of 20 months to 13 years 9 months of age, after which time some limited language acquisition was possible. Tests of dichotic listening showed that both verbal and nonverbal material depended on the right hemisphere. The critical period is not just a period of hemispheric equipotentiality, but one in which there should ensue those stimuli necessary to set in motion a preformed area in the left hemisphere.

The apparent contradiction between the findings with acquired aphasia in children and arguments in favor of an early, probably innate, hemispheric specialization can be resolved if we accept the existence of a critical period during which specific stimuli are required for the development of the functional potentialities of the preformed area. Dependence on the less specialized region will assure function either at an inferior level or at the expense of other functions which it normally subserves.

The hypothesis of a displacement of language representation to the other hemisphere can apply, it would seem, only to a very limited period of time. Subsequently, the situation will be different. As we have seen, both clinical and anatomical evidence exists to show that there is not only a functional but also a structural asymmetry between the hemispheres, present at the earliest age and moreover becoming more accentuated in adulthood. At the same time, it has been proposed (Brown, 1975) that distinct zones become specified within the hemisphere. Thus there will also be an intrahemispheric reorganization among the diverse regions which compose the language zone. Whether these regions have different stages of maturation or represent privileged substrates for certain types of verbal performances, they possess, nonetheless, a general capacity to support all aspects of language.

FINAL REMARKS

During the course of this presentation on the varieties of aphasia, emphasis has been placed on linguistic results and methods as well as on the anatomical location of the lesions responsible for these disorders.

But it is impossible to limit neurolinguistics to a simple application of language disorder studies, to restrict them to the aphasiologist's use of linguistic methods merely to satisfy a technical demand. The linguist, in order to surpass this single role attributed to him, must find several interests in the study of aphasia and then look for ways of verifying or falsifying the language theory that he has adopted. This attitude may have been more prevalent earlier, during participation of linguists in language disorder studies. The implication of this approach was that the various levels of language observed in their studies must correspond to real functioning. A dysfunction corresponding to several precise levels and a general disorder due to the impairment of language—this referring to an integral synthesis of different functions—were sought in the patients studied.

Now the problems are posed differently for us: with aphasic language a set of factors is manifested in which the disturbance, isolated or not, applies to the rules governing the relationships of sound and meaning. Pathological verbal behavior depends on the alteration of such factors as memory, attention, vigilance, perception, and emission.

Thus, after these alterations have been found, it is important to appreciate their degree of interference with the application of grammatical mechanisms. Following an analysis of the aphasic corpus and of tests based on a theory of language, differences must be distinguished between verbal realization in aphasics and that occurring in psychological and psycholinguistic disorders. Finally, the correlations between these "syndromes" and definite lesion sites must also be determined.

Hence the neurolinguistic method must involve exploration of the knowledge and application of rules governing the relationships of sound and meaning as well as exploration of psychophysiological factors that intervene in the usage of these rules. Neurophysiological mechanisms underlie the functioning that is either disturbed or abolished by destruction of cortical zones.

The distinction between these factors and the system of rules clearly relates to that proposed by generative grammar between the model of competence, which has syntactic rules but also semantic and phonological rules, and the model of performance. The model of competence is enacted in the model of performance which contains it, but the performance model also involves the subject and the situation. In other words, disorders of language would not really exist unless the competence model were impaired, but they also would not exist if the only impairment were the diverse components involved in the realization or reception of verbal messages.

Weigl and Bierstwitch (1970) took an analogous position. On the other hand, Whitaker (1970), Goodglass (1976), and others refused to acknowledge this distinction between disorders of competence and performance. Taking as an example agrammatism and referring either to his own results or to those of Zurif *et al.* (1972), Goodglass found that the knowledge of grammatical rules is always to some degree deficient. The fact that recuperation follows the path of previous knowledge does not appear to be a valid argument to him.

The question for us is to determine if the disorder can impair comprehension of the components of the rules (semantic, syntaxic, and phonological) and not just the functioning of these components in diverse verbal performances, which can be impaired differentially according to the lesion and the resulting psychophysiological deficit.

We believe that the collected data argue in favor of the hypothesized integrity of knowledge of the system of rules. Along this line, it should be stressed that a dyssymmetry in the deficits is found to exist when an analysis of the various aphasias is performed, and even a variability of performances along synchronic and diachronic lines is noted. The disappearance of certain obstacles to realization, attained during performance or as a result of recuperation, allows the aphasic patient to use the same rules that he knew before the illness. The control of errors that the aphasic can manifest during his performance, or the recognition of errors presented to him, bears witness to the preservation of syntactic and semantic rules. Similarly, it should be noted that in all the metalinguistic tests the aphasics appeared to treat language as manipulable and could make judgments of grammaticality and acceptability.

Whatever progress is made in defining various types of aphasia, the difference remains enormous between neurolinguistic data, along with proposed models concerning neural substrates and verbal behavior, and actual neurophysiological data. The attempt to align neurophysiology and psychophysiology is, for us, a means of opening new avenues of research. The grouping together of lesions producing the various disorders of language, particularly around the zones of motor emission and sensory reception or even at the zones of polysensory integration, makes it seem more possible to comprehend the mechanisms that underlie the functional organization on which verbal performance depends: decoding of verbal sounds, encoding of phonematic units, and temporal organization of morphematic units according to syntactic rules.

Research on the activity of pyramidal cells during voluntary or conditioned actions in animals suggests the possibility of a specific organization between motor unit discharges and motor activity itself. There is room to allow for such organization in the activity of buccophonatory organs, which permit the encoding of central processes of language and of sensory information and which assure direction and control of the series of centrally chosen articulatory features. The interpretation of these data and those concerning the role of feedback or corollary discharges—still hypothetical—agrees well with models of experimental phonetics of the type elaborated by Liberman *et al.* (1967).

Concerning reception of language, data acquired recently from auditory physiology as well as from animal neuropsychology and experimental phonetics suggest a physiological interpretation of disorders of reception and of verbal comprehension. The work of Liberman *et al.* (1967) implies that the decoding of language sounds cannot be accomplished until information on the encoding process is obtained, whether it be constantly transmitted to the decoding area or stocked in a "memory" controlling this area.

On the basis of clinicoanatomical data, there are arguments suggesting that the aphasic forms in which the disturbance is neither of reception nor of expression depend on the impairment of those associative areas, myelinated late, whose extension is characteristic of the cortex of man. Their function can be to impose an order, both temporal and spatial, on the different activities of zones with more fixed organization, in which the elements respond to specific stimuli. In the case of language, these zones can underlie the mechanisms which permit the application of rules in the production or reception of language.

The relationships of anatomophysiology on the one hand and the introduction of linguistic methods on the other hand have noticeably modified how the problems of aphasia are approached and the direction of research pursued with regard to these problems. Unity or variety in aphasia, the reality of pure aphasia, and the relationships of intellectual disorders and disturbances of language, among other issues, should not be discussed in the same terms as they have been discussed before.

HENRY HÉCAEN

Akelaïtis, A. J. Studies on the corpus callosum. VIII. Study on language functions (tactile and visual lexia and graphia). Unilaterally following section of the corpus callosum. *Journal of Neuropathology and Experimental Neurology,* 1943, *2,* 226–262.

Alajouanine, T. H., and Lhermitte, F. Acquired aphasia in children. *Brain,* 1965, *88,* 653–662.

Alajouanine, T. H., Ombredane, A., and Durand, M. *Le Syndrome de Désintégration Phonétique dans l'Aphasie.* Paris: Masson, 1939.

Alajouanine, T. H., Pichot, P., and Durand, M. Dissociation des altérations phonétiques avec conservation relative de la langue la plus ancienne dans un cas d'anarthrie pure chez un sujet français bilingue. *Encéphale,* 1949, *28,* 245–265

Alajouanine, T. H., Castaigne, P., Lhermitte, F., Escourolle, R., and deRibaucourt, B., Etude de 43 cas d'aphasie post-traumatique. Confrontation anatomo-clinique et aspects évolutifs. *l'Encéphale,* 1957, *46,* 3–45.

Alajouanine, T. H., Lhermitte, F., and de Ribaucourt-Ducarne, B. Les alexies agnosiques et aphasiques. In T. Alajouanine (ed.), *Les Grandes Activités du Lobe Occipital.* Paris: Masson, 1960, 235–265.

Albert, M. L., Sparks, R., von Stockert, T., and Sax, D. A case study of auditory agnosia: Linguistic and nonlinguistic processing. *Cortex,* 1972, *8,* 427–443.

Assal, G., Chapuis, G., and Zander, E. Isolated writing disorders in a patient with stenosis of the left internal carotid artery. *Cortex,* 1970, *6,* 241–248.

Basser, L. S. Hemiplegia of early onset and the faculty of speech with special reference to the effects of hemispherectomy. *Brain,* 1962, *85,* 427–460.

Bastian, H. C. On the various forms of loss of speech in cerebral disease. *British and Foreign Medico Chirurgical Review,* 1869, *43,* 470–492.

Bay, E. Zur Methodik der Aphasie-Untersuchung. *Nervenartz,* 1960, *4,* 145–154.

Benedikt, M. Über Aphasie, Agraphie und verwandte pathologische Zustände. *Wiener Medizinische Presse,* 1865, *6,* 897–899, 923–926, 945–948, 997–999, 1020–1022, 1067–1070, 1094–1097, 1139–1142, 1167–1169, 1189–1190, 1264–1265.

Benson, D. F., and Geschwind, N. The alexias. In P. U. Vinken and G. W. Bruyn (eds.), *Handbook of Clinical Neurology,* Vol. 4, Amsterdam: North-Holland, 1969, pp. 112–140.

Benson, D. F., Sheremata, W. A., Bouchard, R., Segarra, J. M., Price, D., and Geschwind, N. Conduction aphasia. *Archives of Neurology,* 1973, *28,* 339–346.

Benton, A. L., and Joynt, R. J. Early descriptions of aphasia. *Archives of Neurology,* 1960, *3,* 205–221.

Beringer, K., and Stein, J. Analyse eines Falles von "reiner" Alexie. *Zeitschrift für Neurologie und Psychiatrie,* 1930, *123,* 472–478.

Bernhardt, M. Über die spastische cerebrale Paralyse im Kindesalter (Hemiplegia spastisca infantilis) nebst einem Excurse über "Aphasie bei Kindern." *Virchows Archive für Anatomie und Physiologie,* 1885, *102.*

Bisiach, E. Perceptual factors in the pathogenesis of anomia. *Cortex,* 1966, *2,* 90–105.

Blumstein, S. *A Phonological Investigation of Aphasic Speech.* The Hague: Mouton, 1973.

Blumstein, S. E., Baker, E., and Goodglass, H. Phonological factors in auditory comprehension in aphasia. *Neuropsychologia,* 1977, *15,* 19–30.

Bouillaud, J. B., Recherches cliniques propres à démontrer que la perte de la parole correspond à la lésion des lobules antérieurs du cerveau et à confirmer l'opinion de M. Gall sur le siège de l'origine du langage articulé. *Archives Générales de Médecine,* 1825, *3,* 25–45.

Branco-Lefévre, A. F. Contribuiçào paro o estudo da psicopatologia da afasia, em crianças. *Archivos Neuro-Psiquiatria (Sào Paulo),* 1950, *8,* 345–393.

Broadbent, W. H. Cerebral mechanisms of speech and thought. *Medical and Chirurgical Transactions (London),* 1872, 145–194.

Broca, P. Perte de la parole. Ramollissement chronique et destruction partielle du lobe antérieur gauche du cerveau. *Bulletin de la Société d'Anthropologie,* 1861, *2,* 235–237.

Broca, P. Sur le siège de la faculté du langage articulé. *Bulletin de la Société d'Anthropologie,* 1865, *6,* 337–393.

Brown, J. W. On the neural organization of language: Thalamic and cortical relationships. *Brain and Language,* 1975, *2,* 18–30.

Brown, J. W., and Hécaen, H. Lateralization and language representation observations on aphasia in children, left handers and "anomalous" dextrals. *Neurology,* 1976, *26,* 183–189.

Bryden, M. P. Tachistoscopic recognition, handedness and cerebral dominance. *Neuropsychologia,* 1965, *3,* 1–8.

Charcot, J. M. Sur un cas de cécité verbale 154–177. In *Leçons sur les Maladies du système Nerveux III.* Paris. Delahaye et Lecrosnier, 1890.

Chedru, F., and Geschwind, N. Writing disturbances in acute confusional states. *Neuropsychologia,* 1972, *10,* 343–354.

Chescher, E. G. Some observations concerning the relation of handedness to the language mechanism, *Bulletin of Neurological Institute, New York,* 1936, *4,* 556–562.

Chocholle, R., Chedru, F., Chain, P., and Lhermitte, F. Etude psychoacoustique d'un cas de "Surdité corticale." *Neuropsychologia,* 1975, *13,* 163–172.

Cohen, D., and Hécaen, H. Remarques neurolinguistiques sur un cas d'agrammatisme. *Journal de Psychologie,* 1965, *3,* 273–296.

Cohen, D., Dubois, J., Gauthier, M., Hécaen, H., and Angelergues, R. Aspects du fonctionnement du code linguistique chez les aphasiques moteurs. *Neuropsychologia,* 1963, *1,* 165–177.

Collignon, R., Hécaen, H., and Angelergues, G. A propos de 12 cas d'aphasie acquise chez l'enfant. *Acta Neurologica et Psychiatrica Belgica,* 1968, *68,* 245–277.

Conrad, K. Über aphasische Sprachstörungen bei hirnverletzten Linkshändern. *Nervenartz,* 1949, *20,* 148–154.

Conrad, K. New Problems of aphasia. *Brain,* 1954, *77,* 491–509.

Critchley, M. Speech and speech loss in relation to the duality of the brain. In V. Mountcastle (ed.), *Interhemispheric Relations and Cerebral Dominance.* Baltimore: John Hopkins Press, 1962, pp. 208–213.

Crockett, H. G., and Estridge, N. M. Cerebral hemispherectomy. *Bulletin of Los Angeles, Neurological Society,* 1951, *16,* 71–87.

Curry, F. K. W., and Rutherford, D. R. Recognition and recall of dichotically presented verbal stimuli by right and left-handed persons. *Neuropsychologia,* 1967, *5,* 119–126.

Czopf, J. Über die Rolle der nicht dominanten Hemisphäre in der Restitution der Sprache des Aphasischen. *Archive für Psychiatrie und Nervenkrankheiten,* 1972, *216,* 162–171.

Dejerine, J. Sur un cas de cécité verbale avec agraphie suivi d'autopsie. *Mémoires de la Société de Biologie,* 1891, *3,* 197–201.

Dejerine, J. Contribution à l'étude anatomo-pathologique et clinique des différentes variétés de cécité verbale. *Mémoires de la Société de Biologie,* 1892, *4,* 61–90.

Dejerine, J. *Sémiologie des Affections du Système Nerveux.* Paris: Masson, 1914.

Denes, G., and Semenza, C. Auditory modality-specific anomia: Evidence of a case of pure word deafness. *Cortex,* 1975, *11,* 401–411.

Dennis, M., and Whitaker, H. A. Language acquisition following hemidecortication: Linguistic superiority of the left over the right hemisphere. *Brain and Language,* 1976, *3,* 404–433.

Dubois, J., Hécaen, H., Angelergues, R., Maufras du Chatelier, A., and Marcie, P. Etude neurolinguistique de l'aphasie de conduction. *Neuropsychologia,* 1964, *2,* 9–44.

Dubois, J., Mazars, G., Marcie, P., and Hécaen, H. Etude des performances aux épreuves linguistiques des sujets atteints de syndromes parkinsoniens. *l'Encéphale,* 1966, *55,* 496–513.

Dubois, J., Hécaen, H., and Marcie, P. L'Agraphie "pure." *Neuropsychologia,* 1969, *7,* 271–286.

Dubois-Charlier, F. Approche neurolinguistique du problème de l'alexie pure. *Journal de Psychologie Normale et Pathologique.* 1971, *1,* 39–68.

Efron, R. Temporal perception, aphasia and déjà vu. *Brain,* 1963, *86,* 403–424.

Eimas, P., Siqueland, E., Jusczyr, P., and Vigorito, J. Speech perception in infants. *Science,* 1971, *171,* 303–306.

Eisenson, J. Language dysfunctions associated with right brain damage. *Atti del VIIème Congrèsso Internationale de Neurologia,* Rome, 1961.

Exner, S. *Untersuchungen über die Lokalisation der Funktionen in der Grosshirnrinde der Menschen.* Wien. W. Braumaller, 1881.

Faust, C. *Die zerebralen Herdstörungen bei Hinterhauptsverletzungen und ihre Beurteilung.* Stuttgart: G. Thieme, 1955.

Fedio, P. , and Mirsky, A. F. Selective intellectual deficits in children with temporal lobe or centrencephalic epilepsy. *Neuropsychologia,* 1969, *7,* 287–300.

Fedio, P., and van Buren, J. M. Cerebral mechanisms for perception and immediate memory under electrical stimulation in conscious man. Symposium: Human memory and subcortical mechanisms. Annual Meeting of the American Psychological Association, Washington, D.C., 1971.

Fedio, P., and van Buren, J. M. Memory deficits during electrical stimulation of the speech cortex in conscious man. *Brain and Language,* 1974, *1,* 29–42.

Foix, C. Aphasies. In G. Roger, F. Widal, and P. J. Teissier, (eds.), *Nouveau Traité de Médecine.* Paris: Masson, 1928, fasc. XVIII, pp. 135–213.

Foix, C., and Hillemand, P. Rôle vraisemblable du splenium dans la pathogénie de l'alexie pure par lésion de la cérébrale postérieure. *Bulletin et Mémoire de la Société Médicale des Hôpitaux de Paris*, 1925, *49*, 393–395.

French, L. A., Johnson, D. R., Brown, I. A., and van Bergen, F. B. Cerebral hemispherectomy for control of intractable convulsive seizures. *Journal of Neurosurgery*, 1955, *12*, 154–164.

Freud , S. Die infantile Cerebrallähmung. In Nothnagel (ed.), *Specielle Pathologie und Therapie*, Vol. IX. Vienna: Hölder, 1897.

Freund, C. S. Über optische Aphasie und Seelenblindheit. *Archive für Psychiatrie und Nervenkrankheiten*, 1888, *20*, 276–297.

Fromkin, V. A., Krashen, S., Curtiss, S., Rigler, D., and Rigler, M. The development of language in Genie: A case of language acquisition beyond the "critical period." *Brain and Language*, 1974, *1*, 81–108.

Gazzaniga, M. S., and Hillyard, S. A. Language and speech capacity of the right hemisphere. *Neuropsychologia*, 1971, *9*, 451–459.

Gelb, A., and Goldstein, K. *Psychologische Analysen hirnpathologischer Fälle*. Leipzig: Barth, 1920.

Gendrin, 1838. Quoted by J. M. Charcot, 1890.

Geschwind, N. Disconnexion syndromes in animals and man. *Brain*, 1965, *88*, 237–294, 585–644.

Geschwind, N., and Fusillo, M. Color naming defects in association with alexia. *Archives of Neurology*, 1966, *15*, 137–146.

Geschwind, N., and Kaplan, E. A human cerebral deconnection syndrome. *Neurology*, 1962, *12*, 675–685.

Geschwind, N., and Levitsky, W. Human brain, left-right asymmetries in temporal speech regions. *Science*, 1968, *161*, 186–187.

Gloning, I., Gloning, K., Haub, G., and Quatember. Comparison of verbal behavior in right-handed and non right-handed patients with anatomically verified lesion of one hemisphere. *Cortex*, 1969, *5*, 43–52.

Goldstein, K. *Language and Language Disturbances*. New York: Grune and Stratton, 1948.

Goldstein, M. N., Brown, M., and Hollander, J. Auditory agnosia and cortical deafness. Analysis of a case with three years follow up. *Brain and Language*, 1975, *2*, 324–332.

Goodglass, H. Studies on the grammar of aphasics, In S. Rosenberg and J. Koplin (eds.), *Developments in Applied Psycholinguistics Research*. New York: MacMillan, 1968, pp. 177–208.

Goodglass, H. Agrammatism. In H. Whitaker and H. Whitaker (eds.), *Studies in Neurolinguistics*. Vol. 1. New York: Academic Press, 1976.

Goodglass, H., and Quadfasel, F. A. Language laterality in left-handed aphasics. *Brain*, 1954, *77*, 521–548.

Gordinier, H. C. A case of brain tumor at the base of the second left frontal convolution. *American Journal of Medical Sciences*, 1899, *117*, 526–535.

Gosnave, G. Sentence production test in sensory aphasic patients in sentence production: Developments in theory and research. In S. Rosenberg (ed.), *Sentence Production: Developments in Research and Theory*. New York: Halsted Press, 1977, pp. 37–50.

Guiot, G., Hertzog, E., Rondot, P., and Molina, P. Arrest or acceleration of speech evoked by thalamic stimulation in the course of stereotaxic procedure for parkinsonism. *Brain*, 1961, *84*, 363–379.

Guttmann, E. Aphasia in children. *Brain*, 1942, *65*, 205–219.

Haslerud, G. H., and Clark, R. E. On the reintegrative perception of words. *American Journal of Psychology*, 1957, *70*, 97–101.

Head, H. *Aphasia and Kindred Disorders of Speech*, 2 vols. Cambridge: Cambridge, University Press, 1926.

Hécaen, H. Aspects des troubles de la lecture (alexies) au cours des lésions cérébrales en foyer. *Word*, 1967, *23*, 265–287.

Hécaen, H. Essai de dissociation du syndrome de l'aphasie sensorielle. *Revue Neurologique*, 1969, *120*, 229–237.

Hécaen, H. *Introduction à la Neuropsychologie*. Paris: Larousse, 1972.

Hécaen, H. Acquired aphasia in children and the ontogenesis of hemispheric functional specialization. *Brain and Language*, 1976, *3*, 114–134.

Hécaen, H., and de Ajuriaguerra, J. Le problème de la dominance hémisphérique. *Journal de Psychologie*, 1956, 473–486.

Hécaen, H., and de Ajuriaguerra, *Les Gauchers, Prévalence Manuelle et Dominance Cérébrale*. Paris: Presses Universitaires de France, 1963, 171 pp.

Hécaen, H., and Angelergues, R. l'Aphasie, l'apraxie, l'agnosie chez les gauchers. Modalités et fréquence des troubles selon l'hémisphère atteint. *Revue Neurologique*, 1962, *106*, 510–515.

Hécaen, H., and Angelergues, R. Localization of symptoms in aphasia. In A. V. S. de Reuck and M. O'Connor (eds.), *Disorders of Language*. London: Churchill, 1964, pp. 223–246.

Hécaen, H., and Angelergues, R. L'agraphie secondaire aux lésions du lobe frontal. *International Journal of Neurology*, 1966, *5*, 381–394.

Hécaen, H., and Consoli, S. Analyse des troubles du langage au cours des lésions de l'aire de Broca. *Neuropsychologia*, 1973, *11*, 377–388.

Hécaen, H., and Kremin, H. Neurolinguistic research on reading disorders resulting from left hemisphere lesions: Aphasic and "pure" alexias. In H. Whitaker and H. Whitaker (eds.), *Studies in Neurolinguistics*, Vol. 2. Academic Press,, 1976, pp. 269–329.

Hécaen, H., and Marcie, P. Disorders of written language following right hemisphere lesions: Spatial dysgraphia. In S. J. Dimond and J. G. Beaumont (eds.), *Hemisphere Function in the Human Brain*. London: Elek Science, 1974, pp. 345–366.

Hécaen, H., and Piercy, M. Paroxysmal dysphasia and the problem of cerebral dominance. *Journal of Neurology, Neurosurgery and Psychiatry*. 1956, *19*, 194–201.

Hécaen, H., and Sauguet, J. Cerebral dominance in left handed subjects. *Cortex*, 1971, *7*, 19–48.

Hécaen, H., de Ajuriaguerra, J., and David, M. Les déficits fonctionnels après lobectomie occipitale. *Monatsschrift für Psychiatrie und Neurologie*, 1952, *123*, 239–291.

Hécaen, H., Penfield, W., Bertrand, C., and Mamo, R. The Syndrome of apracto agnosia due to lesions of the minor cerebral hemisphere. *Archives of Neurology and Psychiatry*, 1956, *75*, 400–434.

Hécaen, H., Angelergues, R., and Douzenis, J. A. Les agraphies. *Neuropsychologia*, 1963, *1*, 179–208.

Hécaen, H., Dubois, J., and Marcie, P. Aspects linguistiques des troubles de la vigilance au cours des lésions temporales antérointernes droite et gauche. *Neuropsychologia*, 1967, *5*, 311–328.

Hécaen, H., Dubois, J., and Marcie, P. Les désorganisations de la réception des signes verbaux dans l'aphasie sensorielle, *Revue d'Acoustique*, 1968, 287–304.

Heilman, K. M., Coyle, J. M., Gonyea, E. F., and Geschwind, N. Apraxia and agraphia in a left-hander. *Brain*, 1973, *96*, 21–28.

Henschen, S. E. *Klinische und anatomische Beiträge zur Pathologie des Gehirns*. Stockholm: Nordiska Bokhandeln, 1920–1922, pp. 5–7.

Hillier, W. F. Total left cerebral hemispherectomy for malignant glioma. *Neurology*, 1954, *4*, 718–722.

Hoff, H. Die Lokalisation der Aphasie. *Atti del VIIth Congresso Internationale de Neurologia*, Rome, 1961, 555–568.

Hoff, H., Gloning, I., and Gloning, K. Über Alexie. *Wiener Zeitschrift für Nervenheilkunde*, 1954, *10*, 149–162.

Humphrey, M. E., and Zangwill, O. L. Dysphasia in left-handed patients with unilateral brain lesions, *Journal of Neurology, Neurosurgery and Psychiatry*, 1952, *15*, 184–193.

Ingram, D. Cerebral speech lateralization in young children. *Neuropsychologia*, 1975, *13*, 103–105.

Isserlin, M. Über Agrammatismus. *Zeitschrift für die gesamte Neurologie und Psychiatrie*, 1922, *75*, 332–410.

Iwata, M., Sugishita, M., Toyokura, Y., Yamada, R. and Yoshioka, M. Etude sur le syndrome de disconnexion visuo-linguale après la transection du splenium du corps calleux. *Journal of Neurological Sciences*, 1974, *23*, 421–432.

Jackson, H. *Selected Writings*. London: Hodder and Stoughton, t. II, 1931.

Jakobson, R. *Kindersprache, Aphasie und allgemeine Lautgesetze*. Uppsala, 1941.

Jakobson, R., and Halle, M. *Fundamentals of Language*. The Hague: Mouton, 1956.

Jerger, J., Weikers, N. J., Sharbrough, F. W., and Jerger, S. Bilateral lesions of the temporal lobe. *Acta Oto-laryngologica Supplementum 258, Stockholm*, 1969.

Johns, D. F., and Darley, F. L. Phonemic variability in apraxia of speech. *Journal of Speech and Hearing Research*, 1970, *13*, 556–583.

Kennedy, F. Stock-brainedness, the causative factors in the so-called crossed aphasia. *American Journal of Medical Science*, 1916, *152*, 849.

Kimura, D. Speech lateralization in young children as determined by an auditory test. *Journal of Comparative and Physiological Psychology*, 1963, *56*, 899–902.

Kinsbourne, M. The minor cerebral hemisphere as a source of aphasie speech. *Archives of Neurology*, 1971, *25*, 302–306.

Kinsbourne, M., and Rosenfield, D. B. Agraphia selective for written spelling: An experimental case study. *Brain and Language*, 1974, *1*, 215–226.

Klein, R. Über reine Worttaubheit mit besonderer Berücksichtigung der Amusie. *Monatschrift für Psychiatrie und Neurologie*, 1927, *64*, 354–368.

Kleist, K. *Gehirnpathologie*. Leipzig: Barth, 1933.

Kleist, K. *Sensory Aphasia and Amusia*. New York: Pergamon Press, 1962.

Knox, C., and Kimura, D. Cerebral processing of non verbal sounds in boys and girls. *Neuropsychologia*, 1970, *8*, 227–237.

Konorski, J. Pathophysiological analysis of various forms of speech disorders and an attempt of their classification. *Rozprawy Wydzialu Nauk Medycznych*, 1961, *6*, 1–13.

Krashen, S. Lateralization language learning and the critical period: Some new evidence. *Language Learning*, 1973, *23*, 63–74.

Kussmaül, A. *Les Troubles de la Parole*. Traduction française par A. Rue. Paris, 1884.

Lashley, K. S. *Brain Mechanisms and Intelligence*. Chicago: University of Chicago Press, 1923.

Lecours, A. L., and Lhermitte, F. The "pure form" of the phonetic disintegration syndrome (pure anarthria). Anatomoclinical Report of a Historical case. *Brain and Language*, 1976, *3*, 88–113.

Lenneberg, E. *Biological Foundations of Language*. New York: Wiley, 1967.

Levy, J. Psychobiological implications of bilateral asymmetry. In S. J. Dimond and J. G. Beaumont (eds.), *Hemisphere Function in the Human Brain*. London: Elek Science, 1974.

Levy, J., and Trevarthen, C., 1973, quoted by J. Levy, 1974.

Lhermitte, F., and Beauvois, M. F. A visual speech disconnexion syndrome. Report of a case with optic aphasia, agnosic alexia and Colour agnosia. *Brain*, 1973, *96*, 695–714.

Liberman, A. M., Cooper, F. S., Shankweiler, D. P., and Studdert-Kennedy, M. Perception of the speech code. *Psychological Review*, 1967, *74*, 431–461.

Lichteim, L. Über Aphasie. *Deutsche Archive für klinische Medizin*, 1885a, *36*.

Lichteim, L. On aphasia. *Brain*, 1885b, *7*, 433–484.

Liepmann, H., and Pappenheim, M. Über einen Fall von sogenannter Leitungsaphasie. *Zeitschrift für die gesamte Neurologie und Psychiatrie*, 1914, *27*, 1–41.

Luria, A. R. *Traumatic Aphasias*. The Hague: Mouton, 1969.

Marcie, P., Hécaen, H., Dubois, J., and Angelergues, R. Les troubles de la réalisation de la parole au cours des lésions de l'hémisphère droit. *Neuropsychologia*, 1965, *3*, 217–247.

Marie, P. *Travaux et Mémoires*, Vol. 1. Paris: Masson, 1926, pp.1–181.

Marshall, J. C., and Newcombe, F. Syntactic and semantics errors in paralexia. *Neuropsychologia*, 1966, *4*, 169–176.

Maspes, P. E. Le syndrome expérimental chez l'homme de la section du splenium du corps calleux. Alexie visuelle pure hémianopsique. *Revue Neurologique*, 1948, *80*, 100–113.

McFie, J. Intellectual impairment in children with localized post infantile cerebral lesions. *Journal of Neurology, Neurosurgery and Psychiatry*, 1961, *24*, 361–365.

Milner, B. Hemispheric specialization: Scope and limits. In F. O. Schmitt and F. G. Worden (eds.), *The Neurosciences: Third Study Program*. Cambridge, Mass.: MIT Press, 1974a, pp. 75–88.

Milner, B., Branch, C., and Rasmussen, T. Evidence for bilateral speech representation in some non-right handers. *Transaction of the American Neurological Association*, 1966, *91*, 306–308.

Mohr, J. P. Broca's area and Broca's aphasia. In H. Whitaker and H. Whitaker (eds.), *Studies in Neurolinguistics;* Vol. 1, New York: Academic Press, 1976.

Mohr, J. P., Watters, W. C., and Duncan, G. W. Thalamic hemorrhage and aphasia. *Brain and Language*, 1975, *2*, 3–17.

Monrad-Krohn, G. H. Dysprosody or altered "melody of language." *Brain*, 1947, *70*, 405–415.

Moore, W. H., and Weidner, W. E. Bilateral tachistoscopic word perception in aphasic and normal subjects. *Perceptual and Motor Skills*, 1974, *39*, 1003–1011.

Moore, W. H., and Weidner, W. E. Dichotic word-perception of aphasic and normal subjects. *Perceptual and Motor Skills*, 1975, *40*, 379–386.

Nagafuchi, M. Cited by D. Ingram, 1974.

Nielsen, J. M. *Agnosia, Apraxia, Aphasia: Their Value in Cerebral Localization*. New York: Hoeber, 1947.

Niessl von Mayendorff, *Die aphasischen Symptome*. Leipzig: Engelmann, 1911.

Ogle, J. W. Aphasia and Agraphia. *St. George's Hospital Reports*, Vol. II. 1867, pp.83–122.

Ojemann, G. A., Fedio, P., and van Buren, J. M. Anomia from pulvinar and subcortical parietal stimulation. *Brain*, 1968, *91*, 99–116.

Ojemann, G. A., Blick, W. I., and Ward, A. A. Improvement and disturbance of short-term verbal memory with human ventrolateral thalamic stimulation. *Brain*, 1971, *94*, 225–240.

Oldfield, C. Things, words and the brain. *Quarterly Journal of Experimental Psychology*, 1966, *18*, 340–353.

Pelissier, A. *L'Aphasie Motrice "Pure."* Paris: Vigot Frères, 1912.

Penfield, W., and Roberts, L. *Speech and Brain Mechanisms*. Princeton, N.J.: Princeton University Press, 1959.

Pick, A. *Die agrammatischen Sprachstörungen*. Berlin: Springer, 1913.

Pitres, A. Considerations sur l'agraphie. *Revue de Médecine*, 1884, *4*, 855.

Pitres, A. *l'Aphasie Amnésique et Ses Variétés Cliniques*. Paris: Alcan, 1898.

Pötzl, O. *Die optisch-agnostischen Störungen*. Leipzig: F. Deuticke, 1928.

Quensel, F. Die Erkrankungen der höheren optischen Zentren. *Kurzes Handbuch der Ophthalmologie*, 1931, *6*.

Ramier, A. M. Etude des troubles de la dénomination lors des lésions corticales unilatérales. Thèse de IIIème cycle. Paris, Nanterre, 1972.

Rasmussen, T., and Milner, B. The role of early brain injury in determining lateralization of cerebral speech functions. In S. J. Dimond and D. A. Blizzard (eds.), *Evolution and Lateralization of the Brain*. New York: Academy of Sciences, 1977, pp. 355–369.

Riklan, M., and Cooper, I. S. Psychometric studies of verbal functions following thalamic lesions in humans. *Brain and Language*, 1975, *2*, 45–64.

Riklan, M., and Levita, E. *Subcortical Correlates of Human Behavior: A Psychological Study of Basal Ganglia and Thalamic Surgery*. Baltimore: Williams and Wilkins, 1969.

Rössing, H. Zur sprachlichen Leistung der rechten (nicht-dominanten) Hemisphäre. *Zeitschrift für Dialectologie und Linguistik*, 1975, *13*, 172–197.

Rudel, R., Teuber, H. L., and Twitchell, T. E. Levels of impairment of sensorimotor early damage. *Neuropsychologia*, 1974, *12*, 95–108.

Russel, R., and Espir, M. L. E. *Traumatic Aphasia*. Oxford: Oxford University Press, 1961, 177 pp.

Safran, E. M., and Marin, O. S. M. Immediate memory for word lists and sentences in a patient with deficient auditory short-term memory. *Brain and Language*, 1975, *2*, 420–433.

Safran, E. M., Marin, O. S. M., and Yeni-Komshian, G. H. An analysis of speech perception in word deafness. *Brain and Language*, 1976, *3*, 209–228.

Satz, P., Achenbach, K., and Fennelle, E. Correlations between assessed manual laterality and predicted speech laterality in a normal population. *Neuropsychologia*, 1967, *5*, 295–310.

Schiller, F. Aphasia studied in patients with missile wounds. *Journal of Neurology, Neurosurgery and Psychiatry*, 1947, *10*, 183–197.

Schuloff, C., and Goodglass, H. Dichotic listening, side of brain injury and cerebral dominance. *Neuropsychologia*, 1969, *7*, 149–160.

Shallice, T., and Warrington, E. K. Independent functioning of verbal memory stores: A neuropsychological study. *The Quarterly Journal of Experimental Psychology*, 1970, *22*, 261–273.

Shallice, T., and Warrington, E. K. The dissociation between short-term retention of meaningful sounds and verbal material. *Neuropsychologia*, 1974, *12*, 553–555.

Shankweiler, D., and Harris, K. S. An experimental approach to the problem of articulation in aphasia. *Cortex*, 1966, *2*, 277–292.

Shankweiler, D., Harris, K. S., and Taylor, M. L. Electromyographic studies of articulation in aphasia. *Archives of Physiological Medicine and Rehabilitation*, 1968, *49*, 1–8.

Smith, A. Speech and other functions after left dominant hemispherectomy. *Journal of Neurology, Neurosurgery and Psychiatry*, 1966, *29*, 467–471.

Société de Neurologie de Paris. Discussion sur l'aphasie. *Revue Neurologique*, 1908, *1*, 611–636; *2*, 974–1024, 1025–1047.

Sperry, R. W., and Gazzaniga, M. S. Language following surgical disconnection of the hemisphere. In C. H. Millikan and F. Darley (eds.), *Brain Mechanisms Underlying Speech and Language*. New York: Grune and Stratton, 1967.

Spreen, O., Benton, A. L., and Van Allen, M. W. Dissociation of visual and tactile naming in amnesic aphasia. *Neurology*, 1966, *16*, 807–814.

Strub, R. L., and Gardner, H. The repetition déficit in conduction aphasia: Mnestic or linguistic? *Brain and Language*, 1974, *1*, 241–256.

Subirana, A. La droiterie. *Archives Suisses de Neurologie et de Psychiatrie*, 1952, *69*, 321–359.

Subirana, A. Vision neurologique des troubles du langage d'intérêt phoniatrique. Le pronostic des aphasies de l'adulte. *Folia Phoniatrica*, 1956, *8*, 149–197.

Teszner, D., Tzavaras, A., Gruner, J., and Hécaen, H. l'Asymétrie droite-gauche du planum temporale. A propos de l'étude anatomique de 100 cerveaux. *Revue Neurologique*, 1972, *126*, 444–449.

Tissot, R., Mounin, G., and Lhermitte, F. "l'Aggrammatisme." *Etude Neuropsycholinguistique*, Brussels: Dessart, 1973.

Tresher, J. H., and Ford, F. R. Colloid cyst of the third ventricule. *Archives of Neurology and Psychiatry*, 1937, *37*, 959–973.

Trousseau, A. De l'aphasie. *Clinique Médicale de l'Hôtel Dieu de Paris.* Baillière, 1877, p. 669.

Tzortzis, C., and Albert, M. L. Impairment of memory for sequences in conduction aphasia. *Neuropsychologia*, 1974, *12*, 355–366.

van Buren, J. M. Confusion and disturbance of speech from stimulation in vicinity of the head of the caudate nucleus. *Journal of Neurosurgery*, 1963, *20*, 148–157.

van Buren, J. M. The question of thalamic participation in speech mechanisms. *Brain and Language*, 1975, 31–44.

Vilkki, J., and Laitinen, L. V. Differential effects of left and right ventrolateral thalamotomy on receptive and expressive verbal performances and face matching. *Neuropsychologia*, 1974, *12*, 11–19.

Vincent, C., David, M., and Puech, P. Sur l'alexie. Production du phénomène à la suite de l'extirpation d'une tumeur de la corne occipitale du ventricule latéral gauche. *Revue Neurologique*, 1930, *1*, 262–272.

von Monakow, C. *Über die Lokalisation der Hirnfunktionen.* Wiesbaden: Verlag von Bergmann, 1914, 34 pp.

Wada, J., Clark, R., and Hamm, A. Cerebral hemispheric asymmetry in humans. *Archives of Neurology*, 1975, *32*, 239–246.

Warrington, E. K., and Shallice, T. The selective impairment of auditory verbal short-term memory. *Brain*, 1969, *92*, 885–896.

Weigl, E., and Bierwisch, M. Neuropsychology and linguistics: Topic of common research. *Foundations of Language*, 1970, *6*, 1–18.

Weinstein, E., and Keller, N. J. A. Linguistic patterns of misnaming in brain injury. *Neuropsychologia*, 1963, *1*, 79–90.

Weisenburg, T., and McBride, K. E. *Aphasia: A Clinical and Psychological Study.* New York: Commonwealth Fund, 1935.

Wepman, J. M., Bock, R. D., Jones, L. V., and van Pelt, D. Psycholinguistic study of aphasia: A revision of the concept of anomia. *Journal of Speech and Hearing Disorders*, 1956, *21*, 468–477.

Wernicke, C. *Der aphasische Symptomencomplex.* Breslau: M. Cohn et Weigert, 1874, 72 pp.

Wernicke, C. Der aphasische Symptomencomplex. *Die Deutsche Klinik*, 1903, *6*, 487–566.

Westphal, 1874. Cited by Kussmaül, 1884.

Whitaker, H. A. *On the Representation of Language in the Human Mind.* Edmonton: Linguistic Research, Inc., 1971.

Witelson, S. F., and Pallie, W. Left hemisphere specialization for language in the newborn: Neuroanatomical evidence of asymmetry. *Brain*, 1973, *96*, 641–646.

Woods, B. T., and Teuber, H. L. Early onset of complementary specialization of cerebral hemispheres in man. *Transactions of the American Neurological Association*, 1973, *98*, 113–115.

Yamadori, A., and Albert, M. Word category aphasia. *Cortex*, 1973, *9*, 112–125.

Yamadori, A., and Ikumura. Central (or conduction) aphasia in a Japanese patient. *Cortex*, 1975, *11*, 73–82.

Zaidel, E. Language, dichotic listening and the disconnected hemispheres. Paper presented at the Conference on Human Brain Function, UCLA, September 27, 1974.

Zaidel, E. Unilateral auditory language comprehension on the Token Test following cerebral commissurotomy and hemispherectomy. *Neuropsychologia*, 1977*a*, *15*, 1–8.

Zaidel, E. Auditory vocabulary of the right hemisphere following brain bisection or hemidecortication. *Cortex*, 1977*b*, *12*, 191–211.

Zangwill, O. L. Speech and the minor hemisphere. *Acta Neurologica Psychiatrica Belgica*, 1967, *67*, 1013–1020.

Zollinger, R. Removal of the left cerebral hemisphere. *Archives of Neurology and Psychiatry*, 1935, *34*, 1055–1064.

Zurif, E. B., and Bryden, M. P. Familial handedness and left-right differences in auditory and visual perception. *Neuropsychologia*, 1969, *7*, 179–188.

Zurif, E. B., Caramazza, A., and Myerson, R. Grammatical judgments of agrammatic patients. *Neuropsychologia*, 1972, *10*, 405–417.

PART V

General Issues in Brain Mechanisms and Behavior

11

Origins and Mechanisms in the Establishment of Cerebral Dominance

Fernando Nottebohm

A First Look at the Problem

"Cerebral dominance" refers to a gross functional asymmetry between the right and left halves of the brain. In humans, this functional asymmetry seems to be best represented in the hemispheres, or at least it is there that the right and left differences have attracted the greatest clinical attention. Speculations on the origins of this phenomenon differ in considering symmetry or asymmetry as the primitive condition.

Haecker (1927, quoted in Ludwig, 1932, p. 392) stated that "A tendency towards asymmetry and spiral growth seeks expression from the innermost nature of organic matter, but in free moving animals this tendency is almost always overcome by the demands of linear progression and orderly locomotion. However, whenever special conditions of life require an asymmetric or spiral organization—as for example in flatfish or in the shells of foraminifera, snails and cephalopods—then the old spiral developmental tendency breaks through once more." Haecker adds that even in those cases as in *Amphioxus,* where "a symmetric growth tendency seems to be primary and where asymmetry and spiral behavior appear as secondary, . . . these secondary developments can only take place because the tendency towards spiral growth was really available as an old developmental potency in chordates." The example of *Amphioxus* is particularly interesting because it includes components of neural asymmetry: The interior of the oral

Fernando Nottebohm The Rockefeller University, New York, New York 10021.

cavity and the velum are exclusively innervated by the left dorsal spinal nerve (Franz, 1927a, in Ludwig, 1932, p. 222), and locomotion takes the form of clockwise spiral advance (Franz, 1927b). To this, Ludwig (1932, p. 224) comments that if spiral progression was prevalent in earlier epochs, it would account for many of the observed structural asymmetries of the body, but he disagreed with Haecker's tenet of a basic primitive asymmetry that permeated development: "It is not possible to speak of a general tendency of living nature toward asymmetric structure. Rather one should speak of a tendency towards bilateral symmetry typical of all higher animals and which is rarely surrendered. The existence of such a tendency is further substantiated by the fact that when the right or left member of a bilateral pair of organs undergoes atrophy, the surviving member frequently adopts a median position (as in the gonads of *Myxine* and Selachians) or even in some cases adopts a pseudobilateral conformation by developing paired accessory organs (genital tract in snails and nematodes)" (Ludwig, 1932, p. 397).

In principle, bilateral symmetry or asymmetry of organs and functions could be generated by minor variants of the same developmental process. There may often be a small lag in growth between the two halves of the nervous system (Nottebohm, 1972, p. 48; review in Morgan, 1977) so that, for example, processes of cell division, fiber growth, synapse formation, or myelination lead on one side The ontogeny of a majority of systems may ignore these small lags, if they are present at all, so that the ensuing right and left halves end up being mirror images of each other. However, small temporal differences could be seized on by inhibitory influences of the leading side on its trailing counterpart and, in this manner, morphological and functional differences could be magnified. Thus it may be that the mechanisms and potential for developing functional and morphological symmetries and asymmetries are present in the embryonic nervous systems of all animals and that these opportunities are bypassed or exploited in different ways by each species according to the selective pressures that molded its peculiar style of life.

Embryogeny of Left-Right Differences

Embryogeny of a Right and a Left Half

Spemann and Falkenberg (1919) thought that the origin of right-left asymmetries was to be traced to the cytoplasm of the unfertilized egg:

> By whatever meridian the sperm enters the egg, the cytoplasm must always be different on the left and right sides of entry. If it were otherwise, given the well known undifferentiation of the spermatozoon, it would be impossible to provide an explanation of the different development of the left and right sides following fertilization. This implies that the cytoplasm of the egg possesses a bilaterally asymmetrical structure around the ovular axis, to which one can attribute the overt bilaterally asymmetrical development. (p. 398, as quoted in Morgan, 1977, p. 174)

To speak of a right-left axis in the cytoplasm of the unfertilized or fertilized egg, it is already necessary at this stage to demonstrate an anteroposterior axis and a dorsoventral axis. These two axes have been shown to occur in frogs (genus *Rana,* review in Huettner, 1949). While the frog oocyte is still in the ovary, yolk becomes concentrated near one pole, the vegetal pole, while the nucleus moves in the opposite direction toward the animal pole. In future development the animal polar side is destined to produce the anterior end of the embryo, while the vegetal polar portion forms the posterior end. The animal and vegetal hemispheres of the oocyte also differ in that there is a progressive accumulation of black pigment granules in the peripheral ooplasm of the animal hemisphere which lends a black appearance to this region, while the vegetal polar hemisphere remains cream white. At fertilization, peripheral ooplasm flows toward the sperm entrance point. This movement is very pronounced from the region opposite to that of the sperm, so that many of the pigment granules are carried along by it. This causes the formation of a slightly lighter pigmented area (gray crescent) exactly opposite the entrance point of the sperm (Fig. 1).

297

ORIGINS AND
MECHANISMS IN THE
ESTABLISHMENT OF
CEREBRAL
DOMINANCE

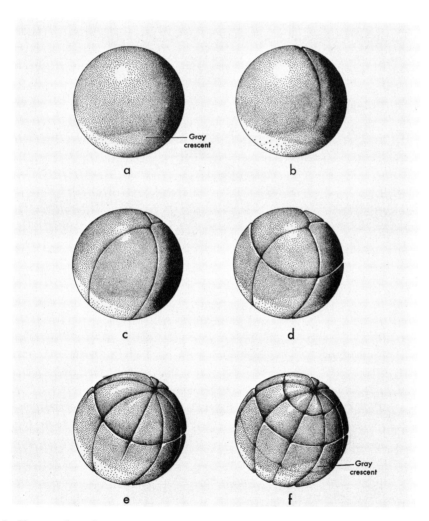

Fig. 1. Cleavages from the zygote of the frog. The yolk-laden vegetal pole is colored lighter, the animal pole darker. The gray crescent is visible before the onset of the first cleavage (from Huettner, 1949, p. 76, with the permission of the Macmillan Co.).

The importance of fertilization in establishing a secondary axis in the frog zygote is controversial. According to Huettner (1949, p. 75),

> As a result of the entrance of the sperm, or some other activation, another axis is laid down, namely the *secondary axis* extending from the center of the gray crescent to the opposite side, to a point below the level of the sperm entrance point. It happens, however, that the secondary axis is not always located in this direction. It is possible that the sperm has nothing to do with the determination of the secondary axis, and that the ovum itself has a fixed inner chemical organization for the axis pattern. That the first cleavage furrow [Fig. 1] coincides with the longitudinal axis passing through the sperm's copulation path, may be due simply to a more liquid ooplasm foreshadowing the first cleavage of the ovum, which is taken by the sperm path because it puts less resistance into its way toward the female pronucleus.* Very often the gray crescent is opposite the sperm entrance point, but in the urodeles the gray crescent makes its appearance before the sperm enters, and in parthenogenetic eggs there seems to be no relationship between parthenogenesis (as for example a pin prick) and bilaterality. This would indicate that the egg has an underlying bilaterality of its own. (p. 75)

The secondary axis determined by the gray crescent intersects the anteroposterior axis determined by the animal and vegetal poles almost at right angles (Fig. 1). The secondary axis is also called the dorsoventral axis, the region of the gray crescent becoming the dorsal side of the future animal and the opposite area the ventral side. The dorsoventral axis establishes the bilateral symmetry of the developing ovum. A perpendicular plane coinciding with the primary and secondary axes divides the ovum into a right and a left half, representing the right and left side, respectively, of the future animal. This plane coincides with the first cleavage plane. Viewed from the side of the gray crescent, the right and left blastomeres are destined to form the right and left sides of the future animal.

The gray crescent of amphibians apparently achieves its role of organizer of the dorsoventral axis by inducing the formation of axial structures such as the notochord and neural tube (Tomkins and Rodman, 1971). A structure akin to the gray crescent of amphibians has not been described in avian and mammalian material, although the zygote of these groups always has an animal and a vegetal pole.

DO GENES DETERMINE RIGHT-LEFT DIFFERENCES IN DEVELOPMENT?

Given that an ovum or zygote has an anteroposterior and a dorsoventral axis, are differences between the right and left sides genetically determined or are they the result of other influences? Morgan (1977) states that there is no known case in which the direction of an asymmetry is determined in an individual by its own genetic material. Collins (1977) similarly claims to be unaware of "any evidence supporting the existence of right and left genes in animal and human populations" (p. 148), although he concedes that asymmetries may be due to an interaction between a genetic determination of the degree of asymmetry and a laterally biased environment.

There are at least two cases where genetic influence on the sense of development of a right-left asymmetry has been clearly established (review in Levy, 1977). In the snail *Limnaea peragra* there is an asymmetry visible as early as the second cell

---

*I.e., unfertilized haploid nucleus of the female egg.

division of the embryo. Instead of occurring at right angles, successive cleavages occur obliquely, with a regular alternation between clockwise and counterclockwise rotation. The cleavage pattern is determined not by the embryo's own genotype but by that of the mother (Sturtevant, 1923), and this cleavage pattern affects the coiling direction of the developing individual. The direction of coiling is affected by a single diallelic locus, dextral coiling being dominant (Srb *et al.*, 1965). If the mother is heterozygous for coiling direction, her progeny will always display dextral coiling. If the progeny, however, have received recessive alleles from both mother and father, the next generation displays sinistral coiling. In this example, the mother's genotype presumably affects direction of coiling indirectly by determining some relevant property of the egg's cytoplasm.

In the second example, an animal's own genotype has been shown to set the direction of asymmetry in an adult anatomical trait. In the fruit fly *Drosophila melanogaster* two loci can produce rotation of the entire abdomen if mutant alleles are present. The direction and extent of the rotation depend on specific alleles (Lindsley and Grell, 1967).

To make a case for genetic control of right-left asymmetries, it does not matter whether these asymmetries are determined by the embryo's own genome or result from cytoplasmic characteristics of the unfertilized ovum determined by the mother's genotype. It is possible that some asymmetries result from an interaction of factors originating from both sources. Although such asymmetries would be heritable and run in families, the probability of their occurrence and the extent of their manifestation would defy a simple Mendelian description. In such cases, testing the extent of genetic control would require careful inbreeding experiments of the kind described by Collins (1977).

Multiple loci might control the occurrence of handedness and hemispheric dominance in humans, but in the absence of strict inbreeding data this point is likely to remain unsettled (review in Levy, 1977, p. 205). Recent experiments by Levy and Reid (1976) show that the direction of cerebral lateralization for spatial and language tasks, as determined by tachistoscopic tests using visual material, can be predicted from a subject's handedness and hand posture during writing (Figure 2).

In subjects with a normal writing posture, the linguistically specialized hemisphere is contralateral to the dominant hand, and the visuospatially specialized hemisphere is ipsilateral; the reverse is true in subjects with an "inverted" hand position during writing. Since anatomical brain asymmetries thought to be related to language function show a strong and comparably biased distribution in adults, neonates, and human fetuses (Cunningham, 1892; Geschwind and Levitsky, 1968; Wada, 1969; Wada *et al.*, 1975; Witelson and Pallie, 1973; review in Rubens, 1977), it seems likely that brain asymmetries for language and handedness precede postnatal environmental influences and therefore have a strong hereditary component. The importance of genetic factors is emphasized by Luria's (1970) finding that the presence or absence of sinistral family members is predictive of the probability of recovery from aphasia following left-hemisphere lesions, in both left- and right-handers: individuals with a history of familial left-handedness are more likely to recover language functions following lesion to the left hemisphere.

Despite the appeal of a simple relation between writing hand posture and hemispheric dominance as reported by Levy and Reid (1976), more recent work suggests that this relation holds only if hemispheric function is tested in the visual domain. Tests using auditory (dichotic) and tactile stimuli do not show a correlation between inferred hemispheric dominance and handwriting posture (Moscovitch and Smith, 1978).

DECODING OF ASYMMETRIES

How do genes influence the direction and extent of anatomical and functional asymmetries of the CNS? Levy (1977) has suggested that since the tertiary asymmetrical structure of proteins is genetically determined, such proteins may provide the readout of right-left asymmetries coded in the genome. This would be so if, during the course of morphogenesis, tertiary asymmetrical proteins brought about morphological asymmetry. This interpretation remains to be tested.

The next step in the readout of genetically coded symmetries would presumably involve asymmetrical patterns of neuronal growth or movement. Heacock and Agranoff (1977) report what may be the first example of this phenomenon: the growing neurite tips of right or left goldfish retina explants kept *in vitro* show a clockwise helicity (Fig. 3). They interpret this growth pattern as a reflection of inherent tendencies not dependent on gravity or other extrinsic factors such as magnetic or Coriolis forces.

Cell formation in the avian embryo occurs initially in the blastoderm, a small disk-shaped mass found in the animal pole of the fertilized egg. Cells detach from the underlying yolk at a point that will become the caudal end of the blastoderm

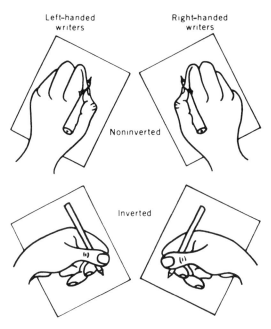

Fig. 2. Typical writing postures of dextrals and sinistrals who write with inverted and noninverted hand positions (from Levy and Reid, 1976, reproduced with the permission of the AAAS).

301

ORIGINS AND
MECHANISMS IN THE
ESTABLISHMENT OF
CEREBRAL
DOMINANCE

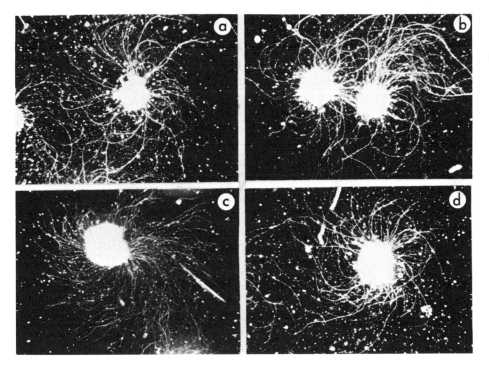

Fig. 3. Explants of goldfish retina on poly-L-lysine-coated tissue culture dishes under dark field illumination after 8 to 12 days *in vitro*. The clockwise pattern of neurite growth demonstrated here was also seen in explants cultured in dishes coated with poly-DL-lysine or poly-D-lysine, regardless of whether the explants came from the right or left eye (from Heacock and Agranoff, 1977, reproduced with the permission of the AAAS).

and give rise to a cavity known as the blastocoel. A crescent-shaped slit opens from the surface into the blastocoel, and its appearance marks the onset of gastrulation.* Cells on both sides of the crescent-shaped slit undergo rapid mitosis and push backward and toward the midline. Eventually, the slit fuses and is pushed forward where it becomes a groove known as the primitive streak (review in Huettner, 1949). By placing vital stains in the area surrounding the formation of the crescent-shaped slit of duck embryos, Lepori (1966b, review in 1969) showed that caudally and medially directed movements on the surface of the blastoderm are more marked on the left than on the right side. During a subsequent stage of development, the primitive streak is markedly shortened, and at this time the tissue on its left side advances slightly over its right counterpart, as shown in Fig. 4 (Lepori 1966a; review in Lepori, 1969). Lepori (1969) also reports that similar processes influence the embryogeny of the avian heart. The avian heart arises from the union of two lateral rudiments, of which the left one is more voluminous in 96% of the cases and moves sooner toward the midline. Interference with the latter movement on the left side leads to a relatively faster movement on the right side and to a heart that shows a displacement towards the left *(situs cordis inversus)*. Lepori (1969) has proposed a unified theory for the ontogeny of anatomical

*Gastrulation is the embryonic stage during which the rudiment of the future alimentary canal is formed.

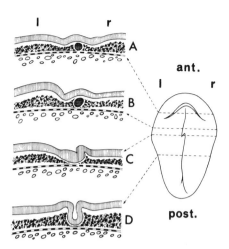

Fig. 4. Duck blastoderm after 23 hr of incubation. Sections A–C were cut at four different rostrocaudal levels. Asymmetries in development can be seen at levels B and C. B corresponds to the level of the neural plaque; C cuts through Hensen's node and shows an asymmetry between the two sides of the primitive streak; l = left; r = right; ant. = anterior; post. = posterior (modified from Lepori, 1969, reproduced with permission from the Monitore Zoologico Italiano).

asymmetries based on the hypothesis that all blastoderm cells, as they begin to move during gastrulation, follow a counterclockwise spiral path (Fig. 5). This would explain why, during formation of the primitive streak, cellular movements converge toward its left side but diverge from its right side. Although Lepori's observations do show differential cell movements in the right and left halves of the embryo, it is not clear whether different rates of cell migration or direction of movement is the primary factor, or whether these are secondary results of different mitotic rates between the right and left embryonic halves. Intriguingly, if the kinds of dynamics represented in Figure 5 are extended to the rostral half of the embryo, then convergence toward the midline would be more marked on the right side, where it could be converted into a right developmental advantage! However, Lepori's model makes no explicit mention of a reversal in the direction of asymmetries as one moves caudorostrally along the embryos longitudinal axis.

Differential rates of cell movement or mitosis may also explain the determination of right-left asymmetries in amphibians. In the newt *Triturus alpestris,* left-side lesions inflicted during the gastrula or neurula* stage frequently result in situs inversus of the heart, gastrointestinal tract, and habenular nuclei of the diencephalon. Situs inversus occurs less frequently after right-side lesions, though the fact that it occurs at all under those circumstances is puzzling. Tissue explants from dorsal neurula-stage embryos reimplanted in the original direction or after 180° rotation also induce situs inversus of gut and heart, with a frequency unrelated to the orientation of the implants. The actual mechanisms involved in the determination of right-left anatomical asymmetries in amphibians and birds remain unclear, although it seems they do not depend on a circumscribed right-left embryonic inducer (review in von Woellwarth, 1950; Lepori, 1969).

*The neurula is the embryonic stage after completion of the neural tube.

303

ORIGINS AND
MECHANISMS IN THE
ESTABLISHMENT OF
CEREBRAL
DOMINANCE

The direction and extent of asymmetry on the various organs of the body do not follow an all-or-nothing rule. Von Woellwarth (1950) described four *T. alpestris* newts with spontaneously occurring situs inversus cordis (from 472 larvae sampled; frequency of occurrence 0.85%). One of these four individuals also showed full situs inversus of the gastrointestinal tract and habenular nuclei of the thalamus; two had a complete situs inversus of the gastrointestinal tract and an attenuated form of situs inversus of the habenular nuclei; the fourth newt showed incomplete inversion of the gastrointestinal tract, and the habenular nuclei were symmetrical. When von Woellwarth induced situs inversus by reimplanting dorsal tissue in the neurula stage or by making one-sided lesions in the gastrula and neurula of *T. alpestris,* he observed that the orientation of the heart, gastrointestinal tract, and habenular nuclei occurred in various possible combinations, so that the outcome could be, respectively, n (normal), n, i (inverse); i, n, n; n, i, i; i, i, n; and n, i, n (Tables 16 and 17 in von Woellwarth, 1950). However, in most cases the various organs shared the sense of asymmetry, and the most frequent result of the reimplantation or lesion experiments was to have n, n, n or i, i, i individuals.

In later experiments, von Woellwarth (1969) has shown that habenular asymmetries develop in *T. alpestris* in the absence of a heart, and therefore cannot be attributed to right-left differences in blood supply. From this, he concludes that the asymmetries evinced by various organs, including the habenula, result from a "general asymmetry-determining factor of the embryo." This factor or a similar one may correspond to that invoked by Lepori (1969) for determining patterns of cell movement in avian embryos and could also account for the spiral growth of neurites of goldfish retinal explants, as described by Heacock and Agranoff (1977).

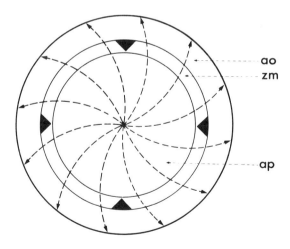

Fig. 5. Dorsal surface of the avian blastoderm illustrating Lepori's interpretation of cell movements. Interrupted lines and arrows represent directions of moving cells, shown to follow a spiral counter-clockwise path. Four solid triangles represent hypothetical caudal tips of the primitive streak. Irrespective of the position of the primitive streak, cellular movements converge toward the left bank and diverge from its right bank; ap = area pellucida; ao = area opaca; zm = marginal zone (from Lepori, 1969, reproduced with permission from the Monitore Zoologico Italiano).

FERNANDO
NOTTEBOHM

Animals that are apparently symmetrical may have asymmetrical behavior. This is not new. Schaeffer (1928) studied the spiraling tendency of blindfolded humans and concluded that mechanisms that produce the spiral path are not in the motor organs but in the central nervous system, and that straight walking, swimming, or driving depends on orienting responses. Many years later, Wilson (1968) noticed that in the absence of visual feedback, flying intact locusts may roll consistently toward the right or left, and that in those cases the roll results from asymmetry in the motor output pattern. In free flight, or in the presence of a simulated horizon, the centrally inherent asymmetrical behavior is corrected by compensatory changes in the motor pattern. Since asymmetries of this type do not show a consistent right or left bias across members of a population, they may be seen as a measure of the difficulty in developing and producing perfectly symmetrical motor outputs.

Somatic and Neural Asymmetries in Invertebrates

In some decapod crustaceans such as the fiddler crab (genus *Uca*), the distal segments of one chela undergo a greater rate of growth than those on the other chela. While the larger chela is used for social signaling, the smaller one is used for feeding (Crane, 1966). In the lobster *(Homarus),* a slow closer muscle serves the larger crusher claw, while a faster closer muscle serves the cutter claw (Jahromi and Atwood, 1971; Govind and Lang, 1974). Since a crusher can develop on either side of the animal, as can the major chela of *Uca,* such a situation should be very useful in analyzing the effects of peripheral asymmetry on the central nervous system. Still another example of asymmetry in decapods is the decalcified and dextrally coiled abdomen of the hermit crab, *Pagurus.* These crabs live in the castoff shells of gastropods, which in most cases also curl to the right. Homologous motoneurons innervating the right and left abdominal musculature differ in size and tonic frequencies (review in Chapple, 1977).

Further examples of asymmetry are provided by gastropod mollusks, the viscera of which undergo a 180° torsion during development, accompanied by a loss of nephridia and gills on the right side as well as alterations in the circulatory system. The evolutionary and developmental conditions which led to this kind of asymmetry are probably also reflected in the gastropod nervous system. Kupfermann and Kandel (1969) described the defensive withdrawal reflex in *Aplysia.* This response involves the simultaneous participation of three organs and is controlled by five cells. These cells are always located in the left half of the abdominal ganglion of this mollusk.

An interesting question is usually one that is hard to answer. Similarly, an observation is more interesting when it fails to match earlier observations or preconceived ideas. Within this framework, the invertebrate examples discussed above are interesting but not striking. What is fascinating about neural asymmetries in vertebrates is that they provide control over a basically symmetrical effector system: Neither our extremities, nor our vocal tract, nor our ears and eyes are grossly asymmetrical, although in the case of the extremities there may be slight differences in length (Ingelmark, 1947; quoted in von Bonin, 1962). In this sense, the gastropod and decapod material is likely to be of limited assistance in understanding the evolutionary significance of neural asymmetry in vertebrates.

HABENULAR ASYMMETRIES IN LOWER VERTEBRATES

For many years, comparative neuroanatomists have realized that the habenular nuclei of lower vertebrates offer examples of marked asymmetry. The habenular nuclei are found in the dorsal anterior diencephalon, under the epiphysis, on either side of the third ventricle. Asymmetrical habenular nuclei have been described in lamprey *(Petromyzon),* sturgeon, eels *(Anguilla anguilla),* newts *(Triturus alpestris* and *T. cristatus),* and frogs *(Rana esculenta, R. temporaria)* (review in Braitenberg and Kemali, 1970; Morgan, 1977). From a statistical viewpoint, the habenular asymmetry in newts (von Woellwarth, 1950) and frogs is a robust phenomenon. In a serial survey of 50 *Rana esculenta* brains, a markedly larger and more lobate left habenular nucleus was found in all cases (Braitenberg and Kemali, 1970). An example of this asymmetry is shown in Fig. 6. Preponderance of the left side has also been described in newts and eels (Braitenberg and Kemali, 1970).

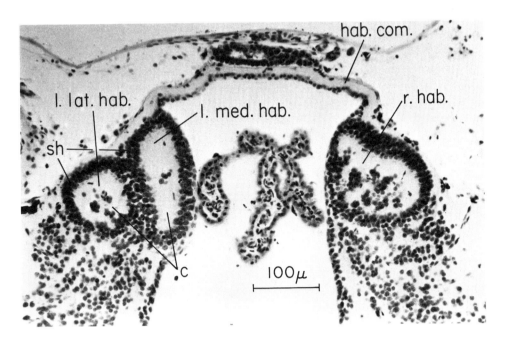

Fig. 6. Nissl stained frontal section of the habenular region in the frog, *Rana esculenta;* l. lat. hab. = left habenular nucleus, lateral part; l. med. hab. = left habenular nucleus, medial part; r. hab. = right habenular nucleus; hab. com. = habenular commissure; sh = shell, and c = core of habenular nuclei. The core consists predominantly of fibers that are not stained by the Nissl procedure (from Braitenberg and Kemali, 1960, reproduced with permission of the *Journal of Comparative Neurology).* Reduced 47% for reproduction.

Asymmetry does not necessarily favor the left side. Lampreys *(Petromyzon)* have a vastly preponderant right habenulopeduncular tract. The fish *Cyclothone acclinidens* and the hagfish *Myxine glutinosa* are credited with a larger right habenular nucleus (review in Braitenberg and Kemali, 1970). In the South African toad *Xenopus laevis,* the habenula is multilobate and shows no obvious morphological asymmetry (Morgan, 1977).

In ammocoetes, the larva of lampreys, the dorsal pineal eye is connected to the right habenula and the ventral pineal eye to the left habenula (Gaskell, 1901, as quoted by Cameron, 1904). To this, Braitenberg and Kemali, 1970, p. 144 add:

> We are not in the possession of the embryological or sufficiently wide comparative material which would enable us to enter a discussion of the relationship between the habenular complex and the pineal organs. This relationship may be invoked to explain asymmetries in the epithalamic region if we will accept that at some stage in evolution two originally paired and bilaterally symmetric organs such as two parietal eyes, each connected to the corresponding half of the epithalamus, shifted their positions rotating around each other to reach positions on the medial plane, ending up either one rostral and one caudal or one dorsal and one ventral. If in this process the connexions with the epithalamus are preserved, at least the fibers should show bilateral asymmetry. If then one of the two parietal organs loses its function or takes over a radically different function from its companion, we are not surprised to find asymmetries in the corresponding central stations.

The "pineal organs" referred to here are also known as the epiphysis cerebri or true pineal, placed posteriorly, and the parapineal organ, placed anteriorly. Although the whole matter of pineal and parapineal asymmetry remains controversial (Holmgren, 1965; Oksche, 1965; Sivak, 1974), it is suggested here that habenular asymmetries may have had their origin in peripheral influences that modified an originally symmetrical part of the sensorium. Habenular asymmetries have not been reported in reptiles, birds, or mammals.

In lower vertebrates, the interpeduncular nucleus receives the main projection from the habenula (Braitenberg and Kemali, 1970). In at least some mammals (rat), the habenula may serve an important role in funneling information from the limbic forebrain to the limbic midbrain (midbrain raphe nuclei) (Wang and Aghajanian, 1977). The apparent loss of habenular asymmetry in higher vertebrates may be related to this important involvement in limbic function.

Hemispheric Asymmetries in Primates

The cerebral hemispheres of the great apes and spinal chord of man offer the only other gross and undisputed examples of anatomical asymmetry in the central nervous system of vertebrates, and even these examples have gained notoriety only in the last 10 or 15 years. As recently as 1962, von Bonin (p. 6) ended a review of the known asymmetries of the human brain by stating: "But all these morphological differences are, after all, quite small. How to correlate these with the astonishing differences in function, such as the speech function on the left side, is an entirely different question, and one that I am unable to answer." As we shall see, the asymmetries can be quite marked, although von Bonin was justified in not wanting to assign to them a causal role.

It has been known for over a century that, in most people, the left hemisphere is dominant for language tasks, and this function is thought to reside predominantly within a ring of cortex that forms the upper and lower banks of the sylvian fissure (Broca, 1865; Wernicke, 1874; Penfield and Roberts, 1959; Luria, 1970). Not surprisingly, the sylvian fissure and structures abutting with it have received the attention of neuroanatomists seeking to relate hemispheric dominance for language function to anatomical asymmetries of the hemispheres. The history of these endeavors is adequately reviewed in three recent publications (Geschwind, 1974; LeMay, 1976; Rubens, 1977). In this chapter, I will only touch on findings of interest to a general discussion of origins and mechanisms in the establishment of cerebral dominance.

The present interest in the anatomical asymmetries of the human brain was prompted, to a large extent, by a report by Geschwind and Levitsky (1968) in which they described a marked anatomical asymmetry between the upper surfaces of the human right and left temporal lobes. Their description focused on the planum temporale, which they defined as that area of cortex lodged between Heschl's gyrus rostrally and the posterior end of the sylvian fossa caudally (Fig. 7). In their survey of 100 adult brains, they found that the left planum temporale was larger in 65% of the cases and the right one in only 11%. Whereas Heschl's gyrus contains the primary auditory cortex which receives the major outflow of the medial geniculate body, the planum temporale contains auditory association cor-

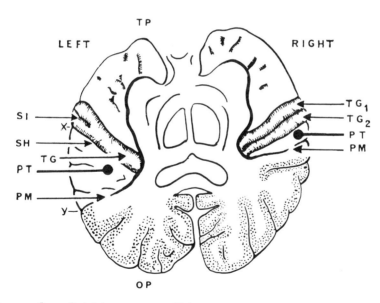

Fig. 7. Upper surfaces of adult human temporal lobes exposed by a cut on each side in the plane of the Sylvian fissure. The sulcus of Heschl (SH) forms the anterior margin of the planum temporale (PT). The posterior margin (PM) is formed on the left side by the end Y of the left Sylvian fissure. In this brain, there is a single transverse gyrus of Heschl (TG) on the left but two on the right (TG₁, TG₂). SI = sulcus intermedius of Beck; TP = temporal pole; OP = occipital pole (from Geschwind and Levitsky, 1968, reproduced with permission of the AAAS).

tex relevant to language processes, including part of the classical area of Wernicke. From these results, Geschwind and Levitsky (1968, p. 187) concluded that "the differences observed are easily of sufficient magnitude to be compatible with the known functional asymmetries."

Geschwind and Levitsky (1968, review in Geschwind, 1974) exposed the planum temporale area by inserting a broad-bladed knife in the sylvian fissure and advancing it along the line of the fissure until the posterior wall was reached. This "posterior wall," which then is taken to be the posterior margin of the planum temporale, may correspond to the end of the sylvian fissure on the left hemisphere but not necessarily on the right one. In a sample of 36 brains, Rubens *et al.* (1976) noticed that in 69% of the cases the right sylvian fissure angulated farther upward than the left one (Fig. 8); in the remaining 11 brains, the difference was less noticeable. As a result, the "posterior wall" of the sylvian fissure as determined by Geschwind and Levitsky (1968) need not correspond with the true termination of the sylvian fissure. According to Rubens (1977, p. 510), the terminal sylvian fissure bend has been regarded as an arbitrary dividing point between temporal and parietal lobes. Sylvian regions posterior to this conventionally belong to the supramarginal gyrus of the parietal lobe. Since it is not yet known how often the auditory association area is limited posteriorly by this terminal upward bend, Rubens (1977, p. 510) argues that "it seems reasonable to question whether gross asymmetry of the planum temporale is a valid indicator of underlying auditory association-cortex asymmetry."

However, Galaburda and Sanides (referred to in Galaburda *et al.,* 1978) have recently mapped the full extent of the several cytoarchitectonic regions contained within the planum temporale and including the portions extending beyond its limits in three serially sectioned brains. They report that the temporoparietal cortex is considerably larger on the left side (Fig. 9). Involvement of the temporo-parietal cortex and its projections may be responsible for the high incidence of comprehension aphasia following lesion of the first temporal gyrus (Luria, 1958), though this interpretation is by no means secure.

Earlier in this chapter I mentioned that the anatomical differences described by Geschwind and Levitsky (1968) are not likely to be the result of postnatal experiental factors. Wada (1969, quoted in Geschwind, 1974) observed similar right-left differences in the size of the planum temporale in newborn humans and in fetal brains and Witelson and Pallie (1973) noted that the left-right difference in the area of the planum temporale was proportionately as large in neonates as in adults. Witelson and Pallie (p. 644) also noted that this anatomical asymmetry "was not as marked for males as for females within the first few days of life"; perhaps a concomitant of the slower maturation of the male nervous system (see p. 329).

The right and left hemispheres of humans differ in still other ways. For example, the left occipital pole is often wider and usually protrudes more posteriorly than the right, whereas the right frontal lobe and the central portion of the right hemisphere more often measure wider than the left. If one frontal pole extends beyond the other, it is usually the right. In left-handed and ambidextrous individuals, the posterior end of the sylvian fissures are more often nearly equal in

309

ORIGINS AND
MECHANISMS IN THE
ESTABLISHMENT OF
CEREBRAL
DOMINANCE

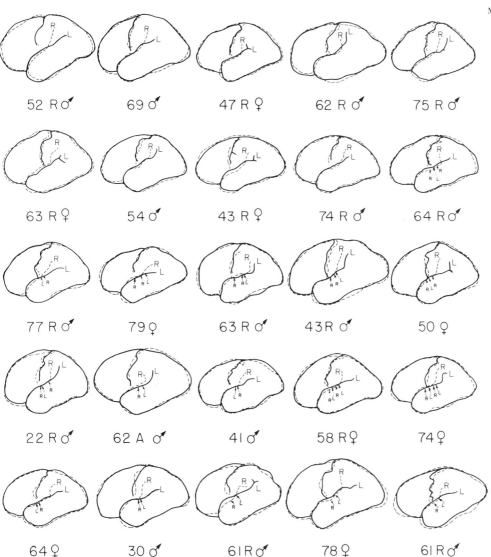

Fig. 8. Comparison of the courses of the right and left Sylvian fissures in 25 adult human brains. To produce this set of drawings, photographic slides of the left lateral and reversed right lateral views of the brain were projected superimposed. The right hemisphere was traced by a dashed line, the left hemisphere by a solid line. The caudal ends of the right and left Sylvian fissures are indicated, respectively, by R and L. Small arrows indicate in some of the brains the juncture of the sulci of Heschl with the upper contour of the temporal lobe, labeled with a small L for the left side and a small R for the right side; there may be one or two sulci of Heschl on each side. Age, handedness when known (right handed = R; ambidextrous = A), and sex are indicated below each drawing (from Rubens *et al.,* 1976, reproduced with the permission of *Neurology*).

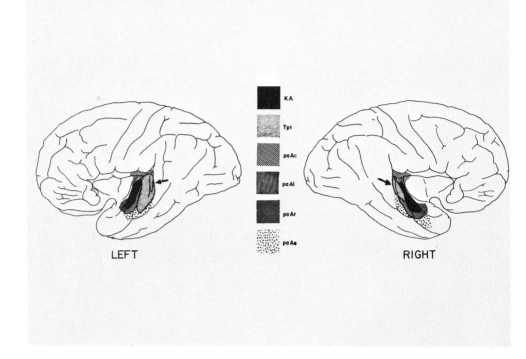

Fig. 9. Cytoarchitectonic areas of the human auditory cortex in one brain. Arrows indicate marked left-right asymmetry of temporoparietal cortex (Tpt), an area thought to be related to language function; KA = koniocortex; pa = subdivisions of the parakoniocortex (from Galaburda *et al.*, 1978, reproduced with permission from the AAAS).

height and the occipital regions are more often equal in width, or the right may be wider (LeMay, 1976).

The biological significance of the right-left anatomical differences observed in the human brain remains unclear. Observations on the sylvian fissures of 17 great apes (orangutan, chimpanzee, and gorilla) revealed that only one individual had the posterior end of the left sylvian fissure higher than the right one; as in humans, the right was higher in the other 16 (Fig. 10). The most striking differences were noted in the ten orangutans included in this group (LeMay, 1976).

Advanced forms of vocal communication are thought to have evolved in complex societies where one individual can assume a variety of social roles and convey subtle nuances of information (Marler, 1965; Green, 1975). If hemispheric asymmetries evolved to process and produce particularly advanced forms of vocal communication, as has been suggested for humans, then one would not expect to find such asymmetries in the orangutan brain. Whereas all other higher primates are sociable, forming groups or at least family parties, orangutans are primarily solitary and their vocal communication does not seem particularly complex (Mackinnon, 1974, Rodman, 1973). It seems reasonable to suggest that anatomical brain asymmetries in humans and apes bear no primary relation to complex forms of vocal communication. Such a conservative view does not exclude the possibility that language evolution seized on preexisting anatomical asymmetries to yield the functional hemispheric dominance observed in modern man.

A recent study by Yeni-Komshian and Benson (1976) adds plausibility to the "conservative" interpretation of primate brain asymmetries. These authors measured the length of the right and left sylvian fissures in brains of humans, chimpanzees, and rhesus macaques. A longer left sylvian fissure was seen in 84% of the humans, in 80% of the chimpanzees, and in 44% of the rhesus monkeys. The mean difference between the lengths of the left and right fissures was 10.2 mm for the human (corresponding to 15% difference) and 2.0 mm (5% difference) for the chimpanzee brains. The rhesus brains showed no significant difference between the left and right fissure lengths.

Cytoarchitechtonic maps of the rhesus (von Bonin and Baily, 1947) and chimpanzee (Bailey *et al.*, 1950) neocortex suggest that in these species, as in humans, the superior surface of the temporal lobe includes an auditory association area homologous to that found in the human planum temporale. From this, Yeni-Komshian and Benson (1976, p. 389) conclude that "sylvian fissure length may be considered an indirect measure of the homolog of the human planum temporale in the chimpanzee and rhesus brain." Actually, there need be no one to one relation between length of the sylvian fissure and volume of the planum temporale. Furthermore, the functional import of right-left differences in length of the sylvian fissure and hypothetical differences in the volume of the planum temporale remains unclear. Both rhesus monkeys and chimpanzees are highly sociable

311

ORIGINS AND
MECHANISMS IN THE
ESTABLISHMENT OF
CEREBRAL
DOMINANCE

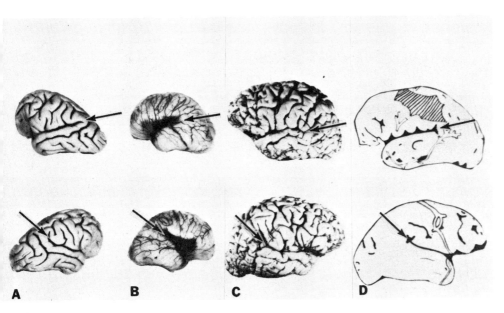

Fig. 10. Lateral views of the right and left hemispheres of (A) orangutan; (B) 16-week human fetus; (C) adult human male; and (D) drawing from the endocranial cast of the La Chapelle-aux-Saints skull of a Neanderthal adult. Arrows indicate the posterior ends of the sylvian fissures, which are higher on the right than on the left (from LeMay, 1976, reproduced with the permission of the New York Academy of Science).

species with vocal repertoires of comparable complexity (Altmann, 1962, 1965; Rowell and Hinde, 1962; van Lawick-Goodall, 1968*a,b,* 1971; Marler, 1976). It is hard to believe that chimpanzees, but not macaques, would need a hypertrophied left planum temporale so as to better meet the requirements of vocal communication. One is tempted to invoke a more general evolutionary progression manifest in pongid apes and further developed in humans, affecting the sylvian fissure and adjacent brain areas. The selective pressures that may have driven this evolutionary progression remain unknown.

Two further examples should underscore the difficulties met when trying to extrapolate functional interpretations from anatomical data. In a sample of 38 skulls of mountain gorillas *(Gorilla g. beringei),* measurements from the anteriormost point of the temporal fossa to the gnathion revealed a longer left side by a mean of 2.7 mm. In 17 of these skulls, the asymmetry was gross (difference of 4 mm or more, roughly 2%) and was accompanied by an obvious lopsidedness of the sagittal crest and heavier toothwear on one side. Similar observations on 138 skulls of the lowland gorilla *(G. g. gorilla)* produced a 0.1-mm-longer right side (which is not significantly different from zero). Groves and Humphrey (1973) emphasize that it would be inappropriate to convert their observations on skull asymmetry to inferences on brain asymmetry. They suggest that the skull asymmetry of mountain gorillas may be a secondary consequence of an asymmetry in the use of the masticatory apparatus, adding (p. 54): "If left-sided chewing is the cause of skull asymmetry in mountain gorillas, it might explain the absence of such asymmetry in lowland gorillas which have less strongly developed masticatory musculature." This, of course, leaves us wondering about the evolutionary significance of left-sided chewing and the minimal neural asymmetry necessary to account for it!

Our last example of anatomical asymmetries concerns the decussation of the pyramids in humans. The pyramidal tracts are the largest of the descending motor pathways in man. Yakovlev and Rakic (1966) looked at a sample of 100 medullae oblongatae of fetuses and neonates. In 87, the decussating bundles of the left pyramid, coming from the left hemisphere, were larger and crossed the midsagittal plane first, i.e., at higher levels, than the decussating bundles of the right pyramid. The significance of this observation remains unclear. In a group of seven adult non-right-handers, Kertesz and Geschwind (1971) found that the left corticospinal crossing occurred first in five cases, while the right crossed first in one case. The pattern of pyramidal crossing showed no significant difference between right-handers and non-right-handers.

RIGHT-LEFT FUNCTIONAL ASYMMETRIES IN THE BRAINS OF PRIMATES

This section is not intended as a survey of the enormous literature on functional asymmetries in the human brain. That material is, to a good extent, covered in Chapters 12–14 of this volume, by Hillyard and Woods, Moscovitch, and Heilman, respectively. I will only dwell on some examples that shed light on the origins and mechanisms in the establishment of cerebral dominance.

There is broad agreement on three kinds of observations: (1) In a majority of humans, skilled manual tasks are conducted by the right hand, under the control

313

ORIGINS AND
MECHANISMS IN THE
ESTABLISHMENT OF
CEREBRAL
DOMINANCE

of the left hemisphere. (2) In most right-handed people, the left hemisphere is dominant for language functions. (3) In most right-handed people, the right hemisphere is dominant for spatial tasks. Why have these functions been captured by their respective hemisphere?

HEMISPHERIC DIFFERENCES IN MOTOR CONTROL

In 1874, Hughlings Jackson noted that in some of the worst cases of aphasia patients were not only speechless but their voluntary power in general seemed much impaired. He gave an example of what he meant by this by describing the performance of such a patient during clinical examination: "I one day tried to examine his eyes, and therefore told him to look in certain directions. The examination was almsot impracticable. He made efforts, but he never did what I told him, whether it was to look in a particular direction or to keep his eyes still. Instead of opening them, he opened his mouth, or screwed up his face, or shut his eyes, and could not be got to look in any particular direction, although he seemed on the alert to act, and was all the time doing something with his muscles" (in Taylor, 1932, p. 136). Following Broca's (1865) lead Jackson suggested that the left hemisphere was the seat for voluntary processes of speech. He was not explicit in extending this left-hemispheric dominance to other motor behaviors, though his observations, quoted above, could have supported such a notion.

In 1908 Hugo Liepmann suggested that apraxia was primarily a movement disorder, a manifestation of the disturbance of a system in the left hemisphere which had to do with the control of "purposive movements, that is, those learned connections of elementary muscle actions" (Liepmann, 1908, p. 19, quoted in Kimura and Archibald, 1974).

More recently Kimura and Archibald (1974) found that patients with left-hemisphere damage were impaired, relative to patients with right-hemisphere damage, on a task in which they copied unfamiliar meaningless movements of the hand and arm. The difficulty in copying the hand movements was unrelated to the presence or absence of hemiplegia, except to the extent that a hemiplegic limb was not testable. The impairment was bilateral and equal on the two hands in cases without hemiplegia. The same patients who showed a movement-copying disorder showed no difficulty in isolated finger flexion or in copying a static hand posture. The movement-copying defect in the left-hemisphere group was not significantly related to verbal impairment. From these and other findings, Kimura and Archibald (1974) conclude that the unique motor functions of the left hemisphere, also for speech, may be related to motor sequencing rather than to symbolic or language function.

Kimura and Archibald (1974) also noted that the same patients that showed difficulty in the movement–copying test showed no obvious difficulty in ordinary daily activities. Perhaps the degree of involvement of the left hemisphere relates to the difficulty of a motor task. Familiar sequences may be less difficult than unfamiliar sequences, and simple movements such as finger flexion easier than more complex sequences. Within such a ranking speech presumably would be at the extreme end of difficulty. One trouble with such an interpretation is that "difficulty" is a subjective measure, in part perhaps related to the voluntary effort and concentration required by a task. The elusiveness of the variable that makes the left hemisphere dominant for some kinds of motor control is emphasized by the fact that though the right hemisphere is unable to speak, it is dominant for singing! (Bogen and Gordon, 1971; Gordon and Bogen, 1974).

Left-hemisphere dominance for motor sequencing may account for cases of aphasia with right-sided paralysis in congenitally deaf persons (review in Lenneberg, 1967, p. 178). None of the four patients involved had oral speech before their stroke; all four used sign language and finger spelling, and in all of them manual language communication was disordered by left-hemisphere lesions.

In a most inspired study, Semmes (1968) noticed that the kind of brain lesion affecting manual performance depended on whether injury was restricted to the right or left hemisphere. Relatively small, focal lesions of the pre- and postcentral sensorimotor areas of the left hemisphere often resulted in marked impairment of the sensory and motor manual tasks controlled by that hemisphere. Comparable injury of nonsensorimotor areas of the left hemisphere did not affect these tasks. The outcome was very different for right-hemisphere lesions. Here placement of injuries in the brain's sensorimotor cortex was not the crucial factor, but size of lesion mattered. Large lesions affecting sensorimotor or nonsensorimotor cortex of the right hemisphere were equally likely to produce decrements in sensory and motor manual tasks. Semmes (1968, p. 11) used these observations to offer a new interpretation of the neural correlates of hemispheric dominance. She proposed that "focal representation of elementary functions in the *left* hemisphere favors integration of *similar* units and consequently specialization for behaviors which demand fine sensorimotor control, such as manual tasks and speech. Conversely, diffuse representation of elementary functions in the *right* hemisphere may lead to integration of *dissimilar* units and hence specialization for behaviors requiring multimodal coordination, such as the various spatial abilities."

It is not clear why focal representation of elementary functions in the left hemisphere should lead to a left-hemisphere advantage in motor sequencing. Yet, this is the conclusion one must draw from integrating the observations of Semmes (1968) and Kimura and Archibald (1974).

In addition to the clinical literature indicating a left-hemisphere dominance for speech production, slow negative potentials which are at a maximum over Broca's area in the left hemisphere have been recorded from normal adult subjects as they spontaneously produced polysyllabic words. These potentials began up to 1 sec before word articulation. Bilaterally symmetrical potentials were seen with analogous, nonspeech control gestures (McAdam and Whitaker, 1971).

No persuasive case has been made for hemispheric dominance for motor control in mammals other than man, although one does find individuals with a right or left hand or paw preference for a particular task (Jung, 1962, p. 269; Warren, 1977).

HEMISPHERIC DIFFERENCES IN THE PROCESSING OF SOUNDS

DICHOTIC TESTS. Hemispheric differences in sensory processes are as strongly marked in humans as hemispheric differences for motor control. So, for example, left, but not right, temporal lobectomy impairs the ability to assimilate verbal auditory material (Meyer and Yates, 1955; Milner, 1958). When different digits are simultaneously presented to the two ears (dichotic listening test) of normal individuals, digits arriving at the right ear are more accurately reported than digits arriving at the left, and this effect occurs in adults as well as in 4-year-old children (Kimura, 1961, 1963). The right ear advantage for verbal material persists even when spoken nonsense sounds or backward-speech sounds are used (Kimura, 1967; Kimura and Folb, 1968). When the sodium amytal test shows that the right hemisphere is dominant for speech, dichotic tests using speech material reveal a left ear advantage (Kimura, 1967).

In 1962, Milner showed that performance on some subtests of the Seashore Measures of Musical Talents is affected by right temporal lobectomy but not by left temporal lobectomy. A right-hemisphere superiority for processing non-speech sounds is confirmed by experiments involving dichotic listening. Dichotic presentation of familiar or unfamiliar melodies yields a left ear advantage, so that a greater proportion of melodies played to the left ear are correctly recognized (Kimura, 1967). Dichotic presentation of hummed melodic patterns or of vocal nonspeech sounds such as laughing, crying, and sighing also elicit a significant left ear superiority. These observations indicate that voice quality *per se* does not independently engage left or right hemisphere mechanisms (King and Kimura, 1972).

The occurrence of a right or left ear advantage in dichotic testing for material thought to be processed by the contralateral hemisphere has been related to the nature of the pathway linking each ear to the two hemispheres. Electrophysiological evidence from studies with cats and dogs suggests that crossed auditory pathways are more effective in conveying information than uncrossed ones (Rosenzweig, 1951; Tunturi, 1946); presumably, this situation also prevails in humans. In humans, inhibition of the uncrossed pathway is believed to occur subcortically. Competition between the two dichotically presented sounds, which accounts for lower dichotic than monotic scores, results from transcallosal competition between the two crossed pathways. Dichotic competition is markedly reduced after section of the corpus callosum (Milner *et al.*, 1968; Zaidel, 1977).

MOTOR THEORY OF SPEECH PERCEPTION. An understanding of the differential auditory processing attributed to the right and left hemispheres is of great importance for reconstructing the conditions that may have led to the marked hemispheric functional asymmetries observed in humans. Words are composed of phonemes or syllables, in themselves empty of meaning. Phonemes are formed by consonants and vowels, jointly referred to as "phones." According to one interpretation, a correct decoding of speech sounds requires that the network in charge of this task know how speech sounds are produced. Phones that are heard as "same" can be shown to have very different sound spectrographic structure depending on the nature of other phones that precede or follow. What those acoustically dissimilar renderings of a same phone have in common is not auditory but articulatory. In normal, fluent speech, coarticulation of phones does not respect word boundaries, and, therefore, even word recognition, it is argued, requires a special speech decoder. Because of its emphasis on articulatory knowledge, this theory has come to be known as the motor theory of speech perception (Liberman *et al.*, 1967; Liberman and Pisoni, 1977). It proposes a special speech processor and places it in the left hemisphere.

Even if one insists that the processing of speech must require a special network not shared with other incoming sounds, there may be alternatives to the motor theory of Liberman *et al.* (1967). Eimas (1974) has posited specialized feature detectors which are finely tuned to restricted ranges of acoustic information in the speech signal. It is possible to selectively adapt such feature detectors and alter the way in which other related speech sounds are perceived (Eimas and Corbit, 1973). Recent observations suggest that such detectors are part of a more general auditory processing system (Tartter and Eimas, 1975). Whether specialized or general purpose, it should be recognized that, for some speech sounds, feature detectors à la Eimas would not seem adequate for decoding the signal into its phonetic components. This, of course, is the basic problem addressed by the motor theory of speech perception.

In a further twist to the adaptation paradigm, adaptation of feature detectors thought to be shared by the articulatory and sensory processing network has been used to support the motor theory of speech perception. In this experiment, subjects utter repetitions of a given consonant-vowel syllable in a whispered voice while listening to white noise through earphones. Sizable auditory adaptation effects are obtained after the repetitive articulation. These effects are virtually identical to the phonetic boundary shifts obtained in perceptual adaptation tests along the same auditorily perceived stimulus series (Cooper, 1975). It would have been interesting to know whether mental repetition of the same consonant-vowel (CV) syllable, trying not to engage efferent pathways, would have had the same effect!

Before leaving the topic of the motor theory of speech perception, I would like to describe an experiment that emphasizes the close intertwining of sensory and motor speech processes. It is possible to match a target tone of varying frequency by computer production of a second tone under the control of transducers that respond to unidirectional movements of the hand, tongue, or jaw. When the target and tracking tones are presented monaurally but to opposite ears, there is a significant right ear advantage only when the tracking tone is controlled by a speech articulator (tongue, jaw) and heard through the right ear; there is no right ear advantage when the tracking tone is hand controlled (Sussman, 1971; Sussman *et al.*, 1974). There is no significant difference between the ears when the task involves amplitude rather than frequency tracking (Sussman *et al.*, 1975). It seems justified to suggest that under the conditions of this experiment the right ear advantage for frequency tracking reflects left-hemisphere integration of auditory and articulatory processes.

There is no reason why the processing of speech sounds should be done in only one manner. Familiarity with the speaker, the context, and the words may obviate the need for an in-depth analytical decoding; instead, the listener may draw on whole-word memories. During language learning, or when speakers use novel accents or intonations or unexpected words, special decoding processes may be brought into action as we grope for a recognizable pattern. The fact that a

317

ORIGINS AND
MECHANISMS IN THE
ESTABLISHMENT OF
CEREBRAL
DOMINANCE

particular way of processing speech sounds can be demonstrated need not negate the occurrence of other parallel strategies. Thus whole-word processing, feature detector networks, and articulatory knowledge may all contribute to the normal perception of spoken language. Each of these processes, in turn, may show different degrees of lateralization.

SENSORY OR MOTOR PRIMACY IN ONTOGENY OF LANGUAGE LATERALIZATION? Does the left-hemisphere dominance for speech tasks emerge as a result of processing or production biases? There are reasons to believe that both biases are present in preverbal infants. I have looked at the patterns of tongue movement during babbling in my two children between the ages of 2 and 5 months. Such observations are easy since infants will often babble as they lie on their backs, holding their mouths partly open so that one can observe the movements of their tongues. During the first weeks of babbling, my boy's tongue deviated dramatically toward the right half of the buccal cavity. This effect was very marked at 4 months of age (Fig. 11) and disappeared one month later. Keeping the tongue in the center seemed to require effort. Deviation toward the right occurred more and more toward the end of a babbling bout, perhaps as a result of fatigue. The tongue remained in the midline during crying or smiling. This boy is now 7 years old and right-handed and has developed language normally. Similar observations repeated on my daughter revealed no consistent asymmetry in tongue movement. I would not report observations on such a small sample were it not that I was impressed by their intraindividual consistency. In the case of my boy, I got the impression that deviation of the tongue to the right (suggesting prevalent left-hemisphere control?) constituted a handicap, even if a fleeting one, for mastery of the early sounds of speech, a price that perhaps some boys, but not girls, have to pay for left-hemispheric dominance of speech processes (see p. 329). In any case, these observations should be repeated. If confirmed, they would suggest a very early onset for the left-hemisphere motor dominance normally underlying speech

*TONGUE	BEHAVIOR**	TONGUE	BEHAVIOR	TONGUE	BEHAVIOR
M1 R1	B	M2 R1	B	R1	B
M2	B	M4 R2	B	M2	B
M1	B	M3	B	M1 R3 L1	B
M4		M6	B	M3 R2	B
M2		M2	B	M1	B
M3		M5	B	M1 R3	B
M4		M5	B	R2	B
M4		R2	B	R1 M2	B
M2	B	R4	B	R2	B
M1	B	R3	B	R6	B
M1	B	R6	B	R6	B
M4	B	R2	B	R4	B
M3	B	R2	B	R2	B
M2	B	M1 R2	B	R2	B
M3	B	R3	B	R2	B
				R3	B

* TONGUE refers to tongue position, which was scored as being in the middle, M, to the right, R, or to the left, L. Each notation on tongue position is followed by number of seconds during which position relative to midline was held and visible. ** BEHAVIOR refers to whether child was babbling, B, or silent, usually smiling.

Fig. 11. Position of tongue with respect to midline during phonation in a 4-month-old boy. All entries recorded over a continuous 1 hr observation period.

control. An equally early onset has been suggested for the lateralized processing of phonetic material, as shown in the next section.

HEMISPHERIC DOMINANCE AND THE CATEGORICAL PERCEPTION OF SPEECH SOUNDS. The way in which infants handle phonetic discriminations is important for developmental and evolutionary reconstructions of hemispheric dominance. Infants 1 and 4 months old are able to discriminate the acoustic cue underlying the adult phonemic distinction between the voiced and voiceless stop consonants /b/ and /p/. More important, these infants show a tendency toward categorical perception: discrimination of the same physical difference is reliably better across the adult phonemic boundary than within the adult phonemic boundary (Eimas *et al.*, 1971). Since categorical perception of phonetic information in adults has been used as one of the arguments for invoking a special, left-hemisphere speech processor, the observations of Eimas *et al.* (1971) suggest that such a special processor is already available at birth. It is only one step further, then, to relate the early occurrence of a special speech processor to the occurrence of anatomical pre- and perinatal brain asymmetries of language-related areas.

Auditory evoked responses (AER) have been used to demonstrate the early occurrence of hemispheric differences in sound processing. Molfese *et al.* (1975) report differences in the AERs recorded from the right and left temporal region of infants, children, and adults; the infants were 1 week to 10 months old. Left hemisphere AERs were larger in amplitude than right hemisphere AERs to speech stimuli for all groups. Nonspeech stimuli produced larger amplitude AERs in the right hemisphere.

The findings of Eimas *et al.* (1971) and of Molfese *et al.* (1975) would seem to lend support to the theory of a special speech processor whose presence in the left hemisphere of infants precedes verbal experience. However, this theory has been challenged on the grounds that other animals also perceive speech sounds in a categorical manner.

Comparison of categorical perception of speech sounds in people and animals involves at least two issues: (1) can categorical perception be achieved? and (2) what is the source of information which determines the position of a boundary between categories? The answer to the first question is affirmative. Categorical perception of speech sounds has been demonstrated in humans, chinchillas (Kuhl and Miller, 1975), and rhesus macaques (Waters and Wilson, 1976). This means that the sensory capability to recognize category boundaries is present in all three species. However, the source of boundary information may differ. Chinchillas have to be trained to respond differently to /t/ and /d/ consonant-vowel syllables: this pair shows an 80-msec difference in voice onset time. Tests with intermediate sounds reveal that the boundary for categorical discrimination falls between 30 and 40 msec, roughly half way between the two end points used in training. A comparable situation applies to the macaques studied by Waters and Wilson (1976). Unlike humans, these monkeys show large shifts in boundary when the range of training stimuli is varied. In these examples with animals, the most parsimonious interpretation would invoke stimulus generalization. A categorical boundary emerges at the meeting point of generalizations induced by the two training stimuli. In some cases, even extensive training fails to induce categorical

319

ORIGINS AND
MECHANISMS IN THE
ESTABLISHMENT OF
CEREBRAL
DOMINANCE

perception of speech sounds, as shown in another experiment with macaques (Sinnott *et al.*, 1976). In a third experiment with macaques, categorical discrimination of synthetic human speech sounds was examined using the cardiac component of the orienting response. This method involves no training with speech sounds. In this case, sounds assigned by human observers to separate phonetic categories were differentiated to a greater extent than sounds assigned to a same phonetic category, although in both situations the test stimuli differed by the same absolute amount (Morse and Snowdon, 1975). Such conflicting observations on macaques are hard to interpret. We may conclude that whereas categorical perception of speech sounds occurs in untrained human infants, engaging preferentially the left hemisphere, similar unreinforced biases are weaker or absent in other mammals.

The observations of Eimas *et al.* (1971) and Molfese *et al.* (1975) suggest that human newborns have a predisposition to treat speech sounds in a special manner. A phenomenon that may be related to this was recently described in birds. Hand-reared swamp sparrows that have had no prior exposure to conspecific song copy synthetic songs made out of conspecific notes, but ignore other similarly structured models composed of the notes of another closely related species (Marler and Peters, 1977). In both examples, we have what may be a predisposition to recognize or treat specially conspecific sounds, and this is manifest in the absence of biases imposed by training and selective reinforcement. The anatomical and physiological basis for such selective processes remains unknown, but could be different for similar perceptual processes induced by training. Of course, we should avoid the "either-or" trap. The processing of conspecific sounds may normally involve some learned and some genetically coded information (Marler, 1976*a*; Streeter, 1976). Genetically coded information may take the form of special signal processors, or manifest itself in the normal interaction of elements within the auditory system, leading to psychoacoustic phenomena of widespread occurrence (Miller, 1977). In the former case, special processors evolve to discriminate special signals; in the latter, special signals evolve to exploit the basic idiosyncrasies of signal processing networks. This theme is likely to remain controversial for many years. We need to learn a lot about the predispositions that auditory pathways in general, and each hemisphere in particular, bring to the processing of sounds in birds, primates, and man.

SPEECH PROCESSING BY THE SUBORDINATE HEMISPHERE OF COMMISSUROTOMY PATIENTS. Patients with unmanageable epilepsy find it very difficult to lead a normal life. Disconnection of the two hemispheres, involving section of the corpus callosum, anterior commissure, hippocampal commissure, and massa intermedia, virtually eliminates epileptic seizures (Bogen and Vogel, 1962). These patients have proved invaluable for study of hemispheric function (Gazzaniga et al., 1962; Gazzaniga, 1970; Sperry, 1974).

Eran Zaidel (1977), a member of Sperry's group at the California Institute of Technology, has used "split-brain" patients to quantify speech comprehension by the right hemisphere. His observations partly support the motor theory of speech perception. Right-hemisphere auditory word recognition in some commissurotomy patients is surprisingly high, corresponding to a mean mental age equivalent of 11.9 years. In these individuals, the performance of both hemispheres shows essentially the same dependency on word frequency as found in normal children and adults. However, the two hemispheres of these patients differ in that the right, mute hemisphere recognizes words using a whole-pattern matching strategy. It has a subnormal and still poorly defined capacity for discriminating phonetic features.

The right hemisphere of the commissurotomy patients studied by Zaidel (1977) does not perform as well as the left one when the words used in word discrimination are presented against a background of noise, suggesting that the right hemisphere is not an efficient signal-from-noise separator in general. It also fails to analyze correctly long, nonredundant sentences where order is important and when the context is not helpful. Zaidel attributes this limitation to a restricted (perhaps as small as three items) short-term verbal memory.

It should be realized that, as a group, "split-brain" patients have in common only a massive loss of interhemispheric connections. The prior history of brain malfunction and damage varies from individual to individual. In those cases where left-hemisphere disturbance started early in infancy, the right hemisphere is more likely to have retained or developed a broad-spectrum language proficiency. When the malfunction that led to commissurotomy started late, then the right hemisphere may perform no better than that of global aphasics. Patient P. S., studied by Gazzaniga, Le Doux, and Wilson (1977), underwent early brain pathology in the left temporal region at the age of 2. Tested after commissurotomy in adulthood, the right and left hemispheres of P. S. showed an ability to rhyme (phonetic analysis), read, spell, and write, and to conduct sophisticated semantic abstractions. The right hemisphere, however, was mute. Gazzaniga and Le Doux (1978) contrast the performance of patient P. S. with that of patient W. S. of the Bogen series, who apparently developed normally through age 30 and, following commisurotomy, showed no signs of right hemisphere language (Gazzaniga and Sperry, 1967). The latter, in all likelihood, is the condition of the right hemisphere in intact people.

LEFT HEMISPHERE ADVANTAGE FOR PROCESSING TEMPORAL INFORMATION

The reaction time to a stimulus delivered to the foot of a man is 25–30 msec slower than the reaction time to a forehead stimulus. Klemm (1925), who made this observation, concluded that the increase in reaction time was a consequence of the extra length of the sensory pathway. Halliday and Mingay (1962, quoted in Efron, 1963a) found that the cortical potentials evoked by toe stimulation occurred approximately 20 msec later than potentials evoked by finger stimulation. They noted that the stimuli delivered to the index finger and toe were not perceived as simultaneous unless the stimulus to the toe preceded the one to the finger by 9 and 17 msec in two subjects studied. Halliday and Mingay concluded that the central nervous system does not correct for the time error produced by the longer pathway and that the perception of simultaneity occurs when two sensory messages reach some point in the central nervous system at about the same time.

Efron (1963*a*) set out to test the hypothesis that the "point in the central nervous system" where temporal discrimination is made is in the hemisphere dominant for speech. He used mild electric shock delivered to the same finger of the right and left hand and light flashes directed at the nasal retina of the right and left eye. The subjects participating in these experiments had to report when two stimuli were perceived as simultaneous. Efron observed a delay of 2–6 msec for the stimuli delivered to the left half of the body (right-hemisphere) in right-handed subjects, and the right half of the body (left-hemisphere) in a few left-handed subjects. He argued that those sensory messages received by the nondominant hemisphere are transferred to the dominant hemisphere by a pathway having a delay of 2–6 msec.

In a second set of experiments, Efron (1963*b*) reasoned that, since the analysis and production of speech demands rich temporal processing, networks engaged in temporal analysis of inputs might be related to those controlling analysis and production of speech. To test this idea, he asked aphasic and nonaphasic brain-damaged patients to indicate which of two visual or auditory stimuli they perceived first. Lesions that impaired discrimination of temporal sequence were all in the hemisphere dominant for speech and were accompanied by some degree of aphasia. Even when the first and second stimuli were separated by intervals of 400–600 msec, the aphasic subjects were still somewhat uncertain as to the correct sequence, and on occasion called the stimuli "simultaneous." From these results, Efron (1963*b*, p. 418) suggested that "we should not look upon the aphasias as unique disorders of *language* but rather as an inevitable consequence of a primary defect in temporal analysis—in placing a 'time-label' upon incoming data." He thought that this deficiency in temporal programming would also affect verbal output: "A disturbance of CNS motor timing mechanisms would be expected to have perhaps more devastating effects on speech than on any other motor function" (p. 418). To this, he added: "It may be precisely because temporal sequencing is performed in this area that the "higher" functions *appear* to reside there" (p. 419).

Efron (1963*b*) divided his aphasic brain-damaged patients into "expressive" (*n* = 6) and "receptive" (*n* = 4) aphasics. Whereas the former had a relatively preserved comprehension of speech, the latter had pronounced difficulty in understanding speech. Paradoxically, though, expressive aphasics had more severe auditory sequencing defects than receptive aphasics. Efron could not resolve this apparent contradiction (see also review by Swisher and Hirsch, 1972). Taken at face value, Efron's (1963*b*) observations suggest that, whereas speech production networks are intimately associated with networks conducting temporal analysis, speech decoding networks have evolved a somewhat greater autonomy.

It is possible that the primary difficulty encountered by Efron's (1963*b*) patients was not a failure to perceive sequencing order but a more basic defect in the processing of rapidly changing acoustic information (Tallal, 1976). In order to accurately report the sequence of two closely spaced sounds, they must be perceived as separate and different. Two sounds may be perceived as different when presented one at a time, yet not be distinguishable as they occur in close proximity. The likelihood of confounding sequencing and discrimination errors is demon-

321

ORIGINS AND
MECHANISMS IN THE
ESTABLISHMENT OF
CEREBRAL
DOMINANCE

strated by the observations of Tallal and Piercy (1973). They noted that developmental dysphasic children who are impaired in their ability to report the temporal sequence of rapidly presented auditory signals also show an equally inferior discrimination of the sound quality of these signals. Tallal and Piercy (1975) argue that the perceptual impairment shown by children with developmental dysphasia is a causal factor in their phonatory difficulties. This, then, might be a case where it is possible to establish a causal link between a form of expressive aphasia and impaired temporal analysis.

More recently, Tallal and Newcombe (1976) studied ten war veterans with left-hemisphere damage. All these subjects showed some degree of dysphasia. There was a high, positive correlation between the degree of language comprehension impairment of these adult aphasics and their ability to respond correctly to rapidly changing acoustic stimuli, regardless of whether the stimuli were verbal or nonverbal. Those patients who had a marked expressive language impairment but who did not have difficulty in receptive language were not impaired in the same perceptual tests. The difference between these results and those of Efron (1963*b*) cannot be reconciled at this time. It should be noted, though, that the tests used were different and that patients in the two studies may have differed in the nature of their brain lesions and accompanying language disorder.

In a related study, Lackner and Teuber (1973) noticed poor temporal judgments with auditory material in patients who had suffered penetrating wounds of the left temporal lobe. These patients showed an impaired ability for resolving temporal separation between clicks. Subjects with left temporal damage who were judged dysphasic were significantly poorer than nondysphasic left-damaged subjects. Echoing Efron's (1963*b*) earlier comments, Lackner and Teuber (1973, p. 413) conclude: "If we assume that the left hemisphere and particularly the left temporal regions are more competent than the right for making fine time discriminations, then we could turn the argument around and suggest that language is 'attracted,' in most of us, to the left rather than right side because of a pre-existing advantage in temporal acuity of the left hemisphere."

It is important to notice that the left hemisphere's superiority for temporal analysis is manifest with visual as well as with auditory material. Efron's (1963*b*) observations in this regard have been confirmed by other studies. For example, left temporal lobectomies significantly impair the capacity for fine resolution of simple visual stimuli separated in time (critical flicker frequency). This effect is much smaller after right temporal lobectomies (Goldman *et al.*, 1968).

The weight of the evidence, of which only a few selected examples on auditory and visual processing have been presented here, has suggested to several authors that the two hemispheres handle information in basically different ways. The left hemisphere is seen as conducting an analytic process, where fine temporal judgements play an important role. The right hemisphere is thought to process information in a more holistic manner, recognizing whole patterns and showing a more direct association between stimuli and responses (Jackson, 1932, Vol. 2, p. 130; Levy-Agresti and Sperry, 1968; Bever and Chiarello, 1974; Gordon and Bogen, 1974). However, it should be realized that the "holistic" and "analytic" labels are verbal handles for processes that still remain very poorly understood.

It is tempting to generalize from Efron's (1963b) speculations on speech and timing mechanisms to suggest that the left hemisphere's proficiency in temporal analysis is one reason why learned motor sequences are controlled by that hemisphere. Motor sequencing of purposeful behavior requires a fine dialogue between brain and muscle and a fine sense of timing. The obvious big question, then, and one for which we have no answers, is whether a comparable dichotomy in the nature of perceptual and motor tasks dominated by each hemisphere occurs elsewhere in the animal kingdom.

323

ORIGINS AND
MECHANISMS IN THE
ESTABLISHMENT OF
CEREBRAL
DOMINANCE

PERCEPTUAL OR MEMORY IMPAIRMENT?

Face recognition is held to be a typical holistic process handled by the right hemisphere (e.g. DeRenzi and Spinnler, 1966; Levy *et al.*, 1972). Yet the immediate recognition of unfamiliar photographed faces is normal in cases of right temporal lobectomy, although poor after a 2-min delay (Milner, 1968). Dee and Fontenot (1973) have shown that the dominance of the right hemisphere for the perception of complex figures of low verbal association arises from hemispheric differences in memory rather than from purely perceptual processes. Complex figures were presented in either the left or the right visual field. After a variable delay (0, 5, 10, or 20 sec), the subject was required to indicate whether or not a new figure was the same as the initial figure. Right-hemisphere superiority was obtained only at the longer retention intervals. A more recent study confirmed the findings of Dee and Fontenot, but in addition showed that comparisons between photographs and caricatures yielded a left-field (right hemisphere) superiority even in a memory-free situation (Moscovitch *et al.*, 1976). From this, the authors concluded that "higher order processes, such as are needed to ... compare caricatures with photographs, require the specialized functions peculiar to the right hemisphere" (p. 401). The right-hemisphere's superiority uncovered by this study was manifest as a 13-msec-shorter delay in reporting the correspondence between photographs and caricatures. It is difficult to decide whether the left-hemisphere's tardiness reflected a difference in higher-order processes or the lack of practice of a hemisphere normally inhibited from conducting such tasks.

In a recent review, Rozin (1976) documents the dissociation of verbal and nonverbal memories. The left temporal lobe and in particular the left hippocampus are seen as playing a major role in establishing the long-term memories of verbal experience. The right hippocampus seems more concerned with establishing long-term memories of nonverbal material (visual, tactile, tonal sequences). What is surprising about these findings is that decoding and short-term memory of sensory information may be little affected by unilateral lesions of the temporal lobe and underlying hippocampus. For long-term memory deficits to occur, the critical temporal lobe structure is the hippocampus: the more hippocampus removed, the more severe the memory deficit (Corsi, 1969, quoted in Milner, 1970). Since encoding of external events into an internal memory representation may often rely on verbal processes, the left hippocampus may have a dominant role in the conversion of short-term to long-term memories, applying to a breadth of material other than the strictly verbal one (review in Signoret and Lhermitte,

1976). Neither right nor left hippocampus seems to be involved in the acquisition of motor skills (Milner, 1970).

It seems clear that one should be careful in distinguishing perceptual from mnemonic hemispheric differences. This distinction has not received sufficient attention in the past. The observations by Milner (1968), Dee and Fontenot (1973), and Moscovitch *et al.* (1976) reported above suggest that the left hemisphere is capable of a kind of visual task thought to require holistic processing and usually assigned to the right hemisphere. There is no evidence that the right hemisphere can process time information as well as the left hemisphere. From this, one may conclude that whereas analytic and holistic processes may coexist in the left hemisphere such coexistence does not normally occur in the right hemisphere. Alternatively, the left hemisphere's short-term recognition of complex visual material may rely on analytic processes which are not encoded verbally and therefore do not lead to formation of long-term memories. This, of course, underscores how poorly we understand what is meant by "analytic" vs. "holistic" perceptual differences! Perhaps it is more descriptive to say that the two hemispheres differ in the kind of temporal analysis they conduct, the type of motor tasks they master, and the nature of material they commit to long-term memory.

Search for Hemispheric Dominance in Macaques

The search for functional hemispheric asymmetries in nonhuman primates is still in its infancy. The species most commonly used has been the rhesus macaque, tested under restrained laboratory conditions. Hamilton (1977) used visual material and large, carefully balanced experimental and control groups. The monkeys were trained and tested before and after section of one or more of the telencephalic commissures. The outcome was unambiguous: "Neither formation of unilateral memories nor differential abilities in learning or performance with the separated hemispheres could be found, which suggests that hemispheric specialization in monkeys, if present, will not be easily detected" (Hamilton, 1977, p. 60).

A conflicting claim has been presented by Doty and Overman (1977) to the effect that the corpus callosum precludes the formation of redundant bilateral engrams. The methodology used by Doty and his group bypasses the normal afferent routes used by visual information. The lateralized stimulus consists of electrical excitation of the striate cortex in one hemisphere. Their observations do not address the question of whether the two hemispheres process stimuli differently or store different kinds of information, and so their work is hard to relate to theories of hemispheric specialization.

Until very recently, Dewson (1977) had been the only one to claim hemispheric specialization for an auditory task in nonhuman primates. His work was conducted with Irus macaques. The paradigm used involved a delayed selective response to a red or green light after hearing a tone or noise stimulus. For example, after hearing a tone, the monkey had to press, after illumination of two response panels, whichever of them was red. Similarly, the correct response to the noise stimulus was to press at whichever of the two panels was lit green. Unilateral surgery involved partial removal of the cortex of the superior temporal gyrus.

There was no histological verification of these lesions, so it is not possible to say whether or not they involved the hippocampus. Four of the five monkeys had undergone unilateral cochlear destruction 2–3 years prior to cortical ablation as part of another experiment. Right or left temporal ablation groups were balanced to incorporate this cochlear variable, as shown in Fig. 12. Figure 12 also offers a synthesis of the experiment's outcome. The animals with right temporal ablation produced correct responses even after delays of 4 sec. Animals with left temporal ablation produced correct responses only at 0-sec delays. In one left temporal individual, it was possible to induce a release of the delay deficit by increasing this delay after each correct response in steps of 0.2 sec. The other individuals were not tested in this manner. One of the monkeys which showed no deficit in delayed response after right temporal lobe ablation showed a deficit after subsequent ablation affecting the left hemisphere. This experiment is not easy to interpret. The groups are very small and seem to have had a complex history. Deficits seem to reflect impairment of a memory function, yet could also have been induced by differential response to the testing apparatus or impatience with the delay paradigm. Since performance could be brought up to normal when delay in testing was augmented by very small steps, memory need not have been the crucial variable. Apparently, in these same animals discrimination between very brief (2–3 msec) acoustic stimuli remained at normal (preoperative) levels regardless of side of temporal ablation (Dewson *et al.*, 1975).

I have emphasized the difficulty in interpreting Dewson's observations because it is tempting to use them as an illustration of the kind of hemispheric

325

ORIGINS AND
MECHANISMS IN THE
ESTABLISHMENT OF
CEREBRAL
DOMINANCE

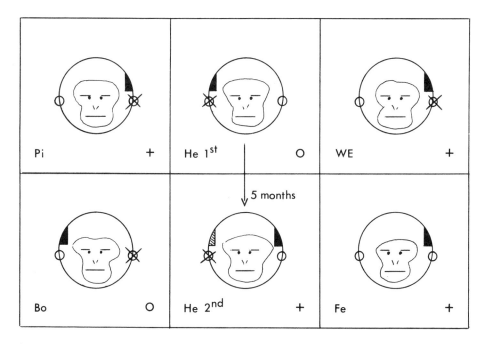

Fig. 12. Representation of experiments and their outcome conducted by Dewson (1977). Darkened areas indicate the side of cortical ablation; crossmarks indicate the side of cochlear destruction; + = presence and 0 = absence of postoperative deficit (reproduced with the permission of Academic Press).

asymmetry that could have preceded human hemispheric dominance for language tasks. This interpretation would be premature. Yet, there is at least one other set of experiments which points in the same general direction suggested by Dewson's work.

Recently, Peterson *et al.* (in press) have produced pilot data that suggest a small but consistent right ear advantage for perception of conspecific sounds in Japanese macaques. Their paradigm involves assigning natural and synthetic macaque sounds to one of the various natural vocalization categories described by Green (1975). The macaques are equipped with earphones and the test stimulus is presented to the right or left ear. The subject has to make a response only if the sound corresponds to the natural vocal category being reinforced. Under those conditions, the five Japanese macaques tested made a significantly greater number of errors when the test stimulus was presented to the left than to the right ear. These results are preliminary. If confirmed, they should suggest a greater left-hemisphere role in the analysis of conspecific sounds, a situation that could be an antecedent to the left-hemisphere language dominance observed in humans.

ONTOGENY OF HEMISPHERIC FUNCTION IN HUMANS

INCOMPATIBILITY OF PROCESSES?

During the early acquisition of language, injury to the right hemisphere affects speech much more frequently than it does in adults (Basser, 1962; Hécaen, 1976). From this, one might infer that during the first few years of life the right hemisphere participates in language functions. The early occurrence of a right hemisphere potential for language is confirmed by the fact that injury to speech areas of the left hemisphere before the age of 6 usually results in an orderly development of language processes by the right hemisphere, so that no permanent dysphasia follows (Milner, 1974; Hécaen, 1976). Milner's interpretation is that "early left-hemisphere lesion leaves the right hemisphere free to develop its innate language capacities, whereas, in the intact brain, these capacities are actively suppressed by the left hemisphere at some critical stage of early development" (Milner, 1974, p. 85). The earlier this derepression occurs, the better. So, for example, syntactic comprehension is modestly affected by prenatal left-hemisphere lesions, but is much more affected by left-hemisphere injury occurring between the first birthday and the age of 5 years (Woods and Teuber, referred to in Teuber, 1975). Goldman (1972) has suggested that there is an asymmetrical maturation of the hemispheres, and that the "noncommitment" of the minor hemisphere at the time of left hemispheric damage is the basis for language compensation by the right hemisphere. Gazzaniga and LeDoux (1978) complement this view by suggesting that as language becomes left lateralized, other functions fill in the vacated synaptic space in the right hemisphere. They add (p. 83): "If a lesion of the left side occurs prior to the time that these other functions have acquired space, recovery is seen. Otherwise, it is not." Although such views make some intuitive sense, there is no evidence that language and "other" functions vie for a same "synaptic space."

It has been argued that even though the two hemispheres are more functionally similar at birth than in adulthood they may not really be equipotential. For example, after perinatal cerebral pathology and subsequent unilateral decortication, syntactic skills are not mediated equivalently by an intact left or right hemisphere. Right hemidecorticates, relative to a left-operated group matched for verbal IQ, show superior comprehension of difficult syntactic material (Dennis and Kohn, 1975). In a separate study, the right or left hemisphere was removed before 5 months of age in infants who had undergone cerebral injury and suffered from seizures. Subsequently, these children acquired language under seizure-free and educationally normal conditions and were tested at 9–10 years of age. Phonemic and semantic abilities were similarly developed by all children; unfortunately, the phonetic tests consisted of words and not of consonant-vowel syllables as would have been required to test phonetic categorical perception. Since none of these children was dysphasic, we may assume that their phonetic processes were adequate to guide normal language production. In these patients, the right but not the left hemisphere was proven deficient in syntactic tasks (Dennis and Whitaker, 1976). It will be remembered that Zaidel (1977) concluded that the syntactic difficulties of the right hemisphere of commissurotomy patients resulted from its shorter memory span for spoken material. This variable could have affected the syntactic performance of the right hemisphere patients tested by Dennis and her colleagues.

Single hemisphere function can also be studied in individuals with agenesis of the corpus callosum. Such a person, as studied by Saul and Sperry (1968; Sperry, 1968, 1970), was found to have speech developed in both hemispheres. At 19 years of age, this individual had an average scholastic record. Although she was first thought to be asymptomatic, further testing showed her to be selectively subnormal on a variety of perceptuomotor, spatial, nonverbal reasoning tasks. These deficits were in contrast to her above-normal scores on tests of verbal intelligence. This case and other examples in the literature are presented as examples of single hemisphere development of language functions at the expense of nonverbal skills (see also Smith, 1972). Perhaps there is here the nub of something important. From an evolutionary viewpoint, language tasks must surely be a recent development. We may safely assume that nonlanguage skills have had a much longer history. What is so insidious about language processes that allows them to thrive during ontogeny at the expense of other skills? What are they taking over? Is it that language processes start earlier, thus maximally exploiting the plasticity of a developing nervous system?

EFFECTS OF "CROWDING"

It is well known that people with most of their cognitive abilities "crowded" into one hemisphere (even though they may have two, as in commissurotomy or callosal agenesis cases) are likely to be lower in general intelligence than the normal population (Saul and Sperry, 1968; Sperry, 1968, 1974; Woods and

327

ORIGINS AND
MECHANISMS IN THE
ESTABLISHMENT OF
CEREBRAL
DOMINANCE

Teuber, 1973; Milner, 1974). It is hard to decide what might be the nature of this "crowding" effect. Is it that there is an incompatibility between "analytic" and "holistic" processes? Is it that verbal and nonverbal memories encroach on each other? Is it that a diversity of attentional mechanisms interfere with each other? This last possibility has been elegantly demonstrated by Okazaki Smith *et al.* (1977). They showed that the normal superiority of the left hand for haptic perception can be reversed by playing music into the left (but not the right) ear. From this, they suggest that the left cerebral hemisphere has full haptic perceptual capability which is subject to right hemisphere interference unless the latter's attentional mechanisms are engaged by contralateral peripheral stimulation.

It is very difficult to weigh the performance of single hemispheres. Ideally, one would like to assume that the "intact" hemisphere is, indeed, intact. Yet, in many cases, the very conditions that led to removal of one hemisphere may have affected the organization of the opposite hemisphere. More basic still, we do not know what it means to the performance of one hemisphere to be deprived of the millions of contacts, some inhibitory, some excitatory, reaching across the corpus callosum or traveling along other pathways. It must mean something since commissurotomy patients are mute for several weeks after callosal section (Bogen, 1976). Similarly, we may expect that commissurotomy and hemispherectomy lead to substantial cell death in the "intact" hemisphere as a normal sequela to severing millions of axons. It may be conservative to assume that although hemispherectomy permits the manifestation of some derepressed functions, in other ways it probably leaves us with a subnormal hemisphere.

It is hard to see how the single hemisphere of a hemispherectomy patient could possibly marshall normal performance on all those tasks for which, in principle, it has the necessary networks. Similar caveats can be voiced for interpreting the performance of patients with callosal agenesis. Agenesis of the corpus callosum is frequently associated with other brain malformations which could play an important role in the production of symptoms (Loeser and Alvord, 1968).

Despite the odds against getting good performance in single hemisphere patients, there is at least one report of a left hemispherectomy for seizures where a 21-year follow-up reveals remarkable preservation of function (Smith and Sugar, 1975). The operation was performed in a 5½-year-old boy. He was tested at 9, 21, and 26 years of age. Performance on verbal and nonverbal tasks was above normal. When last tested, this individual had a full-scale IQ of 116, with a performance IQ of 102 (nonverbal tasks) and a verbal IQ of 126. Unfortunately, this man has not received tests specifically aimed at measuring syntactic (à la Dennis) or phonetic (à la Liberman) competence.

Since the right or left hemisphere of callosal agenesis patients or of patients who underwent early brain damage or hemisperectomy can develop advanced verbal skills, we may infer that in young infants a good many of the networks necessary to learn to speak and to understand speech are available to both hemispheres. Furthermore, there is little in the clinical literature that forces us to accept a basic incompatibility between "holistic" and "analytic" modes of processing sensory inputs. Until conclusive evidence for such incompatibility becomes available, we are equally justified in suggesting that the inferior skills of single hemisphere patients may result from a subnormal single hemisphere, from inter-ference between long-term memory processes, from attentional conflicts, or from a combination of these variables.

329

ORIGINS AND
MECHANISMS IN THE
ESTABLISHMENT OF
CEREBRAL
DOMINANCE

A PRICE TO HEMISPHERIC DOMINANCE?

Women have been reported to excel in verbal ability (fluency, articulation, and perceptual speech). Men are thought to excel in spatial ability (Hobson, 1947; Maccoby, 1966). Boys show right-hemisphere specialization for spatial processing as early as the age of 6 years. Girls show evidence of bilateral representation of spatial processing until the age of 13 (Witelson, 1976). Even as adults, women may show less hemispheric specialization than men (Levy, 1973). Waber (1976) has shown that the difference in verbal and spatial skills between the two sexes is not intrinsic to sexual differences *per se,* but is related to rate of maturation. Regard-less of sex, early-maturing adolescents perform better on tests of verbal than spatial abilities; the late-maturing ones show the opposite pattern. Furthermore, adolescents maturing late are more lateralized for speech than those maturing early. The normal pattern, of course, is for boys to mature later than girls. Waber (1976) argues that differences in mental abilities reflect differences in the organi-zation of cortical function, which in turn are related to differential rates of physical maturation. These are interesting suggestions. In early maturers, the first stages of language development may occur as both the left and then the right hemisphere traverse a critical stage of neural plasticity. This would lead to a substantial, and to some extent lasting, involvement of both hemispheres in language processes. In typical language fashion, this bilateral representation would occur at the expense of nonverbal functions, leading to lower spatial ability scores. Conversely, late-maturing adolescents may have a protracted opportunity to establish language in the left hemisphere. By remaining unilateral, language would control less brain tissue and not encroach* on right hemisphere networks, which can then become the sole domain of nonverbal tasks. The price for a clear-cut hemispheric domi-nance for verbal and nonverbal processes would then be a prolonged maturation.

There is a second kind of price to the "male type" of neural ontogeny, a price that can be measured in terms of malfunction "risks." Language disorders such as stuttering, developmental receptive aphasia, and dyslexia occur more frequently in boys than in girls. For example, the ratio of male to female stutterers is reported to be in the proportion of 3:1 or 4:1. For developmental receptive aphasia, males are affected more than females in a proportion of 5:1 (Brain, 1965, pp. 151, 154). The incidence of developmental dyslexia is approximately 10 times greater in boys than in girls (Benton, 1975). Since boys are thought to have the more marked lateralization for language tasks, this may be a factor leading to increased inci-dence of language pathologies.

The incidence of dyslexia has been related to a bilateral representation of spatial skills (Witelson, 1977). This partial encroachment on the language hemi-sphere may point to the potential risks of lateralization. As long as the left

*Notice that I too have slipped into the untested assumption that language and right-hemisphere functions may compete for a same synaptic space (see p. 327)!

hemisphere is pitched against the right one, and vice versa, each one can preserve its own domain. When two spatial hemispheres vie for attention and for imposing their processing biases, as in dyslexia, then the single language hemisphere is "unbalanced" and its "native" processes are at a disadvantage. If dyslexia resulted merely from the encroachment of spatial skills on language skills, then we would expect to find it as common in women as in men, as well as in single hemisphere patients and in callosal agenesis patients, yet this is not the case.

The problems of dyslexics are not limited to reading difficulties. In relation to normal subjects, dyslexics are significantly inferior in dealing with temporal aspects of nonverbal auditory and visual information. Dyslexics also fare worse than normals in tests of manual dexterity (Zurif and Carson, 1970). The more balanced bilateral representation of verbal and nonverbal skills in the two hemispheres of girls may be a factor in reducing the risk of serious brain malfunction. This view is novel in that it suggests that the exaggerated hemispheric dominance of the male brain, with its accompanying risk of language disorders, may have evolved not to heighten language abilities but to protect spatial skills which normally develop later in ontogeny!

Levy (1969) noted that some left-handed individuals have lower spatial than verbal ability (cf. Nebes, 1971; Miller, 1971), and suggested that this may be due to the higher incidence of bilateral representation of language in sinistrals and the resultant interference with the right hemisphere's processing of spatial information. Subsequently, Levy (1973) has compared sinistrals with women, arguing that in both cases the reduction in spatial abilities may result from a reduction in hemispheric specialization. However, far from being left-handed, women are more consistently right-handed than men (Annett, 1970)! Perhaps the ontogeny of bilateral representation differs between sinistrals, as a group, and women.

If one were to generalize from the examples of Levy (1969) for spatial ability in left-handers, and Witelson (1977) for dyslexia, one would conclude that when a task usually restricted to one hemisphere invades the opposite one the latter's specializations suffer, provided that the invasion is not reciprocal: skills with bilateral representation encroach on skills with unilateral representation. When the invasion is reciprocal, as in women, then the later-developing (spatial) skills suffer. This interpretation is speculative. There is a great need for comparing the effects of unilateral brain lesions in women and men.

Hypoglossal and Hemispheric Dominance in Songbirds

Until very recently, all known examples of hemispheric dominance came from human material. Those who speculated about the evolution of this phenomenon related it to handedness, tool making, and use of weapons, and of course to the emergence of language. Hemispheric dominance was seen as part of the emerging human condition. The first and strong sign that all was not well with this view came with the discovery of left hypoglossal dominance for vocal control in a songbird, the chaffinch (Nottebohm, 1970).

The vocal organ of birds is the syrinx, at the confluence of bronchi and trachea (Fig. 13). Anatomically, the syrinx consists of a right and a left half. These two halves are mirror images of each other. Each of these halves is a functional unit: it has one sound source (the internal tympaniform membrane), and its own air supply, muscular control, and innervation. The tracheosyringealis branch of each hypoglossus innervates the musculature of the ipsilateral syringeal half.

Chaffinches and canaries learn their song by reference to auditory information. Normally, both species copy the song of other conspecifics (Thorpe, 1958; Waser and Marler, 1977), but fail to develop normal song if deafened (Nottebohm, 1968; Marler *et al.*, 1973). In chaffinches and canaries, section of the left hypoglossus or of the tracheosyringealis branch of the left hypoglossus abolishes control over the left syringeal half. After such an operation, most of the components of song disappear: they are replaced by silence or by poorly modulated sounds. Section of the right hypoglossus has a very minor effect on song: most

331

ORIGINS AND
MECHANISMS IN THE
ESTABLISHMENT OF
CEREBRAL
DOMINANCE

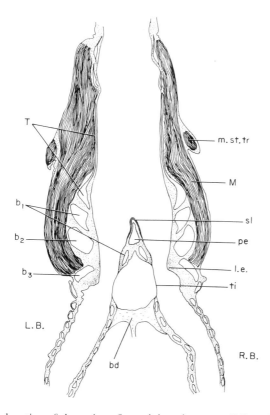

Fig. 13. Longitudinal section of the syrinx of an adult male canary. R.B. and L.B. = right and left bronchi; M = section through the lateral mass of intrinsic syringeal muscles; T = tympanum; b_1–b_3 bronchial half rings; db = bronchidesmus; pe = pessulus; sl = semilunar membrane; l.e. = labium externum; t.i. = internal tympaniform membrane; m.st.tr. = sternotrachealis muscle. Notice that the muscle mass serving the left syringeal half is heavier than its right counterpart.

components of song persist intact. This kind of effect, labeled "left hypoglossal dominance" (Nottebohm, 1970, 1971, 1972, 1977; Nottebohm and Nottebohm, 1976a), is demonstrated in Fig. 14.

During its first breeding season, a male chaffinch learns a repertoire of stereotyped song patterns. No new themes are subsequently added. A chaffinch denied access to conspecific models during that first year develops abnormal song. Subsequent exposure to wild-type song is usually not followed by improvement in singing. Thorpe (1958) called this temporal restriction the "critical period for song learning." If one sections the left hypoglossus of an adult chaffinch after song has been learned, the resulting song loss is permanent. If the same operation is conducted before onset of song learning, such a bird imitates a wild-type model with only its right syringeal innervation intact. This is an important observation. It means that both syringeal halves and their corresponding innervation are equipotential for song learning. Canaries that have the left hypoglossus cut during the first 2 weeks after hatching also develop song of normal complexity under exclusive right hypoglossal control.

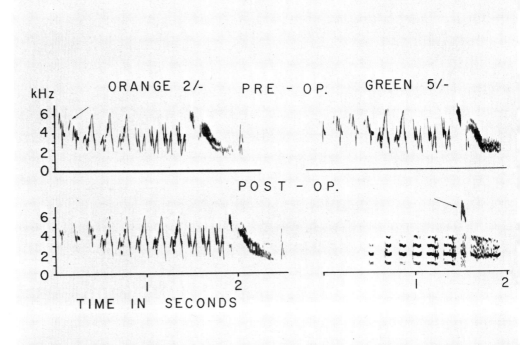

Fig. 14. Sound spectrographic display of the song of two adult male chaffinches. Preoperatively both birds shared the same theme. The right hypoglossus was cut in Orange 2/-, the left hypoglossus in Green 5/-. Both birds were recorded 2 and 4 days after the operation, respectively. In the case of Orange 2/-, the arrow indicates the element lost; for Green 5/-, the arrow indicates the single element that survived the operation (from Nottebohm, 1971, reproduced with the permission of the *Journal of Experimental Zoology*).

333

ORIGINS AND
MECHANISMS IN THE
ESTABLISHMENT OF
CEREBRAL
DOMINANCE

Chaffinch song is testosterone dependent (Collard and Grevendal, 1946; Thorpe, 1958). The critical period for song learning in chaffinches also is testosterone dependent. A chaffinch castrated before the onset of song learning can be made to learn song at 2 years of age, under the influence of exogenous testosterone (Nottebohm, 1969). It is tempting to speculate that in such a bird the potential for reversing hypoglossal dominance would persist for as long as the bird was not made to sing under testosterone therapy. We may have here a molecular handle on reversibility of laterality processes.

Canaries learn a new song repertoire every year (Nottebohm and Nottebohm, 1978). Section of the left hypoglossus in adult canaries that have finished their first season of song learning is followed by development of a new repertoire under exclusive right hypoglossal control (Nottebohm, in press). Thus there is a good correlation between the motor plasticity required for song learning and the plasticity required to switch hypoglossal dominance. However, the new song repertoire developed by adult canaries after left hypoglossal section is less accomplished than that of intact birds.

If the left hypoglossus of young canaries is cut between 17 and 19 days of age, it regrows. Such birds develop a song repertoire of normal complexity under "ambidextrous" (ambisinistrous!) control: approximately half of the song components are controlled by the left hypoglossus, the other half by the right hypoglossus. I have suggested elsewhere that the left hypoglossus and its higher control centers may normally lead in development and thus establish their dominance for song skills (Nottebohm, 1972, p. 48). When this lead is interrupted by nerve section, the right side catches up. If nerve regrowth occurs, both nerves develop song as equal partners! (Nottebohm, in press).

Left hypoglossal dominance may be of wide occurrence among oscine songbirds. To date, it has been described in a total of 16 chaffinches, 49 canaries, and 2 white-crowned sparrows tested in the author's laboratory. Lemon (1973) tested 15 white-throated sparrows, of which 14 showed clear-cut left hypoglossal dominance. In the fifteenth bird, left syringeal denervation had a marked effect on song when recorded 2 days postoperatively. Ten days later, this bird gave a good version of the first half of song, possibly an instance of a young bird relearning song with its right syringeal half. It is impressive that, out of 81 songbirds of four different species tested, results on 80 gave strong evidence of left hypoglossal dominance.

The song control system of canaries includes a well-defined anatomical network (Nottebohm et al., 1976), shown in Fig. 15. The highest vocal control station is the hyperstriatum ventrale, pars caudale, HVc. HVc receives inputs from the telencephalic projection of the auditory system (Kelley and Nottebohm, in press). Bilateral lesion of HVc in adult canaries results in silent song. Such an individual adopts the stance of a singing bird, its throat can be seen to quiver, and the bill is held slightly open, yet no sound or at most some very faint clicks are produced. This performance remains unchanged even a year after operation. If only the left HVc is lesioned, the bird produces audible song which is almost totally lacking in structure and includes virtually no preoperative components. A similar lesion restricted to the right HVc results in the loss of some song components and

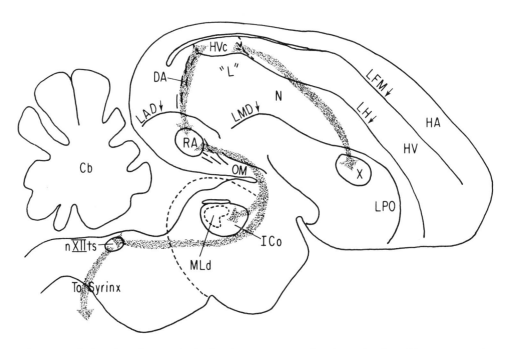

Fig. 15. Sagittal section of canary brain showing structures and pathways implicated in song control. Highest station of the efferent vocal control system is the hyperstriatum ventrale, pars caudale (HVc). HVc projects to the robust nucleus of the archistriatum (RA), which projects to the caudal half of the hypoglossal nucleus (nXIIts). The motoneurons in nXIIts innervate the ipsilateral tracheolateralis, sternotrachealis (see Fig. 13) and intrinsic syringeal musculature. The role of area X of the lobus parolfactorius (LPO), which receives a strong projection from HVc, remains unclear (from Nottebohm *et al.*, 1976, reproduced with the permission of the *Journal of Comparative Neurology*).

the preservation of others; the overall pattern of song delivery in such individuals is well structured (Fig. 16). This observation has now been repeated in five canaries with right HVc lesion and 11 with left HVc lesion. Thus left hypoglossal dominance occurs accompanied by left hemispheric dominance for song control. It is not quite the kind of dominance described in adult humans, where lesions of the right hemisphere usually have no effect on verbal skills. Yet there is an undoubted preeminence for vocal control vested in the left hemisphere of canaries.

Left HVc lesions of adult canaries are followed by gradual recovery of singing performance. When such birds are recorded on the following year, they have developed a new repertoire. Although in many ways this repertoire is less accomplished than that of an intact 2-year-old canary, it does include most of the features of normal song (Nottebohm, 1977). So, much as it is possible to reverse hypoglossal dominance, it also is possible to reverse hemispheric dominance in adult canaries. When the latter phenomenon occurs, the right hypoglossus becomes dominant for song control. Similarly, when the left hypoglossus is sectioned and song is redeveloped under right hypoglossal control, such birds now sing with a right dominant HVc (Nottebohm, in preparation).

Clearly, we have here an invaluable animal model with which to study the neural correlates of cerebral dominance for a learned motor task. This material

335

ORIGINS AND
MECHANISMS IN THE
ESTABLISHMENT OF
CEREBRAL
DOMINANCE

lends itself to study the kinds of neural rearrangements that lead to a reversal of hemispheric dominance. It is not known whether the two hemispheres of canaries have, as is claimed for humans, separate and complementary ways of analyzing sensory inputs. This, too, we hope to explore. Intriguingly, we have not been able to find any gross left-right anatomical asymmetry in the higher stations controlling canary song. The volumes of the right and left HVc or of the right and left robust nucleus of the archistriatum (Fig. 13) are closely comparable. This is important because it suggests that rather gross functional asymmetries can occur in the absence of obvious anatomical asymmetries.

The evolutionary significance of left hypoglossal dominance in birds remains obscure. It is not a necessary condition for vocal learning. Prolific vocal learners such as parrots show no hypoglossal dominance (Nottebohm and Nottebohm, 1976*b*). Conversely, the left hypoglossus of such an archetypal non vocal learner as domestic fowl innervates the right and left musculature of the syrinx, whereas the right hypoglossus innervates only the right syringeal half (Youngren *et al.*, 1974). Unfortunately, we do not know whether in this case the right and left hypoglossi play different roles in vocal control.

Recently, Rogers and Anson (1976) have claimed that the left hemisphere of newly hatched domestic fowl chicks exerts a dominant role in learning visual discriminations and in auditory habituation. This was shown by administering cycloheximide to either hemisphere on day 2 after hatching, and testing with

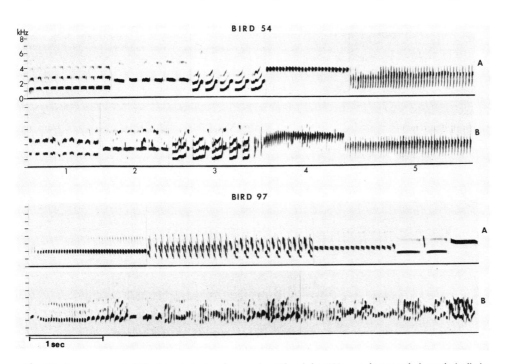

Fig. 16. Song segments (A) of two intact male canaries. The right HVc was destroyed electrolytically in bird 54, the left HVc in bird 97. Both birds were recorded soon after the operation (B). Deficits are more marked following left HVc lesion, involving a virtually total loss of syllable types and phrasing. In bird 54 postoperative syllables 1, 2, 3 and 5 bear a close resemblance to their preoperative counterparts (from Nottebohm *et al.*, 1976, reproduced with the permission of the *Journal of Comparative Neurology*).

visual or auditory material 5–10 days later. Chicks that received cycloheximide in their left hemisphere showed learning deficits. Saline controls or cycloheximide injections into the right hemisphere did not have comparable effects. Cycloheximide inhibits protein synthesis. Its effects would be more severe on the half of the brain that was engaged in laying down learning circuits. Thus the notion of two hemispheres developing at slightly different rates, one leading and one trailing, could explain the differential effect of the drug as well as the preponderance of one hemisphere in learning tests administered at that time. Conceivably, in the adult domestic fowl, both hemispheres fulfill similar roles, although this is not known.

OVERVIEW AND SUMMARY

Anatomical asymmetries between the right and left hemispheres have been described in humans and to a lesser extent in pongid apes. Asymmetries have also been described in the diencephalon of amphibians and some fish. Only in the case of humans have functional asymmetries between the two hemispheres been related to anatomical asymmetries. There is still no evidence that this relation is causal or mandatory except for the fact that anatomical asymmetries are less marked or absent among left-handers, otherwise thought to have less hemispheric lateralization of function (LeMay, 1976). In birds such as canaries that show a marked left hemispheric dominance for vocal control, there is no obvious difference in the size of vocal control areas of the two hemispheres.

Why hemispheric dominance? Levy (1969) has suggested that hemispheric dominance evolved to resolve the incompatibility between the analytic and holistic ways of processing sensory inputs. This is a bold and interesting idea, based on circumstantial evidence from human material. It should be testable in other groups, particularly oscine songbirds and nonhuman primates.

Some time ago I noted that "A behavioral sequence has to commence, and, unless it is rigidly programmed, it must incorporate a continuous decision-making process. Control of the commencement of behavior and decision making might be inefficient under equipotent and simultaneous bilateral representation" (Nottebohm, 1970, p. 953). The need for an executive hemisphere might be particularly acute for learned motor tasks such as speech, manual skills, and birdsong. This view is echoed by Gazzaniga and LeDoux (1978) when they state that "the unilateral representation of the mechanisms by which speech is programmed and executed provides a final cognitive path through which behavior can be organized and controlled" (p. 81). Another related view is expressed by Kimura and Archibald (1974) when they suggest that originally the left hemisphere specialized in the control of sequential motor acts. It is intriguing to think that conditions that favored the emergence of an executive hemisphere may have also led to the sequestering of perceptual and motor processes serving intraspecific communication into that same hemisphere. Whereas Levy (1969) stresses the need to segregate incompatible functions, the view of a dominant executive hemisphere stresses the need for a unified decision-making process. The analytic idiosyncrasies of the left hemsiphere, particularly those involving fine temporal judgments, may be an indispensable part of an executive network!

337

ORIGINS AND
MECHANISMS IN THE
ESTABLISHMENT OF
CEREBRAL
DOMINANCE

Why the left hemisphere and not the right one? Hypothesis: because the left one leads in development. If so, then the common denominator for left hemispheric dominance in avian and human brains is that learned motor tasks and their attendant sensory processes are vested in a more precocial left hemisphere (Nottebohm, 1972). Primacy of control becomes dominance of control and is mirrored by inhibitory processes on the other side. The rest of hemispheric differences may emerge during ontogeny in a complementary manner, exploiting available network space and time.

The "primacy of control" parameter, and by "how much" and for "how long," may be the crucial variables determining most of the observed variations of hemispheric dominance. Much as in amphibians reversal of dominance does not have to affect both halves of the heart, the gut, and the habenula (von Woellwarth, 1950), so the left-right lags in hemispheric development need not affect all circuits in a comparable manner. The hypothesized relation between hemispheric dominance and right-left lags in CNS development fits well with the observations of embryologists such as Lepori (1969), who noted that normally the left side leads in embryonic development.

Most of the speculation on hemispheric dominance has sought to explain why it evolved, but it would be just as interesting to know why it has not evolved in a more marked and widespread manner. The segregation of different functions into separate hemispheres may carry a risk of pathology and substandard performance. The duplication of input processors and memory stores in both sides of the brain may be a good buffer against developmental errors.

The first hundred years in the study of hemispheric dominance focused on clinical data and the human uniqueness of this trait. In the next several decades, we can expect to witness a broad search for the animal and developmental roots of this phenomenon.

REFERENCES

Altmann, S. A. A field study of the sociobiology of rhesus monkeys (*Macaca mulatta*). *Annals of the New York Academy of Science*, 1962, *102*, 338–435.

Altmann, S. A. Sociobiology of rhesus monkeys. II. Stochastics of social communication. *Journal of Theoretical Biology*, 1965, *8*, 490–522.

Annett, M. Handedness, cerebral dominance and the growth of intelligence. In D. J. Bakker and P. Satz (eds.), *Specific Reading Disability*. Rotterdam: Rotterdam University Press, 1970.

Bailey, P., von Bonin, G., and McCulloch, W. S. *The Isocortex of the Chimpanzee*. Urbana: University of Illinois Press, 1950.

Basser, L. S. Hemiplegia of early onset and the faculty of speech with special reference to the effects of hemispherectomy. *Brain*, 1962, *85*, 427–460.

Benton, A. L. Developmental dyslexia: Neurological aspects. In *Advances in Neurology*, Vol. 7. New York: Raven Press, 1975, pp. 1–47.

Bever, T. G., and Chiarello, R. J. Cerebral dominance in musicians and nonmusicians. *Science*, 1974, *185*, 537–539.

Bogen, J. E. Linguistic performance in the short-term following cerebral commissurotomy. In H.

Whitaker and H. A. Whitaker (eds.), *Studies in Neurolinguistics*, Vol. 2. New York: Academic Press, 1976, pp. 193–224.

Bogen, J. E. and Vogel, P. J. Cerebral commissurotomy in man. *Bulletin of Los Angeles Neurological Society*, 1962, *27*, 169.

Brain, L. *Speech Disorders*. London: Butterworths, 1965.

Braitenberg, V., and Kemali, M. Exceptions to bilateral symmetry in the epithalamus of lower vertebrates. *Journal of Comparative Neurology*, 1970, *138*, 137–146.

Broca, P. Sur la faculté du langage articulé. *Bulletin de la Société d'Anthropologie, (Paris)*, 1865, *6*, 377–393.

Cameron, J. On the presence and significance of the superior commissure throughout the vertebrata. *Journal of Anatomy and Physiology*, 1904, *38*, 275–292.

Chapple, W. D. Role of asymmetry in the functioning of invertebrate nervous systems. In S. Harnad, R. W. Doty, L. Goldstein, J. Jaynes, and G. Krauthamer (eds.), *Lateralization in the Nervous System*. New York: Academic Press, 1977, pp. 3–22.

Collard, J., and Grevendal, L. Etudes sur les caractères sexuels des Pinsons *Fringilla coelebs* et *Fringilla montifringilla*. *Gerfaut*, 1946, *2*, 89–107.

Collins, R. L. Toward an admissible genetic model for the inheritance of the degree and direction of asymmetry. In S. Harnad, R. W. Doty, L. Goldstein, J. Jaynes, and G. Krauthamer (eds.), *Lateralization in the Nervous System*. Academic Press: New York, 1977, pp. 137–150.

Cooper, W. E. Selective adaptation to speech. In F. Restle, R. M. Shiffrin, N. J. Castellan, B. Landman, and D. B. Pisoni (eds.), *Cognitive Theory*, Vol. I. Potomac, Md.: Erlbaum, 1975, pp. 24–54.

Corsi, P. M. Verbal memory impairment after unilateral hippocampal excisions. Paper read at the 4th Annual Meeting of the Eastern Psychological Association, April 1969.

Crane, J. Combat, display and ritualization in fiddler crabs (Ocypodidae, genus *Uca*). *Philosophical Transactions of the Royal Society of London, Series B*, 1966, *251*, 459–472.

Cunningham, D. F. *Contribution to the Surface Anatomy of the Cerebral Hemispheres*. Dublin: Royal Irish Academy, 1892.

Dee, H. L., and Fontenot, D. J. Cerebral dominance and lateral differences in perception and memory. *Neurophysiologia*, 1973, *11*, 167–173.

Dennis, M., and Kohn, B. Comprehension of syntax in infantile hemiplegics after cerebral hemidecortication: Left hemisphere superiority. *Brain and Language*, 1975, *2*, 472–482.

Dennis, M., and Whitaker, H. A. Language acquisition following hemidecortication: Linguistic superiority of the left over the right hemisphere. *Brain and Language*, 1976, *3*, 404–433.

DeRenzi, E., and Spinnler, H. Facial recognition in brain damaged patients. *Neurology*, 1966, *16*, 145–152.

Dewson, J. H. Preliminary evidence of hemispheric asymmetry of auditory function in monkeys. In S. Harnad, R. W. Doty, L. Goldstein, J. Jaynes, and G. Krauthamer (eds.), *Lateralization in the Nervous System*. New York: Academic Press, 1977, pp. 63–71.

Dewson, J. H., Burlinghame, A., Kizer, K., Dewson, S., Kenney, P., and Pribram, K. H. Hemispheric asymmetry of auditory function in monkeys. *Journal of the Acoustical Society of America*, 1975, *58*, S66.

Doty, R. W., and Overman, W. H. Mnemonic role of forebrain commissures in macaques. In S. Harnad, R. W. Doty, L. Goldstein, J. Jaynes, and G. Krauthamer (eds.), *Lateralization in the Nervous System*. New York: Academic Press, 1977, pp. 75–88.

Efron, R. The effect of handedness on the perception of simultaneity and temporal order. *Brain*, 1963a, *86*, 261–284.

Efron, R. Temporal perception, aphasia and déja-vu. *Brain*, 1963b, *86*, 403–424.

Eimas, P. D. Linguistic processing of speech by young infants. In R. Schiefelbusch and L. Lloyd (eds.), *Language Perspectives: Acquisition, Retardation and Intervention*. Baltimore: University Park Press, 1974, pp. 55–73.

Eimas, P. D., and Corbit, J. D. Selective adaptation of linguistic feature detectors. *Cognitive Psychology*, 1973, *4*, 99–109.

Eimas, P. D., Siqueland, E. R., Jusczyk, P., and Vigorito, J. Speech perception in infants. *Science*, 1971, *171*, 303–306.

Franz, V. Morphologie der Akranier. *Ergebnisse der Anatomie und Entwicklungsgeschichte* 1927a, *27*, 464–692.

Franz, V. Branchiostoma. In G. Grimpe and E. Wagler (eds.), *Die Tierwelt der Nord- und Ostsee*, Vol. 12, Section b. Leipzig; Akademische Verlagsgesellschaft, 1927b, pp. 1–46.

Galaburda, A. M., LeMay, M., Kemper, T. L. and Geschwind, N. Right-left asymmetries in the brain. *Science*, 1978, *199*, 852–856.

339

ORIGINS AND
MECHANISMS IN THE
ESTABLISHMENT OF
CEREBRAL
DOMINANCE

Gaskell, W. H. On the origin of vertebrates, deduced from the study of Ammocoetes. *Journal of Anatomy and Physiology*, 1901, *35*, 224.

Gazzaniga, M. S. *The Bisected Brain*. New York: Appleton-Century-Crofts, 1970.

Gazzaniga, M. S., and LeDoux, J. E. *The Integrated Mind*. New York: Plenum, 1978.

Gazzaniga, M. S., Bogen, J. E., and Sperry, R. W. Some functional effects of sectioning the cerebral commissures in man. *Proceedings of the National Academy of Sciences, United States of America,* 1962, *48*, 1765–1769.

Gazzaniga, M. S., LeDoux, J. E., and Wilson, D. H. Language, praxis and the right hemisphere: Clues to some mechanisms of consciousness. *Neurology*, 1977, *27*, 1144–1147.

Gazzinga, M. S., and Sperry, R. W. Language after section of the cerebral commissures. *Brain,* 1967, *90*, 131–148.

Geschwind, N. The anatomical basis of hemispheric differentiation. In S. J. Dimond and J. G. Beaumont (eds.), *Hemispheric Function in the Human Brain*. New York: Halsted Press, 1974, pp. 7–24.

Geschwind, N., and Levitsky, W. Human brain: Left-right asymmetries in temporal speech region. *Science*, 1968, *161*, 186–187.

Goldman, P. S. Development determinants of cortical plasticity. *Acta Neurobiologiae Experimentalis*, 1972, *32*, 495–511.

Goldman, P. S., Lodge, A., Hammer, L. R., Semmes, J., and Mishkin, M. Critical flicker frequency after unilateral temporal lobectomy in man. *Neuropsychologia*, 1968, *6*, 355–363.

Gordon, H. W., and Bogen, J. E. Hemispheric lateralization of singing after intracarotid sodium amylobarbitone. *Neurology, Neurosurgery and Psychiatry*, 1974, *37*, 727–738.

Govind, C. K., and Lang, F. Neuromuscular analysis of closing in the dimorphic claws of the lobster *Homarus americanus*. *Journal of Experimental Zoology*, 1974, *190*, 281–288.

Green, S. Variation of vocal pattern with social situation in the Japanese monkey *(Macaca fuscata):* A field study. *Primate Behavior,* 1975, *4*, 1–102.

Groves, C. P., and Humphrey, N. K. Asymmetry in gorilla skulls: Evidence of lateralized brain function? *Nature (London)*, 1973, *244*, 53–54.

Haecker, V. *Goethes morphologische Arbeiten und die neuere Forschung*. Jena, 1927.

Hamilton, C. R. Investigations of perceptual and mnemonic lateralization in monkeys. In S. Harnad, R. W. Doty, L. Goldstein, J. Jaynes, and G. Krauthamer (eds.), *Lateralization in the Nervous System*. New York: Academic Press, 1977, pp. 45–62.

Heacock, A. M., and Agranoff, B. W. Clockwise growth of neurites from retinal explants. *Science,* 1977, *198*, 64–66.

Hécaen, H. Acquired aphasia in children and the ontogenesis of hemispheric functional specialization. *Brain and Language*, 1976, *3*, 114–134.

Hobson, J. R. Sex differences in primary mental abilities. *Journal of Educational Research*, 1947, *41*, 126–132.

Holmgren, U. On the ontogeny of the pineal and parapineal organs in teleost fishes. In J. A. Kappers and J. P. Shade (eds.), *Structure and Function of the Epiphysis Cerebri*. Amsterdam: Elsevier, 1965, pp. 172–182.

Huettner, A. F. *Fundamentals of Comparative Embryology of the Vertebrates*. New York: Macmillan, 1949.

Ingelmark, B. E. Über die Längenasymmetrie der Extremitäten: eine neue röntgenologische Registriermethode. *Uppsala Lakarrfornings Forhandlingar*, 1947, *51*, 17–82.

Jackson, H. On the nature of the duality of the brain. In J. Taylor (ed.), *Selected Writings of John Hughlings Jackson,* Vol. 2. London: Hodder and Stoughton, 1932, pp. 129–145.

Jahromi, S. S., and Atwood, H. L. Structural and contractile properties of lobster leg-muscle fibers. *Journal of Experimental Zoology*, 1971, *176*, 475–486.

Jung, R. Summary of the conference. In V. B. Mountcastle (ed.), *Interhemispheric Relations and Cerebral Dominance*. Baltimore: John Hopkins, 1962, pp. 264–277.

Kelley, D. B., and Nottebohm, F. Projections of a telencephalic auditory nucleus—field L—in the canary. *Journal of Comparative Neurology*, in press.

Kertesz, A., and Geschwind, N. Patterns of pyramidal decussation and their relationship to handedness. *Archives of Neurology (Chicago)*, 1971, *24*, 326–332.

Kimura, D. Cerebral dominance and the perception of verbal stimuli. *Canadian Journal of Psychology,* 1961, *15*, 156–171.

Kimura, D. Speech lateralization in young children as determined by an auditory test. *Journal of Comparitive and Physiological Psychology*, 1963, *56*, 899–902.

Kimura, D. Functional asymmetry of the brain in dichotic listening. *Cortex,* 1967, *3*, 163–178.

Kimura, D., and Archibald, Y. Motor functions of the left hemisphere. *Brain*, 1974, *97*, 337–350.

Kimura, D., and Folb, S. Neural processing of backwards speech sounds. *Science*, 1968, *161*, 395–396.

King, F. L., and Kimura, D. Left-ear superiority in dichotic perception of vocal nonverbal sounds. *Canadian Journal of Psychology*, 1972, *26*, 111–116.

Klemm, O. Über die Wirksamkeit kleinster Zeitunterschiede im Gebeite des Tastsinns. *Archiv für die Gesamte Psychologie*, 1925, *50*, 205–220.

Kuhl, P. K., and Miller, J. D. Speech perception by the chinchilla: Voiced-voiceless distinction in alveolar plosive consonants. *Science*, 1975, *190*, 69–72.

Kupfermann, I., and Kandel, E. R. Neuronal controls of a behavioral response mediated by the abdominal ganglion of *Aplysia*. *Science*, 1969, *164*, 847–850.

Lackner, J. L., and Teuber, H.-L. Alterations in auditory fusion thresholds after cerebral injury in man. *Neuropsychologia*, 1973, *11*, 409–415.

LeMay, M. Morphological cerebral asymmetries of modern man, fossil man and nonhuman primates. In *Origins and Evolution of Language and Speech. Annals of the New York Academy of Sciences*, Vol. 280, 1976, pp. 349–366.

Lemon, R. E. 1973. Nervous control of the syrinx in white-throated sparrows (*Zonotrichia albicollis*). *Journal of Zoology (London)*, 1973, *71*, 131–140.

Lenneberg, E. H. *Biological Foundations of Language*. New York: Wiley, 1967.

Lepori, N. G. 1966a. Asimmetria dei movimenti di convergenza nel balstodisco di Pollo e di Anatra. *Bollettino di Zoologia*, 1966a, *33*, 319–326.

Lepori, N. G. Analisi del processo di accorciamento della linea primitiva nel bastodisco di Pollo e di Anatra. *Acta Embryologiae et Morphologiae Experimentalis*, 1966b, *9*, 61–88.

Lepori, N. G. Sur la genèse des structures asymétriques chez l'embryon des oiseaux. *Monitore Zoologics Italiano (N.S.)*, 1969, *3*, 33–53.

Levy, J. Possible basis for the evolution of lateral specialization of the human brain. *Nature (London)*, 1969, *224*, 614–615.

Levy, J. 1973. Lateral specialization of the human brain: Behavioral manifestations and possible evolutionary basis. In J. Kirger (ed.), *The Biology of Behavior*. Corvallis: Oregon State University Press, 1973.

Levy, J. 1977. The origins of lateral asymmetry. In S. Harnad, R. W. Doty, L. Goldstein, J. Jaynes, and G. Krauthamer (eds.), *Lateralization in the Nervous System*. New York: Academic Press, 1977, pp. 195–209.

Levy, J. and Reid, M. Variations in writing posture and cerebral organization. *Science*, 1976, *194*, 337–339.

Levy, J., Trevarthen, C., and Sperry, R. W. Perception of bilateral chimeric figures following hemispheric deconnection. *Brain*, 1972, *95*, 61–78.

Levy-Agresti, J., and Sperry, R. W. Differential perceptual capacities in major and minor hemispheres. *Proceedings of the National Academy of Sciences of the United States of America*, 1968, *61*, 1151.

Liberman, A. M., and Pisoni, D. B. Evidence for a special speech-perceiving subsystem in the human. In T. H. Bullock (ed.), *Recognition of Complex Acoustic Signals*. Berlin: Dahlem Konferenzen, 1977, pp. 59–76.

Liberman, A. M., Cooper, F. S., Shankweiler, D., and Studdert-Kennedy, M. Perception of the speech code. *Psychological Review*, 1967, *74*, 431–461.

Liepmann, H. *Drei Aufsätze aus dem Apraxiegebiet*. Berlin: Karger, 1908.

Lindsley, D. L., and Grell, E. H. *Genetic Variations of Drosophila melanogaster*. Washington, D.C.: Carnegie Institute of Washington Publication No. 627, 1967.

Loeser, J. D., and Alvord, E. C. Clinicopathological correlations in agenesis of the corpus callosum. *Neurology*, 1968, *18*, 745–756.

Ludwig, W. *Das Rechts-Links-Problem im Tierreich und beim Menschen*. Berlin: J. Springer, 1932 (1970 reprint, Berlin: Springer-Verlag).

Luria, A. R. *Traumatic Aphasia*. Paris: Mouton, 1970.

Maccoby, E. E. *The Development of Sex Differences*. Stanford: Stanford University Press, 1966.

Mackinnon, J. The behaviour and ecology of wild orang-utans (*Pongo pygmaeus*). *Animal Behaviour*, 1974, *22*, 3–74.

Marler, P. Communication in monkeys and apes. In I. DeVore (ed.), *Primate Behavior: Field Studies of Monkeys and Apes*. New York: Holt, 1965, pp. 544–584.

Marler, P. An ethological theory of the origin of vocal learning. In *Origins and Evolution of Language and Speech. Annals of the New York Academy of Sciences*, 1976a, *280*, 386–395.

Marler, P. Social organization, communication and graded signals: The chimpanzee and the gorilla. In P. P. G. Bateson and R. A. Hinde (eds.), *Growing Points in Ethology*. Cambridge: Cambridge University Press, 1976b, pp. 239–280.

Marler, P., and Peters, S. Selective vocal learning in a sparrow. *Science,* 1977, *198*, 519–522.

Marler, P., Konishi, M., Lutjen, A., and Waser, M. S. 1973. Effects of continuous noise on avian hearing and vocal development. *Proceedings of the National Academy of Sciences of the United States of America,* 1973, *70*, 1393–1396.

McAdam, D. W., and Whitaker, H. A. Language production: Electroencephalographic localization in the normal human brain. *Science,* 1971, *172*, 499–502.

Meyer, V., and Yates, A. J. Intellectual changes following temporal lobectomy for psychomotor epilepsy. *Journal of Neurology, Neurosurgery and Psychiatry,* 1955, *18*, 44–52.

Miller, E. Handedness and the pattern of human ability. *British Journal of Psychology,* 1971, *62*, 111–112.

Miller, J. D. Perception of speech sounds in animals: Evidence for speech processing by mammalian auditory mechanisms. In T. H. Bullock (ed.), *Recognition of Complex Acoustic Signals.* Berlin: Dahlem Konferenzen, 1977.

Milner, B. 1958. Psychological defects produced by temporal-lobe excision. *Research Publications, Association for Research in Nervous and Mental Disease,* 1958, *36*, 244–257.

Milner, B. Visual recognition and recall after right temporal-lobe excision in man. *Neuropsychologia,* 1968, *6*, 191–209.

Milner, B. Memory and the medial temporal regions of the brain. In K. H. Pribram and D. E. Broadbent (eds.), *Biology of Memory.* New York: Academic Press, 1970, pp. 29–50.

Milner, B. Hemispheric specialization: Scope and limits. In F. O. Schmitt and F. G. Worden (eds.), *The Neurosciences: Third Study Program.* Cambridge, Mass.: MIT Press, 1974, pp. 75–88.

Milner, B., Taylor, L., and Sperry, R. W. Lateralized suppression of dichotically presented digits after commissural section in man. *Science,* 1968, *161*, 184–186.

Molfese, D. L., Freeman, R. B., and Palermo, D. S. The ontogeny of brain lateralization for speech and nonspeech stimuli. *Brain and Language,* 1975, *2*, 356–368.

Morgan, M. Embryology and inheritance of asymmetry. In S. Harnad, R. W. Doty, L. Goldstein, J. Jaynes, and G. Krauthamer (eds.), *Lateralization in the Nervous System.* New York: Academic Press, 1977, pp. 173–194.

Morse, P. A., and Snowdon, C. T. An investigation of categorical speech discrimination by rhesus monkeys. *Perception and Psychophysics,* 1975, *17*, 9–16.

Moscovitch, M., Scullion, D., and Christie, D. Early versus late stages of processing and their relation to functional hemisphere asymmetry for face recognition. *Journal of Experimental Psychology: Human Perception and Performance,* 1976, *2*, 401–416.

Moscovitch, M., and Smith, L. Differences in neural organization between individuals with straight and inverted hand postures during writing. Paper presented at the International Neuropsychological Society meeting, Minneapolis, Minnesota, February, 1978.

Nebes, R. D. Handedness and the perception of whole-part relationship. *Cortex,* 1971, *7*, 350–356.

Nottebohm, F. Auditory experience and song development in the chaffinch, *Fringilla coelebs. Ibis,* 1968, *110*, 549–568.

Nottebohm, F. The "critical period" for song learning. *Ibis,* 1969, *111*, 386–387.

Nottebohm, F. Ontogeny of bird song. *Science,* 1970, *167*, 950–956.

Nottebohm, F. Neural lateralization of vocal control in a passerine bird. I. Song. *Journal of Experimental Zoology,* 1971, *177*, 229–262.

Nottebohm, F. Neural lateralization of vocal control in a passerine bird. II. Subsong, calls and a theory of vocal learning. *Journal of Experimental Zoology,* 1972, *179*, 35–50.

Nottebohm, F. Asymmetries in neural control of vocalization in the canary. In S. Harnad, R. W. Doty, L. Goldstein, J. Jaynes, and G. Krauthamer (eds.), *Lateralization in the Nervous System.* New York: Academic Press, 1977, pp. 23–44.

Nottebohm, F. Reversal of hypoglossal dominance in canaries following unilateral syringeal denervation. *Journal of Comparative Physiology,* in press.

Nottebohm, F., and Nottebohm, M. Left hypoglossal dominance in the control of canary and white-crowned sparrow song. *Journal of Comparative Physiology,* 1976a, *108*, 171–192.

Nottebohm, F., and Nottebohm, M. Phonation in the orange-winged Amazon parrot, *Amazona amazonica. Journal of Comparative Physiology,* 1976b, *108*, 157–170.

Nottebohm, F., and Nottebohm, M. Relationship between song repertoire and age in the canary, *Serinus canarius. Zeitschrift für Tierpsychologie,* 1978, *46*, 298–305.

Nottebohm, F., Stokes, T. M., and Leonard, C. M. Central control of song in the canary, *Serinus canarius. Journal of Comparative Neurology,* 1976, *165*, 457–486.

Okazaki Smith, M., Chu, J., and Edmonston, W. E. Cerebral lateralization of haptic perception: Interaction of responses to Braille and music reveals a functional basis. *Science,* 1977, *197*, 689–690.

341

ORIGINS AND
MECHANISMS IN THE
ESTABLISHMENT OF
CEREBRAL
DOMINANCE

Oksche, A. Survey of the development and comparative morphology of the pineal organ. In J. A. Kappers and J. P. Shade (eds.), *Structure and Function of the Epiphysis Cerebri.* Amsterdam: Elsevier, 1965, pp. 3–29.

Penfield, W., and Roberts, L. *Speech and Brain Mechanisms.* Princeton, N.J.: Princeton University Press, 1959.

Petersen, M. R., Beecher, M. D., Zoloth, S. R., Moody, D. B., and Stebbins, W. C. Neural lateralization: Evidence from studies of the perception of species—specific vocalizations by Japanese macaques. *Science,* in press.

Riech, F. Epiphyse und Paraphyse im Lebenszyklus der Anuren. *Zeitschrift für vergleichende Physiologie,* 1925, *2,* 524–570.

Rodman, P. S. Population composition and adaptive organization among orang-utans of the Kutai reserve. In R. P. Michael and J. H. Crook (eds.), *Comparative Ecology and Behaviour of Primates.* London: Academic Press, 1973, pp. 172–209.

Rogers, L. J., and Anson, J. M. Hemispheric specialization in chickens. *Proceedings of the Australian Physiological and Pharmacological Society,* 1976, *7,* 92P.

Rosenzweig, M. R. Representations of the two ears at the auditory cortex. *American Journal of Physiology,* 1951, *167,* 147–158.

Rowell, T. E., and Hinde, R. A. Vocal communication by the rhesus monkey *(Macaca mulatta). Proceedings of the Zoology Society of London,* 1962, *138,* 279–294.

Rozin, P. The psychobiological approach to human memory. In M. R. Rosenzweig and E. L. Bennet (eds.), *Neural Mechanisms of Learning and Memory.* Cambridge, Mass.: MIT Press, 1976, pp. 3–48.

Rubens, A. B. Anatomical asymmetries of human cerebral cortex. In S. Harnad, R. W. Doty, L. Goldstein, J. Jaynes, and G. Krauthamer (eds.), *Lateralization in the Nervous System.* New York: Academic Press, 1977, pp. 503–516.

Rubens, A. B., Mahowald, M. W., and Hutton, J. T. Asymmetry of the lateral (sylvian) fissures in man. *Neurology,* 1976, *26,* 620–624.

Saul, R., and Sperry, R. W. Absence of commissurotomy symptoms with agenesis of the corpus callosum. *Neurobiology,* 1968, *18,* 307.

Schaeffer, A. A. Spiral movement in man. *Journal of Morphology and Physiology,* 1928, *45,* 293–398.

Semmes, J. Hemispheric specialization: A possible clue to mechanism. *Neuropsychologia,* 1968, *6,* 11–26.

Signoret, J.-L., and Lhermitte, F. The amnesic syndromes and the encoding process. In M. R. Rosenzweig and E. L. Bennett (eds.), *Neural Mechanisms of Learning and Memory.* Cambridge, Mass.: MIT Press, 1976, pp. 67–75.

Sinnott, J. M., Beecher, M. D., Moody, D. B., and Stebbins, W. C. Speech sound discrimination by monkeys and humans. *Journal of the Acoustical Society of America,* 1976, *60,* 687–695.

Sivak, J. G. Historical note: The vertebrate median eye. *Vision Research,* 1974, *14,* 137–140.

Smith, A. Dominant and non-dominant hemispherectomy. In W. L. Smith (ed.), *Drugs, Development and Cerebral Function.* Springfield, Ill.: Thomas, 1972.

Smith, A., and Sugar, O. Development of above normal language and intelligence 21 years after left hemispherectomy. *Neurology,* 1975, *25,* 813–818.

Spemann, H., and Falkenberg, H. Über asymmetrische Entwicklung und Situs inversus bei Zwillingen und Doppelbindungen. *Wilhelm Roux Archiv für Entwicklungsmechanik der Organismen,* 1919, *45,* 371–422.

Sperry, R. W. Plasticity of neural maturation. *Developmental Biology,* Supplement 2, 1968, 306–327 (27th Symposium). New York: Academic Press.

Sperry, R. W. Cerebral dominance in perception. In F. A. Young and D. B. Lindsley (eds.), *Early Experience in Visual Information Processing in Perceptual and Reading Disorders.* Washington, D.C.: National Academy of Sciences, 1970.

Sperry, R. W. Lateral specialization in the surgically separated hemispheres. In F. O. Schmitt and F. G. Worden (eds.), *The Neurosciences: Third Study Program.* Cambridge, Mass.: MIT Press, 1974.

Srb, A., Owen, R., and Edgar, R. *General Genetics,* 2nd ed. San Francisco: W. H. Freeman, 1965.

Streeter, L. A. Language perception of 2-month-old infants shows effects of both innate mechanisms and experience. *Nature,* 1976, *259,* 39–41.

Sturtevant, A. H. Inheritance and direction of coiling in *Limnaea. Science,* 1923, *58,* 269.

Sussman, H. M. The laterality effect in lingual-auditory tracking. *Journal of the Acoustical Society of America,* 1971, *49,* 1874–1880.

Sussman, H. M., MacNeilage, P. F. and Lumbley, J. L. Sensorimotor dominance and the right-ear advantage in mandibular-auditory tracking. *Journal of the Acoustical Society of America,* 1974, *56,* 214–216.

343

ORIGINS AND
MECHANISMS IN THE
ESTABLISHMENT OF
CEREBRAL
DOMINANCE

Sussman, H. M., MacNeilage, P. F. and Lumbley, J. L. Pursuit auditory tracking of dichotically presented tonal amplitudes. *Journal of Speech and Hearing Research*, 1975, *18*, 74–81.

Swisher, L., and Hirsch, I. J. Brain damage and the ordering of two temporally successive stimuli. *Neuropsychologia*, 1972, *10*, 137–151.

Tallal, P. Auditory perceptual factors in language and learning disabilities. In R. M. Knights and D. J. Bakker (eds.), *The Neuropsychology of Learning Disorders: Theoretical Approaches*. Baltimore: University Park Press, 1976.

Tallal, P., and Newcombe, F. Impairment of auditory perception and language comprehension in residual dysphasia. *Journal of the Acoustical Society of America*, 1976, *59*, 585.

Tallal, P., and Piercy, M. Developmental aphasia: Impaired rate of non-verbal processing as a function of sensory modality. *Neuropsychologia*, 1973, *11*, 389–398.

Tallal, P., and Piercy, M. Developmental aphasia: The perception of brief vowels and extended stop consonants. *Neuropsychologia*, 1975, *13*, 69–74.

Tartter, V. C., and Eimas, P. D. The role of auditory feature detectors in the perception of speech. *Perception and Psychophysics*, 1975, *18*, 293–298.

Teuber, H.-L. Recovery of function after brain injury in man. In *Outcome of Severe Damage to the Central Nervous System*. Ciba Foundation Symposium 34 (new series). Amsterdam: Elsevier–Excerptz Medice–North-Holland, 1975, pp. 159–190.

Thorpe, W. H. Learning of song patterns by birds, with special reference to the song of the chaffinch, *Fringilla coelebs. Ibis*, 1958, *100*, 535–570.

Tomkins, R., and Rodman, W. P. The cortex of *Xenopus laevis* embryos: Regional differences in composition and biological activity. *Proceedings of the National Academy of Sciences of the United States of America*, 1971, *68*, 2921–2923.

Tunturi, A. R. A study on the pathway from the medial geniculate body to the acoustic cortex in the dog. *American Journal of Physiology*, 1946, *147*, 311–319.

van Lawick-Goodall, J. A preliminary report on expressive movements and communication in the Gombe Stream chimpanzees. In P. C. Jay (ed.), *Primates: Studies in Adaptation and Variability*. New York: Holt, Rinehart and Winston, 1968a, pp. 313–374.

van Lawick-Goodall, J. The behaviour of free-living chimpanzees in the Gombe Stream Reserve. *Animal Behaviour Monograph*, 1968b, *1*, 161–311.

van Lawick-Goodall, J. *In the Shadow of Man*. London: Collins, 1971.

von Bonin, G. Anatomical asymmetries of the cerebral hemispheres. In V. B. Mountcastle (ed.), *Interhemispheric Relations and Cerebral Dominance*. Baltimore: Johns Hopkins Press, 1962, pp. 1–6.

von Bonin, G., and Bailey, P. *The Neocortex of Macaca mulatta*. Urbana: University of Illinois Press, 1947.

von Woellwarth, C. Experimentelle Untersuchungen über den Situs inversus der Eingeweide und der Habenula des Zwischenhirns bei Amphibien. *Wilhelm Roux Archiv für Entwicklungsmechanik der Organismen*, 1950, *144*, 178–256.

von Woellwarth, C. Die Ausbildung der Asymmetrie der Nuclei habenulae des Zwischenhirns bei Amphibien in Unabhängigkeit vom Blutkreislauf. *Wilhelm Roux Archiv für Entwicklungsmechanik der Organismen*, 1969, *162*, 306–308.

Waber, D. P. Sex differences in cognition: A function of maturation rate? Science, 1976, *192*, 572–574.

Wada, J. A. Interhemispheric sharing and shift of cerebral speech function. *Excerpta Medica International Congress Series*, 1969, *193*, 296–297.

Wada, J. A., Clarke, R., and Hamm, A. Cerebral hemispheric asymmetry in humans: Cortical speech zones in 100 adult and 100 infant brains. *Archives of Neurology*, 1975, *32*, 239–246.

Wang, R. Y., and Aghajanian, G. K. Physiological evidence for habenula as major link between forebrain and midbrain raphe. *Science*, 1977, *197*, 89–91.

Warren, J. M. 1977. Handedness and cerebral dominance in monkeys. In S. Harnad, R. W. Doty, L. Goldstein, J. Jaynes, and G. Krauthamer (eds.), *Lateralization in the Nervous System*. New York: Academic Press, 1977, pp. 151–172.

Waser, M. S., and Marler, P. Song learning in canaries. *Journal of Comparative and Physiological Psychology*, 1977, *91*, 1–7.

Waters, R. S., and Wilson, W. A. Speech perception by rhesus monkeys: The voicing distinction in synthesized labian and velar stop consonants. *Perception and Psychophysics*, 1976, *19*, 285–289.

Wernicke, C. *Der aphasische Symptomen complex*. Breslau: Max Cohn and Weigert, 1874.

Wilson, D. M. Inherent asymmetry and reflex modulation of the locust flight motor pattern. *Journal of Experimental Biology*, 1968, *48*, 631–641.

Witelson, S. F. Sex and the single hemisphere: Specialization of the right hemisphere for spatial processing. *Science*, 1976, *193*, 425–427.

Witelson, S. F. Developmental dyslexia: Two right hemispheres and none left. *Science,* 1977, *195,* 309–311.

Witelson, S. F., and Pallie, W. Left hemisphere specialization for language in the newborn. *Brain,* 1973, *96,* 641–646.

Woods, B. T., and Teuber, H.-L. Early onset of complementary specialization of cerebral hemispheres in man. *Transactions of the American Neurological Association,* 1973, *98,* 113–117.

Yakovlev, P. I., and Rakic, P. 1966. Patterns of decussation of bulbar pyramids and distribution of pyramidal tracts on two sides of the spinal cord. *Transactions of the American Neurological Association,* 1966, *91,* 366–367.

Yeni-Komshian, G. H. 1976. Anatomical study of cerebral asymmetry in the temporal lobe of humans, chimpanzees, and rhesus monkeys. *Science,* 1976, *192,* 387–389.

Youngren, O. M., Peek, F. W., and Phillips, R. E. Repetitive vocalizations evoked by local electrical stimulation of avian brains. III. Evoked activity in the tracheal muscles of the chicken *(Gallus gallus). Brain Behavior and Evolution,* 1974, *9,* 393–421.

Zaidel, E. Auditory language comprehension in the right hemisphere following cerebral commissurotomy: A comparison with child language and aphasia. In A. Caramazza and E. Zurif (eds.), *Language Acquisition and Language Breakdown: Parallels and Divergencies.* Baltimore: Johns Hopkins University Press, 1977.

Zurif, E. G., and Carson, G. Dyslexia in relation to cerebral dominance and temporal analysis. *Neuropsychologia,* 1970, *8,* 351–361.

12

Electrophysiological Analysis of Human Brain Function

Steven A. Hillyard and David L. Woods

Introduction

Scalp recordings of human brain potentials provide information about underlying brain functions which complements that obtainable from other neuropsychological approaches described in this volume. Like the brain lesion and other neuroanatomical approaches, electrophysiological recordings can assist in the localization of particular sensory, perceptual, and cognitive processes in the brain. This nonintrusive method offers a distinct advantage, however, in that the distribution of brain activity associated with particular behavioral events can be evaluated "on line" in the intact, normally functioning nervous system, rather than inferred on the basis of post-lesion deficits. Electrophysiological studies of brain dysfunctions are also complementary to behavioral tests in that disturbances of the normal spatial and temporal flow of information in the brain can be identified and, in some cases, localized to particular structures.

Two main classes of brain waves can be recorded from surface electrodes in man, the ongoing potential fluctuations of the electroencephalogram (EEG) and the phasic "event-related potentials" (ERPs) which are coupled with specific sensory, motor, or cognitive events. Both types of waves are considered to represent the summated electric fields of large numbers of neuronal membranes acting in synchrony (Regan, 1972). The spectral properties of the EEG have proven useful as indices of certain tonic brain states (Kooi, 1971), but few correlates of phasic perceptual or cognitive processes have been extracted from these ongoing

Steven A. Hillyard and David L. Woods · Department of Neurosciences, University of California, San Diego, La Jolla, California 92093. The preparation of this chapter was supported by grants from NIMH (MH-25594), NASA (NGR 05-009-198), NIH (NS11707-03), and NSF (BNS-7714923).

STEVEN A. HILLYARD
AND DAVID L. WOODS

rhythms. In contrast, a number of different ERPs have been identified in man which correlate closely with specific modes of sensory and cognitive processing. Accordingly, the bulk of this chapter will be devoted to evaluating the burgeoning research on ERPs in the fields of sensory physiology, neurological diseases, human information processing, and cerebral specialization.

TYPES OF EVENT-RELATED POTENTIALS

Event-related brain waves are, by definition, time-locked to some specifiable event, which may be a stimulus input, a response output, or an intermediate stage of sensory or cognitive processing that is more or less directly linked to observable events. Indeed, it may well be that many of the waves being generated continuously in the EEG are, in fact, "event related," if one could only ascertain what the events were.

It is generally necessary to extract the ERPs from the ongoing EEG by computer-averaging procedures, since the latter waves (considered as "noise" in most ERP experiments) are typically larger than the waves of interest. The principle of computer averaging requires that both the waveshape of the ERP and its temporal relationship to the time-locking reference event (stimulus or response event) remain constant from one occurrence to the next. Since the EEG fluctuations are not time-locked to the reference event, they will average out to zero when the ERPs from successive trials are added together by the computer. (See Goff, 1974, for details of recording and averaging techniques.)

The ERPs of the human brain may be classified in various ways. The traditional distinction has been between the early, modality-specific waves that are evoked in the classical sensory pathways by a stimulus, and the later, "nonspecific" waves that are engendered in more widespread areas and are more subject to psychological or cognitive influences. For present purposes, however, it is more appropriate to group ERPs into three categories according to whether they are primarily determined by "exogenous" stimulus events, by "endogenous" cognitive processes, or by some combination of these factors. In the first category are most of the sensory evoked potentials (EPs), which represent the summated electric fields from the synchronous activation of neuronal populations by an external stimulus event. The spatiotemporal configuration of an EP is determined by the integrity and organization of the sensory receptors and pathways involved, and by the physical properties of the stimulus. The EPs are, by definition, rather impervious to variations of the psychological state of the observer. At the other extreme is the class of "endogenous" ERPs, which are coupled with perceptual, cognitive, and motor processes in the brain. Endogenous ERPs are frequently triggered by external stimulus events, but their waveform and timing are determined by the particular cognitive processes activated by the stimulus rather than by its modality or physical properties. Among the endogenous ERPs that have been well studied (Donchin *et al.,* 1978) are the "contingent negative variation" (a slow potential shift which arises during periods of expectancy and response preparation), the "motor potentials" (cortical activity preceding and accompanying voluntary movements), and the P_3 or P_{300} wave (which is correlated with certain decision processes). Intermediate between the purely evoked and the purely emitted ERPs is a class of stimulus-evoked components which may vary in amplitude and/or latency as a function of psychological variables; the "vertex potentials," which are late cortical waves evoked by stimuli in all modalities, have these properties.

Figure 1 illustrates these different classes of ERPs in the auditory modality. The top panel shows the characteristic sequence of components which can be recorded from the scalp following an abrupt sound such as a click. In the first 8 msec after the click are a series of six or seven discrete waves (numbered I–VI) which represent the far fields of evoked neuronal activity in the auditory pathways of the brain stem (Jewett and Williston, 1971). These brain stem EPs are sensitive to stimulus parameters, including intensity, rise time, and repetition rate (Pratt and Sohmer, 1976; Hyde *et al.,* 1976; Hecox *et al.,* 1976), but do not change appreciably with changes of state such as sleep (Amadeo and Shagass, 1973) or deep, barbiturate-induced narcosis (Starr and Achor, 1975). Following the brain

347

ELECTRO-
PHYSIOLOGICAL
ANALYSIS OF
HUMAN BRAIN
FUNCTION

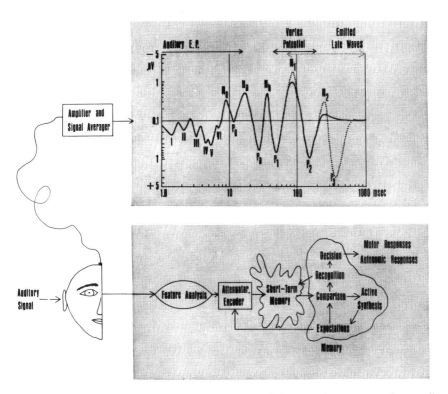

Fig. 1. The dual domains of the ERP approach to neuropsychology. In the upper panel, an auditory signal (click) elicits a stereotyped sequence of evoked and endogenous components at characteristic latencies as indicated on the abscissa. Dotted lines signify ERP components, which vary as a function of information-processing demands. The lower panel illustrates some hypothetical "stages" of processing which may be related to components in the electrophysiological domain, although not necessarily according to their relative positions in this diagram.

stem EP is a series of waves (N_0, P_0, N_a, P_a, N_b) which probably represent a combination of evoked neural activity outside the classical auditory pathway and reflex myogenic activity (Picton *et al.*, 1974; Goff *et al.*, 1978). To date, the primary EP which can be recorded directly from the auditory cortex (Heschl's gyrus) in man (Celesia, 1976) has not been positively identified in scalp recordings.

Between 50 and 250 msec after the stimulus, a series of characteristic cortical waves (P_1, N_1, P_2, N_2) arises which has been termed the "vertex potential" because it is largest at the center of the scalp near the vertex (Fig. 2). Vertex potentials are similar in morphology for visual, auditory, and somatic stimulation (Davis *et al.*, 1972) and, unlike the earlier evoked components, vary in amplitude as a function of alertness level, arousal, and selective attention. Finally, the emitted late wave known as the P_3 or P_{300} (a positive deflection with a latency of around 300 msec, dotted line in Fig. 1) occurs only when the auditory stimulus conveys certain kinds of information that require a decision from the subject (see below).

The lower panel of Fig. 1 depicts a hypothetical sequence of "processing stages" of the sort which have been postulated in various psychological models of human perception and performance (Hillyard and Picton, 1978). One of the basic goals of current psychophysiological research with ERPs is to clarify the relationship between the upper realm of electrophysiological events and the lower realm of psychological constructs which are thought to be operating within the same time frame.

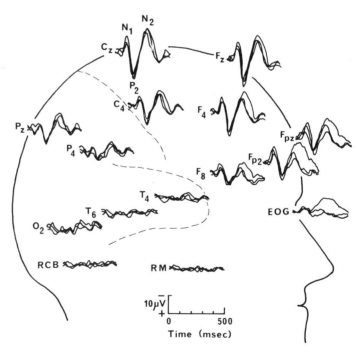

Fig. 2. Scalp distribution of the auditory EP to tone pips presented once every 2.5 sec at 60 dB SL. Electrodes were placed according to the International 10-20 system with a noncephalic (sternocervical) reference. Note that the components of the "vertex potential" (N_1, P_2, N_2) are largest at the vertex (C_z) and midline frontal (F_z) scalp sites. Based on Hillyard and Picton (1978).

SENSORY EVOKED POTENTIALS, PERCEPTUAL DEFICITS, AND
NEUROLOGICAL DISORDERS

349

ELECTRO-
PHYSIOLOGICAL
ANALYSIS OF
HUMAN BRAIN
FUNCTION

Certain EP components can be elicited with a high degree of reliability within a population of normal subjects. Since the "exogenous" EPs are not sensitive to variables of psychological state, deviations from the normal range are strongly indicative of a structural abnormality in the receptor apparatus or sensory pathways. Two varieties of EPs have proven to be especially valuable in assessing the integrity of sensory systems: the auditory brain stem EP and the cortical EP to a patterned visual stimulus.

AUDITORY EPs FROM THE BRAIN STEM

The generators of the successive waves of the auditory brain stem EP have been fairly well localized on the basis of studies of patients with discrete lesions of the brain stem and studies of animals (Jewett, 1970; Buchwald and Huang, 1975; Starr and Hamilton, 1976; Stockard and Rossiter, 1977). Wave I (see Fig. 1) consists of the summated action potentials evoked from fibers of the auditory nerve; wave II most likely originates from the cochlear nuclei, wave III from the superior olivary complex, waves IV and V from the midbrain (probably from the lateral lemniscus and inferior colliculus, respectively), and wave VI from above the midbrain level (perhaps the medial geniculate nucleus). Since the normal range of latency variation of these waves is quite narrow (± 0.2–0.3 msec) in response to a standard click stimulus, delayed or missing components are indicative of dysfunction at specific levels of the brain stem. Thus the flow of auditory information can be "tracked" through the brain stem with a high degree of temporal and spatial resolution.

HEARING DISORDERS. The brain stem EPs provide a sensitive and objective means of assessing hearing deficiences due to impairment of sound conduction to the cochlea, as well as cochlear and retrocochlear disorders (Davis, 1976; Yamada et al., 1975; Galambos and Hecox, 1977; Sohmer and Feinmesser, 1973; Terkildsen et al., 1973). This technique of "brain stem audiometry" involves plotting the latency of the brain stem EPs as a function of stimulus intensity. As shown in Fig. 3, there are characteristic delays and diminution of all components as signal intensity is reduced to near threshold levels. Wave V is typically the most prominent component, and its latency can be readily quantified. In normal individuals, the plot of wave V latency vs. click intensity is highly consistent (Fig. 4, shaded area). Delays of wave V are indicative of the degree of hearing loss, which is tested one ear at a time. This technique can also differentiate between conductive hearing loss, where wave V latency is delayed throughout the intensity range (subject CL, Fig. 4), and sensorineural hearing loss, where the wave V latency is "recruited" into the normal range at high intensities (subject TR).

The brain stem EPs seem to be primarily initiated in the high-frequency (basal) zone of the cochlea in adults (Hecox, 1975) and thus may not be sensitive to selective loss of hearing in the low frequencies (below 1000 Hz). Recent developments, however, indicate that frequency-specific EPs to sinusoidal tones can also be recorded from the brain stem which should enable the evaluation of hearing across the entire frequency spectrum (Suzuki *et al.*, 1977; Huis in't Veld *et al.*, 1977; Stillman *et al.*, 1976; Marsh *et al.*, 1975).

Brain stem audiometry has proven to be of particular value in testing the hearing of very young infants in whom behavioral tests are difficult to apply. The latency/intensity functions for wave V show a steady maturation over the first 2 years of life, and delays of wave V in relation to the age-dependent norms are indicative of hearing disorder (Hecox and Galambos, 1974; Salamy *et al.*, 1975; Schulman-Galambos and Galambos, 1975; Davis, 1976; Mokotoff *et al.*, 1977).

Neurological Disorders. A number of neurological conditions which impinge on the central auditory pathways alter the brain stem EPs in a characteristic fashion. Tumors of the cerebellopontine angle (in or near the auditory nerve), for instance, produce a delay or diminution of all EP components beyond wave I and, in many cases, a delay of wave I itself (Starr and Hamilton, 1976; Rosenhamer, 1977; Terkildsen *et al.*, 1977). EP abnormalities may be present in cases

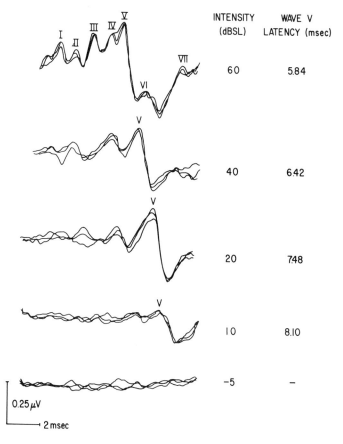

Fig. 3. Brain stem EPs recorded to clicks of different intensities. Note that the latency of all components increases as signal strength is weakened. This is seen most clearly for wave V. From Galambos and Hecox (1977).

351

ELECTRO-
PHYSIOLOGICAL
ANALYSIS OF
HUMAN BRAIN
FUNCTION

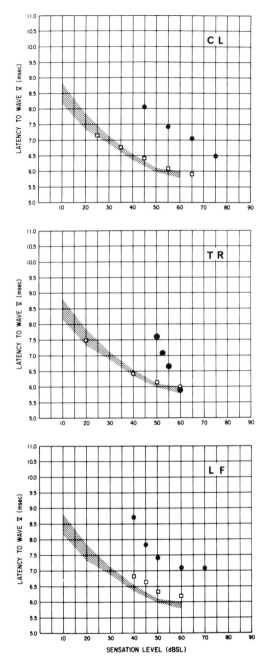

Fig. 4. Progressive shortening of wave V latency as a function of increasing click intensity in three patients with predominantly unilateral hearing loss. The shaded area shows the range of this latency-intensity function in normal hearing adults. □, Wave V latencies for the nonaffected ear; ●, same for affected ear. Patient CL has a conductive loss; TR has a flat sensorineural loss due to Ménière's disease; LF has a sensorineural loss that is severe above 2000 Hz. From Galambos and Hecox (1977).

STEVEN A. HILLYARD
AND DAVID L. WOODS

where a hearing loss is not demonstrable by conventional audiology. Tumors, infarcts, or demyelinating diseases affecting higher levels of the brain stem produce changes in EP components that are diagnostic of the level of the lesion (Starr and Achor, 1975; Stockard and Rossiter, 1977). Thus an infarction affecting the caudal pons leaves waves I and II intact, but the subsequent components are prolonged. With a lesion of the rostral pons or midbrain, waves I, II, and III are normal, but waves IV and V are delayed or absent (Fig. 5), etc.

In patients with suspected multiple sclerosis (MS) or other demyelinating disease, abnormal delays were observed in the brain stem EP components even when no clinical brain stem signs were present (Starr and Achor, 1975; Stockard and Rossiter, 1977). This verification of brain stem pathology through EP recordings was a valuable diagnostic aid in determining whether multiple CNS sites were affected (pointing toward a diagnosis of MS). Recovery of EP latencies toward normal was observed in cases of MS which were clinically improved by treatment with steroids. Thus EP recordings may be used as an objective monitor of the effectiveness of therapeutic regimes for treating MS (as well as other brain stem pathologies).

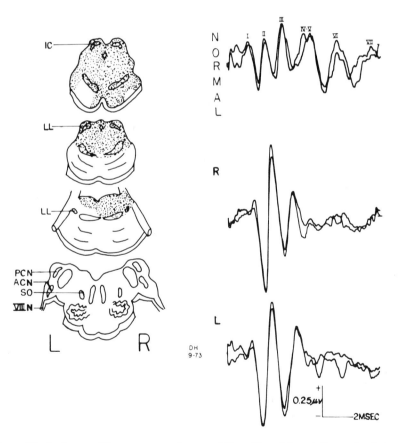

Fig. 5. Loss of the brain stem EP components after wave III to either right or left ear stimulation (lower pair of tracings) in a patient with a tumor involving the midbrain and upper pons (stippled area on cross-sections). Exaggerated wave II is suggestive of a "release" from higher influences due to lesion. From Starr and Hamilton (1976).

Further clinical uses of these auditory EPs from the brain stem include the differentiation between coma of drug or metabolic origin (EPs may be normal) and coma due to structural damage to the brain stem (EPs altered). The permanent absence of waves II–VI is associated with irreversible coma and hence can be used to supplement EEG findings in the determination of "brain death" (Starr, 1976).

353

ELECTRO-
PHYSIOLOGICAL
ANALYSIS OF
HUMAN BRAIN
FUNCTION

VISUAL EPS TO PATTERNED STIMULI

Until recently, the diffuse flash of a stroboscope has been the standard stimulus for clinical and experimental studies of the visual EP in man. The scalp-recorded EP to a diffuse flash is a complicated series of positive and negative deflections, with some components localized over the occipital region and others arising from widely distributed sources (Allison *et al.,* 1977*b*). The clinical applicability of flash EPs has been severely handicapped, however, by the extreme variability of morphology and distribution among subjects. Although some clinical correlations with visual system pathology have been described (Starr, 1977), it has proven very difficult to establish definite criteria of whether or not a given individual's EP is abnormal.

The occipital EP to the onset or reversal of a patterned stimulus (such as a line grating or a checkerboard) is generally more robust and consistent in its componentry across subjects than is the diffuse-flash EP (Halliday *et al.,* 1973). This accords with the well-known receptive field properties of visual cortical neurons, being preferentially activated by linear light-dark boundaries rather than by diffuse light. The use of patterned stimuli also allows for the testing of more complex and naturalistic perceptual functions than is possible with simple flashes.

The EP to a pattern of lines shows orientation specificity, as if it were being generated by a population of cortical "line detector" neurons; the EPs to oblique lines are smaller than those to vertical and horizontal lines (visual anistropy): and the response to lines of a specific orientation or spatial frequency can be "adapted out" by prior exposure (Maffei and Campbell, 1970; Campbell and Maffei, 1970). Visual EPs in man are also indicative of a permanent loss of sensitivity for detecting lines of a particular orientation due to early astigmatism (Freeman and Thibos, 1973), an effect which probably results from a loss of orientation-specific cortical neurons due to improverished visual experience of sharp lines along the axis of the astigmatism (e.g., Blakemore, 1974; Hirsch and Jacobson, 1975). The EPs to check stimuli in man also show binocular and stereoscopic interactions similiar to those observed for single neurons in the visual cortex of animals (Regan, 1972). These findings indicate that scalp-recorded EPs to patterned stimuli in man offer rather direct access to the functioning of binocular, orientation-specific neurons of the occipital cortex.

PATTERN EPS AND VISUAL ACUITY. The occipital EP to a fluctuating checkerboard stimulus is a function of the size of the checks, the retinal eccentricity of their presentation, and, most significantly, the sharpness of focus of the retinal image. For smaller-sized foveal checks (under 20′ of arc), the amplitudes of certain EP components decline progressively as the retinal image is defocused from the emmetropic condition (e.g., Harter and White, 1970; Ludlam and Meyers, 1972).

Using this principle, the amount of refractive (and astigmatic) error in a patient can be determined rapidly (Regan, 1973) and used as a basis for the fitting of corrective lenses. Loss of visual acuity resulting from strabismus (amblyopia ex anopsia) can also be evaluated readily using the pattern-shift EP (Spekreijse *et al.,* 1972; Regan, 1975, 1977). This method may prove especially valuable for objective assessment of improvements in the amblyopia resulting from visual therapy.

Reduced visual acuity caused by insults to the occipital lobe can also be assessed by EPs. In a patient recovering from "cerebral blindness," Bodis-Wollner (1977) found a close parallel between the ability to detect fine gratings (of high spatial frequency) and the appearance of EPs to those gratings.

PATTERN EPs AND COLOR VISION. A reversing checkerboard in which the alternate checks differ in color is a very effective stimulus for selective stimulation of the different cone populations. By recording EPs to such stimuli, the spectral sensitivities of the red, green, and blue cone "channels" can be objectively determined (Regan, 1974). If the adjacent checks are made red and green and equated for luminosity, their reversal provides a purely chromatic (hue) stimulus to the visual system. For color-blind subjects (protanopes or deuteranopes), the EP to this checkerboard drops precipitously when the red-green luminosities are precisely balanced (Regan and Spekreijse, 1974; Estevez *et al.,* 1975). In general, the EPs to colored checkerboards are greatly attenuated when the alternate checks are hues that are confused by the color-blind individual (Kinney and McKay, 1974).

NEUROLOGICAL DISORDERS OF THE VISUAL PATHWAYS. The occipital EP to a reversing checkerboard stimulus (with check sizes ranging between 15' and 50' of arc) has a rather simple morphology, consisting of a prominent positive peak at about 100 msec (depending on subject age and the exact stimulus parameters), preceded and followed by negative peaks. The latency of this positive wave is a very stable feature of this EP, having a standard deviation of the order of 4–7 msec (Halliday *et al.,* 1973; Asselman *et al.,* 1975; Celesia and Daly, 1977). Halliday and co-workers (1972, 1973) were the first to demonstrate that an abnormal delay of this positive component (by more than $2\frac{1}{2}$ standard deviations) was a consistent finding in patients with pathology affecting the optic nerve. Figure 6 (Halliday, 1972) illustrates a delayed positive deflection in the right eye of a patient having multiple sclerosis, in comparison with the normal EP obtained via stimulation of her left eye. This demonstration of optic nerve involvement was instrumental in establishing a diagnosis of multiple sclerosis, since this patient had a variety of other sensory symptoms that were attributable to a hysterical overlay.

In the last 5 years, it has been firmly established that the pattern-shift EP is delayed or greatly attenuated in a variety of disease processes affecting the optic nerve, including compression by tumor, optic atrophy, ischemic neuropathy, demyelination, and optic or retrobulbar neuritis (Asselman *et al.,* 1975; Halliday *et. al.,* 1976; Regan *et al.,* 1976; Celesia and Daly, 1978; Starr *et al.,* 1978). The clinical importance of this EP test derives from its great sensitivity; the major positive wave is often delayed in suspected cases of optic nerve pathology even when the patients' visual functioning is completely normal by standard examinations (visual fields, acuity, fundi). In particular, a delayed pattern-shift EP may give crucial diagnostic information for establishing that multiple demyelinating

355

ELECTRO-
PHYSIOLOGICAL
ANALYSIS OF
HUMAN BRAIN
FUNCTION

lesions are present in suspected cases of multiple sclerosis. Recovery of a delayed or otherwise abnormal EP can also be used to quantify the effects of various therapeutic interventions (Halliday *et al.*, 1976).

Halliday *et al.* have noted that amplitude (rather than latency) changes are more prevalent in cases of optic pathway compression, while longer latencies are characteristic of demyelinating diseases; they suggest that loss of amplitude may result from blocked conduction in nerve fibers, while EP delays may result from slowing of conduction through regions of demyelination.

The evaluation of postchiasmatic lesions of the visual pathway is more complicated, since the latency and morphology of the pattern shift EP are frequently unaltered in patients with substantial homonymous hemianopsia (Asselman *et al.*, 1975; Starr *et al.*, 1978). In such cases, however, the lateral distribution of the EP across the posterior scalp in response to patterned stimulation of the right and left hemifields may be altered (Halliday *et al.*, 1976). The scalp distribution of EPs to hemifield stimulation has been thoroughly studied in normal subjects (Jeffreys and Axford, 1972; Barrett *et al.*, 1976; Shagass *et al.*, 1976), providing a baseline for a more precise localization of postchiasmatic lesions in future studies. Jeffreys and Axford, for instance, have identified specific components of striate and extrastriate origin in the pattern EP.

ERPs and Selective Information Processing

The perceptual experience produced by a given stimulus event does not remain invariant from one presentation to the next, but varies with the momentary state of the subject—his attentiveness, level of arousal, motivation, etc. The

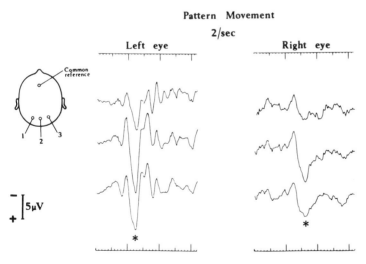

Fig. 6. EPs to a pattern shift recorded from three posterior scalp sites in a patient suspected of having multiple sclerosis. The prominent positive wave of the EP (asterisk) is within the normal latency range when the left eye is stimulated but is delayed for right eye stimulation. Time base: 320 msec total analysis time. From Halliday (1972).

neural processing of a stimulus may be cursory and superficial or detailed and elaborate, depending on how it fits in with the task at hand. Such task-related variations of processing are associated with certain endogenous ERPs appearing on the scalp. Despite our general ignorance of their cerebral origins (Goff *et al.*, 1978), these ERPs offer the only technically feasible approach (at present) to the neurophysiological activities of the human brain as it processes information on a millisecond-to-millisecond basis. In this section, we shall consider how ERP evidence may be used to clarify mechanisms of attention, recognition, decision-making, and other selective cognitive activities, both from physiological and from psychological standpoints.

THEORIES OF SELECTIVE ATTENTION

The normal human brain is equipped with powerful attentional control systems for regulating its responsiveness to selected features of the environment. By definition, selective attentional processes are those which facilitate the processing of one stimulus class in relation to stimuli that are not being attended. Selective processes may be contrasted with arousal and alerting mechanisms which exert a more general facilitatory influence on sensory processing and affect a wide range of inputs nonselectively (Kahneman, 1973). Changes in levels of arousal and wakefulness produce dramatic changes in certain late ERP components (e.g., Picton *et al.*, 1976), but these nonselective effects will not be considered here.

Psychological theories of attention differ according to whether the locus of selectivity is placed at an "early" or a "late" stage of processing. Some models propose an early stage of selection which gives preferential access to stimuli belonging to an attended "channel"* (i.e., stimuli which share some simple cue characteristic such as position in space, pitch, or hue). According to this view, stimuli in unattended channels are rejected after a rapid initial analysis of their channel cues by a hypothesized "filter" or "attenuator" (also known as stimulus set) mechanism (Triesman, 1964; Broadbent, 1970, 1971). Following this initial filtering, material in the attended channel is analyzed along more complex cognitive or semantic dimensions and is compared with stored information in memory. Many variants of this multistage model have been proposed, but all have in common an early "channel selection" mechanism (stimulus set) and a subsequent memory-dependent (response set) mode of selection (e.g., Kahneman, 1973; Keren, 1976).

The theoretical necessity of an "early" mode of selection has been questioned by a number of other authors (e.g., Deutsch and Deutsch, 1963; Moray, 1975; Norman and Bobrow, 1975; Shiffrin *et al.*, 1976). In their formulations, sensory processing becomes selective only at higher memory and decision-making levels and only when the task at hand places a heavy load on the overall processing capacity of the system. Attention is regarded in terms of the selective allocation of "processing resources" to the chosen stimulus or task; when the limited resources

---

*The term "channel" shall be used here to refer to a class of stimuli which have in common such a *simple* sensory cue. In most cases, a channel can be defined as stimuli which fall on a particular zone of receptor surface or a particular receptor population.

357

ELECTRO-
PHYSIOLOGICAL
ANALYSIS OF
HUMAN BRAIN
FUNCTION

are fully occupied, further inputs cannot be processed as effectively. Some models of attention make use of both the hierarchical-stages notion and the concept of resource allocation (Kahneman, 1973).

ERPs and Psychological Constructs

There are a number of ways in which ERPs can contribute to the experimental analysis of attention mechanisms. First, the spatial and temporal localization of ERPs gives an indication of which levels of the sensory pathways participate in stimulus selection. Changes in subcortical EP components, for instance, would provide support for the hypothesis of efferent control (gating) of the peripheral sensory pathways as a mechanism of attention (Hernandez-Peon, 1966). More generally, if distinctive ERP configurations were found to be associated with different modes of attention (e.g., stimulus set selections vs. memory-dependent selections), this would tend to validate such conceptual distinctions. In other words, ERP measures can serve as "converging operations" (Garner *et al.*, 1956), with behavioral measures to strengthen, differentiate, and delimit concepts of selective processing. The temporal relations of ERP components so identified can yield additional clues about the timing and ordering of intermediate stages of information processing, thus cross-validating the inferences that can be made from reaction-time studies (Sternberg, 1969; Vaughan and Ritter, 1973). Finally, ERPs offer a means of measuring the extent and depth of processing of stimuli in an unattended channel, an issue of current theoretical controversy (Moray, 1975; Shiffrin *et al.*, 1976).

Vertex Potentials and Selective Attention

The earliest components that have so far been demonstrated to vary systematically with the direction of attention are the N_1 and P_2 waves of the vertex potential, the former beginning at a latency of about 50 msec in the auditory modality. Picton and Hillyard (1974) reported that the N_1-P_2 evoked by repetitive clicks was enhanced when the clicks were attended (in comparison to when they were ignored), while all the components prior to 50 msec remained stable (Fig. 7). In a more demanding dichotic listening task, Woods and Hillyard (1978) similarly found that the brain stem EPs to right and left ear clicks did not change when attention was switched between the ears. Accordingly, there has been no evidence to date for efferent gating in the human auditory system, despite recent suggestive evidence for such processes in animals (Oatman, 1971; Olesen *et al.*, 1975).

A number of studies over the past 15 years have confirmed that the N_1-P_2 complex is enhanced when attention is shifted to the evoking stimuli (for reviews, see Karlin, 1970; Näätänen, 1975; Hillyard and Picton, 1978). These reviewers have emphasized, however, that most of the earlier studies were not designed properly for demonstrating that these ERP changes were true correlates of selective attention. More recent studies have employed appropriate control procedures, including randomized presentation of relevant and irrelevant stimuli (to rule out the effects of general arousal/alertness), maintenance of a constant peripheral stimulus across conditions, and concurrent recordings of behavioral and ERP measures of attention (for a methodological discussion, see Hillyard and Picton, 1978). Under these controlled conditions, many investigators reported little or no influence on the N_1-P_2 waves of shifting attention from one channel to another, raising doubts about the sensitivity of these waves to selective attention (for reviews, see Näätänen, 1967, 1975).

Wilkinson and Lee (1972) suggested that these negative results might have occurred because the stimuli were delivered so slowly that subjects were not forced to attend selectively to one channel at a time. Following up this idea, Hillyard et al. (1973) loaded subjects so heavily with stimulus information as to make it difficult to attend to all the stimuli at once; sequences of tone pips were presented to the right and left ears in random order at a rapid rate (interstimulus intervals of 100–800 msec). The two channels of tones differed in pitch (800 vs. 1500 Hz) as well as ear of delivery to make them more distinctive. Subjects were required to attend to one ear at a time, reporting the occurrences of occasional "targets" that were slightly higher in pitch. As shown in Fig. 8, the amplitude of the N_1 wave (but not P_2) to attended-channel tones was enlarged by 30–50%, an effect observed consistently in all 20 subjects. Hillyard et al. suggested that this differential N_1 amplitude between attended- and unattended-channel tones might be an electrophysiological sign of a stimulus set (filter) mode of attention.

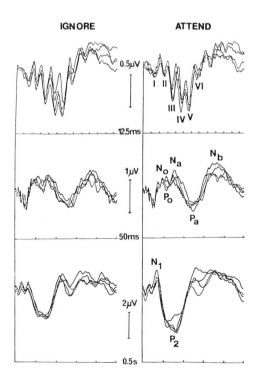

Fig. 7. Averaged ERPs to 60 dB SL clicks presented at 1/sec shown on short (10 msec), medium (50 msec), and long (500 msec) time bases. ERPs on left were taken while the subject read a book, and ERPs on right were obtained when he was listening intently to the repetitive click train, with the goal of detecting an occasional diminution of click intensity. After Picton and Hillyard (1974).

359

ELECTRO-
PHYSIOLOGICAL
ANALYSIS OF
HUMAN BRAIN
FUNCTION

Further studies by Schwent and collaborators (Schwent and Hillyard, 1975; Schwent *et al.*, 1976*a,b*) explored the experimental parameters which optimize the auditory N_1 wave as a measure of attention. They ascertained that the N_1 wave was maximally differentiated between attended and irrelevant channels of input when stimuli were delivered (1) at very rapid rates, (2) from multiple channels, (3) at moderate to low loudness levels, and (4) against a masking background of white noise. These results are consistent with the hypothesis that this mode of attention operates effectively only when the subject's processing resources are severely taxed by competing information in different channels. In the theoretical framework proposed by Kahneman (1973) and by Norman and Bobrow (1975), the interchannel distribution of N_1 may index the allocation of limited attentional resources to the appropriate channel to achieve optimal performance. In support of this idea, we have found that the N_1 wave was allocated equally between two channels in a divided attention task, and the total N_1 output remained constant across conditions of divided and focused attention (Hink *et al.*, 1977).

To test whether the N_1 is a general sign of stimulus set attention, Schwent *et al.* (1976*c*) used different combinations of simple physical cues to distinguish among three channels of tones. In different conditions, the channels were separated by spatial cues alone (one frequency at right, center, and left locations), by pitch cues alone (three different frequencies at a central location), and by both

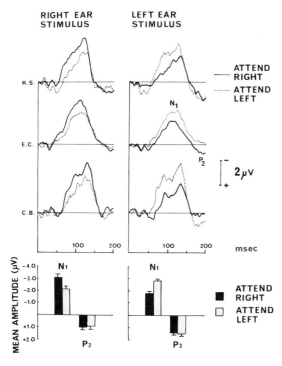

Fig. 8. Averaged ERPs to right ear tone pips (of 1500 Hz) and left ear tone pips (of 800 Hz) delivered in random order to three different subjects. In one condition, subjects attended to right ear tones (solid tracings) and in the other they listened to the left ear tones (dotted tracings). Vertex to mastoid recordings. Lower bar graphs show mean amplitudes (over ten subjects) of N_1 and P_2 components to tones in either ear as a function of direction of attention. From Hillyard *et al.* (1973).

STEVEN A. HILLYARD
AND DAVID L. WOODS

cues together. Subjects attended to one channel at a time, pressing a lever each time they detected an occasional target tone of slightly longer duration. As shown in Fig. 9, focusing attention on a channel enhanced the N_1 wave to the stimuli therein, except for the "center" channels in the single-cue conditions. This failure of selective attention in the central channels was also manifested behaviorally (target detectability was reduced) and was overcome when dual cues were provided (Fig. 9, bottom row). The results of Schwent *et al.* suggest that focusing attention on acoustic channel enhances the N_1 in a similar fashion whether simple pitch or spatial cues define the channels, as would be expected if N_1 were an index of an early, stimulus-set type of attention.

Further studies have indicated that N_1 amplitude provides an index of selective attention between channels of more complex and meaningful sounds such as syllables, environmental sounds, and natural speech (Hink and Hillyard, 1976; Hink *et al.*, 1977, 1978). Again, the critical factor seemed to be that the channels be distinguished by simple physical cues. Thus the focusing of attention on the pitch-spatial attributes of a message was associated with enhancement of the N_1 to all stimuli having those attributes (i.e., belonging to the same channel).

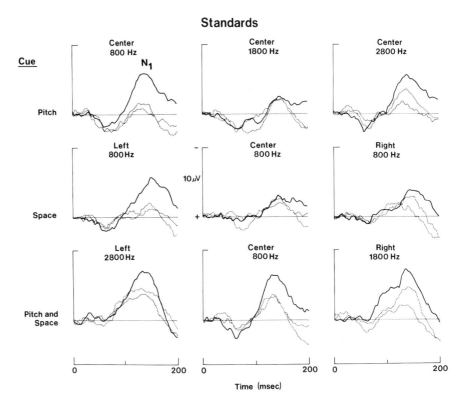

Fig. 9. Effects of channel-selective attention on the N_1 wave to 40-msec (nontarget) tones presented in random order from one of three channels. Top row: ERPs when channels are distinguished only by pitch cues. Middle row: Only spatial cues are present. Bottom row: Both pitch and spatial cues are present. Each group of three overlaid tracings shows ERPs to one channel when it was attended (solid lines) and when attention was directed to another channel (dotted lines). From Schwent *et al.* (1976c).

There is also some evidence that the N_1 wave evoked at the vertex (at 130–170 msec) by somatosensory or visual stimuli may be enhanced when attention is focused on a channel in those modalities (e.g., on a position in visual space or a location on the body) (Debecker, 1967; Eason *et al.*, 1969; Van Voorhis and Hillyard, 1977). It is an intriguing possibility that this incremented negativity in the range of 60–200 msec (depending on modality and stimulus parameters) may represent the activity of a general attentional system for selecting among the available channels of input, if the cues for selection are simple and rapidly analyzable (Hillyard *et al.*, 1978). In contrast, when cues for selection were made more complex (e.g., selections between visual or acoustic patterns presented at a fixed spatial location), the N_1 wave was not differentiated between attended and inattended stimuli (Harter and Salmon, 1972; Chapman, 1973; Hink *et al.*, 1978; Friedman *et al.*, 1975*a*). It remains to be seen, however, what range of stimulus and task situations are conducive to the modulation of N_1 as a function of attention, and whether or not this electrophysiological sign will remain convergent with the behaviorally defined stimulus set mode of attention.

361

ELECTRO-
PHYSIOLOGICAL
ANALYSIS OF
HUMAN BRAIN
FUNCTION

THE P_3 WAVE AND SELECTIVE ATTENTION

In most of the aforementioned studies of multichannel attention, subjects were told to detect infrequent "target" stimuli in one of the channels. The ERP associated with the detection of a target contains a characteristic "P_3" or "P_{300}" component peaking at around 300–400 msec after the stimulus. In the Schwent *et al.* (1976*c*) study, for example, the targets (of slightly longer duration) elicited a P_3 wave when they occurred in an attended channel (Fig. 10, solid lines) but not when attention was shifted away from that channel (dotted lines).

The same type of P_3 wave is emitted on detection of target stimuli of any modality or type, provided that certain conditions are met. First, the subject must be actively attending and discriminating the targets from the nontargets. Second, the targets must require a different response (either overt or covert) or have a different meaning than the nontargets. The specific nature of the response (e.g., counting or lever pressing) does not seem to be very important. Finally, the P_3 is elicited to the target stimulus with an amplitude that is proportional to how unexpectedly it occurs among the nontargets. K. Squires *et al.* (1973, 1975) proposed that P_3 occurs in tasks where the subject is "set" to make a particular response to each of the relevant stimulus alternatives; the P_3 amplitude is then determined by the likelihood of occurrence of that stimulus-response ensemble and the confidence with which the detection is made.

There is no general agreement about the exact properties of the psychological correlates of the P_3 wave. Various authors have suggested that P_3 may be a sign of decision making (Smith *et al.*, 1970), uncertainty resolution (Sutton *et al.*, 1965), delivery of task-relevant information (Sutton *et al.*, 1967), shifting of response strategies (Karlin and Martz, 1973), or readjustment of cognitive strategies in preparation for future trials (Donchin *et al.*, 1978). Here, we only wish to emphasize how the P_3 wave relates to stimulus selection processes. First, it should be noted that P_3 is emitted in the same manner (and with the same posterior scalp distribution) to target stimuli of any modality and complexity. The target cue may be as simple as an intensity shift or as complicated as a number intermixed with letters, one visual pattern among others, or a word that is a synonym of a key word (Chapman, 1973; Donchin *et al.*, 1978). From this, it would appear that identification of a target and emission of P_3 require a rather full analysis of the stimulus in comparison with a reference vocabulary or conceptual categories in memory. Thus P_3 is dependent on selective perceptual processes for identifying particular relevant stimuli in relation to the subject's expectancies and memorized stimulus categories. This type of process seems closely related to Broadbent's "response set" (memory-dependent) mode of selective attention.

If the discrimination of the target from nontarget is made more difficult or complex, there are parallel increases in P_3 latency and in reaction-time (RT) measures of decision speed (Ritter *et al.*, 1972; Donchin *et al.*, 1978). By making target stimuli more unpredictable, however, RTs can be delayed significantly without changing the latency of P_3 (e.g., Karlin and Martz, 1973; K. Squires *et al.*, 1976). This suggests that P_3 is triggered at or near the point of target identification, but before the response is initiated. Thus P_3 latency gives a measure of the speed with which a subject discriminates the target, matches that information against stimulus categories in memory, and arrives at the appropriate decision.

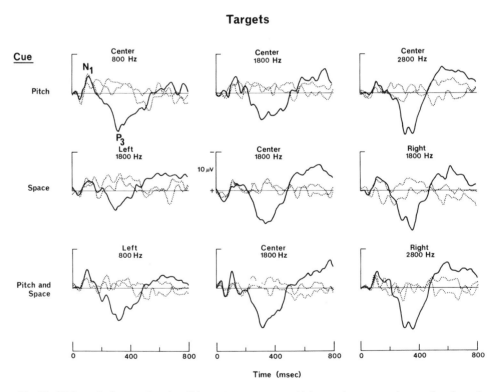

Fig. 10. ERPs to the longer-duration (70-msec) target tones which were interspersed at random in each of the three channels in the Schwent *et al.* (1976c) study. Subjects were required to press a button each time a target was detected. Solid lines are ERPs to targets when the channel was attended and dotted lines are ERPs to the same stimuli when attention was directed to another channel.

ERPs AND "STAGES" OF SELECTION

363

ELECTRO-
PHYSIOLOGICAL
ANALYSIS OF
HUMAN BRAIN
FUNCTION

There is ample evidence that the N_1 and P_3 waves are indices of different selective processes which can be readily dissociated. For instance, these waves are differently affected by the variables of stimulus intensity, repetition rate, and probability. It is also clear that target discriminations within a channel of stimuli can influence P_3 while leaving N_1 invariant, whereas selections between different channels can alter N_1 without affecting P_3 amplitudes (e.g., Harter and Salmon, 1972; Picton *et al.*, 1974). In situations where a subject must select between two (or more) channels and then select out targets within one of the channels, the N_1 and P_3 waves behave as if they were signs of hierarchical stages of selection. That is, all stimuli in the attended channel (targets and nontargets alike) elicit enhanced N_1 waves, but only the attended targets elicit a P_3 wave (Hillyard *et al.*, 1973; Hink *et al.*, 1978).

This ERP configuration suggests that recognition of a target in one channel in the presence of competing inputs from other channels involves two distinct stages of selection. Stimuli are selected first on the basis of their simple physical attributes (stimulus set), with targets and nontargets processed equivalently, as indexed by N_1. Following this initial selection of a channel, stimuli are examined for their target properties in relation to memorized categories (response set). These distinctive properties of the N_1 and P_3 waves thus appear to converge with the Broadbent/Triesman concept of two hierarchically ordered stages of attention. Also consistent with this model is the electrophysiological evidence that stimuli in the rejected channel(s) are not processed so fully as attended material (N_1 waves are smaller and P_3 waves are generally absent in the unattended channels) (Fig. 10), despite Moray's (1975) behavioral evidence to the contrary.

Late Positive ERPs and the Orienting Response

Stimuli which occur as striking deviations from a monotonous background may at times elicit late positive waves (latency 200–400 msec) even though they have not been assigned any task relevance. For instance, if a subject is reading a book and ignoring a background of repetitive tone pips, an occasional shift in their pitch or intensity may elicit an early "P_{3a}" wave (at 220–250 msec) which has a more anterior distribution on the scalp than the P_3 associated with active target detection (N. Squires *et al.*, 1975). Since this P_{3a} was elicited by deviant sounds whether or not they were relevant, N. Squires *et al.* suggested that this wave might be a correlate of "a basic sensory mechanism which registers any change in a background stimulus, perhaps by means of mis-matching a specific neural model (Sokolov) that is established by repetition of the background." This concept was supported by the results of Snyder and Hillyard (1976), who found that isolated stimuli did not elicit a P_{3a} as effectively as did a deviation from a monotonous background. It appears, then, that the P_{3a} may be a sign of an orientation response toward an unexpected shift in a steady acoustic background.

Another variety of P_3 wave was observed when novel visual stimuli were interposed in a monotonous background of numerical stimuli which the subject was counting (Courchesne *et al.*, 1975; Courchesne, 1977). These unrecognizable, jumbled "nonsense shapes" elicited very large P_3 waves (at about 380 msec) that also had a maximum amplitude over the frontal scalp. This frontal P_3 habituated rapidly on repeated presentations of the novel slides, as would be expected if this wave were a component of an orienting response.

CLINICAL RELEVANCE OF ERP APPROACHES

If it can be established that ERPs are signs of particular attentional processes, these measures could be used to characterize deficiencies of attention that are reportedly associated with conditions such as schizophrenia, learning and perceptual disorders, and with normal aging. These are several reasons to believe that ERP assessments of attention might contribute useful information to supplement that obtainable from behavioral testing. Most importantly, the subject's ability to focus (or divide) his attention in a multiple stimulus array can be evaluated without the requirement of obtaining behavioral measures of attention to all the stimulus categories. The capacity for selective processing can thus be probed without the confounding that would arise if discriminative responses had to be made continuously to all stimuli. The assessment of attentional and cognitive functions separate from response output capability would be particularly appropriate for aged or infirm individuals.

Abnormalities of specific components might also provide clues to the qualitative nature of deficient attentional processes. A failure to produce differentiated N_1 waves between attended and irrelevant channels, for instance, would suggest a problem with the early "filtering" process, as the data of Loiselle *et al.* (1977) suggest for a group of children having "minimal brain dysfunction." A small or delayed P_3 wave, on the other hand, would imply processing difficulties at a later stage of memory comparison, recognition, or evaluation. In a person with slowed motor responses, the relative latency of P_3 might indicate whether the problem was with the intermediate cognitive stages or with the final organization and execution of responses.

The two types of P_3 waves that occur to irrelevant stimuli seem particularly appropriate for the assessment of clinical populations, since they can evidently be elicited with minimal cooperation from the subject. The recognition of deviant or novel events requires not only an intact sensory apparatus but also a functioning short- and long-term memory apparatus (to be able to decide what is truly novel in a given context). Thus the presence of these "orienting waves" might make it possible to distinguish between demented patients whose basic sensory and memory processes were diminished and patients with psychiatric or depressive syndromes whose automatic reactions to novelty were still intact.

ERPs, LANGUAGE PROCESSING, AND HEMISPHERIC SPECIALIZATION

The recording of ERPs from the scalp appears to be the only currently feasible method for studying the neurophysiological basis of language processing

365

ELECTRO-
PHYSIOLOGICAL
ANALYSIS OF
HUMAN BRAIN
FUNCTION

in the nonpathological brain. In principle, the behavior of ERPs can dissect the processing of speech into stages of sensory and linguistic analysis, which can be characterized by the latency and spatial distribution of associated components. Since ERPs can be obtained unobtrusively in a natural language context, these processing stages can be evaluated as they occur rather than inferred indirectly from subsequent mediating behaviors. Furthermore, similarities and differences in the cerebral mechanisms engaged during linguistic and nonlinguistic tasks can be examined by applying comparable ERP methodologies to the study of both. For example, equivalent selective processes (by ERP criteria) seem to be involved when attention is focused on any "channel" of auditory input, including speech messages, provided that such a channel is distinguished from competing inputs by pitch cues or spatial position.

Electrophysiological information about normal language processing may help resolve certain inconsistencies in our current knowledge of cerebral specialization. Consider, for example, the partition of cognitive and analytic functions between the hemispheres during the normal processing of speech. While evidence from brain-damaged adult patients suggests that the minor hemisphere has a very limited capacity for understanding speech (Basser, 1962), studies of commissurotomized patients establish that the surgically isolated right hemisphere readily comprehends a variety of linguistic messages (Gazzaniga and Hillyard, 1971; Levy, 1974). The phonetic specialization of the hemispheres in the intact brain (inferred primarily from dichotic listening tasks) appears to be quantitatively small and variable across subjects (e.g., Studdert-Kennedy and Shankweiler, 1970). However, since behavioral results confound hemispheric specialization with an unknown degree of asymmetry in the sensory and transcallosal pathways, they may provide little more insight into normal cortical neurophysiology and interhemispheric integration than does the study of brain-damaged subjects. Electrophysiological measures (EEG and ERPs) of left and right hemisphere function promise to complement and extend the behavioral, clinical, and split-brain approaches. By recording ERPs from the right and left hemispheres, it may become possible to investigate systematically the relative participation and integration of function of the two hemispheres in a variety of tasks. However, before such promises can be realized, deflections within the ERP must be isolated which relate specifically to the information content of a stimulus and the linguistic operations themselves.

BRIEF SURVEY OF PREVIOUS NEUROLINGUISTIC RESEARCH

Despite their promise, the current research literature on ERPs, language processing, and hemispheric specialization presents a confused picture (see Donchin *et al.*, 1977*a,b,* for reviews). A number of earlier investigations found that ERPs to words were larger or more differentiated over the left hemisphere than over the right (Buchsbaum and Fedio, 1969, 1970; Wood *et al.*, 1971; Morrell and Salamy, 1971; Matsumiya *et al.*, 1972; Brown *et al.*, 1973; Teyler *et al.*, 1973; Neville, 1974; Butler and Glass, 1974), but most of these studies can be faulted for improper controls or inappropriate analytic procedures (Friedman *et al.*, 1975*a*;

Galambos *et al.*, 1975). Among the more recent studies, some have also reported a variety of lateral asymmetries in ERPs evoked during language-processing tasks (Molfese *et al.*, 1975; Galin and Ellis, 1975; Brown *et al.*, 1976; Chapman, 1977; Thatcher, 1977; Neville *et al.*, 1977), but others have failed to find such asymmetries in attempted replications of earlier studies (Smith *et al.*, 1975; Mayes and Beaumont, 1977; Tanguay *et al.*, 1977). Although many of these new studies have analyzed their results with more powerful statistical techniques (i.e., discriminant analysis and principal-component analysis) which can identify processing-specific components throughout the ERP wave form, asymmetries have generally been small and variable across subjects. The best-controlled study to date has been that of Wood *et al.* (1971), who compared ERPs to the CV syllable /ba/ in an ongoing stimulus train when it was processed for either phonetic or fundamental frequency cues. They found that the left hemisphere response changed significantly between the two conditions, while the response on the right side did not. The magnitude of these ERP modulations, however, was very small (fractions of a microvolt), and the statistical tests used to establish their significance (multiple Wilcoxen comparisons) have been subsequently criticized by Friedman *et al.* (1975*a*) for possible failure to preserve type I error levels; attempts to replicate these effects have met with mixed success (Wood, 1975; Smith *et al.*, 1975).

Tables 1 and 2 summarize the current body of ERP studies in auditory and visual modalities. Table 3 lists the studies that have investigated ERPs which arise

TABLE 1. VISUAL ERP STUDIES OF LANGUAGE PROCESSING

Authors	Stimuli	Results
Buchsbaum and Fedio (1969, 1970)	Words, dot patterns	Greater left hemisphere ERP changes
Shelburne (1972, 1973)	Letter sequences	No asymmetry in P_3 to words
Marsh and Thompson (1973)	Words, line drawings	No asymmetry in CNV or P_3
Butler and Glass (1974)	Numbers	CNV larger over left hemisphere
Galin and Ellis (1975)	Writing, Kohs Block construction	Flash-probe EPs smaller over the engaged hemisphere
Friedman *et al.* (1975*b*)	Words	No asymmetry in P_3 to words
Marsh *et al.* (1976)	Words, slanted lines	CNV smaller over "engaged" hemisphere
Shelburne (1977)	Letter sequences	No ERP asymmetry, small P_3s in dyslexia
Thatcher (1977)	Letters, dot patterns	Letter matches showed different lateralized factors
Thatcher (1977)	Words, dot patterns	Semantic matches showed asymmetry in P_3
Chapman (1977)	Numbers, letters	Stimulus matches yielded ERP asymmetry at posterior sites
Neville *et al.* (1977)	Dichoptic word pairs, drawings	Larger left hemisphere ERP to words
Kutas and Donchin (1977)	Semantic discrimination	No ERP asymmetry, P_3 latency indexes task difficulty
Mayes and Beaumont (1977)	Writing, Kohs Block construction	Failure to replicate Galin and Ellis (1975)

367

ELECTRO-
PHYSIOLOGICAL
ANALYSIS OF
HUMAN BRAIN
FUNCTION

TABLE 2. AUDITORY ERP STUDIES OF LANGUAGE PROCESSING

Authors	Stimuli	Results
Morrell and Salamy (1971)	Words	Larger ERP over left hemisphere
Wood et al. (1971)	CV syllables	Greater left hemisphere ERP changes between phonetic and acoustic processing
Matsumiya et al. (1972)	Words, environmental sounds	L/R ERP ratio increases with increasing "meaningfulness"
Brown et al. (1973)	Words	Greater left hemisphere lability to perceived changes in meaning
Neville (1974)	Dichotic words, binaural clicks	Shorter left hemisphere latencies to words
Molfese et al. (1975)	Tones, noise bursts, words	Larger left hemisphere ERP to words; larger right hemisphere ERP to tones, noise
Friedman et al. (1975a)	Words, nonspeech sounds	No ERP asymmetry
Wood (1975)	CV syllables	Replicates his previous findings (1971)
Galambos et al. (1975)	Words, tones	No ERP asymmetry
Smith et al. (1975)	CV syllables	Failure to replicate Wood et al. (1971)
Brown (1976)	Words	Replicates his previous findings (1973)
Tanguay et al. (1977)	Words, tones, noise bursts	Failure to replicate Molfese et al. (1975)
Neville et al. (1977)	Dichotic words, melodies	Larger left hemisphere ERP to words
Anderson (1977)	Words	Notes ERP contamination from lateralized eye movements

prior to and during the production of speech. Four general points deserve emphasis: (1) ERP wave forms elicited during linguistic tasks are very similar to those evoked by nonlinguistic stimuli such as tones or patterned flashes of light. Similarly, potentials preceding speech resemble potentials that precede simple nonlinguistic motor acts. (2) There is no consensus about which, if any, of the components of the ERP index hemispheric specialization. (3) There have been few successful replications of studies which have reported task-dependent asymmetries in the distribution of the ERP. (4) Research in neurolinguistics has not converged toward a common set of paradigms—typically, new studies use new electrode placements, data analysis techniques, and tasks.

TABLE 3. ERP STUDIES OF SPEECH PRODUCTION

Authors	Results
McAdam and Whitaker (1971)	Larger CNV over left hemisphere
Morrell and Huntington (1972)	Larger CNV over left hemisphere
Zimmerman and Knott (1974)	Larger CNV over left hemisphere in normals but not stutterers
Grabow and Elliott (1974)	No CNV asymmetry, failure to replicate McAdam and Whitaker (1971)
Low et al. (1976)	Larger CNV over left hemisphere
Anderson (1977)	Notes CNV contamination from lateralized eye movements

STEVEN A. HILLYARD
AND DAVID L. WOODS

It is not surprising that the lateral ERP asymmetries observed in most studies have been either small in magnitude, unreliable, or nonexistent (Galambos *et al.,* 1975; Friedman *et al.* 1975*a,b*). For one thing, the use of long interstimulus intervals (ISIs) and high stimulus intensities has made it likely that the stimulus-bound components of the ERP would be so large that their fluctuations would mask any language-related potentials. In addition, small numbers of responses have typically been summed, so that ERP waveforms contain considerable residual EEG "noise." Perhaps most significantly, the linguistic tasks employed have usually been artificial and easy to perform leisurely such that variable processing strategies could have been used by different subjects. Finally, if ERP signs of language functions are time-locked to the intervening processing operations rather than to the stimulus (as one would expect), then the critical waves might emerge at variable latencies such that the ERP signs at the scalp would be smeared out and attenuated.

Other investigators (Shelburne, 1972, 1973, 1978; Kutas and Donchin, 1978) have employed linguistic paradigms to evaluate ERP signs of more general cognitive functions. Although these studies reported no hemispheric asymmetries, they did find that the P_3 (latency 300–500 msec) can index the timing of certain linguistic decisions. Kutas and Donchin, for example, showed that P_3 latency increased systematically with increasing semantic complexity in a word classification task. Earlier components have also been used to evaluate phonetic processes; for example, the refractoriness of the auditory vertex potential has been correlated with categorical perception (Dorman, 1974).

Lateral asymmetries in the CNV (a sustained DC shift which arises during periods of attention, response preparation, and cognitive activity) have been reported under certain conditions of linguistic analysis (Marsh *et al.,* 1976). Furthermore, several investigators have found that the slow potentials (CNV or Bereitschaftspotential) which precede the articulation of individual words of phonemes are slightly larger over the left than right hemispheres (McAdam and Whitaker, 1971; Zimmerman and Knott, 1974; Low *et al.,* 1976). The validity of some of these asymmetries has been debated, however, because of possible artifactual contamination from extracranial sources (Morrell and Salamy, 1971; Grabow and Elliot, 1974; Grözinger *et al.,* 1975; Anderson, 1977).

The paucity of reliable ERP asymmetries obtained in these different paradigms may reflect several methodological problems. For one thing, the contamination of ERPs by extracranial artifacts is likely to be particularly severe in neurolinguistic studies, since many of the contaminants may themselves have lateralized scalp distributions (e.g., Becker *et al.,* 1973; Anderson, 1977). Moreover, even if a reliable electrophysiological sign of hemispherical specialization can be recorded within a given subject, its reliability across subjects is likely to be limited by population heterogeneity. Such intersubject differences might be expected in the degree and nature of specialization of the cerebral hemispheres. For example, dichotic listening studies reveal that a uniform right-handed population may actually consist of several subpopulations, some with behavioral asymmetries which are consistently opposite to those of the population as a whole and others with no marked asymmetries whatsoever (Porter *et al.,* 1976; Berlin, 1977).

369

ELECTRO-
PHYSIOLOGICAL
ANALYSIS OF
HUMAN BRAIN
FUNCTION

Furthermore, individuals with functionally similar left cerebral dominance may show variations in localization of particular functions within the "dominant" hemisphere. For example, clinical studies reveal that some patients suffer no permanent aphasia after extensive damage to the classical "speech" centers, while others manifest prolonged deficits after damage outside of these areas (Luria, 1963). Even if language functions are localized appropriately on a gross level, variability may be expected in the neuroanatomical configuration of the speech areas (Rubens, 1977). Different spatial relationships between the speech centers and the overlying scalp might change ERP distributions from subject to subject; similar small changes in electrode position over cortical ERP sources are known to change both the polarity and amplitude of the somatosensory evoked response (Allison *et al.*, 1977*a*). Finally, it must be acknowledged that ERPs may turn out to be genuinely insensitive to neurolinguistic processes in the brain, particularly if they occur in small, randomly oriented cells (Golgi type II) or deep within the cortical involutions.

ELECTROPHYSIOLOGY OF NATURAL SPEECH PROCESSING

A new approach would seem to be required if consistent results are to be obtained in neurolinguistic studies. In particular, it seems important to record ERPs while the language-decoding systems are fully engaged by natural spoken messages having a high information content. In this way, the participation of the language-specific brain mechanisms should be enhanced in relation to the ERPs which are determined by the sensory or nonlinguistic aspects of the task. Studies of selective attention (reviewed above) have identified three techniques which optimize the resolution of processing-specific components: (1) processing load should be high, (2) nonspecific (stimulus-bound) ERPs should be attenuated by the use of low-intensity stimuli delivered at a high rate, and (3) EEG noise should be minimized by summing over a sufficient number of individual responses. In collaboration with E. Snyder and R. Galambos we have recently applied these techniques to the investigation of natural speech processing in a task designed to engage linguistic mechanisms on a variety of levels.

METHODS. The stimuli in this experiment consisted of electronically edited words forming a coherent, rhymed poem. The words were read at a moderate rate (approximately 80 WPM) in a monotone and recorded on magnetic tape. Next, all words were edited to have constant rise-fall times (10 and 20 msec, respectively), constant maximum durations (300 msec for monosyllables and 600 msec for polysyllables), and short ISIs (a minimum of 150 msec). Sequences of control tones (400, 1000, and 4000 Hz) were generated that precisely matched the words in loudness (45–55 dB SL), ISIs (mean 250 msec), durations, and rise-fall times. Poems and matched sequences of tones were presented monurally in counterbalanced order. During each 2½-hr experiment, subjects listened to 3000–4000 words and 1600–2000 tones, thus reducing theoretical EEG noise levels to below 0.5 μV. Six male and six female students participated in the experiment; each performed in two experimental sessions on seperate days. All were right-handed.

Poetry was selected for several reasons. First, the analysis of rhyme is reported to be exclusively lateralized to the hemisphere dominant for speech (Levy, 1974). In addition, poetry sounded more natural and required a greater processing effort at this moderate rate of delivery (about half the rate of a normal speech) than did prose. Subjects were instructed to attend closely to each 5–7 min passage, and were required to answer difficult questions on its content.

Scalp electrodes were placed at the vertex, over Wernicke's area, and over its right hemisphere homologue; all referred to the right mastoid process. Vertical and horizontal eye movements were monitored from an electrode beneath the left outer canthus. ERPs were recorded with DC-sensitive amplifiers in order to record the slow components of the word-evoked responses in undistorted form. Previous investigations indicated that the auditory sustained potential (SP, a slow negative component which is evoked by sounds lasting longer than about 200 msec) would be particularly prominent at such short ISIs (Picton and Woods, 1975).

RESULTS. ERPs from two subjects are shown in Fig. 11, averaged over ears, stimuli, and sessions (i.e., there are approximately 8000 monosyllables and 4000 tone responses in each respective tracing). Despite gross differences in task demands and stimulus structure, many of the waveform features were shared by word and tone stimuli, particularly at vertex sites. Although ERPs were small (mean amplitudes for both the N_1 and the SP were less than 3.0 μV, each subject showed reliable N_1 and sustained potential components.

Over all scalp sites, the monosyllables elicited a larger N_1 (by 34%; $P <$ 0.0001) and sustained potential (18% increase; $P < 0.001$) than did the tones. This N_1 difference was largest at left hemisphere derivations in both absolute and relative terms; while N_1 was bilaterally symmetrical during tone presentations, it became asymmetrical during speech (34% larger over left than right hemisphere). Accordingly, the left hemisphere/right hemisphere ratio for N_1 amplitude

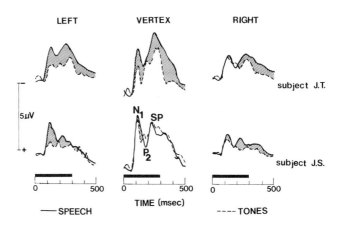

Fig. 11. ERPs from two subjects averaged over all single-syllable words in a passage of poetry and to tone bursts matched for loudness and interstimulus intervals. Subjects were required to answer difficult questions on poetry content, but listened passively to tones.

increased significantly between speech and tone conditions ($P < 0.001$). Sustained potential increases, on the other hand, were more prominent at the lateral sites than at vertex, so that during speech processing the SP distribution increased in breadth but did not change in symmetry.

When individual subjects were examined in detail, two additional patterns emerged. First, the asymmetries seemed to result from the addition of a new component to the ERP rather than a modulation of traditional components. Thus, although N_1 amplitude increased at left hemisphere sites during speech processing, P_2 measures (180–220 msec) actually decreased. This combination of results suggests that the ERP was being negatively modulated throughout the N_1 and P_2 latencies, as may occur during channel-selective attention. As expected, considerable intersubject variability was also observed; most of the mean ERP asymmetries were accounted for by seven of the 12 subjects; the other five subjects showed variable effects.

SOME QUALIFICATIONS. Even if we assume that differences in interhemispheric processing were determining these ERP asymmetries, it is not clear which perceptual, linguistic, or cognitive factors might be responsible. For instance, the asymmetries could reflect an acoustic or a phonetic specialization of one hemisphere or the other (Liberman, 1974); onset components, principally evoked by consonants, were asymmetrically distributed, while the sustained potential, evoked largely by vowels, was distributed symmetrically. The observed asymmetries might also reflect specialization for the decoding of certain syntactic elements such as verbs, the processing of which appears to be particularly lateralized (Gazzaniga and Hillyard, 1971).

Further interpretations of these effects are also possible. It may be the case that stimuli can be shunted to one hemisphere or the other for decoding depending on a subject's cognitive set. For example, some evidence suggests that visuospatial stimuli (generally more accurately processed by the minor hemisphere) can be preferentially processed in the left hemisphere if the subject has a verbal or analytic set (Kinsbourne, 1970; Levy and Trevarthen, 1976). Similarly, electrophysiological studies using nonlinguistic probe stimuli suggest that ERPs to such probes may be asymmetrically distributed when they are embedded in an attended channel of speech, but not when they are in a channel of tones (Hink and Hillyard, 1976). Finally, it is possible that left/right ERP asymmetries increase with increasing task difficulty regardless of the processing strategy required (Matsumiya *et al.*, 1972).

The ERP asymmetries observed in the present study are consistent with results showing the linguistic predominance of the left hemisphere, but, as we have seen, they also lend themselves to alternative interpretations. The current difficulty in deciphering ERP effects is, in a sense, proportional to their potential utility. Because ERPs are sensitive to a broad range of stimulus and processing variables, many controls are necessary before determinants of asymmetries can be unambiguously isolated. Since ERPs remain the only way to examine the neurophysiology of natural speech processing, their interpretation is likely to suffer, for a considerable time, from a lack of converging evidence from other sources.

371

ELECTRO-
PHYSIOLOGICAL
ANALYSIS OF
HUMAN BRAIN
FUNCTION

STEVEN A. HILLYARD
AND DAVID L. WOODS

Allison, T., Goff, W. R., Williamson, P. D., and VanGilder, J.C. On the neural origin of early components of the human somatosensory evoked potential. In J. Desmedt (ed.), *Progress in Clinical Neurophysiology*. Basel: Karger, 1977a.

Allison, T., Matsumiya, Y., Goff, G., and Goff, W. R. The scalp topography of human visual evoked potentials. *Electroencephalography and Clinical Neurophysiology*, 1977b, *42*, 185–197.

Amadeo, M., and Shagass, C. Brief latency click evoked potentials during waking and sleep in man. *Psychophysiology*, 1973, *10*, 244–250.

Anderson, S. A. Language related asymmetries of eye movement and evoked potentials. In S. Harnad, R. Doty, L. Goldstein, J. Jaynes, and G. Krauthamer (eds.), *Lateralization in the Nervous System*. New York: Academic Press, 1977, pp. 403–428.

Asselman, P., Chadwick, D. W., and Marsden, C. D. Visual evoked responses in the diagnosis and management of patients suspected of multiple sclerosis. *Brain*, 1975, *98*, 201–282.

Barrett, G., Blumhardt, L., Halliday, A. M., Halliday, E., and Kriss, A. A paradox in the lateralization of the visual evoked response. *Nature, (London)*, 1976, *261*, 253–255.

Basser, L. S. Hemiplegia of early onset and the faculty of speech with special reference to effects of hemispherectomy. *Brain*, 1962, *85*, 427–460.

Becker, W., Hoehne, O., Iwase, K., and Kornhuber, H. H. Cerebral and ocular muscle potentials preceding voluntary eye movements in man. In W. C. McCallum and J. R. Knott (eds.), *Event-Related Slow Potentials of the Brain: Their Relations to Behavior*. Amsterdam: Elsevier, 1973, pp. 99–104.

Berlin, C. Hemispheric asymmetries in auditory tasks. In S. Harnad, R. Doty, L. Goldstein, J. Jaynes, and G. Krauthamer (eds.), *Lateralization in the Nervous System*. New York: Academic Press, 1977, pp. 303–323.

Blakemore, C. Developmental factors in the formation of feature extracting neurons. In F. O. Schmitt and F. G. Worden (eds.), *The Neurosciences: Third Study Program*. Cambridge, Mass.: MIT Press, 1974.

Bodis-Wollner, I. Recovery from cerebral blindness: Evoked potential and psychophysical measurements. *Electroencephalography and Clinical Neurophysiology*, 1977, *42*, 178–184.

Broadbent, D. E. Stimulus set and response set: Two kinds of selective attention. In D. I. Mostofsky (ed.), *Attention: Contemporary Theory and Analysis* New York: Appleton-Century-Crofts, 1970.

Broadbent, D. E. *Decision and Stress*. New York: Academic Press, 1971.

Brown, W. S., Marsh, J. T., and Smith, J. C. Contextual meaning effects on speech-evoked potentials. *Behavioral Biology*, 1973, *9*, 755–761.

Brown, W. S., Marsh, J. T., and Smith, J. C. Evoked potential waveform differences produced by the perception of different meanings of an ambiguous phrase. *Electroencephalography and Clinical Neurophysiology*, 1976, *41*, 113–123.

Buchsbaum, M., and Fedio, P. Visual information and evoked responses from the left and right hemispheres. *Electroencephalography and Clinical Neurophysiology*, 1969, *26*, 266–272.

Buchsbaum, M., and Fedio, P. Hemispheric differences in evoked potentials to verbal and nonverbal stimuli in the left and right visual fields. *Physiology and Behavior*, 1970, *5*, 207–210.

Buchwald, J. S., and Huang, C.-M. Far-field acoustic response: Origins in the cat. *Science*, 1975, *189*, 382–384.

Butler, S. R., and Glass, A. Asymmetries in the CNV over left and right hemispheres while subjects await numeric information. *Biological Psychology*, 1974, *2*, 1–16.

Campbell, F., and Maffei, L. Electrophysiological evidence for the existence of orientation and size detectors in the human visual system. *Journal of Physiology (London)*, 1970, *207*, 635–652.

Celesia, G. G. Organization of auditory cortical areas in man. *Brain*, 1976, *99*, 403–414.

Celesia, G. G., and Daly, R. F. Visual electroencephalogrphic computer analysis: A new electrophysiological test for the diagnosis of optic nerve lesions. *Neurology*, 1977, *27*, 637–641.

Chapman, R. M. Evoked potentials of the brain related to thinking. In F. J. McGuigan (ed.), *The Psychophysiology of Thinking*. New York: Academic Press, 1973.

Chapman, R. M. Hemispheric differences in averaged evoked potentials to relevant and irrelevant visual stimuli. In J. E. Desmedt (ed.), *Progress in Clinical Neurophysiology. Language and Hemispheric Specialization in Man: Event-Related Potentials*, Vol. 3. Basel: Karger, 1977.

Courchesne, E. Event-related brain potentials. A comparison between children and adults. *Science*, 1977, *197*, 589–592.

373

ELECTRO-
PHYSIOLOGICAL
ANALYSIS OF
HUMAN BRAIN
FUNCTION

Courchesne, E., Hillyard, S. A., and Galambos, R. Stimulus novelty, task relevance and the visual evoked potential in man. *Electroencephalography and Clinical Neurophysiology*, 1975, *39*, 131–143.

Davis, H. Principles of electric response audiometry. *Annals of Otolo-Laryngology*, 1976, *85*, Suppl. 28.

Davis, H., Osterhammel, R., Wier, C., and Gjerdigen, D. B. Slow vertex potentials: Interactions among auditory, tactile, electric and visual stimuli. *Electroencephalography and Clinical Neurophysiology*, 1972, *33*, 537–545.

Debecker, J. Contribution à d'étude physiologique chez l'homme de certains méchanismes cérébraux mis en jeu dans la perception sensorielle. Doctoral dissertation, l'Université Libre de Bruxelles, 1967.

Deutsch, J. A., and Deutsch, D. Attention: Some theoretical considerations. *Psychological Review*, 1963, *70*, 80–90, 1963.

Donchin, E., Kutas, M., and McCarthy, G. Electrocortical indices of hemispherical utilization. In S. Harnad, R. Doty, L. Goldstein, J. Jaynes, and G. Krauthamer (eds.), *Lateralization in the Nervous System*. New York: Academic Press, 1977*a*, pp. 339–384.

Donchin, E., McCarthy, G., and Kutas, M. Electroencephalographic investigations of hemispheric specialization. In J. E. Desmedt (ed.), *Progress in Clinical Neurophysiology. Language and Hemispheric Specialization in Man: Event-Related Potentials*, Vol. 3. Basel: Karger, 1977*b*.

Donchin, E., Ritter, W. R., and McCallum, C. Cognitive psychophysiology: The endogenous components of the ERP. In E. Callaway, P. Tueting and S. Koslow (eds.), *Event-Related Brain Potentials in Man*. New York. Academic Press, 1978.

Dorman, M. F. Auditory evoked potential correlates of speech sound discrimination. *Perception and Psychophysics*, 1974, *15*, 215–220.

Eason, R., Harter, M., and White, C. Effects of attention and arousal on visually evoked cortical potentials and reaction time in man. *Physiology and Behavior*, 1969, *4*, 283–289.

Estevez, O., Spekreijse, H., VanderBerg, T., and Cavonius, C. R. The spectral sensitivities of isolated human color mechanisms determined from contrast evoked potential measurements. *Vision Research*, 1975, *15*, 1205–1212.

Freeman, R., and Thibos, L. Electrophysiological evidence that abnormal early visual experience can modify the human brain. *Science*, 1973, *180*, 876–878.

Friedman, D., Simson, R., Ritter, W., and Rapin, I. Cortical evoked potentials elicited by real speech words and human sounds. *Electroencephalography and Clinical Neurophysiology*, 1975*a*, *38*, 13–19.

Friedman, D., Simson, R., Ritter, W., and Rapin, I., The late positive component (P300) and information processing in sentences. *Electroencephalography and Clinical Neurophysiology*, 1975*b*, *38*, 255–262.

Galambos, R., and Hecox, K. Clincial applications of the human brainstem responses to auditory evoked potentials. In J. Desmedt (ed.), *Auditory Evoked Potentials in Man, Psychopharmacology Correlates of Evoked Potentials*. Basel: Karger, 1977, pp. 1–19.

Galambos, R., Benson, P., Smith, T. S., Schulman-Galambos, C., and Osier, H. On hemispheric differences in evoked potentials to speech stimuli. *Electroencephalography and Clinical Neurophysiology*, 1975, *39*, 279–283.

Galin, D., and Ellis, R. Asymmetry in evoked potentials as an index of lateralized cognitive processes: Relation to EEG alpha asymmetry. *Neuropsychologia*, 1975, *13*, 45–50.

Garner, W. R., Hake, H. W., and Eriksen, C. W. Operationism and the concept of perception. *Psychological Review*, 1956, *63*, 149–159.

Gazzaniga, M. S., and Hillyard, S. A. Language and speech capacity of the right hemisphere. *Neuropsychologia*, 1971, *9*, 273–280.

Goff, W. R. Human average evoked potentials: Procedures for stimulating and recording. In R. F. Thompson and M. M. Patterson (eds.), *Bioelectric Recording Techniques. Part B: Electroencephalography and Human Brain Potentials*. New York: Academic Press, 1974, pp. 102–157.

Goff, W. R., Allison, T., and Vaughan, H. G., Jr. The functional neuroanatomy of event-related potentials. In E. Callaway, P. Tueting and S. Koslow (eds.), *Event Related Brain Potentials in the Man*. New York: Academic Press, 1978.

Grabow, J. D., and Elliott, F. W. The electrophysiologic assessment of hemispheric asymmetries during speech. *Journal of Speech and Hearing Research*, 1974, *17*, 64–72.

Grözinger, B. H., Kornhuber, H., and Kriebel, J. Methodological problems in the investigation of cerebral potentials preceding speech: Determining the onset and suppressing artifacts caused by speech. *Neuropsychologia*, 1975, *13*, 263–270.

Halliday, A. M. Evoked responses in organic and functional sensory loss. In A. Fessard and G. Lelord (eds.), *Activités Évoquées et leur Conditionnement chez l'Homme Normal et en Pathologie Mentale.* Paris: INSERM, 1972, pp. 189–213.

Halliday, A. M., and Michael, E. F. Changes in pattern-evoked responses in man associated with the vertical and horizontal meridians of the visual field. *Journal of Physiology (London)*, 1970, *208*, 499–513.

Halliday, A. M., McDonald, W. I., and Muskin, J. Visual evoked responses in diagnosis of multiple sclerosis. *British Medical Journal*, 1973, *4*, 661–664.

Halliday, A. M., Halliday, E., Kriss, A., McDonald, W. I., and Muskin, J. The pattern-evoked potential in comparison of the anterior visual pathways, *Brain*, 1976, *99*, 357–374.

Harter, M. R., and Salmon, L. E. Intra-modality selective attention and cortical potentials to randomly presented patterns. *Electroencephalography and Clinical Neurophysiology*, 1972, *32*, 605–613.

Harter, M. R., and White, C. T. Evoked cortical responses to checkerboard patterns: Effects of check-size and function of visual acuity. *Electroencephalography and Clinical Neurophysiology*, 1970, *28*, 48–54.

Hecox, K. Electrophysiological correlates of human auditory development. In *Infant Perception: From Sensation to Cognition*, Vol. II. New York: Academic Press, 1975, pp. 151–191.

Hecox, K., and Galambos, R. Brain stem auditory evoked responses in human infants and adults. *Archives of Otolaryngology*, 1974, *99*, 30–33.

Hecox, K., Squires, N., and Galambos, R. Brainstem auditory evoked responses in man. I. Effect of stimulus rise-fall time and duration. *Journal of the Acoustical Society of America*, 1976, *60*, 5, 1187–1192.

Hernandez-Peon, R. Physiological mechanisms in attention. In R. W. Russell (ed.), *Frontiers in Physiological Psychology*. New York: Academic Press, 1966.

Hillyard, S. A., and Picton, T. W. Event-related brain potentials and selective information processing in man. In J. Desmedt (ed.), *Cognitive Components in Cerebral Event-Related Potentials and Selective Attention*. Basel: Karger, 1978.

Hillyard, S. A., Hink, R. F., Schwent, V. L., and Picton, T. W. Electrical signs of selective attention in the human brain. *Science*, 1973, *182*, 177–180.

Hillyard, S. A., Picton, T. W., and Regan, D. M. Sensation, perception and attention: Analysis using ERPs. In E. Callaway, P. Tueting and S. Koslow (eds.), *Event-Related Brain Potentials in Man*. New York: Academic Press, 1978.

Hink, R. F., and Hillyard, S. A. Auditory evoked potentials during selective listening to dichotic speech messages. *Perception and Psychophysics*, 1976, *20*, 236–242.

Hink, R. F., Van Voorhis, S., Hillyard, S. A., and Smith, T. S. The division of attention and the human auditory evoked potential. *Neuropsychologia*, 1977, *15*, 597–605.

Hink, R. F., Hillyard, S. A., and Benson, P. J. Event-related brain potentials and selective attention to acoustic and phonetic cues. *Biological Psychology*, 1978, *6*, 1–16.

Hirsch, H., and Jacobson, M. The perfectible brain: Principles of neuronal development. In M. Gazzaniga and C. Blakemore (eds.), *Handbook of Psychobiology*. New York: Academic Press, 1975.

Huis in't Veld, F., Osterhammel, P., and Terkildsen, K. Frequency following auditory brain stem responses in man. *Scandavian Audiology*, 1977, *6*, 27–34.

Hyde, M. L., Stephens, S. D., and Thornton. A. R. Stimulus repetition rate and the early brainstem responses. *British Journal of Audiology*, 1976, *10*, 41–50.

Jeffreys, D. A., and Axford, J. G. Source locations of pattern-specific components of human visual evoked potentials. I. Components of striate cortical origin. *Experimental Brain Research*, 1972, *16*, 1–21.

Jewett, D. L. Volume-conducted potentials in response to auditory stimuli as detected by averaging in the cat. *Electroencephalography and clinical Neurophysiology*, 1970, *28*, 609–618.

Jewett, D. L., and Williston, J. S. Auditory evoked far fields averaged from the scalp of humans. *Brain*, 1971, *94*, 681–696.

Kahneman, D. *Attention and Effort.* Englewood Cliffs, N.J.: Prentice-Hall, 1973.

Karlin, L. Cognition, preparation and sensory-evoked potentials. *Psychological Bulletin*, 1970, *73*, 122–136.

Karlin, L, and Martz, M. Response probability and sensory evoked potentials. In S. Kornblum (ed.), *Attention and Performance*, Vol. IV. New York: Academic Press, 1973.

Keren, G. Some considerations of two alleged kinds of selective attention. *Journal of Experimental Psychology: General*, 1976, *105*, 349–374.

Kinney, J., and McKay, C. Test of color defective vision using the visual evoked response. *Journal of Optical Society of America*, 1974, *64*, 1244–1250.

375

ELECTRO-
PHYSIOLOGICAL
ANALYSIS OF
HUMAN BRAIN
FUNCTION

Kinsbourne, M. Cerebral basis of asymmetries in attention. *Acta Psychologia,* 1970, *33*, 193–201.

Kooi, K. A. *Fundamentals of Electroencephalography.* New York: Harper and Row, 1971.

Kooi, K. A., Guvener, A. M., and Bagchi, B. K. Visually evoked responses in lesions of the higher optic pathways. *Neurology,* 1965, *15*, 841–854.

Kutas, M., and Donchin, E. Variations in the latency of P300 as a function of variations in semantic categorizations. In D. Otto (ed.), *New Perspectives in Event Related Potentials.* EPA 600 1978.

Levy, J. Psychobiological implications of bilateral asymmetry. In S. J. Dimond and J. G. Beaumont (eds.), *Hemisphere Function in the Brain.* New York: Wiley, 1974, pp. 121–183.

Levy, J., and Trevarthen, C. Metacontrol of hemispheric function in human split-brain patients. *Journal of Experimental Psychology: Human Perception and Performance,* 1976, *2*, 299–312.

Liberman, A. M. The specialization of the langugage hemisphere. In F. O. Schmitt and F. G. Worden (eds.), *The Neurosciences: Third Study Program.* Cambridge, Mass.: MIT Press, 1974.

Loiselle, D. L., Zambelli, A. J., and Stamm, J. S. Auditory evoked potentials as measures of selective attention in older MBD children. Paper read at International Neuropsychological Society, Santa Fe New Mexico, February 1977.

Low, M. D., Wada, J., and Fox, M. Electroencephaographic localization of conative aspects of language production in the human brain. In E. McCallum and J. Knott (eds.), *The Responsive Brain.* Bristol: John Wright, 1976, pp. 165–171.

Ludlam, W. M., and Meyers, R. R. The use of visual evoked responses in objective refraction. *Transactions of the New York Academy of Sciences,* 1972, *34*, 154–170.

Luria, A. R. *Restoration of Function after Brain Injury.* New York: Macmillan, 1963.

Maffei, L., and Campbell, F. W. Neurophysiological localization of the vertical and horizontal visual coordinates in man. *Science,* 1970, *167*, 386–387.

Marsh, G. R., and Thompson, L. W. Effects of verbal and non-verbal psychological set on hemispheric asymmetries in the CNV. In W. C. McCallum and J. R. Knott (eds.), *Event Related Slow Potentials of the Brain.* Elsevier, 1973, pp. 195–200.

Marsh, G. R., Poon, L. W., and Thompson, L. W. Some relationships between CNV, P300 and task demands. In W. C. McCallum and J. Knott (eds.), *The Responsive Brain.* Bristol: J. Wright, 1976, pp. 122–125.

Marsh, J. T., Brown, W. S., and Smith, J. C. Far-field recorded frequency-following responses: Correlates of low pitch auditory perception in humans. *Electroencephalography and Clinical Neurophysiology,* 1975, *38*, 113.

Matsumiya, Y., Tagliasco, V., Lombroso, O. T., and Goodglass, H. Auditory evoked response: Meaningfulness of stimuli and interhemispheric asymmetry. *Science,* 1972, *173*, 790–792.

Mayes, A., and Beaumont, G. Does visual evoked potential asymmetry index cognitive activity? *Neuropsychologia,* 1977, *15*, 249–256.

McAdam, D. W., and Whitaker, H. A. Language production: Electroencephalographic localization in the normal human brain. *Science,* 1971, *172*, 499–502.

Mokotoff, B., Schulman-Galambos, C., and Galambos, R. Brain stem auditory evoked responses in children. *Archives of Otolaryngology,* 1977, *103*, 38–43.

Molfese, D. L., Freeman, R. B., Jr., and Palermo, D. S. The ontogeny of brain lateralization of speech and nonspeech stimuli. *Brain and Language,* 1975, *2*, 356–368.

Moray, N. A data base for theories of selective listening. In *Attention and Performance,* Vol. V. New York: Academic Press, 1975.

Morrell, L. K., and Huntington, D. A. Cortical potentials time-locked to speech production: Evidence for probable cerebral origin. *Life Sciences 11,* 1972, Part I, 921–929.

Morrell, L. K., and Salamy, J. G. Hemispherical asymmetry of electrocortical responses to speech stimuli. *Science,* 1971, *174*, 164–166.

Moushegian, G., Rupert, A. L., and Stillman, R. D. Scalp-recorded early responses in man to frequencies in the speech range. *Electroencephalography and Clinical Neurophysiology,* 1973, *35*, 665.

Näätänen, R. Selective attention and evoked potentials. *Annals of the Finnish Academy of Science,* 1967, *151*, 1–226.

Näätänen, R. Selective attention and evoked potentials in humans—A critical review. *Biological Psychology,* 1975, *2*, 237–307.

Neville, H. Electrographic correlates of lateral asymmetry in the processing of verbal and non-verbal stimuli. *Journal of Psycholinguistic Research,* 1974, *3*, 151–163.

Neville, H. J., Schulman-Galambos, C., and Galambos, R. Evoked potential correlates of functional hemispheric specialization. Presented to the International Neuropsychology Society, Santa Fe, February 1977.

Norman, D. A., and Bobrow, D. G. On data-limited and resource-limited processes. *Cognitive Psychology,* 1975, *7*, 44–64.

Oatman, L. C. Role of visual attention on auditory evoked potentials in unanesthetized cats. *Experimental Neurology,* 1971, *32*, 341–356.

Olesen, T. D., Ashe, J. H., and Weinberger, N. M. Modification of auditory and somatosensory system activity during pupillary conditioning in the paralyzed cat. *Journal of Neurophysiology,* 1975, *38*, 1114–1139.

Penfield, W., and Roberts, L. *Speech and Brain-Mechanisms.* Princeton, N.J.: Princeton University Press, 1959.

Picton, T. W. and Hillyard, S. A. Human auditory evoked potentials. II. Effects of attention. *Electroencephalography and Clinical Neurophysiology,* 1974, *36*, 191–200.

Picton, T. W., and Woods, D. L. Human auditory evoked sustained potentials. *Electroencephalography and Clinical Neurophysiology,* 1975, *38*, 543–544.

Picton, T. W., Hillyard, S. A., Krausz, H. I., and Galambos, R. Human auditory evoked potentials. I. Evaluation of components. *Electroencephalography and Clinical Neurophysiology,* 1974, *36*, 179–190.

Picton, T. W., Hillyard, S. A., and Galambos, R. Habituation and attention in the auditory system. In W. D. Keidel and W. D. Neff (eds.), *Handbook of Sensory Physiology,* Vol. V. pp. 343–387. Berlin: Springer-Verlag, 1976.

Porter, R. J., Jr., Troendle, R., and Berlin, C. I. Effects of practice on the perception of dichotically presented stop-consonant-vowell syllables. *Journal of the Acoustical Society of America,* 1976, *59*, 679–682.

Pratt, H., and Sohmer, H. Intensity and rate functions of cochlear and brainstem evoked responses to click stimuli in man. *Archives of Otolaryngology-Rhinology-Laryngology,* 1976, *212*, 85–92.

Regan, D. *Evoked Potentials in Psychology, Sensory Physiology, and Clinical Medicine.* London: Chapman and Hall, 1972.

Regan, D. Rapid objective refraction using evoked brain potentials. *Investigative Ophthalmology,* 1973, *12*, 669–679.

Regan, D. Electrophysiological evidence for color channels in human pattern vision. *Nature (London),* 1974, *250*, 437–439.

Regan, D. Color coding of pattern responses in man investigated by evoked potential feedback and direct plot techniques. *Vision Research,* 1975, *15*, 175–183.

Regan, D. Speedy assessment of visual acuity in amblyopia by the evoked potential method. *Ophthalmologica,* 1977, *175*, 159–165.

Regan, D., and Spekreijse, H. Evoked potential indications of color blindness. *Vision Research,* 1974, *14*, 89–95.

Regan, D., Milner, B. A., and Heron, J. R. Delayed visual perception and delayed visual evoked potentials in the spinal form of multiple sclerosis and in retrobulbar neuritis. *Brain,* 1976, *99*, 43–66.

Ritter, W., Simson, R., and Vaughan, H. G., Jr. Association cortex potentials and reaction time in auditory discrimination. *Electroencephalography and Clinical Neurophysiology,* 1972, *33*, 547–555.

Rosenhamer, H. J. Observations on electric brainstem responses in retrocochlear hearing loss. *Scandavian Audiology,* 1977, *6*, 1–18.

Rubens, A. B. Anatomical asymmetries of human cerebral cortex. In S. Harnad, R. Doty, L. Goldstein, J. Jaynes, and G. Krauthamer (eds.), *Lateralization in the Nervous System.* New York: Academic Press, 1977, pp. 503–516.

Salamy, A., McKean, C. M., and Buda, F. B. Maturational changes in auditory transmission as reflected in human brain stem potentials. *Brain Research,* 1975, *96*, 361–366.

Schulman-Galambos, C., and Galambos, R. Brainstem auditory-evoked responses in premature infants. *Journal of Speech and Hearing Research,* 1975, *18*, 3, 456–465.

Schwent, V., and Hillyard, S. A. Auditory evoked potentials and multichannel selective attention. *Electroencephalography and Clinical Neurophysiology,* 1975, *38*, 131–138.

Schwent, V. L., Hillyard, S. A., and Galambos, R. Selective attention and the auditory vertex potential. I. Effects of stimulus delivery rate. *Electroencephalography and Clinical Neurophysiology,* 1976a, *40*, 604–614.

Schwent, V. L., Hillyard, S. A., and Galambos, R. Selective attention and the auditory vertex potential. II. Effects of signal intensity and masking noise. *Electroencephalography and Clinical Neurophysiology,* 1976b, *40*, 615–622.

Schwent, V. L., Snyder, E., and Hillyard, S. A. Auditory evoked potentials during multichannel

377

ELECTRO-
PHYSIOLOGICAL
ANALYSIS OF
HUMAN BRAIN
FUNCTION

selective listening: Role of pitch and localization cues. *Journal of Experimental Psychology: Human Perception and Performance,* 1976c, *2*, 313–325.

Shagass, C., Amadeo, M., and Roemer, R. A. Spatial distribution of potentials evoked by half-field of potentials evoked by half-field pattern reversal and pattern onset stimuli. *Electroencephalography and Clinical Neurophysiology,* 1976, *41*, 609–622.

Shelburne, S. A. Visual evoked responses to word and nonsense syllable stimuli. *Electroencephalography and Clinical Neurophysiology,* 1972, *32*, 17–25.

Shelburne, S. A. Visual evoked responses to language stimuli in normal children. *Electroencephalography and Clinical Neurophysiology,* 1973, *34*, 135–143.

Shelburne, S. A. Visual evoked responses to language stimuli in children with reading disabilities. In D. Otto (ed.), *New Perspectives in Event Related Potential Research.* Washington, D.C.: U.S. Environmental Protection Agency, 1978.

Shiffrin, R. M., McKay, D. P., and Shaffer, W. O. Attending to forty-nine spatial positions at once. *Journal of Experimental Psychology: Human Perception and Performance,* 1976, *2*, 14–22.

Smith, D. B. D., Donchin, E., Cohen, L., and Starr, A. Auditory average evoked potentials in man during binaural listening. *Electroencephalography and Clinical Neurophysiology,* 1970, *28*, 146–152.

Smith, T. S., Nielson, B., and Thistle, A. B. Question of asymmetries in auditory evoked potentials to speech stimuli. *Journal of the Acoustical Society of America,* 1975, *58*, 1, 557.

Snyder, E., and Hillyard, S. A. Long-latency evoked potentials to irrelevant deviant stimuli. *Behavioral Biology,* 1976, *16*, 319–331.

Sohmer, H., and Feinmesser, M. Routine use of electrocochleography (cochlear audiometry) on human subjects. *Audiology,* 1973, *12*, 167–173.

Sohmer, H., and Feinmesser, M. Electrocochleography in clinical-audiological diagnosis. *Archives of Otolaryngology-Rhinolaryngology-Laryngology,* 1974, *206*, 91–102.

Sohmer, H., Feinmesser, M., and Szabo, G. Sources of electrocochleographic responses as studied in patients with brain damage. *Electroencephalography and Clinical Neurophysiology,* 1974, *37*, 663–669.

Spekreijse, H., Khue, L. H., and Van der Tweel, L. H. A case of amblyopia. Electrophysiology and psychophysics of luminance and contrast. *Advances in Experimental Medicine and Biology,* 1972, *24*, 141–144.

Squires, K. C., Hillyard, S. A., and Lindsay, P. H. Cortical potentials evoked by feedback confirming and disconfirming an auditory discrimination. *Perception and Psychophysics,* 1973, *13*, 25–31.

Squires, K. C., Squires, N. K., and Hillyard, S. A. Decision-related cortical potentials during an auditory signal detection task with cued observation intervals. *Journal of Experimental Psychology: Human Perception and Performance,* 1975, *104*, 268–279.

Squires, K., Wickens, C., Squires, N., and Donchin, E. The effect of stimulus sequence on the waveform of the cortical event-related potential. *Science,* 1976, *193*, 1142–1146.

Squires, N. K., Squires, K. C., and Hillyard, S. A. Two varieties of long-latency positive waves evoked by unpredictable auditory stimuli. *Electroencephalography and Clinical Neurophysiology,* 1975, *38*, 387–401.

Starr, A. Auditory brain-stem responses in brain death. *Brain,* 1976, *99*, 543–554.

Starr, A. Sensory evoked potentials in clinical disorders of the visual system. *Annual Review of Neuroscience,* 1978, *1*, 103–127.

Starr, A., and Achor, L. J. Auditory brain stem responses in neurological disease. *Archives of Neurology,* 1975, *32*, 761–768.

Starr, A., and Hamilton, A. E. Correlation between pathologically confirmed sites of neurological lesions and abnormalities of far-field auditory brainstem responses. *Electroencephalography and Clinical Neurophysiology,* 1976, *41*, 595–608.

Starr, A., Celesia, G., and Sohmer, H. ERPs and neurological disorders. In E. Callaway, P. Tueting and S. Koslow (eds.), *Event-Related Brain Potentials in Man.* New York: Academic Press, 1978.

Sternberg, S. Memory scanning: Mental processes revealed by reaction time experiments. *American Scientist,* 1969, *57*, 421–457.

Stillman, R. D., Moushegian, G., and Rupert, A. L. Early tone-evoked responses in normal and hearing-impaired subjects. *Audiology,* 1976, *15*, 10–22.

Stockard, J., and Rossiter, V. Clinical and pathologic correlates of brain-stem auditory response abnormalities. *Neurology (Minn.),* 1977, *27*, 316–325.

Studdert-Kennedy, M., and Shankweiler, D. Hemispheric specialization for speech perception. *Journal of the Acoustical Society of America,* 1970, *48*, 2, 579–594.

Sutton, S., Braren, M., and Zubin, J. Evoked potential correlates of stimulus uncertainty. *Science*, 1965, *150*, 1187–1188.

Sutton, S., Braren, M., Zubin, J., and John, E. R. Information delivery and the sensory evoked potential. *Science*, 1967, *155*, 1436–1439.

Suzuki, T., Hirar, Y., and Horiuchi, K. Auditory brain stem responses to pure tone stimuli. *Scandinavian Audiology*, 1977, *6*, 51–56.

Tanguay, P., Taub, J. M., Doubleday, C., and Clarkson, D. An interhemispheric comparison of auditory evoked responses to consonant-vowel stimuli. *Neuropsychologia*, 1977, *15*, 123–131.

Terkildsen, K., Osterhammel, P., and Huis in't Veld, F. Electrocochleography with a far field technique. *Scandinavian Audiology*, 1973, *2*, 141–148.

Terkildsen, K., Huis in't Veld, F., and Osterhammel, P. Auditory brain stem responses in the diagnosis of cerebellopontine angle tumors. *Scandinavian Audiology*, 1977, *6*, 45–50.

Teyler, T. J., Roemer, R. A., Harrison, T. F., and Thompson, R. F. Human scalp-recorded evoked-potential correlates of linguistic stimuli. *Bulletin of Psychonomic Society*, 1973, *1*, 333–334.

Thatcher, R. W. Evoked potential correlates of hemispheric lateralization during semantic information processing. In S. Harnad, R. Doty, L. Goldstein, J. Jaynes, and G. Krauthamer (eds.), *Lateralization in the Nervous System*. New York: Academic Press, 1977, pp. 429–448.

Triesman, A. M. Selective attention in man. *British Medical Bulletin*, 1964, *20*, 12–16.

Van Voorhis, S. T., and Hillyard, S. A. Visual evoked potentials and selective attention to points in space. *Perception and Psychophysics*, 1977, *22*, 54–62.

Vaughan, H. G., Jr., and Ritter, W. Physiological approaches to analysis of attention and performance. In S. Kornblum (ed.), *Attention and Performance*, Vol. IV. New York: Academic Press, 1973.

Wilkinson, R. T., and Lee, M. V. Auditory evoked potentials and selective attention. *Electroencephalography and Clinical Neurophysiology*, 1972, *33*, 411–418.

Wood, C. C. Auditory and phonetic levels of processing in speech perception: Neurophysiological and information-processing analysis. *Journal of Experimental Psychology: Human Perception and Performance*, 1975, *104*, 3–20.

Wood, C. C., Goff, W. R., and Day, R. S. Auditory evoked potentials during speech perception. *Science*, 1971, *173*, 1248–1251.

Woods, D. L., and Hillyard, S. A. Attention at the cocktail party: Brainstem evoked responses reveal no peripheral gating. In D. Otto (ed.), *Multidisiplinary Perspectives in Event-Related Brain Potential Research.*. Washington, D.C.: U.S. Environmental Protection Agency, 1978.

Yamada, O., Yagi, T., Yamane, H., and Suzuki, J.-I. Clinical evaluation of the auditory evoked brain stem response. *Auris-Nasus-Larynx*, 1975, *2*, 97–105.

Zimmerman, G. N., and Knott, J. R. Slow potentials in the brain related to speech processing in normal speakers and stutterers. *Electroencephalography and Clinical Neurophysiology*, 1974, *37*, 599–608.

13

Information Processing and the Cerebral Hemispheres*

Morris Moscovitch

Introduction

An information-processing approach to cerebral function is not altogether new. It would not be distorting the truth too much to say that the initial functional wiring diagrams of the cortex that appeared in the late nineteenth and early twentieth centuries bear more than a superificial resemblance to the flow diagrams that are still in vogue in many circles in cognitive psychology (see Fig. 1). Admittedly, some of the early neurological "localizers" or "diagram makers" had, by our standards, unsophisticated views of psychology and a simplistic notion of the physiological and philsophical problems regarding the localization of function in the nervous system. In fact, some of the functional subsystems, such as writing, reading, and music centers, which they localized in the cortex may remind us more of phrenology than of current information-processing systems. Nevertheless, if we ignore the surface details and terminology of those early functional-anatomical models and attend, instead, to the general assumptions concerning the organization of cognitive processes that underlie them, we will notice a kinship to modern information-processing theory. The early neurologists viewed cognition as the outcome of interactions among functionally and structurally separable subsystems whose

*This chapter is dedicated to the memory of Jack Catlin who died in 1976 at the age of 32. We began our research on information processing and hemispheric specialization together as graduate students (Moscovitch and Catlin, 1970). Although we had never formally collaborated again, Jack remained an excellent colleague and critic and a fine and loyal friend.

Morris Moscovitch   Erindale College, University of Toronto, Mississauga, Ontario M5L 1C6, Canada. The research conducted and reported in this chapter was supported by a National Research Council of Canada Grant No. A 8347.

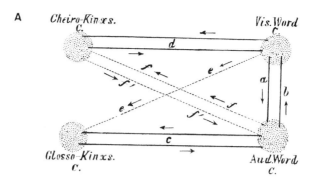

Diagram illustrating the relative positions of the different Word Centres and the mode in which they are connected by Commissures- *a*, the visuo-auditory commissure; *b*, the audito-visual commissures; *c*, the audito-kinæsthetic commissures; *d*, the visuo-kinæsthetic commissures; *e, e*, the visuo-glosso-kinæsthetic commissure; *f, f*, the audito-cheiro-kinæsthetic commissure; *f, f*, the cheiro-kinæsthetic and auditory commissure.

The last three Commissures represent unusual routes for the transmission of stimuli between the Word Centres.

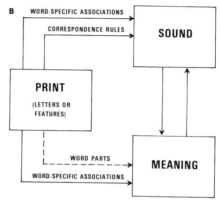

A framework for extracting sound and meaning from print

Fig. 1 Comparison between (A) functional-anatomical diagram (Bastian, 1898) and (B) modern framework for reading (Baron, 1978. Reprinted from *Basic Processes in Reading: Perception and Comprehension*, D. La Berge and S. J. Samuels (eds.). By permission of Lawrence Erlbaum Assoc., Hillsdale, N.J. Copyright, 1978).

operations, to put it in today's terms, transform, decode, classify, interpret, store, retrieve, and produce information. The purpose of their enterprise was to fractionate cognitive behavior into the appropiate subsystems, describe their mode of operation, and determine the nature of their interaction. These assumptions and program of research apply equally well to proponents of the information-processing approach to cognition.

In those early days, there were many neurologists who argued that neither cognition nor the brain was divisible into structural and functional subsystems along the lines proposed by the localizers (Bay, 1962; Goldstein, 1948; Head, 1926; Jackson, 1878; Lashley, 1950). They proposed, instead, that the nervous system was organized according to a hierarchy in which voluntary symbolic behaviors were mediated by the highest levels and stimulus-bound behaviors by the lowest. Generally, they believed that brain damage was not selective, but reduced all functions to a lower level of operation in the hierarchy. For example, normal speech, which is voluntary and abstract, became, according to them, automatic and concrete after brain damage.

Their criticism served only to refine the localization position, not to displace it. Complex functions such as reading, writing, and language were no longer viewed as residing in a portion of the brain known as a reading or writing or language center, but rather were viewed as mediated by a functional system each of whose components had a specific operation to perform that contributed to that function and each of which could be localized to a specific portion of the brain. Moreover, the critics called attention to the fact that brain damage may cause any of these specific subsystems to operate at a different level which would affect the organization of the entire functional system of which that component is a part (see below).

Having discarded many of the more simplistic ideas regarding localization of function, abandoned many, but not all, connectionistic theories, and assimilated new theories and techniques from current human experimental psychology, modern neuropsychology fits even more comfortably than its ancestor into an information-processing approach to human cognition. In addition to sharing with neuropsychology many assumptions regarding the organization of cognitive processes, human information-processing theory has focused its concerns on topics that have traditionally been at the forefront of neuropsychological research, namely, language, reading, perception, memory, and imagery. Through information-processing theory, human experimental psychology has rediscovered its cognitive roots. As a result, cross-fertilization between neuropsychology and experimental psychology is greater than it has been at any time since the turn of the century (James, 1890, but see Hebb, 1949, 1951, and Lashley, 1950, who may be seen as precursors of this era). This does not imply that the two disciplines are in total agreement regarding problems or theory in cognition. The different techniques used by the two disciplines almost ensure that, at the very least, differences in interpretation of some phenomena will occur; sometimes, new techniques will uncover phenomena that would otherwise have remained hidden to the other discipline.

The purpose of this chapter will be to highlight some of the research areas in which cross-fertilization between the two disciplines is very high and indicate, if possible, where advances made in one area might lead to interesting research in another. To avert the possibility that this chapter will provide only a survey of the recent literature (and some timid predictions about the future), I have embedded this review in the framework of an information-processing model of hemispheric asymmetry. By taking such an approach, it will be necessary to limit the scope of the survey to topics involving hemispheric specialization of function. Even then, the area is much too broad to cover fully in a single chapter. As a result, some areas of research, such as memory and language, that are covered in other chapters in this book, will be dealt with only briefly.

The questions we will be concerned with will be (1) at what stage in the information-processing sequence do hemispheric asymmetries emerge? (2) can the structural locus at which this asymmetry appears be specified? (3) what are the consequences of the emergence of such asymmetry on later stages of processing? (4) how can such a functional-neuropsychological approach be applied to cognitive processes such as reading, imagery and attention?

Before beginning to discuss these topics, I want to state my biases concerning neuropsychology clearly. As stated earlier, the value of neuropsychology is that it provides methods for fractionating complex cognitive processes into their constituent components. This dissociation of function is seen most strikingly in cases of brain damage, but may be observed in other circumstances as well. Because it is the pattern of dissociation that is of primary interest to psychologists, it makes little difference from their point of view what structures are responsible for producing that dissociation. It is only significant that lesions "somewhere" selectively affect syntactic but not semantic processing, long-term but not short-term memory; whether "somewhere" refers to the frontal lobes, hippocampus, or pineal gland is irrelevant to psychological theories. Although that claim is valid as far as it goes, to ignore neuroanatomy entirely is foolish and, in the long run, damaging. By specifying the structures that influence different aspects of human cognition, one can then apply the knowledge gained from neuroanatomy, neurophysiology, and comparative studies of these structures to elucidate further the nature of cognitive processes.* Because of these considerations, issues regarding the physical structure of the system mediating cognitive processes will receive some attention. The focus of the chapter, however, will be on functional analysis.

Implicit throughout the chapter is the assumption that the organization of cognitive processes is revealed through dissociation of function and the consequent investigation of the many functional subsystems that analyze, integrate, and produce information. As stated earlier, this assumption is shared by most human experimental psychologists and neuropsychologists. As this chapter will reveal, the data collected so far certainly indicate that this assumption has merit. Whether cognition can be explained by adhering solely to this assumption is a question I would like to consider at the end of the chapter.

Functional Locus of Hemispheric Asymmetries

It is common knowledge, even among educated laymen (Smith, 1975), that the cerebral hemispheres are functionally asymmetrical. The evidence for hemispheric specialization of function is overwhelming. Studies of brain-damaged individuals have shown that damage to the left hemisphere will selectively impair one aspect of cognition, such as language, while sparing others, such as face recognition, whereas damage to the opposite hemisphere will have opposite effects (see recent reviews by Dimond, 1972; Dimond and Beaumont, 1974; Milner, 1974; and almost any issues of any journal on neuropsychology, e.g., *Brain and Language, Cortex,* or *Neuropsychologia*). The functional asymmetry of the hemispheres is also reflected in the performance of normal people. Because sensory projections have privileged access to the contralateral hemisphere, normal people

---

*By comparing the effects of hippocampal damage in humans, rats, and monkeys, a number of investigators (Gaffan, 1974; Nadel and O'Keefe, 1974; O'Keefe and Nadel, in press; Warrington and Weiskrantz, 1973; Winocur and Weiskrantz, 1976) have arrived at fruitful theories explaining memory disorders in humans. Most recently, experiments on rats led Nadel and O'Keefe to propose that cognitive maps are represented in the hippocampus. The implications of this proposal to theories on the role of hippocampus in humans and to theories of human memory in general are far reaching.

have a perceptual bias in favor of information presented to the sensory field contralateral to the hemisphere that specializes in processing that information. Thus words are perceived better in the right visual field and faces, in the left. (For reviews, see Kimura, 1973; Kimura and Durnford, 1974; Moscovitch, 1973, 1976a.) These asymmetries are also manifested in electrophysiological recordings of hemispheric processes. Hemispheric asymmetries in the evoked potential and in the degree of blocking of alpha rhythms are observed on tasks that are mediated primarily by one of the hemispheres (Galin and Ornstein, 1972; Galin and Ellis, 1975; Wood, Goff, and Day, 1971; McAdam and Whitaker, 1971; Molfese *et al.*, 1975; Morrell and Salomy, 1971; but see Mayes and Beaumont, 1977, for contrary evidence).

Despite this proliferation of research on hemispheric specialization, (see *Annals of the New York Academy of Sciences*, 1976, edited by Harnad *et al.*, and 1977, edited by Dimond and Blizard for two major conferences on this topic) and even more speculation about it (see the same *Annals*), there is still a great deal of uncertainty about the exact nature of these functional asymmetries or the range of hemispheric processes over which they apply. The left hemisphere has been variously characterized as a linguistic, voluntary, linear, logical, and sequential processor and the right as a spatial, automatic, synthetic, appositional, holistic processor (Bogen, 1969; Cohen, 1973; Eccles, 1973; Jackson, 1878; Levy, 1974; Ornstein, 1972). Which, if any of these labels, best applies to the two hemispheres is an issue that will be taken up later. In the meantime, we shall discuss a problem more amenable to solution, namely, determining the range of processes for which functional hemispheric asymmetries exist. To answer this question, we need not make a prior commitments to any of the above positions regarding differences between the hemispheres. Nonetheless, we must have some heuristic to guide our search for functional differences and to structure our discussion about the results of the experiments we will discuss. Consequently, for convenience, we will adopt the traditional, conservative assumption which is safe, but almost certainly incomplete, that the left hemisphere specializes in processing verbal information and the right specializes in processing information that cannot be verbalized easily.

The logical first question is: What is the functional and structural locus at which hemispheric asymmetries emerge? To answer the functional question, an information-processing approach will be adopted. The knowledge gained from this approach will then be used to speculate about the structural locus at which the asymmetries appear and to suggest experiments to confirm these predictions.

According to traditional information-processing theory, the form or code in which a stimulus is represented is determined by the transformations which it undergoes through successive stages of processing (see Fig. 2; also Neisser, 1967; Sperling, 1963; Turvey, 1973). The initial stages extract sensory features such as brightness, texture, color, and contour if the stimulus is visual, or loudness, pitch, and clarity if the stimulus is auditory. By representing the stimulus as literally as possible in terms of these low-level, precategorical, "sensory" or "physical" properties, the early stages preserve unbiased information for later ones. Subsequent encoding mechanisms then operate selectively on the information available in the early stages and classify the stimulus in terms of higher-order, more abstract categories. One by-product of such processing is that information that undergoes

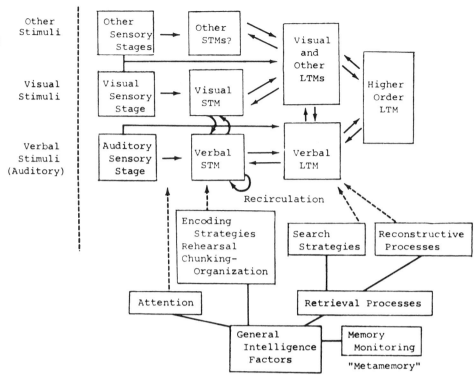

Fig. 2. Hypothetical schematic diagram for information-processing stages. According to this scheme, higher-order relational encoding processes first occur at the interface between sensory and short-term memory (STM). LTM. Long-term memory. From Rozin (1976). Reprinted from *Neurological Mechanisms of Learning and Memory*, M. R. Rosenzweig and E. L. Bennett (eds.). By permission of M.I.T. Press, Cambridge, Mass. (Copyright, 1976).

categorical encoding* is maintained as a relatively stable memory trace. Unless information available in the initial precategorical stages receives the benefit of further encoding, it is lost within a very short time after the stimulus disappears: about 100–200 msec if the stimulus is visual, and about 2 sec if it is auditory. Also, comparable data about other modalities are either unavailable or preliminary.

Within the framework of this information-processing theory, the question

---

*This use of the term "categorical encoding" or "categorical perception" differs somewhat from its more traditonal sense. Generally, the terms refer to the fact that discriminably different stimuli are treated equivalently, that is, they are perceived as belonging to the same category. Our usage merely adds the proviso that those categories be determined by the *relations* among sensory features that comprise the stimulus, or their association to higher-order concepts, rather than by the presence or magnitude of any of those features. Our usage of the term "categorical perception" is somewhat broader than the specialized sense it acquired from studies on speech but is nonetheless compatible with it. There "categorical perception" is said to occur if a sufficient acoustic cue within a speech stimulus is varied in equal steps along a physical continuum and the observer fails to perceive continuous change but rather hears quantal jumps from one category to another. Within the boundaries of the category, all stimuli varying along that continuum are encoded more or less equivalently whereas changes of similar magnitude are highly detectable only across category boundaries. Our use of the term "categorical perception" merely stipulates that these categories be based on relational properties, which indeed they are. Moreover, our usage does not commit us either to a particular method of determining categorical perception or to a particular theory of speech perception, both of which are associated with its specialized sense and both of which may be wrong (Diehl and Rosenberg, 1977; Hanson, 1977; Macmillan *et al.*, 1977; Pisoni and Tash, 1974; Porter and Mirabille, 1977; Repp, 1977).

regarding the locus of hemispheric asymmetries may be rephrased as follows: At which stage in the information-processing sequence do hemispheric asymmetries begin to emerge? Not surprisingly, data from the clinical literature suggest that the functions of the two hemispheres diverge most clearly only at the later, higher-order categorical stages: during the early stages, the two hemispheres process information in a similar fashion. Thus reports of hemispheric asymmetry for the extraction of sensory features such as color, contour, brightness, loudness, pitch, pressure, and touch indicate that asymmetries are either absent or small and inconsistent following unilateral damage (Corkin *et al.*, 1970, 1973; Milner, 1962; Scotti and Spinnler, 1970). In a recent, elegant demonstration of hemispheric similarity in sensory processing, Rotkin, Greenwood, and Gazzaniga (1977) showed that each hemisphere of a split-brain patient shows the same psychophysical power function in scaling pitch and loudness. Higher-order processes that integrate sensory features into more abstract categorical properties, however, are affected differentially by damage to one of the hemispheres. To give an example, the perception and recall of words are impaired more by left than by right hemisphere damage (Luria, 1973; Milner, 1966, 1974) whereas the perception and recall of music (or musical features) are impaired more by right hemisphere damage (Milner, 1962; Gordon, 1974). The perception of the simple acoustic features that compose both speech and music, however, is affected to an equal degree by damage to either hemisphere (Milner, 1962; Gordon, 1974).

A similar picture emerges from studies of normal people. Electrophysiological or perceptual asymmetries consistently in favor of one hemisphere are not usually reported for the detection or discrimination of low-level features such as brightness, contour, loudness, and pitch (Berlucchi *et al.*, 1971; Bradshaw and Perriment, 1970; Filby and Gazzaniga, 1969; Jeeves and Dixon, 1970; Ledlow *et al.*, in press; McKeever and Gill, 1972; Poffenberger, 1912; Wood, 1975; but for contrary results see Longdon *et al.*, 1976; Wada, 1976) even when these features are embedded in verbal (Rabinowicz, 1976; Wood, 1975) or nonverbal (Wood, 1975) contexts or when they are used to distinguish between ostensibly verbal or nonverbal stimuli (Wood, 1975). When higher-order categorical features such as phonemes, words, or facial features must be detected, perceptual and electrophysiological asymmetries are evident (e.g., Moscovitch, 1976a, Moscovith *et al.*, 1976; Patterson and Bradshaw, 1975; Wood *et al.*, 1971).

According to the information-processing framework presented earlier, hemispheric differences in the way a stimulus is processed or represented internally should also vary as a function of the transformation and changes that occur as it is being encoded in memory. The evidence generally supports this notion. Studies of normal and brain-damaged individuals have shown that imposing a delay prior to recognition or recall accentuates hemispheric asymmetries for the identification of a variety of stimuli, including faces (Milner, 1968b; Moscovitch *et al.*, 1976; Patterson and Bradshaw, 1975), nonsense shapes (Dee and Fontenot, 1973; Hatta, 1976a,b), letters (Hines *et al.*, 1973; Rosen *et al.*, 1975), consonant-vowel speech sounds (Donnenfeld *et al.*, 1976), digits (Goodglass and Peck, 1972; Yeni-Komshian and Gordon, 1974), nonsense words (Hannay and Malone, 1976), musical notes (Oscar-Berman *et al.*, 1974), and sentences (Frankfurter and Honeck, 1973; Jarvella and Herman, 1973).

In a series of studies on face recognition, Moscovitch *et al.* (1976) were able to trace the time course for the development of hemispheric differences in the representation of faces by sampling for the existence of perceptual asymmetries at various stages of processing. In one experiment, individuals were presented with a sample face for 500 msec at fixation to ensure that it was received by both hemispheres. Given the long exposure duration, the individual should have had access both to a low-level, short-lived visual trace and to a more stable, higher-order memory representation once the stimulus disappeared. At various intervals after stimulus offset, a face appeared in either the right or the left visual field and the individual had to indicate as quickly as possible whether it matched the sample. A consistent left visual field-right hemisphere superiority emerged only at ISIs of about 100 msec (see Fig. 3a), an interval that approximates the durability of the short-lived, "sensory" visual trace or icon (Coltheart, 1975; Holding, 1975; Turvey, 1973). The initial absence of a left-field advantage suggests that both hemispheres had equal access to the short-lived, precategorical or sensory representation of the sample. For a brief period, sample and test faces would then have been compared on the basis of low-level, "sensory" properties, such as brightness and contour, that are characteristic of this short-term representation. Once this representation decays, the test face could be compared only to the more deeply encoded permanent representation of the sample to which the right hemisphere had preferential access or on which it could operate more efficiently than the left. To confirm this hypothesis, Moscovitch *et al.* (1976) showed that if the short-term trace was degraded prematurely by a visual mask presented during the ISI, a right-hemisphere advantage was noted at even the shortest intervals (see Fig. 3*b*).

Another way of preventing the lower-order trace from participating directly

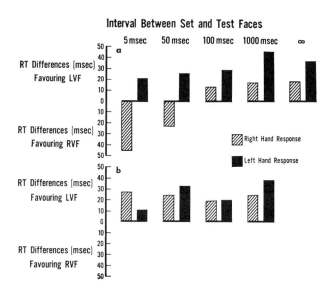

Fig. 3. Average difference in reaction time between the right and left visual fields. The data are broken down by interstimulus interval and responding hand: (a) the interstimulus interval was blank; (b) a mask was present during the interval. From Moscovitch, M., Scullion, D., and Christie, D. *Journal of Experimental Psychology: Human Perception and Performance*, 1976, *2*, 401–416. Copyright 1976 by the American Psychological Association. Reprinted by permission.

in a face comparison task is by requiring the use of higher-order features. An appropriate task is the comparison of caricatures with photographs. The decision that a caricature and a photograph represent the same person cannot be based on the comparison of lower-order "physical" features but must be made with reference to some higher-order abstract or idealized representation of the face. In such a situation, a left field-right hemisphere advantage emerges even when the photograph and caricature are simultaneously available for inspection.

The short duration of the visual trace, its susceptibility to masking by visual noise, and its equal availability to either hemisphere strongly support the notion that this trace represents the results of the very early stages of visual processing. It also raises the possibility that these early processes are peripheral ones, whereas those that distinguish the hemispheres from each other are central. This idea was tested in a study using masking techniques which are presumed to affect selectively either central or peripheral visual processes.

According to Turvey (1973), an unpatterned visual stimulus operates as a peripheral mask by interfering with visual processes involved in extracting physical features of the target. Consequently, the mask is effective only when it is presented to the same eye as the target. Because peripheral masking is sensitive to physical characteristics, such as target and mask energy (luminance × duration), the interstimulus interval at which the target evades the effects of the mask (critical ISI) is inversely proportional to target duration if luminance is kept constant. A plot of this multiplicative function appears in Fig. 4. A central mask, on the other hand, affects target perception by interrupting a central processor that integrates physcial-feature information into relational or patterned information. Consequently, central masking is sensitive to the pattern of the mask rather than its energy and can occur when the target and mask are presented to different eyes. When target duration is plotted against critical ISI for a patterned stimulus, a multiplicative relation is observed at short target duration, suggesting that the mask first interacts with the target in the periphery. At longer target durations, the relation is additive, suggesting that the mask interferes with a central processor that needs a constant amount of time to complete its operation (see Fig. 4).

If the differences between the two hemispheres emerged *only* at the level of the central processor, then a target, be it verbal or nonverbal, would evade the effects of a peripheral mask at the same critical ISI regardless of the visual field to which the target was presented. Visual field differences with regard to the critical ISI would be apparent, however, when a patterned stimulus was used. The central processor in the hemisphere specialized to process the target would complete its operation before its mate in the other hemisphere and thereby escape the effects of the mask sooner.

These predictions were confirmed in a study using three-letter words (CVCs) as targets, a white flash of light as the peripheral mask, and a jumble of straight lines as a pattern mask. The target was presented for durations of 2, 3, 4, 5, 6, 8, 12, 16, 20, and 24 msec in either the right or the left visual field. In one condition it was followed by the peripheral mask and in another by the pattern mask. As Fig. 5a shows, when a peripheral mask was used, the multiplicative masking function and the critical ISI were almost identical for the two visual fields. When the pattern mask interrupted the operations of the central processor, as was the case at

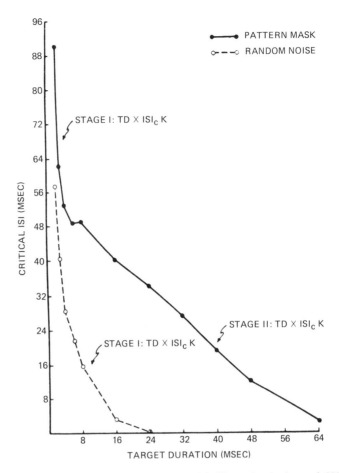

Fig. 4. Relation between target duration and the mean critical interstimulus interval (ISI) for monoptic masking of letter array by random noise and patterns. From Turvey, *Psychological Review*, 1973, *80*, 1–52. Copyright 1973 by the American Psychological Association. Reprinted by permission.

target durations that gave rise to an additive masking function, critical ISIs were consistently shorter in the right visual field. This difference, although small, occurred for all but one of eight subjects and was highly significant ($p < 0.001$; see Fig. 5b). Similar results were obtained in a study by McKeever and Suberi (1974) examining contrast masking functions for laterally displaced letters.

The evidence reviewed in this section indicates that peripheral processes concerned with extraction of physical features of the stimulus are common to both hemispheres. Any cognitive task that can be mediated by these early, low-level processes will be handled equally well by either hemisphere. Hemispheric asymmetries emerge only at the level of a central processor that integrates information from the peripheral channels and represents it in terms of configurational, relational, or categorical properties that reflect the mode of operation peculiar to the processors in each hemisphere. The processors in the right and left hemispheres are presumed to have limited processing capacities, and, by virtue of their differences, they operate relatively, but not totally, independently of each other even at the earliest level at which asymmetries emerge.

This last claim is based on a series of experiments conducted by Moscovitch and Klein. In an earlier study, Klein *et al.,* (1976) had shown that even when words and faces are presented together bilaterally, words are perceived better in the right visual field and faces in the left (see also Hines, 1975; Pirozzolo and Rayner, 1977). This result suggested that the cerebral hemispheres can operate as somewhat separate information-processing channels even under conditions of simultaneous input. To make the case for relative independence and limited capacity even stronger, however, it is necessary to show that each of these channels can be overloaded primarily by material that it is specialized to process. This effect was demonstrated clearly in a study in which subjects were required to identify a foveally presented stimulus in addition to a pair of either words or faces presented in the periphery of each visual field. Recognition of the peripherally presented faces was imparied more if the foveally presented stimulus was a face or a nonsense shape than if it was a word and, conversely, recognition of words in the periphery was impaired most by the foveally presented word (see Fig. 6). Because recognition of faces and nonsense shapes is known to be mediated primarily by the right hemisphere and words primarily by the left, the kind of material-specific perceptual interference noted in this study likely results from competition among the stimuli for hemisphere-specific processing mechanisms that have a limited capacity. Performance in the nonsense shape condition indicates that the effect is

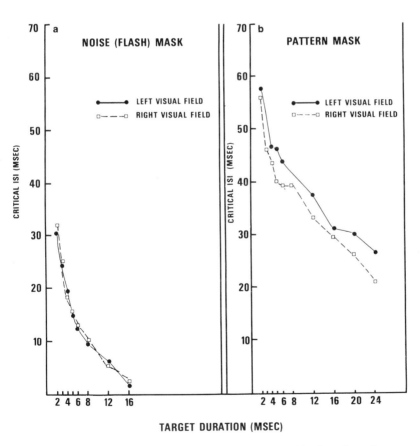

Fig. 5. Relation between target duration and mean critical ISI for masking by noise and patterns when the target and mask appear in the same visual field.

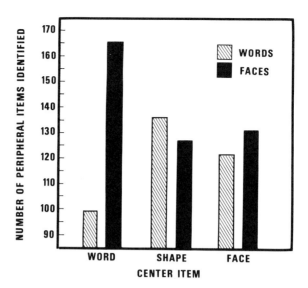

Fig. 6. Number of peripherally presented words or faces that were identified correctly when the foveally presented item was either a word, a shape, or a face.

not due simply to confusion or interference caused by the similarity between the stimulus at the fovea and those at the periphery. If similarity were critical, performance when a central shape was present would be expected to differ significantly from that when a central face was present. Since the perceptual interference effect was almost identical in the two conditions, one can conclude that it results from competition between the two stimuli for a hemisphere-specific processor of limited capacity. It should be noted, however, that the two processors do not operate totally independently of each other. Recognition of the peripheral stimuli is worse whenever any stimulus is present foveally than when none is present. Thus these processors must have processing mechanisms in common, or they require the allocation of attention for their operation, or both. Later experiments have suggested that both are the case, although by far the greatest perceptual interference effects are observed when attentional demands are highest.

These experiments then support the model depicted in Fig. 7. Before we examine the implication that this model has for hypotheses regarding the organization of later information-processing systems in the cerebral hemispheres, let us first determine whether it applies equally well to other modalities.

Somesthesis

The few data available on the somesthetic modality fit easily into the framework provided by the model. Low-level somesthetic features such as touch and pressure seem to be processed equally well by either hemisphere (Corkin *et al.*, 1970, 1973). It is only when these features must be integrated into a higher-order, configurational unit that hemispheric differences in processing occur. Thus the identification of a sequentially presented haptic pattern was better when delivered to the left hand (Nachshon and Carmon, 1975). Similarly, haptic nonsense figures (Milner and Taylor, 1972; Witelson, 1974), braille letters (Hermelin and O'Connor, 1971), shapes (DeRenzi *et al.,* 1971; DeRenzi and Scotti, 1969), tactual closure (Nebes, 1971), and direction of stimulation (Carmon and Benton, 1969; Benton *et al.,* 1973) were identified more accurately by the left hand-right hemisphere. It remains to be seen whether this congruence with the model will be maintained once the operation of the somesthetic system has been analyzed in more detail. For example, the existence of short-lived somesthetic traces comparable to short-term and precategorical acoustic storage in audition has only recently been discovered (Sullivan and Turvey, 1974; Watkins and Watkins, 1974). It would be interesting to know whether these haptic traces are equally accessible to both hemispheres, as the model predicts, or whether the haptic modality is organized differently from the visual and the acoustic ones.

AUDITION

The model's account of the relation between levels of processing and hemispheric asymmetries seems to apply very well to the auditory domain. Research on speech perception suggests that all acoustic signals undergo some common, low-level processing that can be handled equally well by either hemisphere (Studdert-Kennedy and Shankweiler, 1970; Wood, 1974, 1975). The precategorical, acoustic information available from this analysis is then maintained in a short-lasting auditory or echoic trace (Massaro, 1972; Crowder, 1973) that is probably available to both hemispheres as indicated by the absence of an ear advantage in dichotic listening tasks (Darwin, 1974*a,b,* 1975; Shankweiler and Studdert-Kennedy, 1967;

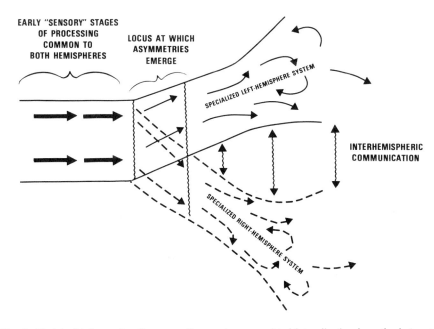

Fig. 7. Model of information flow according to the transmitted-lateralization hypothesis (see text).

Studdert-Kennedy and Shankweiler, 1970). Higher-order processes that are mediated by left-hemisphere mechanisms then integrate the information from the earlier stages of analysis into categorical, phonetic features. This coding process is reflected in the right ear advantage on dichotic tests for such stimuli as stop consonants that show a high degree of categorical perception and leave a poor echoic trace (Liberman, 1974; Pisoni, 1973; Studdert-Kennedy and Shankweiler, 1970). Stimuli that leave a strong echoic trace and that are weakly categorical, such as vowels, usually show a right ear advantage only when the precategorical information is degraded and no longer useful in distinguishing one vowel from another (Darwin, 1974a,b, 1975; Godfrey, 1974; Weiss and House, 1973). Similar processes are presumed to occur in the right hemisphere to extract higher-order, auditory information that is nonlinguistic, such as music (Bever and Chiarello, 1974; Gordon, 1974; Shankweiler, 1966). For both verbal and nonverbal stimuli, then, the model predicts that the magnitude of hemispheric asymmetries will reflect the degree to which precategorical, acoustic information can be shown to influence the perception of even highly categorical stimuli, such as consonants (Pisoni and Tash, 1974).

The model may also help explain some of the discrepancies among studies attempting to obtain a right-ear advantage with monaural linguistic presentation. In general, a right-ear advantage is observed when the task places strong demands on higher-order mnemonic processes which, according to our model, are strongly lateralized. Performance, therefore, is better to monaural right-ear input on tasks that require subjects to remember syntactically complex sentences (Bever, 1971; Frankfurter and Honeck, 1973; Jarvella and Herman, 1973) or to compare a syllable or word to a number of similar items which form the target set (Morais, 1976). When a simple phonetic judgment is required, such as the detection of a single syllable consisting of a stop consonant and a vowel, a monaural right ear advantage may be observed only in conditions in which detection cannot be based on lower-order acoustic (precategorical) information (Morais, 1976; Morais and Darwin, 1974). These conditions, therefore, are similar to ones in which a right-ear advantage for dichotic vowels is obtained. If the monaural stimulus competes with contralateral noise (Springer, 1973), or if comparison with a previous stimulus is based primarily on higher phonetic features (Catlin and Neville, 1976; Morais and Darwin, 1974), a right-ear advantage will emerge. If the monaural signal leaves a strong and clear acoustic trace, either the differences in transmission between the left and right-ear signals to the speech processor may be so reduced that they go undetected, or the simple detection may be based on precategorical information available to both hemispheres (Morais, 1976). The only published study to cause difficulties with this view is by Catlin et al. (1977), who found a monaural right-ear advantage that remained constant whether or not contralateral noise was present. The only interpretation of this result that is consistent with the model is that even the monaural signal was sufficiently degraded so that the subject was forced to rely on phonetic cues in detecting the target stimulus. Under these conditions, adding contralateral noise would not increase the right-ear advantage in a latency task. The validity of this interpretation may be determined by examining how the RT advantage for the right ear is affected by monaural signals that vary systematically in the degree to which they have been degraded.

DISCREPANCIES WITH THE MODEL

Not all studies support the general model. A number of investigators have found that perceptual asymmetries do not exist for the discrimination of low-level features such as brightness (Davidoff, 1975), curvature (Longdon *et al.*, 1976), or simply for the detection of a light (Anzola *et al.*, 1977). In accordance with these findings, other investigators have shown that the detection of these features is affected more by damage to one hemisphere than to the other (Bisiach *et al.*, 1976; DeRenzi and Faglioni, 1965; Howes and Boller, 1975; Scotti and Spinnler, 1970). These findings, however, are often inconsistent in that similar studies fail to confirm them.

Similar inconsistencies are found in tasks in which subjects were asked to discriminate between two simultaneously presented, physically identical letters. Since these physical matches could be made on the basis of low-level features, no perceptual asymmetries should be observed. Many investigators obtained this result (Gazzaniga, 1970; Brooks, personal communication; Ledlow *et al.*, 1972, 1973, 1977; Moscovitch, 1977), although others found a significant left-visual field advantage (Cohen, 1973; Geffen *et al.*, 1972; Gibson *et al.*, 1972; Hellige, 1976; Wilkins and Stewart, 1974). There is no obvious explanation for these discrepancies. One possibility is that slight differences in task demands and stimulus characteristics may force the subject to adopt different strategies. For example, in the letter-matching task the subject has available both lower-level and higher-level information about the stimulus during and immediately following stimulus presentation. Shortly after the stimulus disappears, the subject retains only the information encoded at a higher level. Differences in exposure duration or contrast are known to determine the durability of the lower-order traces once the stimulus disappears. It is significant that the studies that used the shortest exposure durations (Cohen, 1973; Wilkins and Stewart, 1974) and the ones in which the stimuli were degraded (Gibson *et al.*, 1972; Hellige, 1976) found a left-field advantage. Perhaps the relative inaccessibility or transiency of the low-level trace in those studies led the subjects to rely on a more stable higher-order visual representation associated with the right hemisphere. When the low-level trace was long lasting and stable, such differences would not emerge. Similarly, depending on whether accuracy or speed is emphasized or whether discrimination is difficult or easy (Paterson and Bradshaw, 1975), the subject may choose to attend to either high-level or low-level features, respectively, in executing the task. This explanation may apply equally well to studies in which simple features are being detected. If the stimulus is unclear or if speed/accuracy contingencies are of a certain value, individuals may have to use higher-order processes to infer whether a stimulus was indeed present or if it differed to a certain extent from its target (Neisser, 1967).

Admittedly, these explanations are post hoc. But they can be tested easily by varying stimulus or response parameters and seeing what effect they have on perceptual asymmetries. We already know that the size of the right ear advantage for vowels diminishes with increases in discriminability (Godfrey, 1974). There is no reason why this should not also be the case for other stimulus arrays.

The most direct challenge to the model comes from a visual masking study conducted by Cohen (1976) in which she concluded that the persistence of the icon (short-term visual trace), as well as selective sampling from the icon, is different in the left and right visual fields. Because these conclusions argue against the notion that the representation and processing of low-level information is identical in the two visual fields (and the two hemispheres), Cohen's experiment and her arguments will be reviewed in some detail.

An array of six letters was displayed for 100 msec in either the right or the left visual field, and individuals had to report verbally either all the letters (full report) or only those letters that were cued by color and location (partial report). Cuing occurred either 1 sec before the stimulus array or 10 or 50 msec after it. The full report condition produced a right visual field advantage that was especially noticeable if a visual mask was introduced 20 msec after stimulus offset. Since it is presumed that pattern masking effectively terminates processing of the icon, Cohen reasoned that the rate of encoding or readout from the icon in each visual field can be determined by dividing the number of items reported into 120 msec, which was the duration of the trace. This line of reasoning, however, is based on two assumptions; the first is unwarranted and the second is very likely false. The first assumption is that encoding rate is constant and unaffected by the number of items that have already been encoded and stored. The evidence on this point is controversial (Chow and Murdock, 1976; Scarborough, 1972; Sperling, 1963). The second assumption is that the time after stimulus presentation at which higher-order encoding begins is the same in the right and left visual fields. If we assume that in this task encoding is ultimately verbal, then it is likely that items in the right visual field will have more direct access to verbal mechanisms in the left hemisphere than items in the left field. Consequently, right-field items will be encoded earlier and thereby *appear as if* they are being encoded at a faster rate then left-field items. Cohen's calculated estimates of an encoding rate of 22 items/ sec in the right visual field and 18 items/sec in the left are therefore invalid. Since she uses these estimates of encoding rate to calculate iconic persistence and sampling efficiency in the cued condition for each visual field, any conclusions she reaches about these latter two components are also likely to be false (Oscar-Berman *et al.*, 1973, make errors similar to Cohen's in arguing for differences in iconic storage between the two hemispheres).

To demonstrate that low-level representations, such as the icon, are stored or processed differently by the two hemispheres, it is necessary to devise tasks that can be handled on the basis of low-level information. Once successful execution of the task depends on higher-order encoding or response processes that favor one of the hemispheres, a bias is introduced that will necessarily affect the outcome in favor of one of the hemispheres. In essence, this is what happened in Cohen's study. Had her stimuli and responses been neutral, i.e., less verbal, or had she chosen a different procedure, such as matching, to indicate which stimuli were present in the icon, her results and conclusions would probably have been different. By and large, those experiments that fulfilled these criteria support the notion that early, precateogrical information is represented and processed similarly by the two hemispheres. Hemispheric differences emerge only at those levels of processing in which precategorical information is synthesized to form categorical or configurational representations. The problem of specifying the structural locus at which hemispheric asymmetries emerge will be considered in the next section.

SPECULATION ABOUT THE STRUCTURAL LOCUS AT WHICH HEMISPHERIC ASYMMETRIES EMERGE

The designation of an early visual central processing stage as the functional locus at which hemispheric asymmetries emerge provides important clues for determining the structural locus of these asymmetries. Because the operations of this central processing stage seem to be modality specific (Darwin, 1975; Liberman, 1974; Turvey, 1973), it is likely that the structural locus is different for each modality. Let us examine the visual modality first.

We have shown that the differences in hemispheric susceptibility to masking are observed only when a pattern mask interrupts the operation of a central visual process. Because only pattern masking can be effective dichoptically, it suggests that the central processor is found either at or beyond the point at which information from the two eyes converges (Turvey, 1973). Breitmeyer and Ganz (1976) and Weisstein *et al.* (1975) claim that the source of this type of masking is the inhibition exerted by the fast-conducting, transient Y-fiber system on the slower, sustained, pattern-integrating X system. If we extrapolate from animal studies, the evidence suggests that in the majority of cells examined the X and Y systems as well as the input from the two eyes converge primarily in areas 18 and 19 of prestriate cortex (Blakemore, 1975). This suggests that the locus of visual hemispheric asymmetries is either at the prestriate or at the next visual relay in the posterior temporal cortex. The reason for mentioning the posterior temporal cortex as a possibility is that although central masking presumably occurs in the prestriate area (see also Schloterer, 1977) the susceptibility to such masking may be determined by the rate at which the next level integrates prestriate input. Prior to such integration, a pattern mask may prevent the output of the prestriate system from reaching the posterior temporal cortex.

At present, the evidence is inadequate for choosing between prestriate and posterior temporal structures as the locus of visual hemispheric asymmetries.* If the locus were at the level of the prestriate, individuals with unilateral visual cortex damage that spared the posterior temporal lobes would show a pattern of perceptual deficits that depended on the side that was damaged. Individuals with such

---

*It is interesting to note that in monkeys, and presumably in humans, prestriate areas 18 and 19 receive callosal connections only from the visual midline (Berlucchi, 1972). This suggests that stimuli that are presented in the periphery, as they are in experiments on laterality, must reach the appropriate hemisphere via interhemispheric pathways connecting structures anterior to the prestriate. In such cases, hemispheric differences probably emerge at this point or beyond. Moreover, it makes sense that hemispheric asymmetries should emerge at a point at which connections exist for exchanging information between hemispheres.

damage are rare (Perenin and Jeannerod, 1975; Poeppel *et al.*, 1973; Sanders *et al.*, 1974) but nothing is mentioned in the literature about them to indicate that they have impaired specialized left- or right-hemisphere functions. Those patients whose damage extends to posterior temporal-parietal lobe structures, however, do show specific deficits in reading, if the damage is on the left, and in face and object recognition, if the damage is on the right (Geschwind, 1970; DeRenzi *et al.*, 1968; Warrington and James, 1967; Warrington and Taylor, 1973).

Electrophysiological studies, which correlate the pattern of evoked responses to different stimuli under different masking conditions with the operation of specific neural structures, may prove to be a valuable technique for establishing the structural locus of hemispheric asymmetries (Hillyard and Woods, this volume). Despite tremendous advances in electrophysiology, the current techniques have not yet reached the level of sophistication required to solve this problem.

In the auditory domain, the situation is somewhat clearer. Research on auditory neurophysiology, speech perception, and dichotic listening has shown that input from the two ears reaches the hemipsheres primarily via contralateral pathways (Aitken and Webster, 1972; Rosenzeig, 1951) and then converges on a phonetic processor in the left hemisphere (Berlin and McNeil, 1976; Kimura, 1961, 1967; Studdert-Kennedy and Shankweiler, 1970) or on a corresponding processor in the right hemisphere that specializes in decoding complex, nonverbal information (Shankweiler, 1966). Since hemispheric asymmetries in processing auditory information emerge only at the level of these processors, it follows that the structural locus of these asymmetries is at or slightly beyond the sites where input from the two ears converges via interhemispheric pathways in either the right or the left hemisphere. By extrapolating from the work of Pandya *et al.* (1969) on rhesus monkeys, one can assume that there are interhemispheric pathways in the human connecting left and right auditory association cortex (area 22) as well as left and right temporal-parietal cortex (posterior 22 and 39). The latter areas in the left hemisphere are designated as the posterior speech zones (Wernicke's area).

To determine which of these pathways is the primary one used and therefore to locate the phonetic processor in the left hemisphere, Berlin and his colleagues (Berlin and McNeil, 1976; Berlin *et al.*, 1972; Cullen *et al.*, 1974) conducted a series of elegant dichotic speech studies on a normal and brain-damaged population. The brain-damaged population consisted of people with unilateral temporal lobectomies (damage to association cortex), with commissurotomies, or with hemispherectomies. If the specialized left-hemisphere processor were located in the auditory association cortex, or if the pathways relaying left ear input to that processor typically passed through left-hemisphere association cortex, then damage to it would lead to lower than normal scores on a dichotic speech task for both the right and left ears. Instead, he found that *only* right ear performance was impaired. Performance in the left ear was normal. The reverse effect was seen in people with unilateral right temporal damage. On the basis of these results, Berlin and his colleagues concluded that input from the left ear reaches a phonetic processor located in the posterior temporal-parietal cortex via pathways connecting this area to the homotopic region on the right (see Fig. 8). According to the

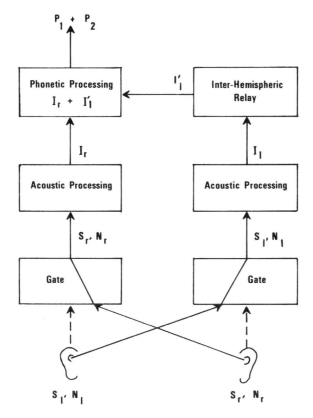

Fig. 8. Flow diagram of speech information processing. S, signal; N, noise; I, extracted information; P, phonemic response (see text). From Cullen et al. (1974). Reprinted by permission of the authors.

model they proposed, patients with commissurotomy or left hemispherectomy should report verbally only the right ear input in dichotic speech tasks. In these patients, the left ear input cannot reach the left hemisphere via callosal pathways and is thereby prevented from competing with the right ear input for access to a limited-capacity phonetic processor. As predicted, Berlin *et al.* found that in these patients' performance on the left ear was near zero whereas performance on the right ear was much better than that of the normal population. Similar results were obtained by Milner *et al.* (1968*b*) and Sparks and Geschwind (1968).

The evidence from these dichotic studies is consistent with earlier suggestions (cited in Geschwind, 1965) that the isolation of a speech processor in Wernicke's area from left and right hemisphere auditory input results in word deafness, a condition in which speech perception is severely impaired relative to the mild impairment in the perception of equally complex nonverbal acoustic information (see also Saffran *et al.*, 1976*a*). Finally, recent evidence regarding the anatomical asymmetries between the left and right hemispheres in the region of the planum temporale (Geschwind and Levitsky, 1968) lends further plausibility to the notion that the structural locus for auditory perceptual asymmetries resides in the posterior temporal-parietal cortex.

Despite all this converging evidence for a posterior-temporal site as the locus of the phonetic processor, there are other studies that suggest that structures in the frontal cortex are also involved in speech processing. Damage to Broca's area (Blumstein *et al.*, 1977*a,b;* Luria, 1970) or to the face area adjacent to it (Taylor *et al.*, 1975) causes severe deficits in phonetic processing, although probably of a different kind from those associated with the posterior speech zones (Blumstein *et al.*, 1977*a,b*). Whether the frontal area receives acoustic information and transforms it into a linguistic code in parallel with the posterior zones or whether it depends on the posterior zone for its linguistic input is a problem left for future research.

If a general principle is to be extrapolated from the dichotic listening studies and, to some extent, from studies on visual perceptual asymmetries, it is that hemispheric asymmetries are first found at sites where input from large portions of the right and left sensory fields converge, usually beyond the first "association" areas. It will be interesting to see whether this prediction is upheld in later research on the visual and auditory systems, as well as on the other sensory modalities for which asymmetries in hemispheric functions are only just beginning to be investigated. (Milner and Taylor, 1972; Witelson, 1974).

INFORMATION PROCESSING BEYOND THE LOCUS AT WHICH HEMISPHERIC ASYMMETRIES EMERGE

If information processing is viewed as a sequence in which higher-order processes operate on input received from lower-order ones, it follows that all processes subsequent to the ones at which hemispheric asymmetries emerge will also reveal hemispherically specialized properties. Put another way, once early, precategorical information has been transformed so that it reflects or is more compatible with the operation of one cerebral hemisphere than the other, then all later transformations of this input will retain hemispherically specialized qualities. For convenience, this hypothesis will be referred to as *transmitted laterlization.* The problem with investigating the merits of this proposal is that our conceptions of what constitutes subsequent processing stages are tied to classes of rival theories that differ from each other in important ways and that are notoriously unstable: compare the many different stages or box models of perception and memory (see Murdock, 1974; Crowder, 1976; Baddeley, 1976) with the levels-of-processing ones (Craik and Lockhart, 1972; Lockhart *et al.*, 1975; Norman, 1976) and with the theories that view perception and memory in terms of operations or skills (Kolers, 1975; Neisser, 1976). Moreover, certain higher cognitive functions that are of concern to neuropsychology, such as perception of temporal order and different aspects of language, either do not fit easily into current information-processing models or are not considered by them at all. If we are willing to live with a little imprecision, it is possible to proceed with our investigation despite these drawbacks. Although we cannot specify with certainty either the nature or the sequence of all higher-order processes, we can agree, in general, which processes in a given theory may be termed postcategorical or postconfigurational—that is, which processes transform or use information that has already been endowed with categorical and a hemispherically-specialized property. According to our hypothesis, all these processes should also show evidence of hemispheric specialization. In this section, we will examine some higher-order processes both in terms of some currently popular information-processing theories and in the light of available neurological evidence. Such an examination will provide at least an initial, crude test of our hypothesis and may also reveal neuropsychological evidence that can help decide between competing theories.

EPISODIC MEMORY

"Episodic memory" is memory for events or episodes. According to Tulving (1973), it is to be distinguished from memory for general information, which he called "semantic memory." Clearly, this distinction is useful in classifying experiments, models, and theories that are concerned primarily with memory for different kinds of information. Whether it is more than a conceptual distinction, that is, whether it refers to two functionally and structurally dissociable memory systems, is debatable (Fedio and van Buren, 1974; Kinsbourne and Wood, 1975; Warrington, 1975; Wilkins and Moscovitch, 1978). For the moment, we have adopted Tulving's terminology for purely classificatory purposes. This section will deal with episodic memory and the next, with semantic.

A class of memory models that were prevalent in the 1960s and that still have many adherents today viewed memory as a series of discrete stores each of which was distinguishably different from the other and each of which held distinguishably different kinds of memories (see Fig. 2). The mode of representation of the stimulus trace and its durability were uniquely determined by, and in a sense defined, the memory store in which it resided. Decoding or transforming operations enabled the stimulus trace to move from one store to the next. According to this class of models, stimulus input was first held in a very short-lasting, precategorical, sensory store known as "sensory memory." Decoding operations transferred the contents of this store into a limited-capacity "short-term memory" (STM) in which some items could be maintained indefinitely but only by active rehearsal. The rehearsal enabled items to be transferred to a permanent "long-term memory" (LTM). Murdock's (1967) conception of this modal "stage" model (see Fig. 9) is still generally accurate, although some details and modifications should be noted. Rehearsal may be neither necessary nor sufficient to transfer

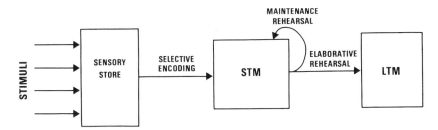

Fig. 9. Slightly revised version of the traditional, basic information-processing stages in human memory.

information to long-term memory (Craik and Watkins, 1973); separate short- and long-term memories are now believed to exist for different modalities (Posner, 1969; Coltheart, 1972; Rozin, 1976); and items in both short and long-term memory can be represented semantically* and phonemically, although not to an equal degree (Bartlett and Tulving, 1974). What has not been modified is the view that different memory stores exist which are related, but separable, from each other.

Although experimental psychologists have questioned the usefulness of this model (see below), neuopsychological research is consistent with the model's compartmentalized approach to memory. According to the "stage" model, hemispheric asymmetries should emerge at the interface between sensory and short-term memory. At this point, stimulus information is no longer represented in terms of precategorical-sensory features but in terms of more abstract, configurational features that, for example, can be used to distinguish verbal from nonverbal material. The evidence presented earlier supports this view and furthermore suggests that sensory and short-term memory can be dissociated neurologically: the former shows no evidence of hemispheric asymmetry, the latter does.

When the transmitted-lateralization hypothesis is examined in terms of the "stages" model, it leads to the prediction that all the memory systems subsequent to the interface between sensory and short-term memory should also show evidence of lateralization. The evidence strongly supports this prediction. Unilateral damage to the anterior, mesial temporal lobe and hippocampus produces deficits primarily in verbal LTM if the damage is on the left and in nonverbal LTM if the damage is on the right (Milner, 1968a, 1971, 1974). Short-term memory remains relatively normal in these circumstances. Lesions in the left parieto-occipital region selectively impair verbal STM but spare LTM (Warrington and Shallice, 1969; Shallice and Warrington, 1970). Patients who display this deficit were traditionally termed "conduction aphasics" (Geschwind, 1970), their identifying symptom being their gross inability to repeat speech while retaining relatively good comprehension and productive capacities. It was Warrington and Shallice's insight to suggest that these patients have a selective impairment of short-term memory. Whereas their immediate recall or recognition of items is poor even when a nonverbal response is required, they seem able to learn a verbal list as quickly as normal people, suggesting an intact long-term memory.

This view was corroborated by Saffran and Marin (1975) by asking individuals to recall a list of words and then plotting the words recalled against the serial position of the word in the original list. Recall of the primary and middle items is believed to be mediated by LTM and that of the most recent items by STM and precategorical acoustical store (PAS) (Crowder and Morton, 1969; Glanzer and Cunitz, 1966). Conduction aphasics were impaired only in their recall of the most

---

*One should not confuse the notion of semantic encoding in long-term memory with semantic memory. The latter refers to memories for general information and, conceptually, it is distinguished from episodic memory. Long-term memory is an aspect of episodic memory, and semantic encoding is the process whereby events are represented in LTM in terms of meaning, i.e., semantically, rather than, say, on the basis of sound, i.e., acoustically or phonetically. As stated earlier, semantic encoding and semantic memory are certainly related, although for the present they are to be kept distinct conceptually.

recent items. This occurred only if the presentation was verbal but not if it was visual, again emphasizing the selective, and lateralized, nature of the STM deficit.

Although these results support the transmitted-lateralization hypothesis, they question one of the basic premises of the "stages" model—namely, that items must pass through STM before they can be stored in LTM. On the basis of their evidence, Warrington and Shallice (1969) suggested that short- and long-term memory are parallel systems to which items can have independent access. Another of Saffran and Marin's (1975) experiments seemed to support this view. Conduction aphasics who were asked to repeat single sentences verbatim were unable to do so even when the sentences were short. They did, however, produce accurate paraphrases, indicating that the sentences had been semantically encoded and retained in LTM.

There are a number of alternative explanations of the findings. First, it is not known how much processing in STM is necessary before an item can be stored in LTM. An STM store whose capacity is reduced may still allow for sufficient processing for the transfer of an item to LTM. Second, it is conceivable that STM is intact but that the retrieval mechanism is impaired so that it is possible only to retrieve items from LTM (Bartlett and Tulving, 1974). Both of these interpretations are compatible with the traditional stage model. A third interpretation stems from Baddeley's view (1976) that STM consists of working memory and a verbal rehearsal loop. It may be that it is the verbal rehearsal loop that is impaired in these patients, suggesting that the classical description that these patients simply have a repetition deficit is correct. All these interpretations derive from the tradition that memory is discontinuous and can be compartmentalized. An alternative view will now be examined.

A "levels-of-processing" approach to memory (Craik and Lockhart, 1972) admits the existence of phenomena that correspond to sensory, short-term, and long-term memory but denies the existence of rigid and discrete memory systems, each with its peculiar processing and storage characteristics. What we term sensory, short-term, and long-term memory is considered by Craik and Lockhart to be a product of the perceptual and encoding operations that a stimulus undergoes. The retention characteristics of the stimulus and its mode of representation are determined by the level at which it is processed. Thus a stimulus that is processed principally at a shallow, sensory level will be remembered poorly (sensory memory?) whereas a stimulus that is processed to a greater, semantic depth will be retained more accurately for a much longer time (in LTM?). Although originally Craik and Lockhart (1972) proposed that stimulus analysis proceeds in a hierarchical manner, from sensory to semantic levels, they have since modified their view (Lockhart *et al.*, 1975). They now allow for a heterarchical processing scheme in which stimulus and task demands determine the order of processing, the amount of elaboration that can occur at any level, and the interaction among different levels (Craik, 1977; Lockhart *et al.*, 1975).

The appeal and strength of a levels of processing approach are its position regarding the relation between mnemonic and encoding processes (Norman, 1976; Craik, 1977). Consequently, we will focus on this aspect of the theory in evaluating it from a neuropsychological perspective. If an individual shows selective memory deficits, the levels approach predicts that he should have correspond-ing deficits in processing and vice versa. One problem with testing this prediction is that the proponents of the levels approach have never clearly specified which processes are required to ensure different degrees of retention. Nonetheless, some rough guesses have been made (Craik, 1977; Craik and Tulving, 1975), and we will go by these.

For example, patients with an inpaired STM would be expected to have processing deficits that were different from those of patients with imparied LTM; similarly, patients with verbal memory impairments would have processing deficits different from those with impairments of nonverbal memory. Unfortunately, there is too little evidence available for an adequate test of the "levels" approach. For example, it would be interesting to know whether patients with selective short-term memory deficits have greater difficulty in processing information at a phonemic than at a semantic level. Do they perform worse at matching words on a phonemic basis, such as finding rhyme pairs, than on a semantic basis, such as finding members of the same lexical category? The evidence that does exist is mainly from studies of patients whose long-term memory is impaired. At best, these studies provide weak support for the "levels" approach and suggest that it must be modified considerably before it can account for the pattern of deficits observed in a clinical population.

Contrary to the predictions derived from the "levels" approach, individuals with severely impaired verbal memory or with global amnesia typically do well on tasks requiring semantic processing. Their verbal IQ scores are in the normal range (Warrington, 1975; Butters and Cermak, 1974; Milner and Scoville, 1957; Teuber *et al.*, 1968; Talland, 1965) and their ability to classify material on the basis of semantic attributes is either intact or only slightly worse than normal (Wilkins and Moscovitch, 1978 Cermak and Reale, 1978; Cermak *et al.*, 1974, 1978). As a result, advocates of a "levels" approach have claimed that although amnesics are capable of processing material semantically, they will not do so ordinarily. Consis-tent with this view are studies showing that Korsakoff amnesics make more phonemic than semantic confusion errors in a recognition memory test (Butters and Cermak, 1975), suggesting that they encode the items phonemically. Their failure to show a spontaneous release from proactive interference (PI) when items from a new semantic category are presented is interpreted by Cermak *et al.* (1974) that Korsakoff amnesics are unable to encode new semantic information automati-cally. Failure to release from PI, however, may have less to do with encoding than with problems at retrieval (Watkins and Watkins, 1975). Moreover, Moscovitch (1976*b*) has shown that patients with left dorsotaleral frontal damage, but no memory deficits, also fail to release from PI, whereas patients with anterior, mesial temporal, and hippocampal damage, whose verbal memory is clearly impaired, show normal release. These results suggest that the Korsakoff amnesic's failure to release from PI is related to his frontal deficits (Oscar-Berman, 1973) rather than to his memory disorder. Corroboration for this view comes from Cermak (1976), who found that an encephalitic amnesic, whose frontal lobes were presumably intact, showed a normal release from PI.

In the task in which confusion errors were examined (Butters and Cermak,

1975), the error rate for both control and Korsakoff patients was so low (a mean of 1 item) that it is difficult to draw any firm conclusion about the encoding process. Moreover, Butters and Cermak draw inferences about the semantic process from performance on a memory task rather than from performance at the time of encoding. This is begging the question. Although the two measures may be related in normal circumstances, the relation is never perfect and may break down entirely in amnesic patients. Subsequent studies by Cermak and his colleagues support this view. Direct tests of Korsakoff amnesics' semantic memory revealed only a mild impairment in the speed with which they retrieved items from "conceptual," but not "lexical," semantic memory (Cermak *et al.*, 1978). Nonetheless, even when they were successfully forced to encode words to a deep, conceptual, semantic level, recall and recognition remained extremely low and were no better than for words encoded at a shallow level. A difference between words encoded at deep and shallow levels did emerge when the list contained only a dozen items and recognition was tested immediately. But even here, they scored no better than 50% correct for deeply encoded items. Since chance performance was 33%, the results only underscore how resistent amnesics' memory is to improvement by such procedures and how poorly a simple level of processing theory accounts for their deficit.

In a similar vein, a study by Wilkins and Moscovitch (1978) conducted on individuals with unilateral temporal lobectomy suggests, as did Cermak *et al.*, (1978) that episodic memory deficits are associated with a very slight deficit in verbal, semantic processing. They asked patients with unilateral right or left temporal lobe excisions to name or classify a series of words or pictures of common objects that were presented successively at a rate of 0.75 sec/item. Only patients with left temporal lobectomy and presumably poor verbal memory performed worse than normal in naming the picture or classifying the pictures or words along a verbal dimension such as living or man-made. They performed normally, however, if they had to classify on the basis of size (e.g., in real life, is the item bigger or smaller than a chair?). Their impaired semantic memory may also account for their difficulty in dividing a list of words into subjective categories (Jaccarino Hiatt, 1978). Whereas normal people construct tightly-knit categories containing very few items, individuals with left temporal lobectomy form larger categories whose members are only loosely related to each other.

It would be parsimonious, and certainly consistent with a "levels" approach, to attribute the verbal memory deficits of patients with left temporal lobectomy to their deficits in verbal, semantic processing. Such a strong conclusion, however, is not warranted by Wilkins and Moscovitch's data. Their patients' semantic deficits, however, appeared only under the stressful conditions produced by Wilkins and Mosovitch's demands for very rapid classification, and even then the deficits were relatively mild compared to ones in episodic memory. Indeed, in a typical episodic memory task the patient will have little problem in classifying the material semantically, yet still perform poorly on recall and recognition (Milner, 1966, p. 115; Cermak and Reale, 1978). Finally, it is worth emphasizing that the greatest semantic processing deficits, as manifested in difficulties of naming and lexical classification, result from damage or stimulation of left posterior temporal and parietal areas (Warrington, 1975; Fedio and Van Buren, 1974). Although some patients with damage to those areas often have poor memory, they do not exhibit the severe episodic memory deficits observed in profoundly amnesic patients whose damage is confined primarily to anterior temporal or limbic structures.

The evidence presented indicates that memory and processing disorders are often associated with each other, but the relation between them is not as strong as a levels approach would predict. In short, there are insufficient grounds for inferring a causal relation between processing and memory deficits. This does not imply that a levels of processing approach should be abandoned. It may be that elaboration of processing at a given level (Craik, 1977; Talland, 1965), distinctiveness of encoding or some higher-order retrieval operations (Moscovitch and Craik, 1976) are critical factors in recall and their impairment is responsible for the memory deficits observed in a clinical population. Alternatively, it is conceivable that an additional consolidation process is necessary before the products of different levels of processing are fixed in memory. Until these possibilities are explored in future experiments, a "stages" model still seems to describe the clinical data best.

Because the status of the levels-of-processing approach in explaining clinical phenomena is uncertain, the transmitted-lateralization hypothesis will not be examined from a levels point of view. Instead, we will proceed directly to a discussion of semantic memory.*

Semantic Memory

As stated earlier, semantic memory refers to our knowledge of general facts, concepts, relations, and rules. Knowledge of history and of mathematical relations, rules of language, the items in our lexicon, cognitive maps, attributes, such as size, of common objects, their class membership—in short, any information or rules for structuring that information that may be shared by members of a society comprises the semantic memory of individual members of a society. The structure of semantic memory (Anderson, 1976; Anderson and Bower, 1974; Collins and Loftus, 1975; Rosch, 1975; Norman and Rumelhart, 1974; Smith *et al.,* 1974; Tulving, 1973), its relation to episodic memory (Lockhart *et al.,* 1975), and the representation of information in semantic memory (Kosslyn and Pomerantz, 1976; Paivio, 1975; Pylyshyn, 1973; Simon, 1972) are topics of some controversy at the moment. What is undisputed, however, is that entry into semantic memory occurs late in the information-processing sequence. According to the transmitted-lateralization hypothesis, then, some aspects of semantic memory will be lateralized to the left hemisphere and others to the right. Insofar as many linguistic processes are lateralized to the left hemisphere, the evidence supporting at least part of this statement is overwhelming and will be summarized briefly (see

---

*This does not mean that all human memory disorders have a single explanation. Disorders of memory are produced by a variety of disturbances (ECS, tumors, anoxia, cerebrovascular accidents, concussions, aging, vitamin B deficiency, encephalopathy) to a variety of structures (hippocampus, mammillary bodies, dorsomedial nucleus of the thalamus, frontal lobes, fornix, cingulate). It is unlikely, given these differences, that all memory disorders, or even the traumatic amnesias, can be traced to a single cause at the psychological level.

Geschwind, 1970; Marin *et al.*, 1976; and Springer, this volume, for a more thorough review). Damage to Broca's area (third frontal convolution) and to Wernicke's area (posterior middle and superior temporal convolutions) produces severe language deficts, the former affecting primarily syntatic processes in comprehension and production and the latter semantic ones (Zurif *et al.*, 1972; Caramazza and Zurif, 1976). Patients who are classified as conduction aphasics according to the Boston Aphasia Inventory (Goodglass and Kaplan, 1972) and who are believed to have left arcuate fasciculus lesions (Geschwing, 1970) also show impaired syntax. Associated with lesions to all these areas is an anomia (difficulty in naming or word finding) whose severity and saliency in comparison with this other symptoms depend primarily on the size and site of lesion, the extent of recovery following damage, and presumably on factors such as the age of the patient (Brown, 1972, Brown and Jaffe, 1975).

Anomia should be of particular interest to the very large group of psychologists whose research on semantic memory focuses on the nature of the internal representation of concepts denoted by single words, i.e., the lexicon. As a number of investigators have observed, a name is not merely a label attached to a simple configuration of perceptual features; it always refers to a concept and thus exists as an integral part of the semantic representation of the objects or concept in question (Brown, 1958; Oldfield, 1966; Vygotsky, 1962). According to this view, disorders in naming will result from any significant disturbance of the set of complex, ordered relations among the semantic and perceptual attributes that constitute the semantic representation of the object or concept. Recent research on anomic patients is consistent with this general view. Individuals who have deficits in naming, but no noticeable perceptual disturbances, seem also to be impaired in classifying these objects according to various categories or according to attributes which a number of objects have in common (Goodglass and Baker, 1976; Dennis, 1976; Warrington, 1975). The disturbance in classification is most severe for items that belong to different, but closely related, categories. As might also be expected, errors in naming most frequently consist of substitutions from a member of the same or related lexical or phonemic categories. Most often, the errors are those of omission and involve low-frequency words more than high-frequency ones. Semantic and phonemic cues help, but name retrieval is cued better by sentences that are semantically constrained and that require the patient to supply the missing word (Goodglass *et al.*, 1976; Marshall *et al.*, 1970). Supplying the missing word itself is the best cue, but even then the patient may not recognize it as appropriate, or, if he does, may be unable to repeat it. Finally, there is recent evidence that disorders of naming could be so selective as to involve only items from a single lexical category, such as body parts (Dennis, 1976).

Aside from these general observations, however, none of the studies on anomia has supplied enough information to derive a picture of the structure of semantic memory, or even of the lexicon, that is sufficiently detailed to help distinguish among a variety of models that have been proposed (Dennis, 1976, comes close). For example, does the dissolution of naming follow a pattern predicted by an ordered feature model, a semantic network model, or a prototype model? What is the relation between the representations of an object that are retained, such as those related to function, and those that are lost, such as those related to category membership? Can the former be used as a peg for sorting related items and thus reconstructing a category? We are far from answering these questions. At present, the quality, variety, and sheer volume of neuropsychological research on verbal semantic memory lag far behind those of the research conducted on a normal population. Hopefully, this imbalance will be rectified in the future since it is a fertile area for research.

It is somewhat unusual to note that almost all disorders of naming or classification are associated with left-sided damage. Presumably, some aspects of the semantic representation of words and objects are nonverbal and mediated primarily by the right hemisphere. Lesser's study (1974) showing impaired semantic skills but normal syntactic and phonological skills in patients with right-hemisphere damage supports this idea. It is significant in this regard that classification according to real-world size was spared in patients with unilateral left temporal damage, but not naming or classification according to a more purely verbal dimension (Wilkins and Moscovitch, 1978). However, the possibility that size classification was mediated by some other region of the left hemisphere, rather than by the corresponding region on the right, was not ruled out. Similarly, Warrington (1975) reports that patients with left-sided damage and severe deficits in semantic memory appreciated that photographs taken from different unusual perspectives represented the same object even though they could not name the object or place it in an appropriate lexical category. This ability to classify and internally represent objects on the basis of higher-order perceptual features is affected most by damage to the right parietal area (Warrington and Taylor, 1973). Whether such functions are integral to the semantic memory system or constitute a stage of processing prior to it is uncertain. Clarification of the status of such visual-spatial operations is important and will be considered again when we discuss imagery. For the moment, it seems safe to assume that orientation in extrapersonal space (Semmes et al., 1963) the internal representation of cognitive maps (Luria, 1973), and perception of some features of faces (Charcot, 1950; DeRenzi and Spinnler, 1966; Hécaen and Angelergues, 1962; Moscovitch et al., 1976; Warrington and James, 1967; Yin, 1970) as well as of objects (Warrington and Taylor, 1973) are mediated primarily by the posterior parieto-occipital zones of the right hemisphere. The relation between these representations and the corresponding verbal, semantic ones remains a central problem in research on semantic memory and hemispheric asymmetry (Paivio, 1975; Pylyshyn, 1973; Kosslyn and Pomrantz, 1976; Moscovitch, 1973; Potter et al., 1977).

Frontal Lobes

Not all hemispheric functions can be accommodated even loosely by the information-processing frameworks discussed in the previous sections. This is especially true of deficits in cognitive function associated with damage to the frontal lobes. Depending on the locus and the extent of the lesion, an individual may show symptoms of motor or cognitive perseveration (Luria, 1973; Milner, 1964), poor fluency (Milner, 1964), or an inability to remember the temporal order of events (Milner, 1974) or may disobey social conventions and be emotionally labile (for review, see Konorski, 1972; Teuber, 1972; Warren and Akert, 1964). Because the symptoms associated with frontal damage in humans have been so diverse, it has been difficult to specify the primary function of the frontal lobe. Some suggestions on this matter are that the frontal lobes are "sources of corollary discharges whereby the organism presets its sensory systems for the anticipated consequences of its own actions" (Teuber, 1972); that the frontal lobes are critical for parsing a sequence of inputs into discrete temporal and spatial events (Pribram, 1971); that the frontal lobes are necessary for the sequential organization of behavior (Luria, 1973); that they are inhibitory structures that mediate the evaluation, and subsequent regulation, of behavioral strategies (Nauta, 1972). The search for a unified view of frontal lobe functions, however, may be misguided. Sufficient neuroanatomical distinctions exist between the various regions of the frontal lobe (Jones and Powell, 1970; Nauta, 1972) that there is no more reason to support that they constitute a unitary system any more than do the various regions of the temporal lobe. At best, a family resemblance may exist among frontal lobe functions (Teuber, 1972), although in such cases one must guard against the possibility that the resemblance exists only in the eye of the beholder.

Clearly, this issue is not going to be resolved here. Instead, the effects of frontal damage will be examined from the perspective of the transmitted-laterality hypothesis. In monkeys (Jones and Powell, 1970; Nauta, 1972), and presumably in man, the frontal lobes receive input from the secondary association cortex of all sensory modalities. Because frontal regions that receive these inputs can be considered to be neurologically upstream from the locus at which hemispheric differences emerge, lateralization of function should be observed for some regions of the frontal lobe. The series of elegant studies conducted by Milner and her students on patients with unilateral frontal damage confirms this prediction (Milner, 1964, 1971, 1974; Jones-Gotman and Milner, 1977; Moscovtich, 1976*b*). A reduction in verbal fluency (e.g., write all the words you can think of beginning with "s" in 5 min) is associated primarily with left supraorbital lesions (Milner, 1964, 1971), whereas a corresponding deficit in nonverbal fluency (e.g., draw all the nonsense figures you can think of) occurs after right supraorbital lesions (Jones-Gotman and Milner, 1977). A similar double dissociation occurs in a test of memory for the temporal order of recent events (Milner, 1974). Individuals are shown two series of cards, one bearing abstract visual designs and the other compound words. At varying intervals in the series, the individual is presented with test cards bearing either two designs or two words, and he must indicate which of the two he saw first. Patients with left frontal damage are impaired only when confronted with the words whereas patients with right frontal damage are impaired on the designs. Impaired performance on the Wisconsin Card Sorting Test, which assesses an individual's ability to switch sets in a hypothesis-testing situation, is greater, and occurs more frequently, following damage to the left than the right dorsolateral frontal cortex (Milner, 1964). More recently, Moscovitch (1976*b*) has found that patients with left, but not right, frontal damage who score poorly on the Wisconsin Card Sorting Test also fail to show a normal "release from PI." Finally, Milner (1965, 1971) has found that right-sided rather than left-sided frontal removals were followed by deficits on certain maze-learning tasks. These deficits, however, did not so much reflect an inability to learn the maze as an unwillingness to obey certain rules. Whether rule-breaking behavior in general is associated more with right than with left frontal damage, or whether it is material specific, remains to be seen.

The review of the evidence on frontal functions, as well as on higher cognitive functions associated with other cortical regions, generally supports the transmitted-lateralization hypothesis. The implications of this hypothesis on models of hemispheric specialization will be examined in the following section.

Transmitted Lateralization and Implications for Models of Hemispheric Organization: Similarities and Differences between Corresponding, Higher-Order Structures in the Left and Right Hemispheres

The previous review of evidence supporting the transmitted-lateralization hypothesis may have left some impressions about hemispheric organizations that were not intended. I will try to correct two of the more salient ones.

The first is that a rigid hierarchical organization exists that requires all information to be transmitted serially and unidirectionally from lower-order systems to progressively higher-order ones. The possibilty that this organizing principle prevails throughout the cerebral hemispheres is remote. Evidence of parallel transmission from a single source to a number of systems and of centrifugal influences of higher-order structures on lower ones suggests that the organization of at least some systems is heterarchical. The transmitted-lateralization hypothesis admits the possiblity of both heterarchical and hierarchical organization, as indeed it must if it is to be viable. Its only critical assumption is that loci exist at which hemispheric asymmetries emerge and from which information is relayed to other systems. Whether information is relayed serially or in parallel is irrelevant.

The second impression is that all areas in one hemisphere that receive or operate on information derived from these loci are functionally and structurally different from the corresponding areas in the other hemisphere. Put another way, this view holds that almost all cortical areas beyond the primary sensory areas show evidence of hemispheric specialization. This impression does not arise merely from the arguments presented in this chapter, but is shared by many neuropsychologists. The primary evidence that goes to create this impression is the fact that unilateral damage of almost all higher-order structures leads to deficits that are different when the damage is on the left than when it is on the right. Although this impression may accurately reflect the true state of things, I wish to consider an alternative view of hemispheric organization that is equally consistent with the available evidence and with the transmitted-lateralization hypothesis.

The alternative is that within each hemisphere there exists a primary group of structures that is fundamentally different on the left from the corresponding group on the right, and whose operation determines the range of specialized capacities of that hemisphere. Associated with this group are a number of secondary, higher-order structures that are the same on the left as on the right. These two sets or groups of structures form a highly integrated system which, when viewed as a whole, is functionally different on the left and on the right.

According to this view, asymmetrical deficits are likely to result after unilateral removal of even those structures that are identical on the two sides because of this close interaction with the primary group of structures. The deficits will reflect the operation of a damaged system that is still different from its homologue on the other side.

Studies on the effects of hippocampal damage will illustrate these points and contrast the two views of hemispheric organization. It is well established that left hippocampal damage leads to verbal memory deficits and right hippocampal damage to nonverbal memory deficits. One explanation for the differential effects on unilateral hippocampal lesions is that the hippocampi are functionally, and presumably structurally, different from each other: the left hippocampus specializes in processing verbal information and the right in processing nonverbal information. It is equally plausible, however, that no fundamental differences exist between the two hippocampi—they are interchangeable. The left and right hippocampi, however, are located within different systems. The different patterns of deficits observed after left and right hippocampal removal are the result of their close association with structures that are indeed different in the left and right hemispheres. Since the hippocampus receives input from cortical structures for which hemispheric asymmetries are likely to exist, the effects of unilateral hippocampal removal on the systems of which they are a part will be different, even if the hippocampus on the left is identical to the one on the right. Put in more functional terms, the operations performed by the left and right hippocampus are very similar, but the data base on which they operate is different. This interpretation is implicit in descriptions of the effects of unilateral hippocampal removal: both serve a mnemonic function, the one for verbal information, the other for nonverbal information (see Milner, 1970, for a similar view regarding the hippocampus and Jones-Gotman and Milner, in press, regarding fluency factors associacited with the frontal lobes).

Because there are few adequate tests for determining similarity between corresponding structures in the two hemispheres, it is difficult to know which view of hemispheric organization is correct. One very crude test is to look for neuroanatomical differences between corresponding structures. These differences have been found for the planum temporale, which is larger on the left (Geschwind and Levitsky, 1968; Tezner et al., 1972; Wada et al., 1975; Witelson and Pallie, 1973), the region of the posterior cortex surrounding the occipital horns, which is larger on the right (McRae et al., 1968; Strauss and Fitz, 1978), and the frontal operculum, which is also larger on the right (Wada et al., 1975). Since the region of the planum temporale includes the auditory association areas and posterior speech zones, and since damage to the right parieto-occipital area causes severe spatial and visual deficits, it is likely that these structural differences are related to functional ones. These regions, in fact, may be considered prime candidates for inclusion into the primary group.

Similar structural differences, however, have not been reported for a variety of structures, the most notable being the hippocampus, anterior mesial temporal lobes, and some regions of the frontal lobe. For each of these structures, the pattern of deficits following unilateral damage suggests an underlying similarity in function between the left and right members. Memory is affected by damage to the hippocampus and mesial temporal lobes, whereas fluency and judgments of relative recency are impaired by damage to different regions of the frontal cortex. What distinguishes left-sided from right-sided damage is whether a verbal or nonverbal analogue of the same task is used. This suggests, again, that the operation of these structures is similar, but that the data bases on which these operations are performed are different.

The fact that gross neuroanatomical asymmetries have not been reported for these structures, however encouraging to our proposal, does not mean that they are functionally similar. Current techniques may simply be too crude to pick up subtle structural differences. For the time being, a functional approach to this problem may prove to be more fruitful.

One such approach is to compare the effects of bilateral with unilateral damage. The argument is that if a structure is fundamentally different on the left from on the right, lateralized deficits associated with unilateral damage should not be greatly aggravated by additional damage to the corresponding structure on the other side. If, however, the two structures perform basically similar functions, the possibilities of compensation by the undamaged side are greatly enhanced. For example, the undamaged structure may have access to information on the contralateral side via the intracerebral commissures and can thereby help operate on such information should damage occur. Consequently, bilateral damage should lead to more severe deficits than unilateral damage even for those functions that appear to be lateralized.

The little evidence that is available is slightly in favor of the second alternative. Bilateral hippocampal and mesial temporal lobe lesions accentuate the memory loss for both verbal and nonverbal material that occurs after unilateral damage to these structures (Jones, 1974; Milner, 1971, 1974). Whereas unilateral damage simply impairs memory for either verbal or nonverbal information, bilateral damage produces a dense amnesia for both. Consistent with this view is the fact that commissurotomized patients typically have impaired verbal and nonverbal memories, possibly because structures like the hippocampus are prevented from having access to information on the contralateral side. In a similar vein, perseveration on verbal and nonverbal tasks seems greater following bilateral frontal damage than perseveration of either kind after unilateral lesions (Luria, 1966). On the other hand, linguistic and spatial functions are likely to be as severely impaired following unilateral posterior left and right hemisphere lesions, respectively, as they would be after bilateral lesions. Significantly, these functions, unlike mnemonic ones, are relatively spared following commissurotomy.

This evidence suggests that two different sets of structures exist within a unified system—a primary set that is fundamentally different on the left than on the right, and a secondary set that is basically similar on the two sides but that, by virtue of its location, is compelled to interact mainly with the primary structures on its side. This is clearly not the final word on the topic. The evidence presented in this section is open to alternative explanations. For example, memory deficits following commissurotomy may result from the reduction of tonic excitation produced by the loss of commissural cells (Milner, 1974). Also, it is possible that some structures, although different on the left and on the right, retain some limited capacity to process information that is usually handled by the other side (Gazzaniga, 1970; Zaidel, 1976, 1977). This possibility makes the interpretation of many studies difficult. However further research will resolve the issues raised in this section, at present it seems prudent to adopt a neutral position—regardless of the status of individual structures, the right and left hemispheric systems which these structures form have fundamental differences between them, not the least of which is their capacity for processing different kinds of information. The system can therefore be treated as a unit, an integrated whole, in later discussion. This approach will be adopted when we examine some hypotheses concerning the nature of hemispheric differences in information processing and their implications for dual-processing theories.

RECAPITULATION

Before we turn to these issues, let us review briefly the major points of the chapter.

1. Information processing at an early, precategorical, and presumably peripheral level is similar in both hemispheres. Thus both hemispheres are equally efficient in extracting and storing information about the "physical" features of the stimulus array.

2. Hemispheric asymmetries in information processing emerge only at a higher level of analysis in which relational or categorical features are represented.

3. The structural locus at which the asymmetry emerges seems to be at the level of second-order association areas for the visual and auditory systems. Presumably this is true of other systems as well, but that will not be known for certain until more information becomes available.

4. From this locus, information is then transmitted either serially or in parallel to a variety of structures that form an integrated functional system, one in the right hemisphere and one in the left. The characteristics peculiar to each system are determined, in part, by the specialized information-processing capacities evident at the locus and, in part, from the specialized operations of the other higher-order structures in that system. From an information-processing point of view, this implies that all processes beyond those at which relational or categorical properties emerge will be functionally lateralized to the left or right hemisphere (transmitted-lateralization hypothesis).

The oldest conceptualization of hemispheric asymmetries, and the one we had adopted for convenience, has been along a verbal-nonverbal dimension. According to this view, the left hemisphere is seen as the primary but not exclusive repository of special-purpose mechanisms necessary to deal specifically with phonological, syntactic, and semantic information that is peculiar to natural speech (Liberman, 1974). Taken further, one could assume that all lateralized left-hemisphere functions are outgrowths or reflections of the operation of these language-specific mechanisms. Presumably, a set of mechanisms that specialize in processing complex, nonverbal information exists primarily in the right hemisphere. If to these assumptions we add another that states that the reflection of hemispheric asymmetries in behavior is determined as much by the cognitive demands of the task as by the stimulus material per se, then this set of assumptions will account for a great deal of the evidence on hemispheric specialization.

Speech, writing, as well as verbally coded information of nonverbal displays such as faces (Levy, 1974; Umilta *et al.,* 1978) or various figures (Dee and Fontenot, 1973; Hannay, 1975) will be processed best by the left hemisphere, whereas nonverbal stimuli or complex nonverbal configurations of verbal material such as shape (Cohen, 1973; Bryden and Allard, 1976) will be processed best by the right hemisphere.

Despite this general success in explaining hemispheric asymmetries in processing, these assumptions have been challenged almost from the moment they were proposed. For Jackson (1878) and his followers (Head, 1926; Goldstein, 1948), the left hemisphere's capacity for processing language was seen as the manifestation of more basic cognitive operations, such as abstract reasoning and the manipulation of symbols, which could be applied to a variety of functions. In support of this proposal they produced evidence showing that left hemisphere damage impairs performance on a variety of tasks that require an "abstract attitude" but that can be considered to be relatively independent of language (Goldstein, 1948). Since then, the number of lateralized functions that cannot be explained easily by invoking a verbal-nonverbal dichotomy have grown and have fostered many other hypotheses on the nature of hemispheric specialization. Because most of the hypotheses, old and new, have much in common, only two will be discussed—the sequential-processing hypothesis and the analytic-holistic hypothesis. These two were chosen because they are representative of this class of hypothesis and yet are sufficiently distinctive to be differentiated easily from each other.

SEQUENTIAL-PROCESSING HYPOTHESIS

Because temporal, sequential information is characteristic of language, a number of investigators have suggested that the perception and production of temporal sequences, even if they are not linguistic, are mediated primarily by the left hemisphere. Research on a variety of nonverbal tasks strongly supports this view.

Using normal people, Efron (1963*a*) has shown that judgments of temporal order of two brief tactile stimuli are mediated primarily by the left hemisphere. Mills (1977) has obtained similar results using nonverbal auditory stimuli. In addition, she found that judgments about brief, temporal intervals, even when they are not sequential, are mediated by the left hemisphere. Studies on a clinical population corroborated Efron and King's findings. Patients with left-hemisphere damage, especially if they are aphasic, are unable to determine the temporal order of two tones until they are separated by an interval that is much greater than that required by normal people or by people with right-hemisphere damage (Efron, 1963*b;* Lackner and Teuber, 1973). Essentially similar results were obtained by Carmon and Nachson (1971) in a task requiring patients with left- or right-sided damage to indicate manually the sequence in which a series of lights were presented. As with speech, the identification of temporally patterned, nonverbal stimuli (such as Morse code) yields a right ear advantage on dichotic listening tasks (Halperin *et al.,* 1973; Papcun *et al.,* 1974). Using a tactile analogue of the dichotic listening task, Nachson and Carmon (1975) found that the right hand could identify a sequence of taps delivered to the fingers better than the left.

On the motor end, the evidence that sequencing requires the integrity of the left hemisphere comes primarily from the work of Kimura, Milner, and their colleagues (Kimura, 1973; Kimura and Archibald, 1974; Lomas and Kimura, 1976; Mateer and Kimura, 1977; Milner, 1976). Taken together, their studies show that initiation, production, or memory of a sequence of manual or oral movements, but not the individual movements in the sequence, was impaired most by left-hemisphere anesthetization, damage, or interference.

The evidence on the lateralization of sequential and temporal processing indicates that the nature of hemispheric specialization cannot be explained only in terms of a verbal-nonverbal dichotomy. Moreover, it suggests that temporal sequencing operations play an important role in language comprehension and production. To go beyond this and propose that it is primarily on the basis of temporal sequencing operations that left hemisphere functions, such as language, are distinguished from right hemisphere ones is unwarranted. First, as Poeck and Huber (1977) rightly noted, there is more to language, and even speech, than the production and analysis of temporal sequence. It is impossible to understand normal and aphasic language without reference to the organization of the lexicon and to the contextual factors and rules that govern the choice and determine the order of items in an utterance. None of these, nor other left hemisphere functions, such as memory for verbal information, can be interpreted simply by invoking the operation of a temporal, sequential processor, however important that processor might be for some motor and perceptual aspects of linguistic behavior. Second, some activities that are ostensibly sequential are mediated primarily by the right hemisphere. Typically, haptic information is gathered sequentially as the fingers move over the object. Nevertheless, haptic perception is better with the left hand than with the right (Witelson, 1974). Music, which is organized in temporal sequences, is often perceived better by the right ear than the left (Kimura, 1963; Shankweiler, 1966). Finally, the case could even be made that visual perception of the sort mediated by the right hemisphere consists of sequential information gathered from successive eye movements or successive movements of the perceived object.

To counter such arguments, a number of investigators have proposed that these right hemisphere tasks are only ostensibly sequential—their characteristic feature is that they are spatial. By that, I take it to mean that information, however derived, must ultimately be organized with reference to spatial coordinates. This analysis makes sense when applied to perception of objects by vision and by touch (DeRanzi *et al.*, 1968; DeRenzi and Scotti, 1969). However, it is difficult to see how it applies to the perception of music. Undismayed by this apparent difficulty, and wishing to accommodate data from the auditory modality, Gordon (1974) proposed that it might be better to consider spatial functions as nontemporal. According to Gordon, musical stimuli are nontemporal if they are not distinguished primarily on the basis of time and rhythm factors. Chords, which yield a reliable left ear advantage, are considered to be nontemporal. The classification of melodies would depend on their composition, which explains why a left ear advantage for melodies is not found consistently.

As ingenious as Gordon's explanation is, it doesn't provide specific enough guidelines for determining which tonal sequences are "temporal" and which are not. Too much of the decision is left to intuition.

An alternative proposal, however, was to distinguish stimuli on the basis of a holistic-analytic dimension. Those stimuli that are amenable to holistic processing will show a left ear-right hemisphere advantage, whereas those that require analysis will show a right ear-left hemisphere advantage. Despite the fact that distinctions along an analytic-holistic dimension are intuitive at best, it has become a popular way to characterize processing differences between the left and right hemisphere. We will now turn to a discussion of this hypothesis.

ANALYTIC-HOLISTIC HYPOTHESIS

According to the analytic-holistic hypothesis, the left hemisphere specializes in analyzing complex stimulus configurations into discrete features whereas the right hemisphere takes into account the holistic properties of the stimulus configuration and constructs a meaningful gestalt. The clearest evidence supporting this view is descriptive and somewhat anecdotal. Drawings of patients with some forms of left-hemisphere damage will reflect the holistic processing of the intact right hemisphere. These patients retain the general outline or shape but omit specific details (Gardner, 1974). Patients with damage to some right-hemisphere areas, however, include minute details of identifying features in their drawings, but seem unable to construct the general shape or organization in which these details must be embedded. Similar accounts are given of patients with a severe prosopagnosia that results primarily from right-hemisphere damage (Charcot, in James, 1950; Hécaen and Angelergues, 1962). Such patients can distinguish one person from another only on the basis of salient features, such as a moustache or glasses or a hat rather than by the general configuration of the face. Once the feature is removed, the person becomes unrecognizable. Levy *et al.* (1972) report that the left hemisphere of commisurotomized patients uses a similar, analytic strategy in learning to recognize faces and complex shapes, whereas the right hemisphere immediately apprehends these complex configurations as a gestalt.

All the other evidence for the analytic-holistic hypothesis is much more inferential and derived, at times, from experiments that produce inconsistent results and that are difficult to replicate. One strategy followed in almost all the experiments is based on the intuitive notion that a stimulus is apprehended more rapidly if it is processed holistically than if it must be analyzed feature by feature. The right hemisphere should therefore complete these perceptual tasks before the left. Two experiments conducted on split-brain patients seem to support this idea. In the first experiment, Zaidel and Sperry (1973) had split-brain patients perform a tactual version of Raven's Progressive Matrices Test. The subject was presented with a series of tactual patterns and had to indicate which of two test patterns that he felt with either the right or the left hand best completed the series. Although the subjects could perform the task with either hand, they were much faster with the left, leading the authors to suggest that the right hemisphere handled the task holistically and the left analytically. In a similar type of experiment, Levy (1974) asked split-brain patients to match an unfolded, two-dimensional design, which they felt with the right or left hand, to a folded, three-dimensional visual representation of it. Of the six patients tested, only the three without right-hemisphere damage scored above chance with their left hands. Only one of the three was able to score above chance with his right hand, but the correlation between the scores of the two hands on different items of the set was only marginally significant. Because the sets which the right hand found easier contained blocks whose features could be easily described but difficult to visualize, whereas the reverse was true for the sets which the left hand found easier, Levy suggested that the hemispheres used different strategies in conducting the task. Later experiments with chimeric figures (see below) led Levy to conclude that the left hemisphere used an analytic strategy and the right a holistic one.

The results of these two experiments support the idea that the two hemispheres go about their tasks in different ways. It does not follow, however, that the best description of their performance is along analytic-holistic lines. For example, it may be that the left hemisphere simply cannot process complex nonverbal haptic information as efficiently as the right (Milner and Taylor, 1972) or that its nonverbal memory is so poor that it cannot store that information for a sufficiently long time to make the necessary match unless it can encode the information verbally. Operating under such constraints, the left hemisphere may focus on picking up information about easily named features. Such explanations can account for Levy's and Zaidel and Sperry's results without recourse to vague analytic-holistic dichotomies.

A number of investigators have attempted to find evidence for the analytic-holistic hypothesis by showing that serial processing is characteristic of the left hemisphere and parallel processing, of the right. The rationale behind this is that analytic strategies are likely to require serial, item-by-item processing whereas holistic strategies may be more amenable to processing all features simultaneously. Cohen (1973) presented normal subjects with arrays of two to five items either in the right or the left visual field and asked subjects to indicate whether all the items were the same or different. She found that "same" response latencies increased with the number of letters when the array was presented to the right visual field (left hemisphere) but remained more or less constant when it was presented to the left visual field (right hemisphere). This result is consistent with the analytic-holistic hypothesis. Unfortunately, it is the only result in Cohen's experiments that is. When shapes were used, or when a "different" response was required, both hemispheres processed the information in an identical manner. Later attempts to replicate Cohen's results met with varying success. White and White (1975) found that shapes and letter arrays are processed in parallel regardless of which visual field receives them. Because response latencies favored the right hemisphere in all conditions, they assumed that the results reflected primarily right hemisphere processes. Stillman (personal communication), on the other hand, found that the items in the array were always processed serially.

Serial processing is the rule if a test item presented to either the right or the left visual field must be matched against a memory set consisting of one to items (Klatzky and Atkinson, 1971; Moscovitch, 1972). In these cases, the hemisphere that is favored is determined by whether the match is verbal or visual, rather than by the matching process. Serial processing also describes right-hemisphere performance in matching two black and white grids for identity. Gross (1972) found that response latencies increased linearly as the similarity between the grids increased, but favored the right hemisphere in all the "similarity" conditions.

Seamon (1972) reported a study in which he asked subjects to remember a set of words by rehearsing them individually or by constructing an integrated image of the objects represented by the words. He then presented a probe and asked subjects to indicate whether the probe was in the set. Response latencies to the probe increased linearly with the number of items in the rehearsal condition but remained constant in the imagery condition. Seamon and Gazzaniga (1973) modified this study by presenting the probe to the right or the left visual field and found that latencies favored the left hemisphere in the rehearsal condition and the right hemisphere in the imagery condition. Rothstein and Atkinson (1975), however, could not replicate Seamon's (1972) original results thereby casting some doubt on the paradigm's usefulness for inferring something about the processing modes of the two hemispheres.

Overall, the evidence on serial and parallel processing suggests that they do not provide a basis for distinguishing between the two hemispheres. This is unfortunate since the serial-parallel dichotomy provided one of the clearest operational definitions for differentiating analytic from holistic processes*. Without a clear way of determining which strategies or processes are analytic and which are holistic, the distinction can serve only a heuristic purpose. This can be

---

*It should be noted that a traditional parallel-process model is still a feature model. That is, before processing or comparison can occur, single features must be isolated or identified, procedures that presumably are analytic. We are then faced with the contradiction that parallel-processing, which is the hallmark of a holistic approach, requires an analytic strategy to isolate the features that are to be processed. The only way around this problem is to propose another class of parallel-process models or to abandon the idea that there is a strong correspondence between analytic-holistic strategies and serial-parallel processing. I thank Dr. Carlo Umilta for this observation.

beneficial if the analytic-holistic distinction is used to gain insight into otherwise puzzling data and thus generate ideas for future research. All too often, however, the analytic-holistic hypothesis is invoked as an explanation when simpler, clearer explanations exist (see Gordon's, 1975, comments on Bever and Chiarello, 1974; also, apply the stages-of-processing approach suggested in this chapter to Bever *et al.'s,* 1976, results).

None of the dichotomies reviewed in this section adequately accounts for the functional differences between the left and right hemispheres. Perhaps the correct dichotomy has yet to be discovered. Alternatively, it may be that there is no single principle that describes the organization of the left and right hemispheres. The hope of finding such a principle seems to be derived from the notion that in each hemisphere higher-order structures form a unified or closely integrated system. The notion of a hemispheric system, however, need not imply the existence of a single, unifying principle; it only implies that the structures that form the system are highly interrelated and operate in concert on any given task, with each component in the system contributing its specialized function. Depending on the demands of the task, the organization of the system at the time the task is attempted, and a host of other internal and external factors, the operation of different structures will be emphasized, which, in turn, will bias the operation of the entire system now in one way, now in another. According to this view, the organizing principle, to some extent, is situationally determined. Under some conditions, the operation of the hemispheric systems may best be described along a verbal-nonverbal dimension, under others along an analytic-holistic one, and so on.

Whether the operation of the hemispheres is best described by a single principle, or a multiplicity of them, is a problem that is not likely to be resolved soon. What is not at issue is that two fundamentally different systems exist that are capable of processing information somewhat independently of each other. Some further consequences of having two systems operate on identical data will be examined in the next section.

DUAL PROCESSING

In the real world, stimulus input is not usually restricted to one hemisphere. Typically, the same auditory information is received by both ears, and, since both eyes focus and scan any visual stimulus that catches an individual's attention, the same visual information is directed to both hemispheres. It is only somesthetic information that is sometimes received initially by only one hemisphere simply because objects may be manipulated by only one hand. Even in such instances, however, both hemispheres are likely to receive simultaneously some information about the object that is being manipulated since the normal tendency is to look at the object, or to shake it or tap it to hear what it is made of, or even to smell it. In fact, information about most objects that catch our attention is often received via more than one sensory modality. Given these circumstances, and because the early processing stages are similar in the two hemispheres, the information they receive about the stimulus complex will be very similar up to the point at which hemispheric asymmetries emerge. Beyond that point, the information that is picked up and encoded from the same input, or the form in which that information is represented, is different in the left than in the right hemisphere. This is the sense in which the term "dual processing" will be used for the moment. A related but more general sense of the term (Paivio, 1969, 1971) will be introduced later.

Since each stimulus is received by the higher-order, specialized processing systems in each hemisphere, all stimuli should undergo dual processing. The degree to which this occurs, however, will depend on the nature of the stimulus material and the task demands. Some stimuli may be highly lateralized in the sense that only the specialized mechanisms of one hemisphere are capable of processing the stimulus to any significant degree and storing and using the subsequent information. Speech and highly complex visual stimuli that are difficult to verbalize fall into this category. Other types of stimuli, which are easily represented visually and verbally, such as pictures of common objects, or the objects themselves, seem to be processed and encoded by the specialized mechanisms of either hemisphere as indicated by the difficulty of obtaining evidence for large and consistent hemispheric asymmetries for processing such stimuli (Dee and Fontenot, 1973; White, 1969; DeRenzi, 1968). To prove that dual processing indeed occurs, however, it is also necessary to show that each hemisphere picks up different information about these stimuli. A few recent experiments demonstrate this point elegantly.

The most dramatic demonstration of dual processing is provided by Levy and her co-workers' studies of commissurotomized patients (Levy, 1974; Levy and Trevarthen, 1976; Levy *et al.*, 1972). In these studies, split-brain patients were shown chimeric stimuli formed by joining two half pictures, each representing a different object, and each being projected to a different hemisphere. The patients were then asked to match the chimeric stimuli with test pictures in free vision. The chimeric and test stimuli were alike either in function (e.g., cake, knife, and fork) or in appearance (e.g., cake and hat). When matching instructions were ambiguous, the left hemisphere matched by function and the right, by appearance. When the instructions specified that functional or structural matches be made, left-hemisphere control (primarily right-hand pointing) was elicited for the former and right-hemisphere control for the latter. Using similar techniques, Levy and Trevarthen (1977) also showed that phonetic matches or name matches were controlled by the left hemisphere, even for such complex configurations as faces or nonsense shapes. Appearance matches, however, were typically controlled by the right hemisphere, although the left hemisphere encoded information, albeit poorly, along these dimensions. These studies indicate that both hemispheres have access to similar, low-level information that is then processed differently by the two higher-order hemispheric systems. The right-hemisphere processes and encodes information on the basis of appearance, whereas the left concentrates primarily on functional and nominal aspects of the input.

Experiments on individuals with unilateral brain damage support this interpretation. Jaccarino (1975) asked individuals with right- or left-temporal lobectomy to remember a group of pictures of a number of common objects, which included a cup or house. They were then tested for recall and recognition both immediately and after 1 day. Immediate recall scores were lower than those of a normal control group for only the left temporal group. When tested 1 day later, both groups of patients recalled fewer items than the control group, suggesting that immediate recall was mediated primarily verbally whereas delayed recall may require a visual component that is mediated by the right hemisphere. In favor of this interpretation is the fact that patients with left temporal damage, despite their poor recall, were somewhat better than the right temporal and control group at recognizing the correct picture among five similar alternatives.

In another study, Moscovitch (1976c) presented a similar group of patients with a randomly ordered set of 16 drawings of common objects, each of which belonged to one of four lexical and shape categories. The lexical categories were furniture, vehicle, animal, and clothing. The shape category was determined by the axis along which the drawing was made: vertical, horizontal, oblique left, and oblique right. Thus a drawing of a bear drawn in an upright posture would belong to the lexical category "animal" and the shape category "vertical"; a pair of pants drawn along a similar axis would belong to the same shape category as the bear, but to a different lexical category, and so on. In testing normal people for free recall of the names of drawings, Frost (1972) found evidence of clustering according to both lexical and shape categories. Despite modifying her procedure somewhat, Moscovitch confirmed her results with normal people. Individuals with unilateral right temporal lobectomy, however, clustered only according to the lexical category, whereas those with left temporal damage clustered primarily according to shape. Similar biases in clustering could be created in normal people by presenting a verbal or nonverbal interference task at the time the pictures are presented (Moscovitch, 1977). Asking an individual to name or recognize a word or nonsense shape at the same time as he is encoding each drawing interferes selectively with the verbal or nonverbal representation of the drawing in memory. Consequently, in the verbal interference condition the clustering is primarily by shape, whereas in the nonverbal interference condition the clustering is primarily lexical.

These dual-processing effects are not restricted only to purely pictorial stimuli. Jones (1974) found that imagery instruction helped patients with left temporal lesions to improve their verbal memory for concrete words but not for abstract ones. Similar effects of imagery as a memonic aid are reported by Patten (1972). However, the right temporal-lobe patients in Jones's (1974) study were not impaired in comparison to a control group. In a later study, however, Jones-Gotman and Milner (1978) were successful in demonstrating that if a large series of words was used, individuals with right temporal damage did indeed recall fewer imaged, concrete word pairs than a normal individual but recalled an equal number of abstract words.

Further suggestive evidence for dual hemispheric processing of concrete words, but not of abstract ones, comes from observations of individuals with semantic or phonemic dyslexia that results from left hemisphere damage (Marshall and Newcombe, 1973; Saffran *et al.,* 1976b; Shallice and Warrington, 1975). Analysis of these individuals' reading errors indicates a preponderance of semantic confusions. For example, they read "marriage" as "wedding," "brown" as "green." Further tests indicated that they lack a phonemic representation for the word but retain a semantic one. More interestingly from our point of view is that these semantic errors occur primarily for concrete words which, at times, are also read correctly. These patients fail utterly in attempting to read abstract words, often producing no response at all. It has been suggested on the basis of these results that concrete words have direct access to a semantic (perhaps visual) representation in the right hemisphere and that it is on the basis of this representation that reading occurs. Some evidence in favor of this interpretation is that those concrete words that have a high imagery value are read best of all.

The results of studies of perceptual asymmetry in normal people are also consistent with this interpretation. The right visual field superiority for word recognition is reduced if concrete words are used (Hines, 1976) and reduced still further if those words are high in imagery value (Marcel and Patterson, 1978). If a same-different reaction time procedure is used, perceptual asymmetry for high-imagery concrete words are small or absent even when the subject is asked to decide whether the item belongs to a particular lexical category (Bradshaw and Gates, 1978; Day, 1977). Abstract words, however, show the usual right-field advantage*. These results are similar to ones obtained with split-brain patients whose right hemisphere gives evidence of comprehending some concrete nouns better than all other verbal material (Gazzaniga, 1970; Zaidel, 1973). Its ability to understand the phonemic representation of the noun is grossly deficient, if it exists at all (Levy, 1974).

Finally, a very interesting and dramatic dissociation between phonemic and semantic aspects of reading occurs in some Japanese patients who have two writing systems, a syllabically based phonemic one, *kana*, and a semantically based, ideographic one, *kanji*. Lesions, presumably to the anterior portions of the left hemisphere, selectively impair reading of *kana,* whereas lesions to more posterior portions of the left hemisphere impair reading of both types of material (Sassanumo, 1975). That both kinds of reading are impaired by posterior left hemisphere lesions does not necessarily imply that ordinarily all reading of *kanji* is mediated by that region. It may merely be necessary for the organization of input-output relations to the semantic system. One line of experimentation that may be useful in determining whether semantically based reading is mediated by the right hemisphere in readers of *kanji* and in phonemic dyslexics is to see if on tests of visual-perceptual asymmetry they show a left rather than a right visual field advantage. Preliminary studies by Bogio (personal communication) show this pattern of results. An alternative approach would be to demonstrate that concurrent nonverbal tasks disrupt the phonemic dyslexic's ability to read even concrete words by interfering with right hemisphere pictorial processes.

Evidence for dual hemispheric processing of pictures, and even of faces,

*One should be careful not to exaggerate the laterality differences between concrete and abstract words in normal people. They are typically small and difficult to obtain (personal observation) and, except for Day's (1977) study, both types of words produce a right field–left hemisphere advantage. This suggests that it is only under special circumstances that the right hemisphere's presumed competence in processing concrete words is fully manifested in performance (Moscovitch, 1976a).

words, and letters (Cohen, 1973; Geffen *et al.*, 1973), is substantial. Its relevance for more general theories of *dual encoding,* however, is unclear. In recent years, there has been a growing controversy on the nature of mental representation. One side believes that there are at least two forms of mental representation that differ fundamentally from each other (Cooper and Shepard, 1973; Kosslyn and Pomerantz, 1977; Paivio, 1969, 1971, 1975). One type of representation is verbal, abstract, and amodal whereas the other form is nonverbal, perception like, and therefore analogue. The other side maintains that all knowledge or meaning is represented neither in verbal nor nonverbal form, but rather in terms of abstract propositions specifying relations between entities (Chase and Clark, 1972; Pylyshyn, 1973). The arguments on both sides have been presented elegantly and in great detail and will not be reviewed here. For our purposes it is sufficient to note that the controversy has focused on imagery and is concerned not about the content of the imaginal representation but about the form that representation takes. According to one view, the image one has of a horse standing in a field, or of a familiar face, is represented in a visual, analogue form that is fundamentally different from the form in which a linguistic utterance describing the scene or face is represented. Proponents of the opposite view might easily concede that the "image" contains a great deal of information that the utterance does not, but would maintain that both are represented in terms of similar abstract propositions describing relations among entities.

Evidence from neuropsychological research is not likely to resolve this controversy. For example, one might suspect that the existence of dual hemispheric processing would tip the scales in favor of the multiple-representation point of view. However, advocates of the single-representation view could argue that the evidence merely suggests that the two hemispheres are specialized to process and store different kinds of information. The form in which that information is represented, however, is identical on the two sides. Nor is their claim as farfetched as it first seems. If information in the left and right hemispheres were represented in fundamentally different forms, these differences might preclude exchange of information between the two hemispheres unless a third, abstract code existed that encompassed both of them (Moscovitch, 1973; Pylyshyn, 1973). Kosslyn and Pomerantz (1977), however, note that all that is needed for such an exchange to occur is a set of transformation rules that specify how information from one system can be mapped in terms of the other. "These rules would take the form of processes or routines, which when applied to information coded in one form would produce a corresponding representation in another form."

A solution to this controversy is unlikely so long as it depends on proving that words and images are (or are not) simply phenomenological manifestations of similar abstract propositions. On the other hand, a more pragmatic or functional approach suggests a rather clear-cut, although certainly not one-sided, view of the status of words, images, and abstract representations. According to this approach, the form in which information appears to be represented is determined by the demands of the task and the type of data collected by the investigator. If an individual is tested for his ability to remember discrete events, such as unrelated words, sentences, faces, or pictures—or if he is asked to make judgments about particular attributes, such as size or category membership, of real-world objects—then distinctions between perceptually based (images) and verbal-amodal codes are likely to be useful, and even necessary, for explaining his performance. This is true of behavioral (Kolers, 1975; Kosslyn and Pomerantz, 1977) as well as neuropsychological experiments (Jaccarino, 1975; Jones, 1974; Moscovitch, 1976c; Wilkins and Moscovitch, 1978). If, however, the subject's knowledge of or memory for the meaning or implications of events is tested, then the evidence is likely to show that he relies on an abstract representation of these events in performing the task (Marschark and Paivio, 1977; Potter *et al.,* 1977).

ATTENTION

Were all stimuli or tasks handled primarily by either one hemisphere or the other, but not both, the problem of attention would be of little concern to neuropsychologists interested in hemispheric specialization. Stimulus processing would be based entirely on predetermined and fixed correspondences between stimulus properties and hemispheric mechanisms. Stimulus properties alone would then determine the direction of perceptual asymmetries. But as the previous section emphasized, many stimuli may be processed by both hemispheres either spontaneously or through training. Whether the stimulus or task is handled primarily by the left or right hemisphere, or both, is often influenced by attentional factors—that is, by cognitive strategies that are under the individual's control. Given this state of affairs, it is critical to understand how attentional processes interact with hemispheric ones. Before we can take up this issue, we will review briefly the major points common to most current theories of attention.

PRINCIPLES OF ATTENTION THEORY*

The term "attention" typically refers to a control process that enables the individual to select, from a number of alternatives, the task he will perform, or the stimulus he will process, and the cognitive strategy he will adopt to carry out these operations. In addition, the term "attention" implies that a certain effort or intensity is required in exercising the capacity for selection and in supporting the ensuing operations. Energy or effort is required to prime or facilitate the structures involved in processing a given task. Both dimensions, selectivity and effort, are critical aspects of attention. Thus, in reading a passage while simultaneously listening to another one, a person may choose to attend to (selectively process) only the written material and the amount of attention (effort) the task requires varies depending on the stimuli themselves (emotional, difficult, or neutral passage), task demands, alertness, etc. Finally, and most importantly, attention is limited, although not fixed. That is, it is impossible to attend fully to a limitless number of stimuli or tasks simultaneously. (If it were possible, selection would not be necessary.) In the above example, there is a cost to attending to the written material—

*The ideas in this review are derived primarily from Kahneman (1973), Posner (1975), and Posner and
  Snyder (1975), although they are not always identical with the views of these authors.

the spoken material is not processed as well and may consequently be comprehended or remembered poorly.

Attention or processing capacity is limited because the structures required to
process information and the effort needed to maintain such activities are finite.
Structural limitations are evident when common mechanisms are needed to
perform two or more different tasks. Competition for these mechanisms leads to
interference and a reduction in performance level of all the tasks. Focusing
attention on one task gives it privileged access to those mechanisms and ensures
that at least its level of performance remains relatively high while the performance
of the others will suffer accordingly. Even if the tasks do not compete for common
structures, they may nonetheless interfere with each other if the attention (effort)
that each demands exceeds the amount available to the individual. The amount of
attention (effort or energy) allocated to one task reduces the amount available to
the others and prevents them from being performed efficiently. How much
attentional capacity is available as well as how it is allocated is determined by the
physiological state of the individual, his expectancies and intentions, by the overall
demands of the task, and by the moment-to-moment shifts in demand as the task
is being performed.

Hemispheric Priming

Up until now, it has been assumed that perceptual asymmetries arise because
stimuli presented to one sensory field have more direct access to the hemisphere
that specializes in processing them than do stimuli presented to the opposite
sensory field. This model is a structural model in which information is viewed as
flowing passively from the sensorium to central processing mechanisms. Even if it
is acknowledged that cognitive strategies rather than stimulus material per se
determine the direction and magnitude of perceptual asymmetries, the framework of a passive structurally determined system is still retained. The strategy
"sets" the system to operate in one or another mode and, information is then
shuttled through as passively as it had been before. This view may not be wrong
and has much in common with current notions that attention primes the structures required to process some information, organizes the sequence of processing,
and then allows information to flow through with only minor adjustments being
made as processing occurs (Kahneman, 1973; Logan, 1978). Before we return to
such a notion, another model will be explored.

As an alternative to the structural, direct-access model, a number of investigators have proposed that perceptual asymmetries arise because individuals attend
to (selectively process) input in one sensory field (Inglis, 1965; Treisman and
Geffen, 1968). That such attentional shifts correspond so closely to know hemispheric asymmetries seemed puzzling. To explain this coincidence, Kinsbourne
(1970) proposed that expecting to engage in verbal or nonverbal activities, or
actually being engaged in such activities, primes left and right hemisphere structures, respectively. That is, attention (energy or arousal) is allocated to the hemisphere involved in processing verbal or nonverbal information, which in turn
causes attention (selective perception) to shift toward the sensory field contralat-

eral to the primed hemisphere. As evidence, Kinsbourne and his associates (Kinsbourne, 1970, 1973, 1975) showed that priming the left hemisphere with a verbal memory task leads to a right visual field advantage in the perception of material that was otherwise neutral with respect to laterality. Similarly, priming the right hemisphere with a nonverbal memory task reverses perceptual asymmetry for the same material. When fixation does not have to be maintained at a specific point, as it does in tachistoscopic tasks, Kinsbourne (1972) was able to show that verbal and nonverbal tasks cause the eyes to move in a direction contralateral to the primed hemisphere. Kimura (1973) observed a similar effect for arm and hand movements (gestures) during speech. Attention drawn to the structures mediating these cognitive acts overflows and primes adjacent motor structures.

Since he advanced his hypothesis, a great deal of research has been devoted to testing Kinsbourne's attentional model against the more traditional "direct access" one. Some studies support aspects of it (Hellige and Cox, 1976; Klein *et al.*, 1976; Morais and Bertelson, 1975; Morais and Landercy, 1977; Rosen *et al.*, 1975; Spellacy and Blumstein, 1970) while others do not (Berlucchi *et al.*, 1974; Geffen *et al.*, 1972, 1973; Klein *et al.*, 1976; Moscovitch, 1976*a;* Schwartz, 1978) and, in some cases, do not even replicate Kinsbourne's own findings (Boles, 1977; Gardner and Branski, 1976). Taken together, these studies suggest that the "attentional" influences of this type on perceptual asymmetries may be present, but they are weak and unreliable, and show their greatest effect for material that is not strongly lateralized.

It is not our purpose, however, to debate the merits of the "attention" and "direct access" models. Since it was first proposed, the "attention" model has been modified considerably to account for the findings that were contrary to its earliest predictions (e.g., follow the evolution of expectancy, prestimulus, and poststimulus factors in Kinsbourne, 1970, 1973, 1975, and Ledlow *et al.* (in press) and Swanson *et al.* (1978). The direct access model, on the other hand, has not changed as much since its inception primarily because it can still account for those findings in which attentional factors are minimally involved. Nonetheless, it is clear that some modifications are necessary if it is to remain viable. Even a strict structural model must make some provisions for attentional variables if only to account for such obvious effects as altering an expected right-ear advantage by deliberately attending only to the left-ear input. Even split-brain patients who fail to report verbally messages presented to the left ear in a dichotic task can learn to report a large percentage of them with practice (Sparks and Geschwind, 1968). As stated by Klein *et al.* (1976), the purpose now is not to determine whether one of the models is right, but to understand how attentional and structural factors interact to produce perceptual asymmetries and, in the long run, to process information.

In its strong form, Kinsbourne's hypothesis leaves little room for incorporating the structural aspects of the direct access model. Klein *et al.* (1976), however, suggested that priming may operate by facilitating structures in one hemisphere so that stimulus inputs that have direct access to that hemisphere will be processed either more quickly or more accurately than they would be otherwise. The same outcome may be achieved by more indirect means if priming causes the subject to process the stimulus material in a mode that is consistent with the cognitive capacities of the primed hemisphere. Thus priming, induced by the expectancy generated by task demands, can cause material that is capable of being dually processed to be handled primarily by one or the other of the hemispheres. By amalgamating factors of both the attentional and direct access model, Klein *et al.*'s (1976) proposal can claim much of the explanatory power of both theories and extend their application to new phenomena. First, it accounts for the improved performance of the hemisphere subordinate for a particular task if that hemisphere had been primed prior to initiation of that task (Hellige and Cox, 1976; Klein *et al.*, 1976). Second, it predicts that the effect of priming induced by expectancy or concurrent tasks will vary inversely according to how strongly lateralized the stimulus material and perceptual tasks are (Hellige and Cox, 1976; Kinsbourne, 1975; Klein *et al.*, 1976). Third, it can account for the presence of perceptual asymmetries in situations in which neither hemisphere is primed relative to the other prior to the presentation of the stimulus. In these circumstances, it is primarily principles of direct access that operate to yield perceptual asymmetries (Berlucchi *et al.*, 1974; Cohen, 1972; Geffen *et al.*, 1973; Moscovitch, 1976a; Goodglass and Calderon, 1977). Finally, research conducted in the framework of a direct access model has shown that perceptual asymmetries emerge only at late, higher-order processing stages. The combined attentional–direct access model would then predict that lateralized, hemispheric priming would affect only the later stages of processing. Some recent evidence suggests that this is indeed the case (Rosen *et al.*, 1975).

There are some anomalous findings that even the "combined" model would not have predicted but that are not inconsistent with it. In most circumstances, priming effects induced by expectancy and concurrent activity facilitate the operation of structures specialized to process the expected or auxiliary task. In some instances, however, this rule seems not to hold. Expectancies sometimes lead to priming of the left hemisphere even when it is not the most qualified to execute a particular task; and concurrent tasks often require so much attention (effort) that rather than prime the hemisphere to handle other tasks more efficiently they interfere with its execution of any other tasks. The latter, seemingly paradoxical, phenomenon follows directly from the principles of general attention theory and will be dealt with in the next section. The present discussion will concern only the effects of expectancy.

The anomalous effects of expectancy are seen most clearly in Levy and Trevarthen's study of split-brain patients. The reader will recall that most split-brain patients who were asked to match chimeric figures with pictures in free vision exhibited left-hemisphere control when matching by function and right-hemisphere control when matching by appearance. In one of the four patients, however, the left hemisphere assumed control even when the individual was instructed to match by appearance and even though its capacities in this regard were inferior to the right hemisphere's. It is critical to note, however, that once it assumed control the left hemisphere matched the items according to appearance, albeit relatively poorly. In another patient, the left hemisphere would occasionally wrest control from the right hemisphere and make functional matches despite the fact that the individual was instructed to match by appearance. Only when the individuals were forced to respond with the left hand did the right hemisphere become fully dominant. Similar right-hemisphere intrusions, however, were not noted when the individuals were requested to match by function. In all cases, the left hemisphere assumed complete control.

These results illustrate that hemispheric priming effects elicited by expectancy do not always coincide with the specialized capacities of the hemisphere. The left hemisphere may become primed and assume dominance even in situations in which its capacities for executing the task are inferior to the right hemisphere's. This display of arrogance by the left hemisphere was considered by Gazzaniga (1975) to be a source of difficulty in testing the right-hemisphere's capacity in split-brain patients.

Two studies of priming in normal people indicate that the phenomenon is not limited to commissurotomized patients. In the first study, Klein and Smith (in preparation) asked individuals to determine whether a pair of words or a pair of pictures presented to the left or the right visual field represented objects from the same superordinate category (e.g., a car and a train are both vehicles). Decision latencies were shortest for words presented in the right visual field and for pictures presented in the left visual field. Presenting the individual with the name of the category to which one of the items belonged prior to its appearance reduced response latencies to right-field pairs more than to left-field ones in the word condition. This is consistent with the notion that such advance knowledge primed the semantic network in the hemisphere that mediated this task. Perception of items that had direct access to that hemisphere would then be facilitated more than usual. Significantly, "priming" affected both visual fields equally in the picture condition, suggesting that the left hemisphere was primed at least as much as the right even though it was less qualified to execute the picture task.

Cohen (1975) reports a similar finding in a study on mental rotation. Individuals were required to indicate whether a letter that was rotated various degrees from the upright position was a "normal" or "backward" version of the letter. Without foreknowledge of the letter or the degree of rotation, response latencies were shorter to letters appearing in the left visual field than in the right, indicating a right-hemisphere superiority for this mental rotation task. When the individual was given advanced knowledge of either the letter or the letter and the degree of rotation, performance improved more for right-field stimuli than for left ones and led to a reversal in laterality, suggesting that these expectancies predominantly primed the left hemisphere and enabled it to control performance even though its capacity for mental rotation was inferior to the right hemisphere's.

In a similar vein, Marin and Saffran (1975) report a case of an individual who could not perform a perceptual task because his damaged left hemisphere assumed control of it. Only when he was asked to keep silent or count out loud, an activity that presumably occupied the left hemisphere and forced it to relinquish control, could the patient then perform the task with his healthy right hemisphere.

These findings, as well as some others discussed in Moscovitch (1976a), lend some credence to the old idea that the left is indeed the dominant hemisphere in the sense that it will assume control of a task even in situations where its capacity to handle the task is inferior to the right hemisphere's (Levy and Trevarthen, 1976). Why this should be the case is not known. One possibility is that instructions and advanced information were delivered verbally and that verbal input alone is sufficient to prime the left hemisphere (Bowers and Heilman, 1976). If, in addition, the left-hemisphere's ability for dealing with the task is limited, then left-hemisphere dominance, although not necessarily left-hemisphere superiority, would be established. If this is the case, then it should be possible to attenuate or even reverse this tendency by establishing expectancies nonverbally. Thus, in Cohen's (1975) study, right-hemisphere superiority might have been maintained by giving the subject advanced knowledge of the orientation and the letter visually rather than verbally. Alternatively, it is possible that people in Western society tend to encode material verbally whenever the opportunity presents itself. Such a tendency would be enhanced if the subject were permitted to prepare himself for a task such as Cohen's, Klein and Smith's, and Marin and Saffran's that could be accomplished easily with a verbal strategy. This hypothesis would be easy to test. Whatever the explanation of this phenomenon, the attention–direct access model could easily explain the changes in perceptual asymmetries that accompany it. Once priming occurs, the stimuli that have direct access to the primed hemisphere are processed better than they would be otherwise and may even be given an advantage over stimuli presented to the opposite, superior, but less primed, hemisphere.

INTERFERENCE

An auxiliary task may prime a hemisphere and facilitate performance of other tasks done concurrently only under optimal conditions. These conditions seem to be ones in which the auxiliary task draws a sufficient amount of effort to prime related structures in the same hemisphere yet not too much to deprive the other task of its needs. If each of the concurrent tasks requires a great deal of attention or if the tasks compete for common processing mechanisms, then the auxiliary task will interfere with whatever other task is done concurrently. Thus concurrent verbal activity facilitates simple motor responses such as undirected eye and hand movements (Kimura, 1973; Kinsbourne, 1972) and simple manual responses (Bowers and Heilman, 1976) that are executed by the hemisphere mediating the verbal task. If the motor response is a complex one that requires some effort to execute, such as rapid, rhythmic, or sequential fingertapping, or dowel balancing, then concurrent verbal activity will interfere primarily with the right hand's performance whereas concurrent nonverbal activity, such as humming, will interfere somewhat with the left hand's performance (Hicks, 1975; Hicks et al., 1975; Kinsbourne and Cook, 1971; Lomas and Kimura, 1976). That interference is greatest when concurrent tasks are mediated by the same hemisphere indicates that competition for common processing mechanisms is as much the source of interference as is competition for limited attentional (effort) capacity. In fact, it may be that structural interference and capacity interference interact so that the greater the competition for common mechanisms, the greater the amount of effort needed to support the concurrent activities (Logan, personal communication).

This kind of lateralized interference is very severe in split-brain patients. A verbal task such as reading or whistling will greatly disrupt, or even halt, concurrent fingertapping or card sorting by the right hand, but not by the left, whereas humming or whistling a tune will have a similar effect on left-hand but not right-hand performance (Kreuter *et al.*, 1972; Franco, 1977). Why split-brain patients should be so affected by this kind of interference has not yet been determined. One possibility is that they have less attentional capacity than normal (Dimond, 1976). A second is that the commissures are needed to allocate attentional capacity to the unoccupied hemisphere. A third possible explanation is that in normal people the organization and programming of the motor task may be assumed by the unoccupied hemisphere, which then would merely transmit commands to the motor region of the occupied one in the case where motor movements and cognitive tasks are executed by the same hemisphere. Since such transmission is precluded by commissurotomy, the unoccupied hemisphere is prevented from sharing the workload in split-brain patients. Until more is known about the role of the cerebral commissures in concurrent processing and in allocating attention the merits of these proposals will remain in doubt.

Similar interference effects are observed in perceptual tasks. Dimond (1974) reviews many studies showing that tachistoscopic perception of two simultaneously presented stimuli is enhanced if each is presented to different visual fields than if they are presented to the same field. Dimond argues that presenting the stimuli to different fields directs them to different hemispheres, reduces structural interference, and thereby improves performance. Structural interference will occur even if stimuli are presented to different visual fields so long as they require the same hemispheric mechanisms for their analysis. Hines (1975) showed that perception of nonsense shapes is less accurate if they are presented bilaterally, one to each visual field, than if each shape presented unilaterally or in combination with words such that a word is presented to one field and a shape to the other. Under bilateral presentation the two nonsense shapes compete with each other for access to right-hemisphere mechanisms. Such competition is absent in the unilateral condition and reduced in the word-shape condition where the single shape has privileged access to the right hemisphere because the word is processed primarily by the left hemisphere. Moscovitch and Klein (1977) reached similar conclusions on the basis of studies of material-specific interference in which subjects were required to identify a central stimulus prior to identifying peripheral ones. If the central stimulus was processed by the same hemisphere as the peripheral ones, then the peripheral stimuli were identified more poorly than if the central and peripheral stimuli consisted of items that were processed by different hemispheres. Moscovitch and Klein also showed that such interference effects are greatest in those situations in which attention is required. If the central shape is present, but ignored by the individual, then material-specific interference effects are barely observable.

Finally, the fact that attempting to identify any central item, regardless of its nature, will interfere to some extent with the perception of any peripheral one, suggests that the interference effects are not purely structural, but also result from competition for limited attentional (effort) capacity.

Taken together, these results argue against the notion of a single processing bottleneck and support the idea of Allport et al., (1972) that information processing involves "a number of special computers [processors and stores] operating in parallel" and, in some cases, each having a limited capacity. The specialized left- and right-hemisphere systems may be considered as two such "computers" and knowledge of their capabilities may serve as a convenient heuristic for predicting the degree of interference and facilitation among concurrent tasks. Moreover, these studies also indicate that both systems draw on a limited attentional (effort) capacity available to the individual, confirming Kahneman's (1973) position that an attention model is incomplete unless it incorporates principles regarding the allocation of attentional capacity.

Automatic Processing

According to Posner (Posner, 1975; Posner and Snyder, 1975), processes are automatic if their activation receives no allocation of attention (effort). Posner has proposed three operational criteria for automaticity—the process occurs "without intention, without giving rise to conscious awareness, and without interference with other ongoing activities" (Posner and Snyder, 1975). The third criterion needs to be qualified since the lack of intentionality, the first criterion, is often demonstrated by showing that an automatic process indeed interferes with other tasks (Conrad, 1974; Dyer, 1973; Warren, 1972, 1974). Presumably, the lack of interference criterion applies only to those situations in which competition for common processing mechanisms (structural interference) is minimal. Even then, Posner's criteria for automaticity may be too rigid. For example, some processes may fulfill one of the criteria but not the others (Logan, 1978). Alternatively, the interference criterion may be met if task A is paired with task B, but not if it is paired with task C. Or task A may not interfere with either B or C, but be disrupted by one of them. Would such tasks or processes be considered automatic? As Kahneman (1973) observed, all processes require at least a minimal attentional capacity to be activated. Posner's criteria for automaticity should perhaps be considered as ideal ones that are rarely realized but which may be approached with practice. The notion of relative, rather than absolute, automaticity would be more correct and more useful for our purposes: the more automatic a process or skill is, or becomes, the less attention it requires.

With this point of view in mind, we may examine the question of automaticity in relation to hemispheric processes. Bradshaw et al. (1971, 1972) found that delayed auditory feedback disrupts speech more if the input is to the right ear than the left, whereas the opposite is true for rhythmic tapping. Were the subject able to completely suppress processing the delayed feedback, his speech or tapping would not be disrupted. Such input, however, gets processed automatically (unintentionally) and intrudes on ongoing behavior. That the disruptive effects of delayed auditory feedback are lateralized merely suggests that automatic activation is achieved more easily if the input has direct access to the structures that process it. Presumably, the less-direct input is sufficiently degraded by the time it reaches those structures that its ability to activate them is reduced. This interpretation is consistent with the results of other laterality studies on the disruptive effects of unintentionally processed material. Heilman *et al.* (1977) found that discrimination of monaural tonal sequences was less disrupted by speech input if both stimuli were presented to the left ear than if they were presented to the right. The opposite result was obtained when tonal sequences were paired with music. Here, too, irrelevant input was more difficult to ignore, and was consequently more disruptive if it had direct access to the hemisphere that ordinarily processed it. Cohen and Martin (1975) reached a similar conclusion regarding lateralized response mechanisms on the basis of their studies on dichotic "Stroop" effects in which the disruptive effects of producing responses inconsistent with perceptual categories (respond "high" to a low-pitched tone and "low" to a high-pitched tone) are greater with input to the right than the left ear.

These studies indicate that as a result of automaticity, perceptual asymmetries are produced or magnified by the presence of material which the individual makes no attempt to process. Automatic processing, however, may sometimes have opposite effects. A number of investigators have noted that perceptual asymmetries become attenuated over successive trials (Hellige, 1976; Kallman and Corballis, 1975; Ward and Ross, 1977). Although performance improves overall, the effect is greater for input directed to the inferior sensory field. Since it is known that skills or processes become more automatic with practice, the attenuation may result from progressively greater automation of processes dealing with input from the inferior sensory field. Although this interpretation has never been tested, it is a simple matter to do so. To assess the amount of attention required for processing input to either sensory field, the subject's performance on a concurrent, auxiliary task may be monitored. If the above interpretation, is correct, practice on the perceptual asymmetry task should lead to greater improvement on the auxiliary task when the input is in the inferior field than when it is in the dominant field. If this prediction is confirmed, it would be interesting to determine exactly which processes become more automatized. For example, the processes involved in transferring degraded input from the inferior field to the dominant hemisphere may have become more efficient. Alternatively, it may be the case that the inferior hemisphere has developed or improved its own methods of dealing with that input so the advantage of transferring it to the other hemisphere would be diminished. The fact that practice diminishes perceptual asymmetries only in those situations in which the set of items to be perceived is small and predictable favors the latter possibility.

Aside from these studies, there are few others that deal even indirectly with automatic processing. It would be interesting to know, for example, how much attention is devoted to encoding different aspects of material that can be dually processed. Subjects seem aware of encoding pictures verbally, but often are unaware of encoding or even being influenced by the spatial qualities of the material, although such influences can be demonstrated (Frost, 1972; Moscovitch,

1976*c*). Do these subjective impressions coincide with the true attentional demands that such verbal and nonverbal processes require? Research along these lines would provide a start for resolving issues regarding hemispheric control of consciousness. In situations where the hemispheres are simultaneously processing different aspects of the same input, and the individual is free to attend to either aspect, it may be that only the outcome of left hemisphere processes reaches conscious awareness (see previous discussions of priming and "dominance" relevant to this issue). Even if this were found to be the case, it would not endorse Eccles's (1973) view that consciousness resides in the left hemisphere. Should the individual wish, he could become aware of information represented in the right hemisphere.

It is clear from the studies reviewed in this section on attention that no theory on hemispheric and perceptual asymmetries would be complete without considering the role of attentional factors. These studies, however, are also a forceful reminder of how fragile and labile perceptual asymmetries can be. Here, as in all matters requiring "attention," there is both a benefit and a cost to using it. On the one hand, attentional factors help account for many discrepancies in studies of hemispheric asymmetries, which, in turn, may be helpful in deriving general principles regarding the interaction of control and structural factors. On the other hand, "attentional" explanations are too "flexible" and, like attention itself, may be allocated too easily to explain away results that are contrary to predicted outcomes. When this occurs, there is the danger that studies of perceptual asymmetries will have lost their usefulness as tools for understanding hemispheric organization and will themselves become the object of investigation.

Rather than end this section on a pessimistic note, let us consider very briefly an area of investigation that has barely been tapped but that holds some promise for understanding attentional processes.

ATTENTION AND BRAIN DAMAGE

In some sense, a great many of our skills can be considered relatively automatic. That is, they are handled efficiently and with little effort, their execution requires only slight conscious awareness, and, often, they may be completed without our intention. One has only to consider walking, driving, riding a bicycle, reading, and even speaking to realize that this is the case. Indeed, the smooth efficient, integrated, almost effortless functioning of mental processes may be the hallmark of a healthy nervous system. This does not imply that these skills, or a great many processes that mediate them, do not require any attention; it merely suggests that the attentional demands are relatively small.

This point is highlighted if we examine the behavior of some individuals with focal cortical damage. For these individuals, tasks that are mediated by the damaged area and that were ordinarily trivial to perform prior to the damage now require tremendous effort. The activity becomes voluntary and conscious in the extreme. This point is best illustrated by Brodal (1973), who describes his experiences following a stroke to the motor region of the right hemisphere:

It was a striking and repeatedly made observation that the force needed to make a scarcely paretic muscle contract is considerable. The expression "force" in this connection refers to what one, for lack of a better expression, might call force of innervation. Subjectively, this is experienced as a kind of mental force, a power or will. . . . The greater the degree of paresis of such a muscle, the greater was the mental effort needed to make it contract and to oppose voluntarily even a very weak counter force. On the other hand, only a slight mental effort was needed to bring about a fairly good contraction of a muscle able to work with about half or a little less of its full force.

This force of innervation is obviously some kind of *mental* energy . . . the result of which is seen as a contraction of the muscle(s) in question. The expenditure of this mental energy is very exhausting. . . . (p. 677)

Similar observations were made by Moss (1972), who seemed objectively to have fully recovered from aphasia, but nonetheless continued to feel that he expended a much greater than normal amount of effort to find the proper words to express his thoughts. The correct words no longer came to him "automatically" and easily, but rather their retrieval required constant attention and often a conscious search.

It would be rash to derive general principles of attention on the basis of these subjective reports. There is good reason, however, to believe that these experiences are representative of many individuals with brain damage and, moreover, that they are too robust to disappear on formal investigation. If, for the moment, we take these subjective reports at face value, they suggest the following interesting questions. Do functions ever return to their former state of relative automaticity, or do processes that mediate them always require more than a normal amount of attention to be activated? Would performance on concurrent tasks be a sensitive indication of the degree of recovery? Is an increased amount of attention allocated to all processes affected by brain damage? It is conceivable, for example, that even slight impairments in some functions are noted by the individual and added attention is allocated to the processes mediating them, whereas other functions may become grossly impaired by comparison before the individual is aware of any change that would necessitate a greater allocation of attention. Once a deficit is noted, however, is attention allocated to all processes mediating that function, only to those that are impaired, or only to processes of which we are conscious regardless of whether or not they are the ones that are impaired? Would processes to which attention is barely allocated, or allocated after long delays, be those which would be considered automatic under ordinary circumstances? What is it that becomes less automatic following brain damage—the organization of specific processes that combine to mediate a function, or the elicitation or release of those processes, or both? (See Brodal, 1973, pp. 679–680, for relevant observations.) Does the loss of an area mediating one process make more attention available to other processes? Are the effects of increased attention on performance following brain damage similar to those of increased arousal? Are there areas that primarily demand attention (effort), others that allocate it, and still others that supply it, or are such divisions merely conceptual ones that have no structural correlate?

These questions are not directed specifically to issues regarding the relation between attention and hemispheric asymmetries. Answers to these questions, however, should increase our understanding of attentional processes in general and thereby advance our knowledge of their interaction with hemispheric and perceptual asymmetries in particular.

Taking Stock

This chapter has dealt primarily with perceptual rather than motor skills, and with cortical rather than subcortical process as manifested in an "average" young adult population rather than in a variety of people of different ages and with different skills. Research on motor skills, subcortical functions, and individual differences is quite active and likely to become even more so in the future. Whether an information-processing approach to these problems will prove valuable remains to be seen.

For the problems and phenomena reviewed in this chapter, the partnership between information-processing theory and neuropsychology has been successful and lucrative for both. The theoretical constructs and experimental paradigms derived from information-processing theory helped clarify and explain existing neuropsychological phenomena and sometimes even helped discover new ones. Examples of this include studies determining the functional (and perhaps structural) locus at which hemispheric asymmetries emerge, the analysis of conduction aphasia in terms of deficits in short-term or working memory, studies of phonemic dyslexia, the notion of transmitted lateralization and the concept of dual processing, dozens of experiments on perceptual asymmetry, as well as the groundwork for neuropsychological research on attention and semantic memory.

Each successful application of information-processing theory to neuropsychological problems both fortified the theory and moved it forward. The discovery that hemispheric asymmetries emerged only at higher, categorical stages of processing and that brain damage could selectively impair either short- or long-term memory is one of the strongest pieces of evidence that processing is discontinuous and can be properly described by some form of "stage" model. Evidence of the selective effects of left and right hemisphere damage on processing, storing, and retrieving different kinds of information may provide some useful insights for theories of dual encoding, whereas new research on anomia, on phonemic dyslexia, and on the various forms of aphasia continue to extend our knowledge of the normal organization of semantic memory, reading, and language, respectively (see Marin *et al.*, 1976, and in this volume).

Just as the achievements are similar, so are the drawbacks of information-processing theory and neuropsychology. Both are highly successful in fractionating complex behaviors into simpler components. The synthesizing of these components back in to a unified system, however, has eluded both disciplines. For example, although there is some information on how linguistic utterances are comprehended and produced when either a syntactic or a semantic processor is impaired, there is hardly an inkling of how both processors operate in concert under normal circumstances. Similarly, we know the effects of left or right hemisphere damage in information processing, but we know nothing of how left or right hemisphere information is integrated.

A similar complaint could be leveled against information-processing theory. Artificial experimental procedures, such as masking or the requirement to process or remember disconnected events, do indeed help isolate components of the information-processing sequence. Normal, everyday perception, however, seems to be much more continuous and contextually bound than these experiments suggest. Suggestions as to how each of these components is integrated to produce normal, continuous perception and memory either have serious flaws (Turvey, 1977) or seem not to provide good explanations for the range and type of cognitive phenomena observable outside the laboratory (Neisser, 1976).

To abandon the information-processing enterprise as a reaction to such criticism seems wrong, particularly because the fit between neuropsychological data and information-processing theory is so good. The components suggested by the theory seem to have a neuropsychological reality. In their interaction with the real world and not merely in a laboratory setting, patients with various kinds of brain damage behave as if one of the components identified by information-processing theory were impaired. What is needed, then, is not an entirely new theory, but a framework that will incorporate knowledge about the operation of discrete components and, at the same time, indicate how they might be integrated to produce continuous, unified cognitive functions.

Acknowledgments

I thank Danny Klein, Gordon Logan, Jill Moscovitch, and Bernard Schiff for the valuable comments, criticisms, and suggestions they made in numerous discussions and after reading earlier drafts of this chapter.

REFERENCES

Aitken, L. M., and Webster, W. R. Medial geniculate body of the cat: Organization and responses to tonal stimuli of neurons in ventral division. *Journal of Neurophysiology*, 1972, *35*, 365.

Allport, D. A., Antonis, B., and Reynolds, P. On the division of attention: A disproof of the single channel hypothesis. *Quarterly Journal of Experimental Psychology*, 1972, *24*, 225–235.

Anderson, J. R. *Language and Thought*. Hillsdale, N.J.: Erlbaum, 1976.

Anderson J. R., and Bower, G. H. *Human Associative Memory*. New York: Wiley, 1974.

Anzola, G. P., Bertolini, G., Buchtel, H. A., and Rizzolatti, G. Spatial compatibility and anatomical factors in simple and choice reaction times. *Neuropsychologia*, 1977, *15*, 295–302.

Baddeley, A. D. *The Psychology of Memory*. New York: Basic Books, 1976.

Baron, J. Mechanisms for pronouncing printed words: Use and acquisition. In D. La Berge and S. J. Samuels (eds.), *Basic Processes in Reading: Perception and Comprehension*. Hillsdale, N.J.: Erlbaum, 1978.

Bartlett, J. C., and Tulving, E. Effects of temporal and semantic encoding in immediate recall and upon subsequent retrieval. *Journal of Verbal Learning and Verbal Behavior*, 1974, *13*, 297–309.

Bastian, H. C. *Aphasia and Other Speech Defects*. London: H. K. Lewis, 1898, p. 235.

Bay, E. Aphasia and non-verbal disorders of language. *Brain*, 1962, *85*, 411–426.

Benton, A. L., Levin, H. S., and Varney, N. R. Tactile perception of direction in normal subjects. *Neurology*, 1973, *23*, 1248–1250.

Berlin, C. I., and McNeil, M. R. Dichotic listening. In N. J. Lass (ed.), *Contemporary Issues in Experimental Phonetics*. New York: Academic Press, 1976.

Berlin, C. I., Lowe-Bell, S. S., Cullen, J. K. Jr., Thompson, C. L., and Stafford, M. R. Is speech "special"? Perhaps the temporal lobectomy patient can tell us. *Journal of the Acoustical Society of America,* 1972, *52*, 702–705.

Berlucchi, G. Anatomical and physiological aspects of visual functions of the corpus collosum. *Brain Research,* 1972, *37*, 371–392.

Berlucchi, G. Cerebral dominance and interhemispheric communication in normal man. In F. O. Schmitt and F. G. Worden (eds.), *The Neurosciences: Third Study Program.* Cambridge, Mass.: MIT Press, 1974, pp. 65–69.

Berlucchi, G., Heron, W., Hyman, R., Rizzolatti, G., and Umilta, C. Simple reaction times of ipsilateral and contralateral hand to lateralized visual stimuli. *Brain,* 1971, *94*, 419–430.

Berlucchi, G., Brizzolara, D., Marzi, C., Rizzolatti, G., and Umilta, C. Can lateral asymmetries in attention explain interfield differences in visual perception? *Cortex,* 1974, *10*, 177–185.

Bever, T. G. The nature of cerebral dominance in speech behaviour of the child and adult. In R. Huxley and E. Ingram (eds.). *Language Acquisition: Model and Methods.* New York: Academic Press, 1971.

Bever, T. G., and Chiarello, R. Cerebral dominance in musicians and non-musicians. *Science,* 1974, *185*, 537–539.

Bever, T. G., Hurtig, R. R., and Handel, A. B. Analytic processing elicits right ear superiority in monaurally presented speech. *Neuropsychologia,* 1976, *14*, 175–182.

Blakemore, C. Central visual processing. In M. S. Gazzaniga and C. Blakemore (eds.), *Handbook of Psychobiology.* New York: Academic Press, 1975.

Blechner, M. J., Day, R. S., and Cutting, J. E. Processing two dimensions of nonspeech stimuli: The auditory phonetic distinction reconsidered. *Journal of Experimental Psychology: Human Perception and Performance,* 1976, *2*, 257–266.

Blumstein, S. E., Baker, E., and Goodglass, H. Phonological factors in auditory comprehension in aphasia. *Neuropsychologia,* 1977a, *15*, 19–30.

Blumstein, S. E., Cooper, W. E., Zurif, E. B., and Caramazza, A. The perception and production of voice-onset time in aphasia. *Neuropsychologia,* 1977b, *15*, 371–384.

Bogen, J. E. The other side of the brain. II. An appositional mind. *Bulletin of the Los Angeles Neurological Societies,* 1969, *34*, 135–162.

Boles, D. B. Laterally biased attention with concurrent verbal load: multiple failures to replicate. Paper based on an M.A. thesis submitted to the Department of Psychology, University of Oregon, Eugene, Oregon, 1977.

Bowers, D., and Heilman, K. Material specific hemispheric arousal. *Neuropsychologia,* 1976, *14*, 123–127.

Bradshaw, J. L., and Gates, E. A. Visual field differences in verbal tasks: Effects of task familiarity and sex of subject. *Brain and Language,* 1978, *5*, 166–187.

Bradshaw, J. L., and Perriment, A. D. Laterality effects and choice reaction time in a unimanual two-finger task. *Perception and Psychophysics,* 1970, *7*, 185–188.

Bradshaw, J. L., Nettleton, N. C., and Geffen, G. Ear differences and delayed auditory feedback: Effects on a speech and music task. *Journal of Experimental Psychology,* 1971, *91*, 85–92.

Bradshaw, J. L., Nettleton, N. C., and Geffen, G. Ear asymmetry and delayed auditory feedback: Effect of task requirements and competitive stimulation. *Journal of Experimental Psychology,* 1972, *94*, 269–275.

Breitmeyer, B. G., and Ganz, L. Implications of sustained and transient channels for theories of visual pattern masking, saccadic suppression, and information processing. *Psychological Review,* 1976, *83*, 1–36.

Brodal, A. Self observations and neuroanatomical considerations after a stroke. *Brain,* 1973, *96*, 675–694.

Brown, J. *Aphasia, Apraxia, and Agnosia: Clinical and Theoretical Aspects.* Springfield, Ill.: Thomas, 1972.

Brown, J. W., and Jaffe, J. Hypothesis on cerebral dominance. *Neuropsychologia,* 1975, *13*, 107–110.

Brown, R. How shall a thing be called? *Psychological Review,* 1958, *65*, 14–21.

Bryden, M. P., and Allard, F. Visual hemifield differences depend on typeface. *Brain and Language,* 1976, *3*, 191–200.

Butters, N., and Cermak, L. S. Some comments on Warrington and Baddeley's report of normal short-term memory in amnesic patients. *Neuropsychologia,* 1974, *12*, 283–285.

Butters, N., and Cermak, L. S. Some analyses of amnesic syndromes in brain-damaged patients. In R. L. Isaacson and K. H. Pribram (eds.), *The Hippocampus,* Vol. 2. New York: Plenum, 1975.

Caramazza, A., and Zurif, E. B. Dissociation of algorithmic and heuristic processes in language comprehension: Evidence from aphasia. *Brain and Language,* 1976, *3*, 572–582.

Carmon, A., and Benton, A. L. Tactile perception of direction and number in patients with unilateral cerebral disease. *Neurology*, 1969, *19*, 525–532.

Carmon, A., and Nachshon, I. E. Effect of unilateral brain damage on perception of temporal order. *Cortex*, 1971, *7*, 410–418.

Catlin, J., and Neville, H. The laterality effect in reaction time to speech stimuli. *Neuropsychologia*, 1976, *14*, 141–143.

Catlin, J., VanDerveer, N. J., and Teicher, R. D. Monaural right-ear advantage in a target identification task. *Brain and Language*, 1977, *3*, 470–481.

Cermak, L. S. The encoding capacity of a patient with amnesia due to encephalitis. *Neuropsychologia*, 1976, *14*, 311–326.

Cermak, L. S., and Reale, L. Depth of processing and retention of words by alcoholic Korsakoff patients. *Journal of Experimental Psychology: Human Learning and Memory*, 1978, *4*, 165–174.

Cermak, L. S., Butters, N., and Moreines, J. Some analysis of the verbal encoding deficits in alcoholic Korsakoff patients. *Brain and Language*, 1974, *1*, 141–150.

Cermak, L. S., Reale, L., and Baker, E. Alcoholic Korsakoff patients' retrieval from semantic memory. *Brain and Language*, 1978, *5*, 215–226.

Charcot, cited in W. James, *Principles of Psychology*, Vol. 2. New York: Dover, 1950, pp. 58–60.

Chase, W. G., and Clark, H. H. Mental operations in the comparison of sentences and pictures. In L. Gregg (ed.), *Cognition in Learning and Memory*. New York: Wiley, 1972.

Chow, S. L., and Murdock, B. B. Jr. Concurrent memory load and the rate of readout from iconic memory. *Journal of Experimental Psychology: Human Perception and Performance*, 1976, *2*, 179–190.

Cohen, G. Hemispheric differences in a letter classification task. *Perception and Psychophysics*, 1972, *11*, 137–142.

Cohen, G. Hemispheric differences in serial versus parallel processing. *Journal of Experimental Psychology*, 1973, *97*, 349–356.

Cohen, G. Hemispheric differences in the utilization of advance information. In P. M. Rabbit and S. Dornic (eds.), *Attention and Performance V*. London: Academic Press, 1975.

Cohen, G. Components of the laterality effect in letter recognition: Asymmetries in iconic storage. *Quarterly Journal of Experimental Psychology*, 1976, *28*, 105–114.

Cohen, G., and Martin, M. Hemisphere differences in an auditory Stroop Test. *Perception and Psychophysics*, 1975, *17*, 79–83.

Collins, A. M., and Loftus, E. A spreading activation theory of semantic processing. *Psychological Review*, 1975, *82*, 407–428.

Coltheart, M. Visual information-processing. In P. C. Dodwell (ed.), *New Horizons in Psychology*, Vol. 2. London: Penguin Books, 1972.

Coltheart, M. Iconic memory: A reply to Professor Holding. *Memory and Cognition*, 1975, *3*, 42–48.

Conrad, C. Context effects in sentence comprehension. *Memory and Cognition*, 1974, *2*, 130–138.

Cooper, L., and Shepard, R. N. Chronometric studies of the rotation of mental images. In W. G. Chase (ed.) *Visual Information Processing*. New York: Academic Press, 1973.

Corkin, S., Milner, B., and Rasmussen, T. Somatosensory thresholds: Contrasting effects of post-central gyrus and posterior parietal-lobe excisions. *Archives of Neurology*, 1970, *23*, 41–58.

Corkin, S., Milner, B., and Taylor, L. Bilateral sensory loss after unilateral cerebral lesion in man. *Transactions of the American Neurological Association*, 1973, *98*, 25–29.

Craik, F. I. M. Depth of processing in recall and recognition. In S. Dornic and P. M. A. Rabbitt (eds.), *Attention and Performance VI*. New York: Academic Press, 1977.

Craik, F. I. M., and Lockhart, R. S. Levels of processing: A framework for memory research. *Journal of Verbal Learning and Verbal Behaviour*, 1972, *11*, 671–684.

Craik, F. I. M., and Tulving, E. Depth of processing and the retention of words in episodic memory. *Journal of Experimental Psychology: General*, 1975, *104*, 268–294.

Craik, F. I. M., and Watkins, M. J. The role of rehearsal in short-term memory. *Journal of Verbal Learning and Verbal Behavior*, 1973, *12*, 599–607.

Crowder, R. G. Representation of speech sounds in precategorical acoustic storage. *Journal of Experimental Psychology*, 1973, *98*, 14–24.

Crowder, R. G. *Principles of Learning and Memory*. Hillsdale, N.J.: Erlbaum, 1976.

Crowder, R. G., and Morton, J. Precategorical acoustic storage (PAS). *Perception and Psychophysics*, 1969, *5*, 365–373.

Cullen, J. K., Jr., Berlin, C. I., Hughes, L. F., Thompson, C. L., and Samson, D. S. Speech information flow: A model. *Proceedings of a Symposium on Central Auditory Processing Disorders*. Omaha: University of Nebraska Medical Center, 1974, pp. 108–127.

Darwin, C. J. Ear differences and hemispheric specialization. In F. O. Schmitt and F. G. Worden (eds.), *The Neurosciences: Third Study Program*. Cambridge, MIT Press, 1974, pp. 57–63.

Darwin, C. J. Speech perception. In E. C. Carterette and M. P. Freedman (eds.), *Handbook of Perception*, Vol. 7. New York: Academic Press, 1975.

Davidoff, J. B. Hemispheric differences in the perception of lightness. *Neuropsychologia*, 1975, *13*, 121–124.

Davis, A. E., and Wada, J. A. Hemispheric asymmetry: Frequency analysis of flash and click evoked responses to non-verbal stimuli. *Electroencephalography and Clinical Neurophysiology*, 1974, *37*, 1–9.

Day, J. Right-hemisphere language processing in normal right-handers. *Journal of Experimental Psychology: Human Perception and Performance*, 1977, *3*, 518–528.

Dee, H. L., and Fontenot, D. J. Cerebral dominance and lateral differences in perception and memory. *Neuropsychologia*, 1973, *11*, 167–174.

Dennis, M. Dissociated naming and locating of body parts after left anterior temporal lobe resection: An experimental case study. *Brain and Language*, 1976, *3*, 147–163.

DeRenzi, E. Nonverbal memory and hemispheric side of lesion. *Neuropsychologia*, 1968, *6*, 181–189.

DeRenzi, E., and Faglioni, P. The comparative efficiency of intelligence and vigilence tests in detecting cerebral damage. *Cortex*, 1965, *1*, 410–433.

DeRenzi, E., Faglioni, P., and Spinnler, H. The performance of patients with unilateral brain damage on face recognition. *Cortex*, 1968, *4*, 17–33.

DeRenzi, E., and Scotti, G. The influence of spatial disorders in impairing tactual discrimination of shapes. *Cortex*, 1969, *5*, 53–62.

DeRenzi, E., Scotti, G., and Spinnler, H. Perceptual and associative disorders of visual recognition. *Neurology*, 1969, *19*, 634–642.

DeRenzi, E., and Spinnler, H. Facial recognition in brain-damaged patients. *Neurology*, 1966, *16*, 145–152.

DeRenzi, E., Faglioni, P., and Scotti, G. Judgement of spatial orientation in patients with focal brain damage. *Journal of Neurology, Neurosurgery, and Psychiatry*, 1971, *34*, 489–495.

Diehl, R. L., and Rosenberg, D. M. Acoustic feature analysis in the perception of voicing contrasts. *Perception and Psychophysics*, 1977, *21*, 418–422.

Dimond, S. *The Double Brain*. London: Churchill Livingstone, 1972.

Dimond, S. J. Depletion of attentional capacity after total commissurotomy in man. *Brain*, 1976, *99*, 347–356.

Dimond, S., and Beaumont, J. (eds.). *Hemisphere Function in the Human Brain*. London: Elek Scientific Books, 1974.

Dimond, S., and Blizard, D. (eds.). Conference on evolution and lateralization of the brain. *Annals of the New York Academy of Sciences*, 1977, *299*.

Donnenfeld, H., Rosen, J. J., MacKavey, W., and Curcio, F. Effects of expectancy and order of report on auditory asymmetries. *Brain and Language*, 1976, *3*, 350–358.

Dyer, F. N. The Stroop phenomenon and its use in the study of perceptual, cognitive, and response processes. *Memory and Cognition*, 1973, *1*, 106–120.

Eccles, J. C. *The Understanding of the Brain*. New York: McGraw-Hill, 1973.

Efron, R. The effect of handedness on the perception of simultaneity and temporal order. *Brain*, 1963a, *86*, 261–284.

Efron, R. Temporal perception, aphasia, and deja vu. *Brain*, 1963b, *86*, 403–424.

Fedio, P., and Van Buren, J. M. Memory deficits during electrical stimulation of the speech cortex in conscious man. *Brain and Language*, 1974, *1*, 29–42.

Filby, R. A., and Gazzaniga, M. S. Splitting the normal brain with reaction time. *Psychonomic Science*, 1969, *17*, 335–336.

Fontenot, D. J., and Benton, A. L. Tactile perception of direction in normal subjects. *Neuropsychologia*, 1971, *9*, 83–88.

Franco, L. Hemispheric interaction in the processing of concurrent tasks in commissurotomy subjects. *Neuropsychologia*, 1977, *15*, 707–710.

Frankfurter, A., and Honeck, R. P. Ear differences in the recall of monaurally presented sentences. *Quarterly Journal of Experimental Psychology*, 1973, *25*, 138–146.

Frost, N. Encoding and retrieval in visual memory tasks. *Journal of Experimental Psychology*, 1972, *95*, 317–326.

Gaffan, D. Recognition impaired and association intact in the memory of monkeys after transection of the fornix. *Journal of Comparative and Physiological Psychology*, 1974, *86*, 1100–1109.

Galin, D., and Ellis, R. R. Asymmetry in evoked potentials as an index of lateralized cognitive processes: Relation to EEG alpha asymmetry. *Neuropsychologia,* 1975, *13*, 45–50.

Galin, D., and Orstein, R. Lateral specialization of cognitive mode. *Psychophysiology,* 1972, *9*, 412–418.

Gardner, E. B., and Branski, D. M. Unilateral cerebral activation and perception of gaps: A signal-detection analysis. *Neuropsychologia,* 1976, *14*, 43–54.

Gardner, H. *The Shattered Mind.* New York: Random House, 1974.

Gazzaniga, M. S. *The Bisected Brain.* New York: Appleton-Century-Crofts, 1970.

Gazzaniga, M. S. Brain mechanisms and behavior. In M. S. Gazzaniga and C. Blakemore (eds.), *Handbook of Psychobiology.* New York: Academic Press, 1975.

Geffen, G., Bradshaw, J. L., and Nettleton, N. C. Hemispheric asymmetry: Verbal and spatial encoding of visual stimuli. *Journal of Experimental Psychology,* 1972, *95*, 25–31.

Geffen, G., Bradshaw, J. L., and Nettleton, N. C. Attention and hemispheric differences in reaction time during simultaneous audio-visual tasks. *Quarterly Journal of Experimental Psychology,* 1973, *25*, 404–412.

Geschwind, N. Disconnexion syndromes in animals and man. *Brain,* 1965, *88*, Part I (237–294), Part II (585–644).

Geschwind, N. The organization of language and the brain. *Science,* 1970, *170*, 940–944.

Geschwind, N., and Levitsky, W. Human brain: Left-right asymmetries in temporal speech region. *Science,* 1968, *161*, 186–187.

Gibson, A. R., Dimond, S. J., and Gazzaniga, M. S. Left-field superiority for word matching. *Neuropsychologia,* 1972, *10*, 463–466.

Glanzer, M., and Cunitz, A. R. Two storage mechanisms in free recall. *Journal of Verbal Learning and Verbal Behavior,* 1966, *5*, 351–360.

Godfrey, J. J. Perceptual difficulty and the right-ear advantage for vowels. *Brain and Language,* 1974, *1*, 323–336.

Goldstein, K. *Language and Language Disturbances.* New York: Grune and Stratton, 1948.

Goodglass, H., and Baker, E. Semantic fields, naming, and auditory comprehension in aphasia. *Brain and Language,* 1976, *3*, 359–374.

Goodglass, H., and Caulderon, M. Parallel processing of verbal and musical stimuli in right and left hemispheres. *Neuropsychologia,* 1977, *15*, 397–407.

Goodglass, H., and Kaplan, E. *The Assessment of Aphasia and Related Disorders.* Philadelphia: Lea and Febiger, 1972.

Goodglass, H., and Peck, E. A. Dichotic ear order effects in Korsakoff and normal subjects. *Neuropsychologia,* 1972, *10*, 211–217.

Goodglass, H., Kaplan, E., Weintraub, S., and Ackerman, N. The "tip-of-the-tongue" phenomenon in aphasia. *Cortex,* 1976, *12*, 145–153.

Gordon, H. W. Auditory specialization of the right and left hemispheres. In M. Kinsbourne and W. L. Smith (eds.), *Hemispheric Disconnection and Cerebral Function.* Springfield, Ill.: Thomas, 1974.

Gordon, H. W. Hemispheric asymmetry and muscial performance, *Science,* 1975, *189*, 68–69.

Gross, M. M. Hemispheric specialization for processing of visually presented verbal and spatial stimuli. *Perception and Psychophysics,* 1972, *12*, 357–363.

Halperin, Y., Nachshon, I., and Carmon, A. Shift of ear superiority in dichotic listening to temporally patterned nonverbal stimuli. *Journal of the Acoustical Society of America,* 1973, *53*, 46–50.

Hannay, H. J., and Malone, D. R. Visual field effects and short-term memory for verbal material. *Neuropsychologia,* 1976, *14*, 203–209.

Hannay, J. Real or imagined incomplete laterization of function in females. *Perception and Psychophysics,* 1976, *19*, 349–352.

Hanson, V. L. Within-category discriminations in speech perception. *Perception and Psychophysics,* 1977, *21*, 423–430.

Harnad, S. R., Steklis, H. D., and Lancaster, J. (eds.). Origins and evolution of language and speech. *Annals of the New York Academy of Sciences,* 1976, *280*.

Hatta, T. Asynchrony of lateral onset as a factor in differences in visual field. *Perceptual and Motor Skills, 1976a, 42*, 163–166.

Hatta, T. Hemisphere asymmetries in the perception and memory of random forms. *Psychologia, 1976b, 19*, 157–162.

Head, H. *Aphasia and Kindred Disorders of Speech.* Cambridge: Cambridge University Press, 1926.

Hebb, D. O. *The Organization of Behavior.* New York: Wiley, 1949.

Hebb, D. O. The role of neurological ideas in psychology. *Journal of Personality,* 1951, *20*, 39–55.

Hécaen, H., and Angelergues, R. Agnosia for faces (prosopagnosia). *Archives of Neurology,* 1962, *7*, 24–32.

Heilman, K., Bowers, D., Rasbury, W. C., and Ray, R. M. Ear asymmetries on a selective attention task. *Brain and Language*, 1977, *4*, 390–395.

Hellige, J. B. Changes in same-different laterality patterns as a function of practice and stimulus quality. *Perception and Psychophysics*, 1976, *20*, 267–273.

Hellige, J. B., and Cox, P. J. Effects of concurrent verbal memory on recognition of stimuli from the left and right visual fields. *Journal of Experimental Psychology: Human Perception and Performance*, 1976, *2*, 210–221.

Hermelin, B., and O'Connor, N. Functional asymmetry in the reading of Braille. *Neuropsychologia*, 1971, *9*, 431–435.

Hicks, R. E. Intrahemispheric response competition between vocal and unimanual performance in normal adult human males. *Journal of Comparative and Physiological Psychology*, 1975, *89*, 50–60.

Hicks, R. E., Provenzano, F. J., and Rybstein, E. D. Generalized and lateralized effects of concurrent verbal rehearsal upon performance of sequential movements of the fingers by the left and right hands. *Acta Psychologica*, 1975, *39*, 119–130.

Hines, D. Independent functioning of the two cerebral hemispheres for recognizing bilaterally presented tachistoscopic visual-half-field stimuli. *Cortex*, 1975, *11*, 132–143.

Hines, D. Recognition of verbs, abstract nouns, and concrete nouns from the left and right visual half-fields. *Neuropsychologia*, 1976, *14*, 211–216.

Hines, D. Differences in tachistoscopic recognition between abstract and concrete words as a function of visual half-field and frequency. *Cortex*, 1977, *13*, 66–73.

Hines, D., Satz, P., and Clementino, T. Perceptual and memory components of the superior recall of letters from the right visual half-fields. *Neuropsychologia*, 1973, *11*, 175–180.

Holding, D. H. Sensory storage reconsidered. *Memory and Cognition*, 1975, *3*, 31–41.

Howes, D., and Boller, F. Simple reaction time: Evidence for focal impairment from lesions of the right hemisphere. *Brain*, 1975, *98*, 317–322.

Inglis, J. Dichotic listening and cerebral dominance. *Acta Oto-laryngologica*, 1965, *60*, 231–238.

Jaccarino, G. Dual encoding in memory: Evidence from temporal-lobe lesions in man. Unpublished M.A. thesis. McGill University, 1975.

Jaccarino Hiatt, G. Impairment of cognitive organization in patients with temporal-lobe lesions. Unpublished Ph.D. Thesis, McGill University, 1978.

Jackson, H. On the affections of speech from disease of the brain. *Brain*, 1878, *1*, 304–330.

James, W. *Principles of Psychology*, 1890. Reissued, New York: Dover, 1950.

Jarvella R. J., and Herman, S. J. Speed and accuracy of sentence recall: Effects of ear presentation, semantics, and grammar. *Journal of Experimental Psychology*, 1973, *79*, 111–113.

Jeeves, M. A., and Dixon, N. F. Hemisphere differences in response rates to visual stimuli. *Psychonomic Science*, 1970, *69*, 408–412.

Jones, E. G., and Powell, T. P. S. An anatomical study of converging sensory pathways within the cerebral cortex of the monkey. *Brain*, 1970, *93*, 793–820.

Jones, M. K. Imagery as a mnemonic aid after left temporal lobectomy: Contrasts between material-specific and generalized memory disorders. *Neuropsychologia*, 1974, *12*, 21–30.

Jones-Gotman, M., and Milner, B. Design fluency: The invention of nonsense drawings after focal cortical lesions. *Neuropsychologia*, 1977, *15*, 653–674.

Jones-Gotman, M., and Milner, B. Right temporal-lobe contribution to language-mediated verbal learning. *Neuropsychologia*, 1978, *16*, 61–71.

Kahneman, D. *Attention and Effort*. Englewood Cliffs, N.J.: Prentice-Hall, 1973.

Kallman, H. J., and Corballis, M. C. Ear asymmetry in reaction time to musical sounds. *Perception and Psychophysics*, 1975, *17*, 368–370.

Kimura, D. Cerebral dominance and the perception of verbal stimuli. *Canadian Journal of Psychology*, 1961, *15*, 166–171.

Kimura, D. Speech lateralization in young children as determined by an auditory test. *Journal of Comparative and Physiological Psychology*, 1963, *56*, 899–902.

Kimura, D. Functional asymmetry of the brain in dichotic listening. *Cortex*, 1967, *3*, 163–178.

Kimura, D. Manual activity during speaking. I. Right-handers. *Neuropsychologia*, 1973, *11*, 45–50.

Kimura, D., and Archibald, Y. Motor functions of the left hemisphere. *Brain*, 1974, *97*, 337–350.

Kimura, D., and Durnford, M. Normal studies on the function of the right hemisphere in vision. In S. J. Dimond and J. G. Beaumont (eds.), *Hemisphere Function in the Human Brain*. London: Elek Scientific Books, 1974.

Kinsbourne, M. The cerebral basis of lateral asymmetries in attention. *Acta Psychologica*, 1970, *33*, 193–201.

Kinsbourne, M. Eye and head turning indicates cerebral lateralization. *Science*, 1972, *176*, 539–541.

Kinsbourne, M. The control of attention by interaction between the cerebral hemispheres. In S. Kornblum (ed.), *Attention and Performance IV*. New York: Academic Press, 1973, pp. 239–256.

Kinsbourne, M. The mechanism of hemispheric control of the lateral gradient of attention. In P. M. A. Rabbit and S. Dornic (eds.), *Attention and Performance V*. New York: Academic Press, 1975.

Kinsbourne, M., and Cook, J. Generalized and lateralized effects of concurrent verbalization on a unimanual skill. *Quarterly Journal of Experimental Psychology*, 1971, *23*, 341–345.

Kinsbourne, M., and Wood, F. Short-term memory processes and the amnesic syndrome. In D. Deutsch and A. J. Deutsch (eds.), *Short-term memory*. New York: Academic Press, 1975.

Klatzky, R. L., and Atkinson, R. C. Specialization of the cerebral hemispheres in scanning for information in short-term memory. *Perception and Psychophysics*, 1971, *10*, 335–338.

Klein, D., Moscovitch, M., and Vigna, C. Attentional mechanisms and perceptual asymmetries in tachistoscopic recognition of words and faces. *Neuropsychologia*, 1976, *14*, 55–66.

Kolers, P. A. Memorial consequences of automatized encoding. *Journal of Experimental Psychology: Human Learning and Memory*, 1975, *1*, 689–701.

Konorski, J. (ed.). Symposium on the frontal granular cortex and behavior held in Jablonna near Warszawa, Poland, August 1971. Published in *Acta Neurobiologica Experimentalis*, 1972, *32*.

Kosslyn, S. M., and Pomerantz, J. R. Imagery, propositions, and the form of internal representation. *Cognitive Psychology*, 1977, *9*, 52–76.

Kreuter, C., Kinsbourne, M., and Trevarthen, C. Are deconnected cerebral hemispheres independent channels? A preliminary study of the effect of unilateral loading on bilateral finger tapping. *Neuropsychologia*, 1972, *10*, 453–461.

Lackner, J. R., and Teuber, H.-L. Alterations in auditory fusion thresholds after cerebral injury in man. *Neuropsychologia*, 1973, *11*, 409–416.

Lashley, K. S. In search of the engram. *Society of Experimental Biology Symposium No. 4: Physiological Mechanisms in Animal Behavior*. New York: Cambridge University Press, 1950.

Ledlow, A., Swanson, J. M., and Carter, B. Specialization of the cerebral hemispheres for physical and associational memory comparison. Paper presented at the Midwestern Psychological Association Meeting, Cleveland, Ohio, 1972.

Ledlow, A. S., Swanson, J. M., and Levy, J. Hemispheric differences in RT experiments: Transcallosal transfer of information or shift of attention? Cited in Levy (1974).

Ledlow, A., Swanson, J. M., and Kinsbourne, M. Lateral differences in reaction time and evoked potentials: A localization of structural and attentional effects. *Journal of Experimental Psychology: Human Perception and Performance*, in press.

Lesser, R. Verbal comprehension in aphasia: An English version of three Italian tests. *Cortex*, 1974, *10*, 247–263.

Levy, J. Psychobiological implications of bilateral asymmetry. In S. J. Dimond and G. Beaumont (eds.), *Hemisphere Function in the Human Brain*. London: Elek Scientific Books, 1974.

Levy, J., and Trevarthen, C. Metacontrol of hemispheric function in human split-brain patients. *Journal of Experimental Psychology: Human Perception and Performance*, 1976, *2*, 299–312.

Levy, J., and Trevarthen, C. Perceptual, semantic, and phonetic aspects of elementary language processes in split-brain patients. *Brain*, 1977, *100*, 105–118.

Levy, J., Trevarthen, C., and Sperry, R. W. Perception of bilateral chimeric figures following hemispheric deconnexion. *Brain*, 1972, *95*, 61–78.

Liberman, A. M. The specialization of the language hemisphere. In F. O. Schmitt and F. G. Worden (eds.), *The Neurosciences: Third Research Program*. Cambridge, Mass.: MIT Press, 1974, pp. 43–56.

Lockhart, R. S., Craik, F. I. M., and Jacoby, L. L. Depth of processing in recognition and recall: Some aspects of a general memory system. In J. Brown (ed.), *Recognition and Recall*. London: Wiley, 1975.

Logan, G. D. Attention in character classification: Evidence for the automaticity of component stages. *Journal of Experimental Psychology: General*, 1978, *107*, 32–63.

Lomas, J., and Kimura, D. Intra hemispheric interaction between speaking and sequential manual activity. *Neuropsychologia*, 1976, *14*, 23–33.

Longden, K., Ellis, C., and Iverson, S. D. Hemispheric differences in the discrimination of curvature. *Neuropsychologia*, 1976, *14*, 195–202.

Luria, A. R. *Higher Cortical Functions in Man*. New York: Basic Books, 1966.

Luria, A. R. *Traumatic Aphasia*. The Hague: Mouton, 1970.

Luria, A. R. *The Working Brain*. London: Penguin, 1973.

Macmillan, N. A., Kaplan, H. L., and Creelman, C. D. The psychophysics of categorical perception. *Psychological Review, 1977, 84*, 452–471.

Marcel, T., and Patterson, K. Word recognition and production: Reciprocity in clinical and normal studies. In J. Requin (ed.), *Attention and Performance VII*. Hillsdale, N.J.: Erlbaum, 1978.

Marin, O. S. M., and Saffran, E. M. Agnosic behavior in anomia: A case of pathological verbal dominance. *Cortex, 1975, 11*, 83–89.

Marin, O. S. M., Saffran, E. M., and Schwartz, M. F. Dissociations of language in aphasia: Implications for normal functions. *Annals of the New York Academy of Sciences, 1976, 280*, 868–884.

Marschark, M., and Paivio, A. Integrative processing of concrete and abstract sentences. *Journal of Verbal Learning and Verbal Behavior, 1977, 16*, 217–232.

Marshall, J. C., and Newcombe, F. Patterns of paralexia: A psycholinguistic approach. *Journal of Psycholinguistics, 1973, 2*, 175–199.

Marshall, M., Newcombe, F., and Marshall, J. C. The microstructure of word-finding difficulties in a dysphasic subject. In G. B. Flores d'Arcais and W. J. M. Levelt (eds.), *Advances in Psycholinguistics*. Amsterdam-London: North-Holland Publishing Co., 1970.

Massaro, D. W. Preperceptual images, processing time, and perceptual units in auditory perception. *Psychological Review, 1972, 79*, 124–145.

Mateer, C., and Kimura, D. Impairment of nonverbal oral movements in aphasia. *Brain and Language, 1977, 4*, 262–276.

Mayes, A., and Beaumont, G. Does visual evoked potential asymmetry index cognitive activity? *Neuropsychologia, 1977, 15*, 249–256.

McAdam, D. W., and Whitaker, H. A. Language production: Electroencephalographic localization in the normal brain. *Science, 1971, 172*, 499–503.

McKeever, W. F., and Gill, K. M. Interhemispheric transfer time for visual stimulus information varies as a function of the retinal locus of stimulation. *Psychonomic Science, 1972, 26*, 308–310.

McKeever, W. F., and Huling, M. P. Lateral dominance and tachistoscopic word recognition performance obtained with simultaneous bilateral input. *Neuropsychologia, 1971, 9*, 15–20.

McKeever, W. F., and Suberi, M. Parallel but temporally displaced visual half field metacontrast functions. *Quarterly Journal of Experimental Psychology, 1974, 26*, 258–265.

McRae, D. L., Branch, C. L., and Milner, B. The occipital horns and cerebral dominance. *Neurology, 1968, 18*, 95–98.

Mills, L. Left-Hemispheric specialization in normal subjects for judgements of successive order and duration of nonverbal stimuli. Unpublished doctoral thesis, University of Western Ontario, 1977.

Milner, B. Laterality effects in audition. In V. B. Mountcastle (ed.), *Interhemispheric Relations and Cerebral Dominance*. Baltimore: Johns Hopkins University Press, 1962.

Milner, B. Some effects of frontal lobectomy in man. In J. M. Warren and H. Akert (eds.), *The Frontal Granular Cortex and Behaviour*. New York: McGraw-Hill, 1964, pp. 313–334.

Milner, B. Visually guided maze learning in man: Effects of bilateral hippocampal, bilateral frontal, and unilateral cerebral lesions. *Neuropsychologia, 1965, 3*, 317–338.

Milner, B. Amnesia following operation on the temporal lobe. In C. W. M. Whitty and O. L. Zangwill (eds.), *Amnesia*. London: Butterworth, 1966.

Milner, B. Brain mechanisms suggested by studies of temporal lobes. In C. H. Millikan and F. L. Darley (eds.), *Brain Mechanisms Underlying Speech and Language*. New York: Grune and Stratton, 1967.

Milner, B. Preface: Material specific and generalized memory loss. *Neuropsychologia, 1968a, 6*, 175–179.

Milner, B. Visual recognition and recall after right temporal-lobe excision in man. *Neuropsychologia, 1968b, 6*, 191–209.

Milner, B. Pathologie de la mémoire. In *La Mémoire*. Paris: Presses Universitaires de France, 1970, pp. 185–212.

Milner, B. Interhemispheric differences and psychological processes. *British Medical Bulletin, 1971, 27*, 272–277.

Milner, B. Hemispheric specialization: Scope and limits. In F. O. Schmitt and F. G. Worden (eds.), *The Neurosciences: Third Research Program*. Cambridge, Mass.: MIT Press, 1974, pp. 75–89.

Milner, B. Hemispheric asymmetry and the control of gesture sequences. *Proceedings of the 21st International Congress of Psychology* (Paris), 1976, p. 149.

Milner, B., and Scoville, W. B. Loss of recent memory after bilateral hippocampal lesions. *Journal of Neurology, Neurosurgery, and Psychiatry, 1957, 20*, 11–21.

Milner, B., and Taylor, L. Right-hemisphere superiority in tactile pattern-recognition after cerebral commissurotomy: Evidence for nonverbal memory. *Neuropsychologia, 1972, 10*, 1–15.

Milner, B., Corkin, S., and Teuber, H.-L. Further analysis of the hippocampal amnesia syndrome. *Neuropsychologia*, 1968a, *6*, 215–234.

Milner, B., Taylor, L., and Sperry, R. W. Lateralized suppression of dichotically presented digits after commissural section in man. *Science*, 1968b, *161*, 184–185.

Molfese, D., Freeman, R. B., Jr., and Palermo, D. S. The ontogeny of brain lateralization for speech and nonspeech stimuli. *Brain and Language*, 1975, *3*, 356–368.

Morais, J. Monaural ear differences for reaction time to speech with a many-to-one mapping paradigm. *Perception and Psychophysics*, 1976, *19*, 144–148.

Morais, J., and Bertelson, P. Spatial position versus ear of entry as determinant of the auditory laterality effects: A stereophonic test. *Journal of Experimental Psychology: Human Perception and Performance*, 1975, *1*, 253–262.

Morais, J., and Darwin, C. J. Ear differences for same-different reaction times to monaurally presented speech. *Brain and Language*, 1974, *1*, 363–374.

Morais, J., and Landercy, M. Listening to speech while retaining music: What happens to the right-ear advantage? *Brain and Language*, 1977, *4*, 295–308.

Morrell, L. K., and Salomy, J. G. Hemispheric asymmetry of electrocortical responses to speech stimuli. *Science*, 1971, *174*, 164–166.

Moscovitch, M. Choice reaction-time study assessing the verbal behaviour of the minor hemisphere in normal adult humans. *Journal of Comparative and Physiological Psychology*, 1972, *80*, 66–74.

Moscovitch, M. Language and the cerebral hemispheres: Reaction-time studies and their implications for models of cerebral dominance. In P. Pliner, T. Alloway, and L. Krames (eds.), *Communication and Affect: Language and Thought*. New York: Academic Press, 1973, pp. 89–126.

Moscovitch, M. On the representation of language in the right hemisphere of right-handed people. *Brain and Language*, 1976a, *3*, 47–71.

Moscovitch, M. Differential effects of unilateral temporal and frontal lobe damage on memory performance. Paper presented at the International Neuropsychological Society Meeting, Toronto, 1976b.

Moscovitch, M. Verbal and spatial clustering in free recall of drawings following left or right temporal lobectomy: Evidence for dual encoding. Paper presented at the Canadian Psychological Association Meeting, Toronto, 1976c.

Moscovitch, M. Selective interference effects on verbal and spatial clustering in free recall of drawings: Evidence for dual encoding. Paper presented at the meeting of the Canadian Psychological Association, Vancouver, B. C., June, 1977.

Moscovitch, M., and Catlin, J. Interhemispheric transmission of information: Measurement in normal man. *Psychonomic Science*, 1970, *18*, 211–213.

Moscovitch, M., and Craik, F. I. M. Depth of processing, retrieval cues, and uniqueness of encoding as factors in recall. *Journal of Verbal Learning and Verbal Behavior*, 1976, *15*, 447–458.

Moscovitch, M., and Klein, D. Material specific interference effects and their relation to functional hemispheric asymmetries. Paper presented at the International Neuropsychological Society Meeting, Santa Fe, New Mexico, 1977.

Moscovitch, M., Scullion, D., and Christie, D. Early vs. late stages of processing and their relation to functional hemispheric asymmetries in face recognition. *Journal of Experimental Psychology: Human Perception and Performance*, 1976, *2*, 401–416.

Moss, C. S. *Recovery with Aphasia*. Urbana: University of Illinois Press, 1972.

Murdock, B. B., Jr. Recent developments in short-term memory. *British Journal of Psychology*, 1967, *58*, 421–433.

Murdock, B. B., Jr. *Human Memory: Theory and Data*. Hillsdale, N.J.: Erlbaum, 1974.

Nachshon, I., and Carmon, A. Hand preference in sequential and spatial discrimination tasks. *Cortex*, 1975, *11*, 121–131.

Nadel, L., and O'Keefe, J. The hippocampus in pieces and patches: An essay on modes of explanation in physiological psychology. In R. Bellairs and E. G. Gray (eds.), *Essays on the Nervous System: A Festschrift for Professor J. Z. Young*. Oxford: Clarendon Press, 1974.

Nauta, W. J. H. Neural associations of the frontal cortex. *Acta Neurobiologica Experimentalis*, 1972, *32*, 125–140.

Nebes, R. D. Superiority of the minor hemisphere in commissurotomized man for the perception of part-whole relations. *Cortex*, 1971, *7*, 333–349.

Neisser, U. *Cognitive Psychology*. New York: Appleton-Century-Crofts, 1967.

Neisser, U. *Cognition and Reality*. San Francisco: Freeman, 1976.

Norman, D. A. *Memory and Attention*, 2nd ed. New York: Wiley, 1976.

Norman, D. A., and Rumelhart, D. E. *Explorations in Cognition.* San Francisco: Freeman, 1975.

O'Keefe, J., and Nadel, L. *The Hippocampus as a Cognitive Map.* London: Oxford University Press, in press.

Oldfield, R. C. Things, words, and the brain. *Quarterly Journal of Experimental Psychology,* 1966, *18*, 340–353.

Ornstein, R. E. *The Psychology of Consciousness.* San Francisco: Freeman, 1972.

Oscar-Berman, M. Hypothesis testing and focusing behavior during concept formation by amnesic Korsakoff patients. *Neuropsychologia,* 1973, *11*, 191–198.

Oscar-Berman, M., Goodglass, H., and Cherlow, D. G. Perceptual laterality and iconic recognition of visual materials by Korsakoff patients and normal adults. *Journal of Comparative and Physiological Psychology,* 1973, *82*, 216–231.

Oscar-Berman, M., Goodglass, H., and Donnenfeld, H. Dichotic ear-order effects with non-verbal stimuli. *Cortex,* 1974, *10*, 270–277.

Paivio, A. Mental imagery in associative learning and memory. *Psychological Review,* 1969, *76*, 241–263.

Paivio, A. *Imagery and Verbal Processes.* New York: Holt, Rinehart and Winston, 1971.

Paivio, A. Perceptual comparisons through the mind's eye. *Memory and Cognition,* 1975, *3*, 635–647.

Pandya, D. N., Hallett, M., and Mukherjee, S. K. Intra- and interhemispheric connections of the neocortical auditory system in the rhesus monkey. *Brain Research,* 1969, *14*, 49.

Papcun, G., Krashen, S., Terbeek, D., Remington, R., and Harshman, R. Is the left hemisphere specialised for speech, language and/or something else? *Journal of the Acoustical Society of America,* 1974, *55*, 319–327.

Patten, B. M. The ancient art of memory. *Archives of Neurology,* 1972, *26*, 25–31.

Patterson, K., and Bradshaw, J. L. Differential hemispheric mediation of nonverbal visual stimuli. *Journal of Experimental Psychology: Human Perception and Performance,* 1975, *1*, 246–252.

Perenin, M. T., and Jeannerod, M. Residual vision in cortically blind hemifields. *Neuropsychologia,* 1975, *13*, 1–8.

Pirozzolo, F. J., and Rayner, K. Hemispheric specialization in reading and word recognition. *Brain and Language,* 1977, *4*, 248–261.

Pisoni, D. B. Auditory and phonetic memory codes in the discrimination of consonants and vowels. *Perception and Psychophysics,* 1973, *13*, 253–260.

Pisoni, D. B., and Tash, J. Reaction times to comparisons within and across phonetic categories. *Perception and Psychophysics,* 1974, *15*, 285–290.

Pizzamiglio, L., and Parisi, D. Studies on verbal comprehension in aphasia. In G. B. Flores d'Arcais and W. J. M. Levelt (eds.), *Advances in Psycholinguistics.* Amsterdam: North-Holland, 1970.

Poeck, K., and Huber, W. To what extent is language a sequential activity? *Neuropsychologia,* 1977, *15*, 359–364.

Poeppel, E., Held, R., and Frost, D. Residual function after brain wounds involving the central visual pathways in man *Nature (London),* 1973, *243*, 295–296.

Poffenberger, A. T. Reaction time to retinal stimulation with special reference to the time lost in conduction through nerve centres. *Archives of Psychology,* 1912, *13*, 1–73.

Porter, R. J., and Mirabile, P. J. Dichotic and monotic interactions between speech and nonspeech sounds at different stimulus onset asynchronies. *Perception and Psychophysics,* 1977, *2*, 408–412.

Posner, M. I. Abstraction and the process of recognition. In G. H. Bower and J. T. Spence (eds.), *The Psychology of Learning and Motivation,* Vol. 3. New York: Academic Press, 1969, pp. 43–100.

Posner, M. I. Psychobiology of attention. In M. S. Gazzaniga and C. Blakemore (eds.), *Handbook of Psychobiology.* New York: Academic Press, 1975.

Posner, M. I., and Snyder, C. R. R. Attention and cognitive control. In R. Solso (ed.), *Information Processing and Cognition: The Loyola Symposium.* Potomac, Md.: Erlbaum, 1975.

Potter, M. C., Valian, V. V., and Faulconer, B. A. Representation of a sentence and its pragmatic implications: Verbal, imagistic, or abstract. *Journal of Verbal Learning and Verbal Behavior,* 1977, *16*, 1–12.

Pribram, K. H. *Languages of the Brain.* Englewood Cliffs, N.J.: Prentice-Hall, 1971.

Pylyshyn, Z. W. What the mind's eye tells the mind's brain: A critique of mental imagery. *Psychological Bulletin,* 1973, *80*, 1–24.

Rabinowicz, B. H. A non-lateralized auditory process in speech perception. Unpublished M.A. thesis, University of Toronto, 1976.

Repp, B. H. Dichotic competition of speech sounds: The role of acoustic stimulus structure. *Journal of Experimental Psychology: Human Perception and Performance,* 1977, *3*, 37–50.

Rosch, E. Cognitive representation and semantic categories. *Journal of Experimental Psychology: General,* 1975, *104*, 192–233.

Rosen, J., Curicio, F., McKavey, W., and Herbert, J. Superior recall of letters in the right visual field with bilateral presentation and partial report. *Cortex*, 1975, *11*, 144–154.

Rosenzweig, M. R. Representation of the two ears at the auditory cortex. *American Journal of Physiology,* 1951, *167*, 147–158.

Rothstein, L. D., and Atkinson, R. C. Memory scanning for words in visual images. *Memory and Cognition*, 1975, *3*, 541–544.

Rotkin, L., Greenwood, P., and Gazzaniga, M. S. Psychophysics with the "splitbrain" patient: Perceptual asymmetries and verbal mediation in sensory judgments. Paper presented at the Eastern Psychological Association Meeting, New York, 1977.

Rozin, P. The psychobiological approach to human memory. In M. R. Rosenzweig and E. L. Bennett (eds.), *Neurological Mechanisms of Learning and Memory.* Cambridge, Mass.: MIT Press, 1976.

Saffran, E. M., and Marin, O. S. M. Immediate memory for words lists and sentences in a patient with deficient auditory short-term memory. *Brain and Language*, 1975, *2*, 420–433.

Saffran, E. M., Marin, O. S. M., and Yeni-Komshian, G. H. An analysis of speech perception in word deafness. *Brain and Language,* 1976*a*, *3*, 209–228.

Saffran, E. M., Schwartz, M. F., and Marin, O. S. M. Semantic mechanisms in paralexia. *Brain and Language,* 1976*b*, *3*, 255–265.

Sanders, M. D., Warrington, E. K., Marshall, J., and Weiskrantz, L. "Blindsight": Vision in a field defect. *Lancet,* 1974, April, 707–708.

Sasanumo, S. Kana and kanji processing in Japanese aphasics. *Brain and Language*, 1975, *2*, 369–383.

Scarborough, D. L. Memory for brief visual displays of symbols. *Cognitive Psychology*, 1972, *3*, 408–429.

Schloterer, G. Changes in visual information processing with normal aging and progressive dementia of the Alzheimer type. Unpublished Ph.D. thesis, University of Toronto, 1977.

Schwartz, G. E., Davidson, R. J., and Maer, F. Right hemisphere lateralization for emotion in the human brain: Interaction with cognition. *Science,* 1975, *190*, 286–288.

Schwartz, M. Visual field effects with chimeric faces. Paper presented at the meeting of the International Neuropsychological Society. Minneapolis, Minnesota, February, 1978.

Scotti, G., and Spinnler, H. Colour imperception in unilateral hemisphere-damaged patients. *Journal of Neurology, Neurosurgery, and Psychiatry,* 1970, *33*, 22–28.

Seamon, J. G. Imagery codes and human information retrieval. *Journal of Experimental Psychology,* 1972, *96*, 468–470.

Seamon, J. G., and Gazzaniga, M. J. Coding strategies and cerebral laterality effects. *Cognitive Psychology,* 1973, *5*, 249–256.

Semmes, J., Weinstein, S., Ghent, L., and Teuber, H.-L. Correlates of impaired orientation in personal and extrapersonal space. *Brain,* 1963, *86*, 747–772.

Shallice, T., and Warrington, E. K. Independent functioning of verbal memory stores: A neuropsychological study. *Quarterly Journal of Experimental Psychology,* 1970, *22*, 261–273.

Shallice, T., and Warrington, E. K. Word recognition in a phonemic dyslexic patient. *Quarterly Journal of Experimental Psychology,* 1975, *27*, 187–199.

Shankweiler, D. Effects of temporal-lobe damage on perception of dichotically presented melodies. *Journal of Comparative Psychology,* 1966, *62*, 115–119.

Shankweiler, D., and Studdert-Kennedy, M. Identification of consonants and vowels presented to the right and left ears. *Quarterly Journal of Experimental Psychology,* 1967, *19*, 59–63.

Simon, H. A. What is visual imagery? An information processing interpretation. In L. W. Gregg (ed.), *Cognition in Learning and Memory.* New York: Wiley, 1972.

Smith, A. *Powers of Mind.* New York: Ballantine, 1975.

Smith, E. E., Shoben, E. J., and Rips, L. J. Comparison processes in semantic memory. *Psychological Review,* 1974, *81*, 214–241.

Sparks, R., and Geschwind, N. Dichotic listening in man after section of neocortical commissures. *Cortex,* 1968, *4*, 3–16.

Spellacy, F., and Blumstein, S. The influence of language set and ear preference in phoneme recognition. *Cortex,* 1970, *6*, 430–439.

Sperling, G. A model for visual memory tasks. *Human Factors*, 1963, *5*, 19–31.

Sperry, R. W. Lateral specialization in the surgically separated hemispheres. In F. O. Schmitt and F. G. Worden (eds.), *The Neurosciences: Third Study Program.* Cambridge, Mass.: MIT Press, 1974.

Springer, S. Ear asymmetry in a dichotic detection task. *Perception and Psychophysics,* 1971, *10*, 239–241.

Springer, S. P. Hemispheric specialization for speech opposed by contralateral noise. *Perception and Psychophysics,* 1973, *13*, 391–393.

Strauss, E., and Fitz, C. Occipital horn asymmetry in children. Paper presented at B.A.B.B.L.E. Conference, Brock University, St. Catherines, Ontario, 1978.

Studdert-Kennedy, M., and Shankweiler, D. Hemispheric specialization for speech perception. *Journal of the Acoustical Society of America*, 1970, *48*, 579–594.

Sullivan, E. V., and Turvey, M. T. On the short-term retention of serial tactile stimuli. *Memory and Cognition*, 1974, *2*, 600–606.

Swanson, J. M., Ledlow, A., and Kinsbourne, M. Lateral asymmetrics revealed by simple reaction time. In M. Kinsbourne (ed.), *Hemispheric Asymmetry of Function*. New York: Cambridge University Press, 1978.

Talland, G. A. *Deranged Memory*. New York: Academic Press, 1965.

Taylor, L., Milner, B., and Darwin, C. J. Verbal disabilities associated with lesions of the left face area. In preparation. Summarized in *The 17th International Symposium of Neuropsychology* (G. Ettlinger. H.-L. Teuber, and B. Milner). *Neuropsychologia*, 1975, *13*, 125–133.

Teszner, D., Tzavaras, A., Gruner, J., and Hécaen, H. R. L'asymétrie droite-gauche du Planum temporale. A propos de l'étude anatomique de 100 cerveaux. *Revue Neurologique*, 1972, *126*, 444–449.

Teuber, H.-L. Unity and diversity of frontal lobe functions. *Acta Neurobiologia Experimentalis*, 1972, *32*, 615–656.

Teuber, H.-L., Milner, B., and Vaughn, H. G., Jr., Persistent anterograde amnesia after stabwound of the basal brain. *Neuropsychologia*, 1968, *6*, 267–282.

Treisman, A., and Geffen, G. Selective attention and cerebral dominance in perceiving and responding to speech messages. *Quarterly Journal of Experimental Psychology*, 1968, *20*, 139–150.

Tulving, E. Episodic and semantic memory. In E. Tulving and W. Donaldson (eds.), *Organization of Memory*. New York: Academic Press, 1972, pp. 382–404.

Turvey, M. On peripheral and central processes in vision: Inferences from an information-processing analysis of masking with patterned stimuli. *Psychological Review*, 1973, *80*, 1–52.

Turvey, M. T. Contrasting orientations to the theory of visual information processing. *Psychological Review*, 1977, *84*, 67–88.

Umilta, C., Brizzolara, D., Tabossi, P., and Fairweather, H. Factors affecting face recognition in the cerebral hemispheres: Familiarity and naming. In J. Requin (ed.), *Attention and Performance VII*, Hillsdale, N.J.: Lawrence Erlbaum, 1978.

Vygotsky, L. S. *Thought and Language*. Cambridge, Mass.: MIT Press, 1962.

Wada, J., Clark, R., and Hamm, A. Cerebral hemispheric asymmetry in humans. *Archives of Neurology*, 1975, *32*, 239–246.

Ward, T. B., and Ross, L. E. Laterality differences and practice effects under central backward masking conditions. *Memory and Cognition*, 1977, *5*, 221–226.

Warren, J. M., and Akert, K. *The Frontal Granular Cortex and Behaviour*. New York: McGraw-Hill, 1964.

Warren, R. E. Stimulus encoding and memory. *Journal of Experimental Psychology*, 1972, *94*, 90–100.

Warren, R. E. Association, directionality, and stimulus encoding. *Journal of Experimental Psychology*, 1974, *102*, 151–158.

Warrington, E. K. The selective impairment of semantic memory. *Quarterly Journal of Experimental Psychology*, 1975, *27*, 635–657.

Warrington, E. K., and James, M. An experimental investigation of facial recognition in patients with unilateral cerebral lesions. *Cortex*, 1967, *3*, 317–326.

Warrington, E. K., and Shallice, T. The selective impairment of auditory verbal short-term memory. *Brain*, 1969, *92*, 885–96.

Warrington, E. K., and Taylor, A. M. The contribution of the right parietal lobe to object recognition. *Cortex*, 1973, *7*, 152–164.

Watkins, M. J., and Watkins, O. C. A tactile suffix effect. *Memory and Cognition*, 1974, *2*, 176–180.

Watkins, O. C., and Watkins, M. J. Build-up of pro-active inhibition as a cue-overload effect. *Journal of Experimental Psychology: Human Learning and Memory*, 1975, *104*, 442–452.

Weiss, M. J., and House, A. S. Perception of dichotically presented vowels. *Journal of Acoustical Society of America*, 1973, *53*, 51–58.

Weisstein, N., Ozog, G., and Szoc, R. A comparison and elaboration of two models of metacontrast. *Psychological Review*, 1975, *82*, 315–343.

White, M. J. Laterality differences in perception: A review. *Psychological Bulletin*, 1969, *72*, 387–405.

White, M. J. Hemispheric asymmetries in tachistoscopic information-processing. *British Journal of Psychology*, 1972, *63*, 497–508.

White, M. J., and White, K. G. Parallel-serial processing and hemispheric functions. *Neuropsychologia*, 1975, *13*, 377–381.

Wickens, D. Encoding categories of words: An empirical approach to memory. *Psychological Review,* 1970, *77,* 1–15.

Wilkins, A., and Moscovitch, M. Selective impairment of semantic memory after temporal lobectomy. *Neuropsychologia,* 1978, *16,* 73–79.

Wilkins, A., and Stewart, A. The time course of lateral asymmetries in visual perception of letters. *Journal of Experimental Psychology,* 1974, *102,* 905–908.

Winocur, G., and Weiskrantz, L. An investigation of paired-associate learning in amnesic patients. *Neuropsychologia,* 1976, *14,* 97–110.

Witelson, S. F. Hemispheric specialization for linguistic and nonlinguistic tactual perception using a dichotomous stimulation technique. *Cortex,* 1974, *10,* 1–17.

Witelson, S. F., and Pallie, W. Left hemisphere specialization for language in the newborn: Neuroanatomical evidence of asymmetry. *Brain,* 1973, *96,* 641–646.

Wood, C. C. Parallel processing of auditory and phonetic information in speech perception. *Perception and Psychophysics,* 1974, *15,* 501–508.

Wood, C. C. Auditory and phonetic levels of processing in speech perception: Neurophysiological and information-processing analysis. *Journal of Experimental Psychology: Human Perception and Performance,* 1975, *104,* 3–20.

Wood, C. C., Goff, W. R., and Day, R. S. Auditory evoked potentials during speech perception. *Science,* 1971, *173,* 1248–1251.

Yeni-Komshian, G. H., and Gordon, J. F. The effect of memory load on the right ear advantage in dichotic listening. *Brain and Language,* 1974, *1,* 375–382.

Yin, R. K. Face recognition by brain-injured patients: A dissociable ability. *Neuropsychologia,* 1970, *8,* 395–402.

Zaidel, E. Linguistic competence and related functions in the right cerebral hemisphere of man following commissurotomy and hemispherectomy. Unpublished doctoral thesis, California Institute of Technology, Pasadena, 1973.

Zaidel, E. Auditory vocabulary of the right hemisphere following brain bisection of hemidecortication. *Cortex,* 1976, *12,* 191–211.

Zaidel, E. Unilateral auditory language comprehension of the Token Test following cerebral commissurotomy and hemispherectomy. *Neuropsychologia,* 1977, *15,* 1–18.

Zaidel, D. and Sperry, R. W. Performance on the Raven's coloured progressive matrices test by subjects with cerebral commissurotomy. *Cortex,* 1973, *9,* 34–39.

Zurif, E., Caramazza, A., and Myerson, R. Grammatical judgements of agrammatic aphasics. *Neuropsychologia,* 1972, *10,* 405–417.

14

The Neuropsychological Basis
of Skilled Movement in Man

KENNETH M. HEILMAN

DEFINITION OF THE PROBLEM

There are many ways of investigating the neuropsychological basis of skilled movements—ablation, stimulation, electrophysiological recording (EEG and single cell), and neurochemistry. Although some stimulation and EEG (evoked potential and contingent negative variations) studies have been performed in man, much of what we know about the neuropsychology of skilled movement comes from the studies of patients with such disorders.

Disorders of skilled movement may be caused by diseases that affect muscles, the myoneural junction, peripheral nerves (afferent and efferent), the spinal cord, brain stem, cerebellum, basal ganglia, and cortex. Defects in some of these areas, however, produce disorders of skilled movement because these defects cause weakness (muscle, myoneural junction, peripheral nerves, spinal cord, or brain stem) or sensory loss (receptor, peripheral nerves, cord, brain stem, thalamus, or primary sensory cortex). Disorders of skilled movements not associated with weakness or sensory loss can be induced by diseases that affect either the basal ganglia or the cerebellum. The functions of the cerebellum and basal ganglia have not been completely elucidated. It appears, however, that the cerebral cortex alone cannot execute a coordinated skilled movement. The cerebellum and basal ganglia are reciprocally linked to the motor cortex to form a loop (Kornhuber, 1972) that may act as a servomechanism, with the subcortical structures acting as comparators. The cerebellum would be important in rapid movements (ballistic,

KENNETH M. HEILMAN   Department of Neurology, College of Medicine, University of Florida, and Veterans Administration Hospital, Gainesville, Florida 32610.

phasic), and the basal ganglia would be important in slow movements (tonic). In addition to causing loss of skilled movements, disorders of the basal ganglia and cerebellum manifest themselves by changes in posture and tone, tremors, dysmetrias, and other forms of stereotypic movement abnormalities. Although disorders of the subcortical structures can produce abnormalities of skilled movement, the scope of this chapter will be confined to disorders of skilled movement that are unassociated with abnormality of tone and posture or stereotyped movements and to disorders of skilled movement caused by cortical defects.

Asanuma (1975) showed that when an area 4 neuron is stimulated by low levels of current, only the motor neuron pool going to one muscle is activated. His findings suggest that muscles are represented separately and independently at different cortical loci. Since this chapter is primarily concerned with movements and acts and not with control of muscles, the function of primary motor cortex will also not be discussed in detail.

DISORDERS OF SKILLED MOVEMENT (APRAXIA) FROM CALLOSAL LESIONS

Disorders of skilled movement not caused by weakness, deafferentation, abnormality of tone or posture, abnormal movements, intellectual deterioration, poor comprehension, or uncooperativeness were termed "apraxia" by Steinthal (1871). Although in 1866 Hughlings-Jackson (cited in Taylor, 1932) described patients who were unable to perform voluntary skilled movements in the absence of weakness, it was primarily Liepmann (Liepmann and Maas, 1907; Liepmann, 1908) who initiated interest in apraxia as disorders of skilled movement. Liepmann and Maas (1907) studied a patient with right hemiplegia. When this patient attempted to carry out verbal commands with his left hand, he performed poorly. On postmortem examination he was found to have a lesion in the left basis pontis, which accounted for his right hemiplegia, and an infarction of the corpus callosum, which spared the splenium of the corpus callosum. Several years before Liepmann's studies, Broca (1863) reported eight right-handed patients with aphasia. All eight patients had their lesion in the left hemisphere. Broca's observations as well as Wernicke's (1874) indicated that language is mediated by the left hemisphere. Because language is decoded in the left hemisphere and because it is the primary motor area in the right hemisphere that controls the distal muscles in the left arm, a lesion of the callosum, similar to that which Liepmann and Maas reported, could produce abnormalities of skilled movement because this lesion disconnected the language area of the brain from the motor areas, which are responsible for carrying out the command. When the patient reported by Liepmann and Maas was tested by having him imitate skilled movements, his performance remained poor. When an object was placed in this patient's hand, skilled movements were still poor. Interestingly, this patient was able to detect the normal movement when it was performed by the examiner. Because this patient's primary visual area, visual association area, primary somesthetic area, somesthetic association area, and premotor and motor areas were all intact in his right hemisphere, a disconnection between the language areas in the left hemisphere and motor areas in the right hemisphere should have allowed him to use an object correctly and to imitate. Since the patient described by Liepmann and Maas could not imitate or use an object, they concluded that the left hemisphere contains not only language but also motor engrams that control all purposeful skilled movements. Lesions of the corpus callosum therefore not only disconnect the language hemisphere from the hemisphere controlling the left hand but also separate motor engrams in the left hemisphere from those in the right hemisphere.

Ettlinger (1969) noted that there were no reports of apraxia in experimental animals similar to the apraxia reported by Liepmann. He therefore concluded that the defect seen in man by Liepmann and others was produced because language was mediated by the left hemisphere, the left hand was controlled by the right hemisphere, and a lesion of the corpus callosum disconnected language from movement.

Gazzaniga et al. (1967) studied patients who had had a callosal section. When their nondominant upper extremity was tested, several of those patients were unable to perform in response to command but could imitate and use objects. These observations support Ettlinger's theory that right-handed humans cannot carry out commands with their left hand because they have a disconnection between the left hemisphere, which mediates comprehension of the command, and the right hemisphere, which controls the left hand.

Geschwind and Kaplan (1962) also reported a patient with callosal dysfunction who was unable to carry out commands with the left hand but was able to imitate and use objects. Later, after reviewing several other cases of corpus callosum disconnection, Geschwind (1965) remarked that the independence of the right hemisphere in nonlanguage function which was manifested by his patient was unusual and may have been an exception.

Perhaps, unlike Liepmann and Maas's patient, who probably had visuokinesthetic motor engrams restricted to his left hemisphere, the patients reported by Gazzaniga et al. (1967) and Geschwind and Kaplan (1962) had bilateral engrams. One suspects that if these patients either were to undergo hemispherectomy or were to have an extensive lesion of the left hemisphere and if they recovered language and could be tested for apraxia, they would not be apraxic. Recovery of function will be discussed later in this chapter.

DISORDERS OF SKILLED MOVEMENT (APRAXIA) FROM LEFT HEMISPHERE LESIONS

Liepmann noted not only that lesions of the callosum induce apraxia of the left hand but also that lesions of the left hemisphere may cause a similar disorder. Unlike the patients with apraxia associated with a callosal lesion, patients with left hemisphere lesions often have associated aphasia. Liepmann termed apraxia of the left hand caused by left hemisphere lesions "sympathetic apraxia." Because with this disorder patients are most often aphasic, it is commonly assumed that the inability to carry out commands properly is caused by a comprehension disorder; however, if one observes the movements of these patients it is obvious that they comprehend the command and are trying to perform the correct act. The main problem appears to be that the movements of these patients are often awkward, incomplete, and poorly sequenced. To demonstrate that they comprehend the commands, they may use body parts as objects.

Goldstein (1948) argued that aphasia is part of a generalized disturbance in symbolic behavior and is caused by left hemisphere dysfunction. Whereas aphasia is a disturbance of verbal symbolization, apraxia is a defect of nonverbal symbolization (e.g., gesture and pantomime) (Goldstein, 1948). Patients with ideomotor apraxia perform poorly to command and imitation, but they improve with the use of the actual object. These facts lend support to the postulate that apraxia is a defect in nonverbal symbolization. However, several studies lend support to Liepmann's hypothesis that the left hemisphere controls skilled movements and that destruction of the engrams, or separation of these engrams from the motor areas controlling the extremity, causes abnormalities of skilled movement. Goodglass and Kaplan (1963) tested apraxic aphasic patients and control aphasic subjects with the Wechsler Adult Intelligence Scale and used the performance-scaled score as a measure of intellectual ability. They also tested their subjects' ability to gesture and perform simple and complex pantomimes. The apraxic aphasics performed poorer on these motor skills than did their intellectual counterparts in the control groups. No clear relationship emerged between the severity of aphasia and the degree of gestural deficiency, and the apraxic aphasic patients were less able to imitate than were the nonapraxic controls.

Although Goodglass and Kaplan believed that their results supported Liepmann's hypothesis, they noted that their apraxic aphasic subjects did not have any difficulty in handling objects. Liepmann, however, thought apraxic patients were clumsy with objects; and Geschwind (1965) noted that although such patients may improve with the actual handling of objects, their actions nevertheless remain clumsy. Clumsiness of the left hand on handling objects is difficult to quantify, and if apraxia is in part a disconnection from or destruction of the area containing motor memories then brain-damaged apraxic patients should differ from nonapraxic patients. In 1973 I reported studies of apraxic aphasics and nonapraxic aphasics who were given a rapid fingertapping task with their left hand. The apraxic aphasic group performed significantly poorer than did the nonapraxic aphasic group. The severity of the apraxic disorder also correlated with performance on the tapping task. Similar results had previously been reported by Wyke (1967), who did not test for apraxia but also used a repetitive nonsymbolic movement to test patients with disease of either the right or the left hemisphere. She demonstrated that patients with left hemisphere disease performed more poorly with their ipsilateral hand than did those with right hemisphere disease. Wyke concluded that "ipsilateral control does not exist from the right hemisphere"; however, her results also support Liepmann's hypothesis the left hemisphere contains the motor memories that help control the right hemisphere via the corpus callosum. Kimura and Archibald (1974) studied the ability of left hemisphere-impaired aphasics and right hemisphere-impaired controls to copy unfamiliar, meaningless motor sequences. The performance of aphasic apraxic patients with left hemisphere impairment was poorer than that of the controls, which again supported Liepmann's hypothesis.

There are studies, however, that tend to refute Liepmann's hypothesis that apraxia is a disorder of skilled movements and not a form of asymbolia. Pieczuro and Vignolo (1967), for example, studied 35 patients with lesions of the right hemisphere and 70 with lesions of the left hemisphere by testing manual dexterity on a screwing task. These patients' performance of the task was impaired by lesions in either hemisphere, and the severity of the apraxia was independent of manual dexterity. I am not certain why Pieczuro and Vignolo's study is discrepant from Wyke's (1967, 1968), Kimura and Archibald's (1974), and mine (1973, 1975). Perhaps the strongest support for Liepmann's hypothesis that apraxia is a disorder of skilled movements comes from Liepmann's own observations that only 14 out of 20 apraxic patients were aphasic. Goodglass and Kaplan (1963) and my colleagues and I (Heilman *et al.*, 1973; Heilman, 1974) also have described similar patients. In addition, aphasic patients are often not apraxic (Heilman, 1973, 1975).

Because a poor correlation exists between the severity of symbolic disorders (asphasia) and disorders of skilled movements and because even nonsymbolic movements are poorly performed by apraxics, there is little evidence to support the hypothesis that apraxia is a disorder of symbolic behavior.

ACQUISITION OF SKILL BY THE LEFT HEMISPHERE

If, as Liepmann proposed, the left hemisphere contains motor engrams and apraxia is produced by a disconnection of these engrams from the primary motor area, then performance of patients with ideomotor apraxia should not only be defective in pantomime (Goodglass and Kaplan, 1963), meaningful imitation (Goodglass and Kaplan, 1963), meaningless imitation (Kimura and Archibald, 1974), meaningful use of actual objects (Kimura and Archibald, 1974), and meaningless use of actual objects (Heilman, 1973, 1975) but should also be defective in acquisition and retention of new motor skills. To test acquisition and retention of motor skills, my associates and I (Heilman *et al.*, 1975) studied nine right-handed hemiparetic patients with apraxia and aphasia and eight right-handed hemiparetic controls with aphasia but without apraxia. These subjects were given six trials on a rotary pursuit apparatus (five acquisition trials and one retention trial). All subjects used their left, nonparetic hand. The performance of the control group on the sixth trial was significantly better than on the first trial; however, there was no significant difference between the first and sixth trials in the apraxic group, which suggested that these patients had a defect in motor learning. The defect appeared to be caused by a combined defect of both acquisition and retention. Wyke (1971) studied patients with either right or left hemisphere disease. Her subjects were given motor acquisition tasks that required bimanual coordination. Although patients with left hemisphere disease demonstrated acquisition, it was less than that of those with right hemisphere disease.

Since Wyke did not separate her left hemispheric group into apraxic and nonapraxic patients, one could not be certain whether apraxic patients would have demonstrated poorer learning than the nonapraxic patients with left hemisphere impairment. Nevertheless, these motor learning studies provided further support to Liepmann's hypothesis and support our observations.

Although we have provided evidence that motor engrams are stored in the left hemisphere of right-handed subjects, this evidence has been based solely on ablative studies. If engrams are stored in the left hemisphere, then one would expect the right hand to be able to acquire new skills more rapidly than the left hand. In addition, skills learned by the left hand should benefit the right hand's performance more than would skills acquired by the right hand benefit the left hand. To study acquisition and transfer of skills, Hicks (1974) instructed subjects to print inverted and reversed letters. Taylor and I (1977) instructed subjects to press a given sequence of buttons. Although Hicks's study used letters and ours used a visuospatial array, both studies showed not only that the right hand learns faster than the left but also that, once a skill is acquired, the right hand retrieves this engram better than does the left hand. Some earlier studies (Briggs and Brogden, 1953; Meier and French, 1965) also supported these observations.

Role of the Right Hemisphere in Skilled Movement

Although I have provided evidence that motor engrams are stored in the left hemisphere, I have not explained why some right-handed aphasic patients are not apraxic. Possibly some of these patients have a small lesion or their lesion missed some critical area. I have, however, seen patients with large lesions who were not apraxic but others with small lesions who were severely apraxic. And of patients who had lesions in the same area, some were apraxic and some nonapraxic. Although the size and locus of a lesion undoubtedly determine the presence or absence of apraxia as well as its severity, they appear not to be the only determinants. While studying apraxic patients with the rotary pursuit apparatus, my associates and I tested a right-handed patient with a large frontoparietal lesion of the left hemisphere; this patient was also aphasic, apraxic, and hemiplegic (right side). Although this patient was apraxic, his acquisition of skill on the rotary pursuit apparatus was similar to the acquisition of nonapraxic controls. Several weeks later he was brought before a large class of medical students. When the lecturer tried to demonstrate the apraxic disturbance, the patient's performance was flawless.

The mechanism for recovery of function in the patient is unknown. However, I postulate that the right hemisphere contains the engrams for motor skills. Some patients with left hemisphere lesions are not apraxic because the lesion did not destroy motor engrams or disconnect these engrams from the motor areas, but possibly other patients are aphasic and hemiplegic but not apraxic because their right hemisphere has taken over function for the left. This hypothesis is similar to the one first proposed by Kleist (1916) to explain why certain patients with lesions of the left hemisphere recover language function.

In right-handed patients almost all cases of apraxia are from left hemisphere lesions (Geschwind, 1965; Goodglass and Kaplan, 1963; Hécean and de Ajuriaguerra, 1964; Hécean and Sanguet, 1971). Rarely does a patient with apraxia have lesions on the right side, and almost all of these patients are left-handed (Hécean and Sanguet, 1971). Apraxia appears to be rare in left-handed patients and usually results from bilateral disease. Evidence points to familially left-handed patients having bilateral function and therefore more of a regression of functional defects (Hécean and Sanguet, 1971), including apraxia (Heilman *et al.*, 1973). Some right-handed patients with large lesions of the left hemisphere possibly either recover from apraxia or never manifest symptoms of apraxia. These patients may have a higher incidence of familial left-handedness, which allows them to encode engrams on the right side. However, this hypothesis also has not been tested.

LEFT HEMISPHERE MECHANISMS USED IN THE PROCESSING OF SKILLED MOVEMENTS

Movements can be initiated by stimuli such as commands, imitation, and use of an object. Geschwind (1965) proposed that language elicits motor behavior by using a neural substrate like that proposed by Wernicke (1874) to explain language processing (Fig. 1). Auditory stimuli travel along auditory pathways and reach Heschl's gyrus (primary auditory cortex). From Heschl's gyrus, the auditory message is relayed to the posterior superior portion of the temporal lobe (auditory association cortex). On the left side, this area is called Wernicke's area and appears to be important in language comprehension. Wernicke's area is connected to the premotor areas (motor association cortex) by the arcuate fasciculus, and the motor association area on the left is connected to the primary motor area on the left. When someone is told to carry out a command with his right hand, he uses Wernicke's reflex arch. Geschwind (1965) proposed that if a command must be carried out with the left hand, since it is rare to find fibers that run obliquely in the corpus callosum, fibers either cross from Wernicke's area to the auditory association area on the other side or cross from the premotor areas on the left side to the premotor areas on the right side and then to the motor areas on the right side. Geschwind postulated that the connections between the motor association areas

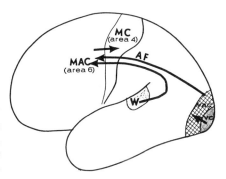

Fig. 1. Geschwind's schema. Lateral view of left side of brain. W, Wernicke's area, AF, Arcuate fasciculus; MAC, motor association cortex; MC, motor cortex, VAC, visual association cortex; VC visual cortex. The arrows indicate major connections of the areas shown.

are the important active pathway. He believed that disruptions in Wernicke's reflex arch and its connection to the right premotor area explain most of the apraxic disturbances. It may now be worthwhile to explore whether or not lesions in Wernicke's schema can indeed explain the variety of apraxic disturbances seen by neurologists. Lesions in Heschl's gyrus, Wernicke's area, or the connections between Heschl's gyrus and Wernicke's area cause defects in comprehension; therefore, although aphasic patients fail to carry out commands, their defect is not one of performance of skilled movements but rather that of a comprehension defect.

Patients with severe comprehension disturbances and an inability to follow commands often can perform whole-body commands (stand, sit, turn around) or midline commands (close your eyes, stick out your tongue). Geschwind has postulated that there may be connections between Wernicke's area and a group of pontine nuclei (Türck's bundle), which may be used in whole-body commands, but it is not clear how with the destruction of Wernicke's area these pontine nuclei could comprehend language. Unlike the distal extremity, which is completely innervated from the contralateral hemisphere, midline muscles have both contralateral and ipsilateral innervation (Kuypers and Brinkman, 1973). The right hemisphere of right-handers is capable of some language comprehension (Gazzaniga, 1970). Although Gazzaniga demonstrated that nouns are more easily comprehended than verbs, perhaps analogous to motor innervation, verbs that deal with midline function are more likely to be encoded bilaterally than are verbs that do not rely on midline function. To my knowledge, however, this hypothesis has not been tested.

Because lesions of the callosum would separate the right primary motor areas from the engrams of the left hemisphere, they would therefore compromise not only the ability to perform in response to commands but also the ability to imitate and to use an object. Lesions that destroy the left motor association cortex (premotor areas) would also destroy the callosal pathway from the left to the right motor association cortex; therefore, a lesion in the left motor association cortex would induce a defect similar to that induced by a lesion in the body of the corpus callosum (sympathetic dyspraxia). Lesions of the left motor association cortex are often associated with right hemiplegia, so the right side of most of these patients cannot be tested. If, however, these patients were not hemiparetic, they would probably be apraxic on the right. According to Geschwind's (1965, 1967) schema, lesions of the arcuate fasciculus should disconnect the posterior language areas, which are important in comprehension, from the motor association cortex, which is important in encoding motor engrams. Based on this schema, patients with parietal lesions, which spare motor association cortex, should be able to comprehend commands but not perform skilled movements in response to command. Theoretically, however, these patients should be able to imitate, but they cannot. They also have difficulty with the use of objects (Heilman, 1975). Geschwind noted that fibers passing from visual association cortex to motor cortex also pass anteriorly via the arcuate fasciculus. He proposed that the arcuate fasciculus of the left hemisphere is dominant for these visuomotor connections.

There is no evidence to support this hypothesis; however, perhaps even more important, even if one assumed that the left arcuate fasciculus was dominant for visuomotor connections and that this dominance explained why these patients cannot imitate, it could not explain why these patients are clumsy when they use objects or perform other somesthetic motor tasks (Heilman, 1973). One would also have to assume that the arcuate fasciculus also carries somesthetic motor impulses and that the left fasciculus is again dominant. An alternative hypothesis that may explain why patients with a parietal lesion cannot properly imitate or use an object is that visuokinesthetic motor engrams are stored in the dominant parietal cortex. These engrams help program the motor association cortex as to what movements are necessary; and the motor association cortex programs the motor cortex, which innervates the specific muscle motor neuron pools needed to carry out the skilled act. The motor association cortex programs movements (more than one muscle) and visuokinesthetic engrams in the parietal cortex program sequences of movements in space needed to perform skilled acts (see Fig. 2). The schema postulated in Fig. 2 not only explains why patients with parietal lesions are unable to perform skilled acts in response to command, to imitate, or to use objects but also explains another type of apraxia.

In 1973, I described three unusual patients who had neurological signs and symptoms usually associated with left angular gyrus dysfunction (i.e., anomia, constructional apraxia, agraphia, alexia, and other elements of Gerstmann's syndrome). Unlike the usual patients with ideomotor apraxia who move clumsily and use body parts as objects, these patients hesitated to make any movements and often appeared as if they did not understand the command. They could, however, demonstrate both verbally and by picking out the correct act (from several performed by the examiner) that they did understand the command. Unlike patients with ideomotor apraxia, these patients were able to both imitate and use actual objects flawlessly; because of this, their engrams for motor sequences and engrams for movements apparently were intact. What seemed to be defective in these patients was the ability of language to elicit the correct motor sequences. I have postulated that patients had a disconnection between language-decoding areas and the area containing the visuokinesthetic motor engrams for acts (see Fig. 2).

The patients with callosal lesions reported by Geschwind and Kaplan (1962) and Gazzaniga *et al.* (1967) could not perform with their left hand in response to command. These patients could imitate and use objects and therefore were behaviorally similar to the patients with left hemisphere angular gyrus lesions (Heilman, 1973) who could perform with neither hand. If normal performance on imitation and use of an object suggests that visuokinesthetic motor engrams are intact and connected to premotor and primary motor areas, then patients with callosal lesions and those with angular gyrus lesions must have had a disconnection between language areas and the area where visuokinesthetic motor engrams are stored. In patients with callosal lesions, these engrams were presumably in both hemispheres, whereas comprehension of commands was being mediated by the left hemisphere. In patients with angular gyrus lesions, both comprehension of the commands and the visuokinesthetic engrams were being mediated by the left hemisphere, and the angular gyrus lesion disconnected language areas from these engrams. An alternative hypothesis is that in patients with angular gyrus lesions the right hemisphere was mediating language comprehension, the left hemisphere contained the visuokinesthetic engrams, and the angular gyrus lesions disconnected the language processing from these engrams.

DeRenzi *et al.* (1968) have described several patients who were unable to use an object. These patients, however, could correctly perform in response to command and could imitate. Neither we nor Geschwind (1967) have ever seen the type of patient reported by DeRenzi *et al.*, who unfortunately did not test these patients for agnosias but nevertheless doubted that this could be the explanation. In addition, almost all of the patients had a defect in comprehension, and possibly they did not comprehend what was wanted by the examiner or they had other conceptual disorders. My colleagues and I have seen severely demented patients, similar to those described by Marcuse (1904) and Pick (1905), who when given a goal that requires a series of acts (i.e., clean the pipe, put tobacco in the pipe, light the pipe, and smoke it) have difficulty with sequencing these acts. These demented patients often forget what their goal was and how to get to it. When tested verbally (e.g., what were you supposed to do and how do you go about it?), their verbal performance was just as poor as their motor performance.

Theoretically, the motor behavior of patients with destroyed parietal areas where acts are programmed (the visuokinesthetic motor engrams) should be similar to motor behavior seen in patients with this parietal area disconnected from motor association areas; that is, both should have difficulty with performing a skilled act in response to command, with imitating, and with use of an object. Patients, however, in whom engrams for skilled acts are retained but motor association is disconnected or motor association cortex is destroyed should be able to differentiate (recognize) a correctly skilled act from a poorly performed one, but patients who have destroyed these visuokinesthetic motor engrams should not be able to make this differentiation. In addition, when they perform poorly, their

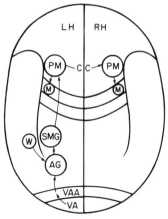

Fig. 2. Author's schema. View from top of brain. W, Wernicke's area; VA, primary visual area; VAA, visual association area; AG, angular gyrus; SMG, supramarginal gyrus; PM, premotor area (motor association cortex); M, motor cortex; CC, corpus callosum; LH, left hemisphere; RH, right hemisphere. The arrows indicate major connections of the areas shown.

poor performance should not trouble them, because their defect is in the terminal portion of a feedback system.

As has been mentioned, Liepmann and others have noted that patients with ideomotor apraxia are able to select a correct or incorrect movement performed by the examiner. This appears to provide evidence contrary to our schema; however, in most of these recognition tests the tester asks the patient to indicate if the act performed by the examiner is the target act (tell me if this is how you use a screwdriver). The tester then performs a well-coordinated, skilled act (e.g., brushing hair) and will ask the patient, "Am I using a screwdriver?" Since each of the acts performed by the tester has a different semantic content, the examiner is testing the comprehension of the question "What does this act mean?" Comprehension of pantomime may be processed by an area different from that used to process visuokinesthetic engrams. When a patient with ideomotor apraxia performs poorly, he does not make an inappropriate movement—that is, when asked to use a screwdriver, he does not brush his hair. His movements are correct in intent but, as previously stated, are clumsy. Since a patient with ideomotor apraxia does not perform inappropriate acts, it is not surprising that he can recognize inappropriate acts. As would be expected, an apraxic patient also can match an examiner's movement to a picture (Kimura and Archibald, 1974). Pictures, unlike a sequence of movements, are static and can probably be mediated by matching iconic memories.

To test whether patients with ideomotor apraxia have difficulty discriminating clumsy from normal movements, we (Heilman and Valenstein, in preparation) showed films of pantomimed acts (flipping a coin without the coin). Although this study has not been completed, it appears that ideomotor apraxics rarely select the inappropriate act as the correct one, but often they will pick the clumsy act or the act using a body part as an object. These preliminary observations suggest that some patients with ideomotor apraxia do have a defect in the comprehension of pantomimed acts. We have also noted that ideomotor apraxics seldom recognize that their poor performance is in error (anosognosia).

Unlike patients with parietal lesions, patients with destruction of motor association cortex or disconnection of motor association cortex from these visuokinesthetic engrams (callosal lesions) should be able to recognize the correct act; when they make errors, they should be able to recognize their errors. Although many apraxic patients have Broca's aphasia, Mohr *et al.* (1975) have demonstrated that most of these patients have lesions that extend into the parietal region. Therefore, Broca's aphasics do not have lesions restricted to their motor association cortex. The ideal patient to test would be one with callosal disconnection from an anterior cerebral artery infarction or from a lesion confined to the left premotor cortex. Unfortunately, we have not tested such a patient.

A patient who is apraxic because of destruction of premotor areas or separation of premotor areas from the primary motor area should not only recognize the proper and coordinated performance of skilled acts but should also recognize his own errors.

Typically, the patient with ideomotor apraxia improves by actually using an object, but why is not known. Liepmann thought that using the actual object required somesthetic motor connections. Somesthetic motor connections are bilateral and may be intact either in both hemispheres with posterior lesions or in the right hemisphere in large left hemispheric lesions.

Patients with lesions anterior to the motor cortex have what Liepmann termed "limb-kinetic apraxia." Theoretically, a lesion of the left frontal lobe would destroy motor engrams (for movements) of the right hand and disconnect visuokinesthetic engrams and language from the left side. The patient with such a defect should not be able to perform with either hand in response to a command. Use of objects will be performed better with the left hand than the right; and if the patient has visuokinesthetic engrams encoded in his right hemisphere, he should be able to imitate with his left hand better than with his right. If visuokinesthetic engrams are only in his left hemisphere, as previously mentioned, both hands will imitate poorly. Because frontal lesions are often associated with pyramidal tract lesions in area 4 (primary motor area), it would explain why some of the preceding conditions have not been reported for the right hand. A lesion in the right frontal lobe should produce a picture where the right hand performs normally in response to a command, imitates, and uses objects. The left hand, however, should be unable to respond to a command, to imitate, or to use objects. Even with more simple movements, the left hand should be clumsy. Dr. R. T. Watson has demonstrated such a patient to me. Even with such simple movements as picking up a coin, the patient was more clumsy than is usually seen with disconnection and ideomotor apraxia. The patient, however, had an extensor plantar response and slightly increased reflexes on the right side, so we could not be certain that this patient's lesion did not affect area 4 or the pyramidal tract. As with the ideomotor limb apraxias previously discussed, the patients performed poorly not only to command but also to imitation. These patients may improve somewhat with use of objects.

SKILLED MOVEMENTS USED IN SPEECH AND WRITING

Skilled movements are used not only to gesture and to manipulate objects but also to express language. Regarding speech, some authors have classified certain types of nonfluent aphasias as apraxias of speech (Johns and Darley, 1970; Deal and Darley, 1972). Buccofacial apraxia was first described by Hughlings-Jackson (1932). When these patients are asked to blow out a match, stick out their tongue, suck on a straw, or perform other similar commands, they often have difficulty performing these movements. DeRenzi *et al.* (1966) have noted that 90% of Broca's aphasics have buccofacial apraxia. Because there are patients with nonfluent aphasia but who do not have buccofacial apraxia, buccofacial apraxia would seem unlikely to be causing this aphasic disturbance. It can be argued, however, that speech requires finer coordination than does response to a command (e.g., blow out a match), and therefore the slow, badly articulated speech of the nonfluent aphasic may still be caused by an apraxic disturbance. Buccofacial apraxia and Broca's aphasia often coexist, but they can also be completely dissociated, which suggests that the association cortex that mediates facial praxis is not the same as the area that mediates the organization of movements important in speech. Patients may have conduction aphasia with or without buccofacial apraxia. Those with conduction aphasia with buccofacial apraxia may have fluent speech, so if buccofacial apraxia is supposed to be causing the nonfluent disorders of Broca's aphasia, how can it also be causing the fluent aphasia seen in conduction aphasia? I have also examined a patient with aphemia (nonfluent aphasia with intact writing skills) who did not have buccofacial apraxia. Therefore, although patients with Broca's aphasia or aphemia or both may have disorders of programming movements needed for speech, buccofacial apraxia is not causing the nonfluent speech. I do not wish to embark on a discussion of language disorders; but besides having faulty motor programming, patients with Broca's aphasia have other language disorders, including comprehension disorders, which suggest that this aphasic disorder is more than an apraxic disturbance.

Agraphia is most commonly associated with aphasia, and in most patients with agraphia the disorder of language cannot be separated from the disorder of movement. There have been several cases, however, where disorders of writing have not been associated with language disorders. Most of these case reports have been in left-handed patients. We (Heilman *et al.*, 1973) described a left-handed man who had been taught to write with his right hand. The patient developed a left hemiplegia. Although the patient was not aphasic, he lost the ability to write with his right (nonparetic) hand. He also had an ideomotor apraxia of his right hand. Liepmann and Maas (1907), Geschwind and Kaplan (1962), and Gazzaniga *et al.* (1967) have all shown that right-handed patients with callosal lesions have agraphia and apraxia of their left hand but not of the right hand. In patients with callosal dysfunction, because the left hand/right hemisphere is deprived of either language or motor engrams or both, we cannot be certain if the agraphia in left-hand performance is caused by the loss of language or a loss of motor engrams. Nielsen (1946) had a left-handed patient who probably had a callosal lesion; he could not write with his right hand but could with his left hand. I do not know which hemisphere mediated language in this patient, but this man's agraphia may have been an example of the converse of the preceding patients with callosal lesions. Also in 1973, we described a patient who had a large lesion in the region of the left hemisphere which usually mediates language. Since the patient was not aphasic, language had to be mediated by the opposite (right) hemisphere. As suggested previously, Liepmann thought that manual dominance (handedness) reflected the ability of one hemisphere to learn and store motor tasks more readily than the other. Because the patient we described was left-handed and language was mediated by the left hemisphere, skilled motor movements were possibly mediated by the right hemisphere. Assuming that this patient was "left-brained" for language and speech and right-brained for handedness, it would follow that when he wrote with his right hand (as he was accustomed to doing), impulses must have traversed the callosum twice (linguistic material was transferred to the right hemisphere to arouse the appropriate visuokinesthetic motor engrams; then these engrams were transferred back to the left motor region, which controls the right hand). If he wrote with his left hand, impulses would have to traverse the callosum only once. A callosal section in this man would have caused apraxia and agraphia of the right hand, because the right hand would be disconnected from the motor engrams, and agraphia of the left hand, because it would be disconnected from the language areas. We have also reported a similar clinical picture in right-handers (Heilman *et al.*, 1975). These patients illustrated that normal writing requires not only language skills but also motor skills and that destruction or separation of the motor engrams from primary motor areas produces a disorder of writing in the absence of a disorder of language.

References

Asanuma, H. Recent developments in the study of columnar arrangement of neurons within the motor cortex. *Physiological Reviews,* 1975, *55*, 143–156.

Briggs, G. E., and Brogden, W. J. Bilateral aspects of the trigonometric relationships of precision and angle of linear pursuit movements. *American Journal of Psychology,* 1953, *66*, 472–478.

Broca, P. Localisation des fonctions cérébrales siege du langage articulé. *Bulletin de la Société de Anthropologie,* 1863, *4*, 200–204.

Deal, J. L., and Darley, F. L. The influence of linguistic and situational variables on phonemic accuracy in apraxia of speech. *Journal of Speech and Hearing Research,* 1972, *15*, 639–653.

DeRenzi, E., Pieczuro, A., and Vignolo, L. Oral apraxia and aphasia. *Cortex,* 1966, *2*, 50–73.

DeRenzi, E., Pieczuro, A., and Vignolo, L. Ideational apraxia: A quantitative study. *Neuropsychologia,* 1968, *6*, 41–52.

Ettlinger, G. Apraxia considered a disorder of movements that are language dependent: Evidence from a case of brain bisection. *Cortex,* 1969, *5*, 285–289.

Gazzaniga, M. *The Bisected Brain.* New York: Appleton-Century-Crofts, 1970.

Gazzaniga, M., Bogen, J., and Sperry, R. Dyspraxia following division of the cerebral commissures. *Archives of Neurology,* 1967, *16*, 606–612.

Geschwind, N. Disconnexion syndromes in animals and man. *Brain,* 1965, *88*, 237–294, 585–644.

Geschwind, N. The apraxias in phenomenology of will and action. In E. W. Straus and R. M. Griffith (eds.), *The Second Lexington Conference on Pure and Applied Phenomenology.* Pittsburgh: Duquesne University Press, 1967, pp. 91–102.

Geschwind, N., and Kaplan, E. A human cerebral disconnection syndrome. *Neurology,* 1962, *12*, 675–685.

Goldstein, K. *Language and Language Disturbances.* New York: Grune and Stratton, 1948.

Goodglass, H., and Kaplan, E. Disturbance of gesture and pantomime in aphasia. *Brain,* 1963, *86*, 703–720.

Hécean, H., and deAjuriaguerra, J. *Left-Handedness.* New York: Grune and Stratton, 1964.

Hécean, H., and Sanguet, J. Cerebral dominance in left-handed subjects. *Cortex,* 1971, *7*, 19–48.

Heilman, K. M. Ideational apraxia—A re-definition. *Brain,* 1973, *96*, 861–864.

Heilman, K. M. Apraxia and agraphia in a right-hander. *Cortex,* 1974, *10*, 284–288.

Heilman, K. M. A tapping test in apraxia. *Cortex,* 1975, *11*, 259–263.

Heilman, K. M., Coyle, J. M., Gonyea, E. F., and Geschwind, M. Apraxia and agraphia in a left-hander. *Brain,* 1973, *96*, 21–28.

Heilman, K. M., Schwartz, H. D., and Geschwind, N. Defective motor learning in ideomotor apraxia. *Neurology,* 1975, *25*, 1018–1020.

Hicks, R. E. Asymmetry of bilateral transfer. *American Journal of Psychology,* 1974, *87*, 667–674.

Hughlings-Jackson, J. In J. Taylor (ed.), *Selected Writings of John Hughlings-Jackson.* London: Hodder and Stoughton, 1932.

Johns, D. F., and Darley, F. L. Phonemic variability in apraxia of speech. *Journal of Speech and Hearing Research,* 1970, *13*, 556–583.

Kimura, D., and Archibald, Y. Motor functions of the left hemisphere. *Brain,* 1974, *97*, 337–350.

Kleist, K. Über Leitungsaphasie und grammatische Störungen. *Monatsschrift für Psychiatrie und Neurologie,* 1916, *40*, 118–121.

Kornhuber, H. H. Cerebral cortex, cerebellum, and basal ganglia: An introduction to their motor functions. In F. O. Schmitt and F. G. Worden (eds.), *The Neurosciences: Third Study Program.* Cambridge, Mass.: MIT Press, 1972, pp. 267–280.

Kuypers, H. G. J. M., and Brinkman, J. Cerebral control of contralateral and ipsilateral arm, hand and finger movements in a split-brain rhesus monkey. *Brain,* 1973, *96*, 653–674.

Liepmann, H. Du linke Hemisphäre und das Handeln. *Drei Aufsätre dem Aufsätze dem Apraxiegebeit.* Berlin: Karger, 1908, pp. 17–50.

Liepmann, H., and Maas, O. Fall von linksseitiger Agraphic und Apraxie bei rechtsseitiger Lähmung. *Journal für Psychologie und Neurologie,* 1907, *10,* 214–227.

Marcuse, H. Apraktische Symptome bei einem Fail von seniler Demenz. *Zentralblatt für Nowenheilkunde und die Psychiatrie,* 1904, *27,* 737–751.

Meier, M. J., and French, L. A. Lateralized defects in complex visual discrimination and bilateral transfer of reminiscence following unilateral temporal lobectomy. *Neuropsychologia,* 1965, *3,* 261–272.

Mohr, J. R., Funkenstein, H. H., Finkelstein, S., Pessin, M. S., Duncan, G. W., and Davis, K. Broca's area infarction versus Broca's aphasia. *Neurology,* 1975, *25,* 349.

Nielsen, J. *Agnosia, Apraxia, Aphasia* (reprint 1946 ed.). New York: Hafner, 1965.

Pick, A. *Studien über motorische Apraxia und ihre nahestehende Erscheinungen.* Leipzig: Deuticke, 1905.

Pieczuro, A., and Vignolo, L. A. Studio sperimentale sull'aprassia ideomotoria. *Sistema Nervoso,* 1967, *19,* 131–143.

Steinthal, H. *Abriss der Sprachwissenschaft.* Berlin: 1871.

Taylor, H. G., and Heilman, K. M. Asymmetries in the acquisition and transfer of distal motor performance. Presented before the International Neuropsychological Society, Santa Fe, New Mexico, February 1977.

Wernicke, C. *Der aphasische Sumptomenkomplex.* Breslau: Cohn and Weigart, 1874.

Wyke, M. Effect of brain lesions on the rapidity of arm movement. *Neurology,* 1967, *17,* 1113–1120.

Wyke, M. The effect of brain lesions in the performance of an arm-hand precision task. *Neuropsychologia,* 1968, *6,* 125–134.

Wyke, M. The effects of brain lesions on the learning performance of a bimanual coordination task. *Cortex,* 1971, *7,* 59–71.

PART VI

Disorders of Psychological Processes Following Brain Damage

15

Cerebral Mechanisms of Information Storage: The Problem of Memory

Murray Glanzer and Elisabeth O. Clark

Introduction

Recently one of those rare events has occurred in which developments in two separate fields—the experimental psychology of memory and physiological psychology—have yielded congruent information. We will consider those developments here. The chapter will be organized into two main sections: first, a review of some theory in the psychology of memory, which will center on multiple-store models, since those models have clear relevance to current physiological findings; second, a review of work on the effects of brain damage and brain stimulation on memory. Both sections will be concerned wholly with work on human subjects. There is, of course, a large literature on the physiology of memory in other species, including studies specifically concerned with the role of the limbic system (Drachman and Ommaya, 1964; Gaffan, 1976; Isaacson, 1975; O'Keefe, Nadel *et al.*, 1975). Although the work is suggestive, it does not establish effects in other species that closely parallel the effects found in man. More generally stated, it remains to be established that homologous brain structures, in the several species studied, are carrying out closely related memory functions. A more optimistic view may be found in Iversen (1973) and Weiskrantz (1966).

Murray Glanzer and Elisabeth O. Clark   Department of Psychology, New York University, New York, New York 10003. This chapter was written under Grant GB-3208 from the National Science Foundation. Elisabeth O. Clark holds a predoctoral fellowship from the National Institutes of Mental Health.

MURRAY GLANZER
AND ELISABETH O.
CLARK

During the first half of this century the psychological study of memory centered on a view of learning as the fixing or associating of ideas, or, later, of responses to stimuli. Forgetting was viewed as the disruption of these associations by the learning of new associations or the rearousal of old associations. This general approach to forgetting was labeled "interference theory."

The view of memory as the setting up and disruption of associations never became productive in relation to physiological work. It ran, moreover, into unsolved problems in the interpretation of critical data during the 1950s and 1960s. At the present time, the theory does not play a central role in work on memory, although some of its concepts are still applied. For a recent summary of the work on association and interference theory, see Horton and Turnage (1976).

A different type of theory has developed in the last 20 years that has been productive in relation to physiological work. This has been labeled multiple-stage, multiple-process, or multiple-store theory. It arose in part out of a view of organisms as information-processing systems, a view stimulated by advances in information theory and communication engineering. The information-processing approach was extensively presented by Broadbent (1958). It also arose in part out of the physiological theorizing of Hebb (1949). A full review of the work on multiple-store models of memory may be found in Horton and Turnage (1976) and Murdock (1974).

We will briefly outline a simplified form of the theory. A more detailed exposition of the theory, its mathematical structure, and its empirical supports may be found in Atkinson and Shiffrin (1968) and Glanzer (1972). Critical reviews of the theory may be found in Murdock (1974) and Postman (1975).

According to this theory an item of information goes through at least three stages or processes: sensory store, short-term store, and long-term store.

1. Sensory store: Preliminary processing that converts the input into a sensation and holds it briefly (for approximately 250 msec) at that level. This store is also referred to as the "iconic store." Extensive experimental work has been carried out on the characteristics of this stage. A summary of some of this work may be found in Neisser (1967).

2. Short-term store: A second stage of processing that converts the information into more fully meaningful units and that holds it for longer periods of time. This is also referred to as "primary memory." It has been at times identified with attention. Again, extensive experimental work has been carried out on the characteristics of this stage. The current information about it is that it is limited in capacity, is modality specific, and loses items primarily by displacement. It is limited in capacity to a few units. It is modality specific in that it demonstrates differences in the way material entering through different sense modalities is stored. It loses items primarily by displacement: presentation of new items removes all trace of earlier items. The thoroughness of displacement in short-term store is seen when you look up a telephone number which you plan to use in dialing. If you are interrupted before dialing, even briefly, by conversation, a

complete loss of that stored number will occur. Work on short-term store has been carried out in a variety of experimental situations. Some of them are the following:

467

CEREBRAL
MECHANISMS OF
INFORMATION
STORAGE: THE
PROBLEM OF MEMORY

    a. Free recall—The subject is given a list of words and is asked to recall them in any order.

    b. Fixed order recall—The same task as above but with the requirement to recall items in the order presented. This is also referred to as an immediate memory task.

    c. Probe recall—The subject is given a list of items and is then asked to give a specified item out of the list, e.g., the third item.

    d. Distractor (recall) task—The subject is given a small set of items, e.g., three letters, and then given a distractor task for varying periods of time followed by a request to recall the set of items (Peterson and Peterson, 1959).

All the tasks above are recall tasks. There are also several recognition tasks in which the subject is given a list of items and is asked at some point whether an item has been presented in the list or not. These tasks may be used to separate out short-term store from long-term store. In free recall, for example, a serial position effect is seen when the probability of recall is plotted against the position of the item in the presentation list. The standard curve is as presented in Fig. 1 (Glanzer and Cunitz, 1966). It has a beginning peak, a relatively flat middle section, and a marked end peak. The end peak of this curve is interpreted as evidence of items

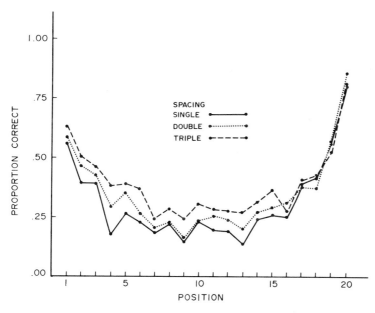

Fig. 1. A serial position curve is a plot of the proportion of recalls for each list word as a function of its position in the presentation. The serial position curves shown here were obtained for free recall with three different list presentation rates (spacing): one word every 3 sec (single), every 6 sec (double), every 9 sec (triple). The separation at all positions except the end is standard. From Glanzer and Cunitz (1966).

held in short-term store. Averaging the number of words that are represented by that rise gives, under a variety of conditions, the same number (Glanzer and Razel, 1974). This is evidence of the limited capacity noted above. Requiring that the subject do something before recall is permitted removes the end peak. Figure 2 shows the effect on a serial position curve of requiring the subject to carry out a rehearsal-blocking task before recalling the list items. This is the displacement effect spoken about earlier. If the presentation is auditory, the end peak will be higher than if the presentation is visual. This effect reflects the modality-specificity of the short-term store. While an item is held in short-term store two different activities are carried out. One is simple maintenance rehearsal of the item which keeps it available. The other is processing to copy information in the item into long-term store. The effectiveness of the copying or registration procedure hinges on the existence of organization in memory that is appropriate for the item; the meaningfulness of the item, a related aspect; and the extent to which the subject explores the meaning of the item, also referred to as "depth of processing."

3. Long-term store: Once information is transferred to long-term store, it may or may not be responded to correctly on subsequent tests. The stored information may be destroyed, or it may be present but not retrievable. Recent work has favored the second alternative. This fits the recent emphasis on search processes, retrieval cues, and retrieval strategies in long-term store. The recovery of information from long-term store can be blocked in a number of ways. It can be blocked in the experimental situation by imposing a second task on the subject while the material to be remembered is presented. When this is done in free recall, the early part of the serial position curve, which reflects long-term store, is lowered. The end peak, which reflects short-term store, is relatively unaffected. Figure 3 shows such an effect (Silverstein and Glanzer, 1971). In this case it is

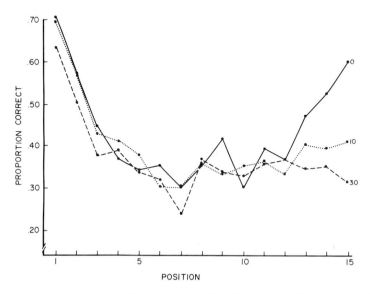

Fig. 2. Serial position curves obtained for free recall with either no delay (0), 10 sec, or 30 sec filled delay before recall. From Glanzer and Cunitz (1966).

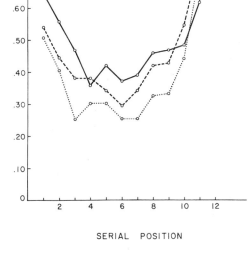

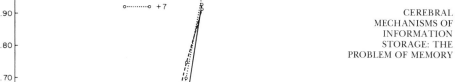

469

CEREBRAL
MECHANISMS OF
INFORMATION
STORAGE: THE
PROBLEM OF MEMORY

Fig. 3. Serial position curves obtained for free recall with a concurrent adding task imposed on the subject during list presentation. The concurrent task varied in difficulty from easy (+1), to medium in difficulty (+4), to very difficult (+7). From Silverstein and Glanzer (1971).

reasonable to assume that the loss is due to the blocking of transfer from short-term store to long-term store. In other cases, it is reasonable to assume that the blocking occurs in the retrieval of the information from long-term store.

Recovery of information from long-term store can also be blocked by brain damage.* This blocking is called "anterograde amnesia," amnesia in which the subject can retain new information for brief periods of time but is unable to retain it for longer periods of time. Anterograde amnesia appears in several syndromes: transient global amnesia, herpes encephalitis amnesia, senile dementia, temporal lobe amnesia, and the Korsakoff syndrome. Since extensive research has been carried out on the temporal lobe and Korsakoff syndrome amnesias, this work will be considered in detail below. An example of the free recall performance of a group of amnesic patients is presented in a study by Baddeley and Warrington (1970) (see Fig. 4). Again, the portion of the curve that reflects long-term store, the early part of the serial position curve, is lowered. The end peak of the curve, which reflects short-term store, is unaffected.

---

*There is a dispute in the literature as to whether amnesia reflects a blocking of transfer to long-term store or retrieval from long-term store. We will therefore use the phrase "either transfer to or retrieval from" repeatedly in this chapter. We believe that it is not possible to determine, at present, which of those two functions may be impaired in cases of amnesia. This point is more fully discussed later in the text.

Before leaving the free recall task we should emphasize the following. The serial position curve is analyzed into two parts. The early and middle positions reflect long-term store. The last few positions reflect short-term store. The effects on these two parts are distinct. In anterograde amnesia the effect is on long-term store—either transfer to long-term store or retrieval from long-term store.

The literature is plagued by the use of the phrase "short-term memory" to describe effects on long-term store. A patient whose immediate memory is normal but who cannot learn anything new despite hundreds of trials is confusingly described in that usage as having a defect of short-term memory.

The data presented above have all been based on the free recall task and the serial position curve obtained from it. Another task that is frequently used in multiple-store analysis of performance is the distractor task. In this task a short sequence of items is presented to the subject, who is then required to carry out a rehearsal-blocking task, i.e., distractor, for a specified delay period, and then asked to recall the sequence in order. What is plotted is the number of recalled items as a function of delay, the time spent on the rehearsal-blocking task. This curve shows a rapid decline followed by a gradual leveling off to an asymptote. The initial part of this curve primarily reflects short-term store. The asymptote reflects long-term store. Again, the distinction between the two components has not been kept clear in the literature.

When amnesic subjects are compared with normal subjects on a distractor task, they will show divergent curves for recall with delay that go to different asymptotes. Examples of such curves may be found in Cermak *et al.* (1971) and Milner (1973).

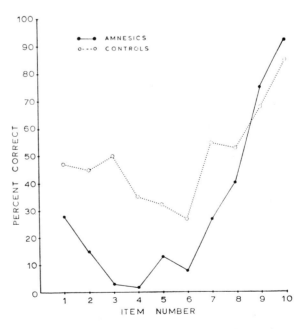

Fig. 4. Serial position curves obtained for free recall by amnesic subjects and normal control subjects. From Baddeley and Warrington (1970).

The multiple-stage model outlined above has been criticized by theorists who prefer a "continuous" system of memory. A continuous system of memory does not distinguish between stages or stores. An example of such a continuous system is found in the depth-of-processing proposal by Craik and Lockhart (1972). However, we believe that, particularly for any linkage with physiological data, a multiple-store model has special advantages. The discussion of the amnesias is clearly focussed in terms of a multiple-store model. It permits an easy development of further physiological theory, e.g., the role of the Papez circuit.

471

CEREBRAL
MECHANISMS OF
INFORMATION
STORAGE: THE
PROBLEM OF MEMORY

A Review of Related Work on the Effects of Brain Damage and Brain Stimulation on Memory

In this section we will cover two types of amnesia for which we have considerable information concerning physiological bases. We will also review some studies in which the relation between physiological factors and memory deficits is explored further.

Temporal Lobe Amnesia

In a series of studies of patients who have undergone temporal lobectomy, Milner and her co-workers have established a clear set of findings concerning the effects on memory of temporal lobe lesions and the critical locus that produces those effects (Milner, 1965a, 1970, 1971; Milner et al., 1968; Scoville and Milner, 1957).

We will consider first the bilateral temporal lesions. Depending on the specific structures affected, this type of lesion may result in a severe, permanent anterograde amnesia. Short-term store as evidenced by performance on immediate memory tasks is unimpaired. Delayed responses can be made by these subjects only if they are permitted to use the still intact maintenance rehearsal capability of short-term store, as when they are given verbalizable material (Sidman et al., 1968). Either transfer of new material to long-term store or retrieval from long-term store of new material is, however, blocked. In general, the subject cannot learn anything new. He cannot learn a list of numbers or words, remember new personal experiences, or recognize people even though he sees them repeatedly. There are a few types of learning which still seem possible, as will be noted below. The patient with this type of amnesia cannot, however, function by himself in a normal environment.

In addition to the anterograde amnesia the bilateral patients show some retrograde amnesia. They cannot recall some information that was learned before the brain damage occurred. Other functions that involve only the storing or retrieval and use of old information are, however, unimpaired. Problem solving and intelligence, as tested on standard intelligence tests, seem unaffected. Skills learned before surgery are also unaffected.

Evidence collected on both bilateral and unilateral lesions indicates that the critical area in these cases is the hippocampus. When the hippocampus is spared, the amnesia does not appear (Milner, 1968b, 1970).

There are, as noted above, a few types of learning that are still evident with hippocampectomy-produced amnesia (Corkin, 1965, 1968; Milner *et al.*, 1968). It is not clear why these are spared. They are mirror drawing, rotary pursuit, tracking and tapping tasks, and simple visual and tactual maze learning. All of these could be classified as motor learning tasks. Also spared is some perceptual learning of incomplete pictures. Milner *et al.* note, moreover, that there is evidence of some minimal learning about places, people, and important events even in an extreme case, Milner's patient H. M. We repeat, however, that the overall impairment of learning is so severe that the patient cannot function in a normal environment.

Unilateral hippocampal lesions produce a very different pattern of impairment. First, the impairment is slight when compared with the impairment produced by bilateral lesions. The subject can still function in a normal environment. Special testing is needed to bring out the defect.

Second, the unilateral hippocampal lesions produce a specialized memory deficit. Lesions on the left produce a deficit in verbal memory. Lesions on the right produce a deficit in what might be termed "nonverbal" memory. This term covers visuospatial memory and memory for nonverbalizable shapes and displays. Milner (1968a) emphasizes the point that these are material-specific, not modality-specific, lateralized deficits. Memory for words is impaired in left hippocampectomized patients whether the words are presented aurally or visually.

The simplest data in support of the claimed lateralization are the following from Milner (1973). When a distractor task is given with verbal material (trigrams), the effects can be seen in the depression of performance for the left temporal patients. Right temporals show no effect. Moreover, the extent of the deficit in the left temporals is clearly related to the amount of the left hippocampus removed. When a parallel distractor task is given with nonverbal material (spatial location), there is a depression in performance for right temporal patients and none for left temporals. Again, the extent of the deficit in the right temporals is clearly related to the amount of the right hippocampus removed.

Data from a number of tasks that can be labeled either verbal or nonverbal show the same lateralization. Among the tasks defined as nonverbal is the learning of block-tapping sequences (Milner, 1971), the recognition of recent occurrence of unfamiliar faces (Milner, 1968b), and visually guided maze learning (Milner, 1965b). A study by Gerner *et al.* (1972) adds data in support of these distinctions. On a verbal paired associates task with a multiple-choice recognition test, the left temporal patients made more errors than the normal control subjects. The right temporal patients did not. On a parallel nonverbal nonsense figure paired associates task, the right temporal patients made more errors than the normal control patients. The left temporal patients were close to the normal control subjects in performance. Other data from commissurotomized patients lend support to the assignment of verbal memory to the left hemisphere and nonverbal to the right hemisphere (Milner, 1973).

473

CEREBRAL
MECHANISMS OF
INFORMATION
STORAGE: THE
PROBLEM OF MEMORY

Not only are the effects of unilateral lesions less severe than the effects of bilateral lesions, but also they are not as persistent over time. Scoville and Milner (1957) and Milner (1968*a*) have stated that the effects of the unilateral lesions are temporary. Blakemore and Falconer (1967) have presented data on the effect of unilateral temporal lobectomy both on intelligence test performance and on memory over a 10-year period. Patients with left temporal lobectomy show a marked drop in the verbal IQ from which they recover within a year. They also show a marked drop in verbal learning and need 5 years or more to recover from this decrement. Patients with right temporal lobectomy show a transitory drop in performance IQ and no effect on verbal learning. The recovery period may, however, be more protracted than those data indicated. Newcombe (1969) found that men who suffered unilateral focal missile wounds of the brain still showed measurable signs of impairment in verbal memory and learning 20 years later. The impairment was lateralized: subjects with left hemisphere damage did worse than subjects with right hemisphere damage. The data did not, however, support differential effects of loci within the hemispheres, e.g., temporoparietal vs. frontal.

An explanation of the recovery that does occur is that the undamaged hemisphere compensates for damage to the other hemisphere by taking over its functions. Data in support of this idea are found in the case of visually guided maze learning mentioned above (Milner, 1965*b*). Unilateral right temporal lesions have an effect. Unilateral left temporal lesions do not. Bilateral lesions, which damage the right temporal lobe and presumably block possible compensation by also damaging the left temporal lobe, produce the most severe deficit.

In summary, the multiple-store theory of memory and the data on the effects of hippocampectomy fit nicely. With hippocampectomy short-term store functions normally. Long-term store is impaired. Either transfer of new information in or retrieval of newly transferred information is blocked. The data on the association of verbal memory deficits with left hemisphere lesions and nonverbal memory deficits with right hemisphere lesions add an interesting detail to a multiple-store view. Long-term store is material specific and is lateralized. Short-term store, by contrast, is modality specific. That fact has been well established with normal subjects (Murdock and Walker, 1969).

Further discussion of theoretical implications will be held until we have summarized relations between other specific brain lesions and psychological function, in particular the Korsakoff syndrome and relations between brain stimulation and memory.

KORSAKOFF SYNDROME

The Korsakoff syndrome has as its most striking characteristics a severe anterograde amnesia and a limited retrograde amnesia.* In these characteristics it is very similar to the temporal lobe amnesia discussed above. The physiological

*Some writers (Brion, 1969, p. 30) include confabulation as one of the symptoms of the Korsakoff syndrome. Two extensive studies of Korsakoff patients indicate, however, that this symptom is not characteristic of the stable phase of the disorder, which we are discussing here (Victor *et al.*, 1971, pp. 58–62; Talland, 1965, p. 57).

basis of the Korsakoff syndrome is, however, bilateral damage to the mammillary bodies (Brierly, 1966), usually accompanied by lesions to the medial thalamus and hypothalamus (Ojemann, 1966).* Brion (1969) emphasizes the fact that the Korsakoff syndrome is associated with bilateral lesions. In this respect it resembles the association of anterograde amnesia with bilateral hippocampal lesions. The syndrome usually occurs as a result of prolonged alcoholism, which induces a thiamine (vitamin B_1) deficiency. This in turn produces lesions of the mammillary bodies and other parts of the limbic system. The Korsakoff syndrome has, however, also been reported in cases in which there has been thiamine deficiency without alcoholism, in cases in which there have been tumors in areas near the mammillary bodies, e.g., the third ventricle, and in toxic or cerebral degenerative conditions.

This disorder has occurred with considerable frequency in the past, and a large number of patients with the syndrome have been studied in detail. There are an extensive study by Talland (1965) and a series of studies by Cermak and Butters and their associates cited below. Talland carried out comprehensive testing of Korsakoff patients in a variety of areas—verbal and motor skills, perception, intelligence, and reasoning. The results give us a much fuller picture of the Korsakoff patient than we have for other types of anterograde amnesia. Clinical observation, including Talland's, indicates that Korsakoff patients are apathetic. It has not been determined, however, whether this emotional and motivational state is a cause of the memory defect, whether it is a result of the memory defect, or whether both the memory defect and the emotional and motivational characteristics are determined by some other factor. Talland's data also indicate that in each of the areas of perception, cognition, and skill tested there is some evidence of deficiency. The same question arises about the relation of each of these deficiencies to the memory defects—whether the deficiency is a cause, a result, or a correlate of the memory defect, with both symptoms determined by other factors.

We do not know at this point whether fuller testing of hippocampal patients would give the same pattern of deficits in other aspects of psychological functioning. There are, however, reports that indicate that this may very well be the case. Both Milner's patient, H. M. (Milner *et al.*, 1968), and Talland's Korsakoff patients have particular difficulty with the Gottschaldt Hidden Figures Test. H. M. is slower in simple reaction time tests than normal control subjects (Corkin, 1968); Talland's Korsakoff patients are consistently and significantly slower than control subjects on a variety of tests of speed of motor response, although his piecemeal analysis of the data understates the size of the effect. Milner's patient, H. M., appears relatively unmotivated, at least with respect to food and sex (Milner *et al.*, 1968); Korsakoff patients are apathetic and unmotivated, as noted above. Also in support of the identity of symptoms is the fact that motor learning is relatively intact in Korsakoff patients (Brooks and Baddeley, 1976) as it is in hippocampectomy patients (Corkin, 1968).

*The majority of recent writers consider lesions of the mammillary bodies as necessary and sufficient for the production of the amnesia. Victor *et al.* (1971, p. 173), however, argue on the basis of their data that lesions of the medial dorsal nuclei of the thalamus, not the mammillary bodies, are critical.

475

CEREBRAL
MECHANISMS OF
INFORMATION
STORAGE: THE
PROBLEM OF MEMORY

Some of the recent investigations of anterograde amnesia have assumed, at least implicitly, an identity of the hippocampal and Korsakoff syndromes by lumping patients of both types in an undifferentiated amnesia category for study (e.g., Baddeley and Warrington, 1970). If it eventually turns out that the several types grouped together do share the subsidiary deficits as well as the anterograde amnesia, the grouping will have been justified.

Talland presents a considerable amount of data that support the claim that Korsakoff patients have special difficulty in learning, in particular learning for retention. Although the tasks are not ideal for separating short-term and long-term store components, they do show the characteristics of unimpaired short-term store and difficulty in either registering in or retrieving from long-term store. For example, one of the tasks, a variant of the distractor task, consisted of the presentation of a sentence to the subjects followed by an immediate recall, a 5-min interview that served as an interpolated task, and a second recall. In this task, the Korsakoff patients dropped from a score of 4.81, out of 5 possible, to a score of 0.94. The control subjects went from 4.38 to 3.88.

Data that separate out the effects of short-term and long-term store more clearly are found in the work of Cermak and Butters and their collaborators, most of which is summarized in a paper by Cermak and Butters (1973). Cermak *et al.* (1971) have used the distractor task and have demonstrated that the loss of trigrams or words over an 18-sec interval follows a different and lower course for the Korsakoff patient than for control subjects. We would emphasize that the curves are going to different asymptotes and that they therefore indicate a difference in either registration or retrieval from long-term store. Cermak *et al.* also see a short-term store defect in those data that we do not see. The fact that the curves separate as they go to different asymptotes does not imply that less information is held in short-term store or that information is being lost faster from short-term store. To establish those points requires, at a minimum, a demonstration that the rates of decline differ, taking into account the different asymptotes.

Subsequent studies in that paper and in other papers by Cermak and Butters are concerned with a psychological analysis of the memory defect in Korsakoff patients. They do establish that the Korsakoff patients are different from the control subjects in the way in which they handle semantically meaningful or semantically related material (Cermak *et al.*, 1973, 1974, 1976). The patients do not seem to respond to the semantic characteristics of the material presented to them and therefore do not take advantage of those characteristics the way normal subjects do. There are, however, results reported by Baddeley and Warrington (1973) that do not agree with this generalization. Baddeley and Warrington found that their amnesic patients, mostly Korsakoff patients, made use of semantic groupings in free recall.

In a related argument, Butters *et al.* (1973) propose that the Korsakoff memory deficit is specific to verbal material and present some data to support that proposal. The data are not completely convincing. A later study by DeLuca *et al.* (1975) clearly contradicts that proposal. Memory for both verbal and nonverbal material is affected in Korsakoff patients. At this point, we cannot say that the Korsakoff patients show a specific inability to make use of semantic relations in words or a specific inability in the handling of words. Indeed, on the basis of Milner's findings with bilateral temporal patients we would expect that these bilaterally damaged patients should suffer an overall deficit rather than a material-specific deficit.

Cermak *et al.* (1971) also attempt to separate out how much of the Korsakoff memory deficit is due to impaired registration and how much to impaired retrieval. On the basis of comparing retention with recall and recognition tests, they conclude that both types of impairment are involved (Cermak *et al.*, 1971, p. 314). The issue that they raise is a complex one and cannot be settled by the comparison that they use. Comparison of recognition and recall involves a translation of data from one class of responses to another. It also involves a theoretical decision about the role of retrieval in recognition. Both of these complications make the use of comparisons of recall with recognition questionable.

There has been a wealth of theorizing about the Korsakoff syndrome. Talland summarizes 32 theoretical proposals concerning the syndrome which he groups as theories of cognitive derangement, affective inhibition of recall, insufficiency of conative function, defective field structure, and neurological theories. Talland also considers in detail and rejects two specific theories. One was proposed by van der Horst concerning an impairment in the sense of time. The other was proposed by Claparède concerning an impairment in referring experiences to the self.

Talland proposes that the amnesia is due to reduced activation of some critical memory process that results in reduced registration activity and reduced retrieval activity. In Talland's terms (p. 320), there are "reduced activation and premature closure." We have mentioned this proposal specifically because it concurs with other proposals in the literature and because we believe that it furnishes the basis for a general theory which covers a range of amnesias.*

In general, the data on the Korsakoff syndrome fit well into the multiple-store model. As indicated above, the Korsakoff patient's performance is very much like that of the hippocampectomized patient. The theoretical analysis that applies to one applies equally well to the other.

ALCOHOLIC BLACKOUT

Alcoholic blackout is an amnesia that occurs during heavy drinking. It is associated with the later stages of alcoholism (Goodwin, 1970). A series of investigations by Goodwin and others has established a number of points concerning the blackout. These points are set forth in reports of studies (Goodwin, 1971; Goodwin *et al.*, 1970, 1973; Ryback, 1970) and in review papers (Goodwin *et al.*, 1969; Goodwin and Hill, 1973; Ryback, 1971).

The course of a blackout is as follows. An alcoholic starts a period of heavy drinking, taking in a large amount of alcohol during a short period of time. A complete anterograde amnesia occurs during which the subject functions very

---

*E. E. Coons suggested that the administration of an activating drug such as amphetamine may counter the low activation level that characterizes Korsakoff patients. It may also relieve their amnesia. Our search of the literature did not discover any published reports of use of a drug in this way.

much like a bilateral hippocampectomized or Korsakoff patient. He can retrieve information registered earlier in long-term store. General cognitive functioning seems unimpaired. He can enter and retrieve new information from short-term store. During the blackout, he cannot, however, enter new information or retrieve it from long-term store. This period of alcoholic blackout may last from several hours to several days. The subject usually closes out this period with sleep. When he wakes, the information presented to him during the blackout cannot be recovered. For example, Goodwin et al. (1970) induced blackouts experimentally. During the blackouts, the subjects could recall information about their childhood, do arithmetic computations, carry out conversations. They could also recall items shown to them if asked a minute later. If, however, asked 30 min later they could neither recall nor recognize the item. This loss was permanent. When tested 24 hr later, after recovery from the blackout, i.e., after remission of the anterograde amnesia, there was no recovery of the lost information. Goodwin (1971) distinguishes the blackout effect from grayout, which he considers a state-dependent effect. Grayout is a partial failure to recall events that can be remedied by furnishing reminders to the subject. The blackout effect covers spans of time completely and cannot be countered by cueing.

477

CEREBRAL
MECHANISMS OF
INFORMATION
STORAGE: THE
PROBLEM OF MEMORY

The blackout is of particular interest because it is one of the few ways in which severe but temporary anterograde amnesia can be produced. Ryback (1970) has speculated on the relation of blackout to a disruption of function in the Papez circuit, referring specifically to hippocampal function. Goodwin et al. (1970) have theorized concerning individual differences in metabolism in determining the susceptibility to blackout. They have shown that the likelihood of a blackout can be predicted from past blackouts. Their data also suggest that the rate of increase of blood alcohol during drinking may be a key factor. They suggest that these relations may stem from individual differences in the efficiency of metabolizing alcohol.

Another possibility, we believe, is that the blackout is a sign of partial damage to the mammillary bodies. Blackout, in this view, is a precursor of the Korsakoff syndrome. This relation is supported by the association between blackout and duration and severity of alcoholism reported by Goodwin et al. (1969).

We suggest the following eclectic hypotheses on the basis of the available information on both the Korsakoff syndrome and the blackouts:

1. That the Korsakoff syndrome is the end point on a continuum of increasing memory impairment correlated with increasing physiological damage.
2. That blackouts are the product of a composite of chronic physiological effects, i.e., the physiological damage referred to above, and a temporary effect, probably due to inefficiency in metabolizing alcohol.

These two hypotheses lead to the assertion that alcoholics should show memory deficits before the Korsakoff syndrome appears. There is, indeed, some evidence to support this assertion (Illchysin and Ryback, 1976). The pre-Korsakoff deficit may be the subtler deficit found in the unilateral hippocampectomized patients, who are still able to function in a normal environment. The hypotheses also lead to the assertion that the autopsy of alcoholics should reveal brain damage, e.g., either partial damage to the mammilary bodies or unilateral damage to the mammillary bodies. We have found, however, no published reports that can be used to evaluate this assertion.

DIRECT STIMULATION

Over 40 years ago, Papez (1937) designated a circuit that is of critical importance in motivation and emotion. The circuit includes the neocortex, the hippocampus, the fornix, the mammillary bodies, the anterior nucleus of the thalamus, and the cingulate gyrus of the cortex. The units in that circuit also have a critical role in human memory. A flow chart of the units that are important in memory is shown in Fig. 5.*

Fedio, Ommaya, and others have used direct electrical stimulation on several parts of the circuit[†] and have measured the effect of the stimulation on verbal and nonverbal memory. The verbal memory task was the recall of names of pictured objects. The nonverbal memory task was the recognition of nonsense figures. The procedure in the verbal memory task was as follows.

The subject saw a picture which he named. Four seconds later, another picture was presented which the subject also named. He then recalled the name of the preceding picture. With such an arrangement it is possible to determine the effect of the stimulation on the retrieval alone, or on the registration and retrieval, and, assuming that the physiological effect of the stimulation stops with the end of the stimulation, the effect of the stimulation on the registration alone. For example, the subject saw and recalled a series of seven pictured objects. Stimulation occurred during the presentation of the third and fourth pictures. This meant that item 2 was presented without the stimulation but recalled with the stimulation (stimulation on retrieval alone). Item 3 was both presented and recalled with the continuing stimulation. Item 4 was presented with stimulation but recalled without it (stimulation on registration alone). The testing of the nonverbal material was not set up to permit this separation.

Fedio and Ommaya (1970) demonstrated that stimulation of the left cingulum resulted in a decrease in verbal recall. The decrease was slight when the stimulation occurred during registration alone. It was greater when the stimulation occurred during retrieval alone and greatest when the stimulation spanned both the registration and retrieval. This pacing and coordination of testing and stimulation represent a promising technique for the analysis of the circuit's working. Application of the same analytic technique in a subsequent study of the cingulum, unfortunately, does not give exactly the same results (Ommaya and Fedio, 1972).[‡] Application of the technique to the pulvinar (Ojemann and Fedio,

---

*The figure gives a highly simplified representation. The output of the cingulum, for example, goes first to the subicular and entorhinal cortex (Raisman *et al.*, 1965). The fibers from the entorhinal cortex go to the hippocampus, while those from the subicular cortex pass through the hippocampus and end in the mammillary bodies (Swanson and Cowan, 1975).

[†]The stimulation was part of the testing carried out to guide surgery for the relief of intractable pain, epilepsy, parkinsonism, motion disorders, etc.

[‡]There is no effect at all when stimulation occurred during registration alone in this study.

1968) and to the ventrolateral thalamus (Ojemann *et al.*, 1971*a*), moreover, gives a complicated pattern of results.

There is another more general problem in the form of the memory test used in these direct stimulation studies. Since at most one new item intervenes between presentation and testing, it is impossible to say whether the effects observed are on short-term store or long-term store or both. The technique requires development. It remains promising.

The memory decrement observed above occurred only during left cingulum stimulation. No effect on verbal memory was observed during right cingulum stimulation. The authors gave memory tests to the same patients after bilateral lesions of the cinguli. They found no effect on verbal memory or intelligence test performance. An earlier study of bilateral cingulotomy found only evidence of a transitory effect on memory (Whitty and Lewin, 1960). On the basis of this absence of a strong or permanent effect, Fedio and Ommaya suggest (p. 90) that the cingulum stimulation has its effect on the hippocampus, which receives input from the cingulum. This leaves something of a puzzle. Some effect of cingulotomy on memory would still be expected if impulses from the cingulum to the hippocampus are involved in memory.

Ommaya and Fedio (1972) complete the picture of the effects of cingulum stimulation. They showed again that left cingulum stimulation, but not right cingulum stimulation, produces a decrement in verbal memory. They also showed a parallel effect of right cingulum stimulation on nonverbal memory. Right cingulum stimulation, but not left cingulum stimulation, produces a decrement in the recognition of nonsense forms.

In the same study, Ommaya and Fedio carried out memory tests during unilateral stimulation of the hippocampus. They found no memory effects there.

479

CEREBRAL
MECHANISMS OF
INFORMATION
STORAGE: THE
PROBLEM OF MEMORY

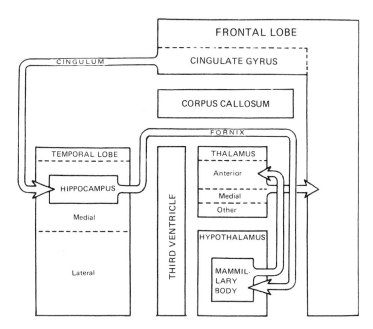

Fig. 5. Schematic diagram of the brain structures involved in memory. From Ojemann (1966).

Chapman *et al.* (1967) did, however, find an effect with bilateral stimulation of the hippocampus. V. H. Mark in the discussion section of that paper (p. 53) also reported effects of bilateral stimulation. Ommaya and Fedio suggest that they found no effect because it is the hippocampal gyrus, not the hippocampus, that plays the key role in memory. They cite papers by McLardy (1970) and Gol and Faibish (1967) in support of this argument. McLardy's argument, however, is contradicted by Penfield's (1974) finding of amnesia in a patient who had bilateral hippocampal damage but normal hippocampal gyri. It seems more likely that, for some reason, the hippocampus requires bilateral stimulation to show an effect.

Ojemann and Fedio (1968) examined another part of the Papez circuit in a study of the effects of stimulation on the thalamus. They found that with a verbal memory test stimulation of the left pulvinar resulted in a decrement in recall. Stimulation of either the right pulvinar or the left lateral thalamus outside the pulvinar had no effect. Fedio and van Buren (1975) complete the picture with respect to lateralization. They show again that stimulation of the left pulvinar, but not the right pulvinar, has an effect on verbal memory. They show in addition that stimulation of the right pulvinar, but not the left pulvinar, has an effect on nonverbal memory. The picture with respect to these nuclei is, however, more complicated than in the case of cingulum stimulation because pulvinar stimulation also produces naming and perceptual errors.* We could find no evidence in the literature that lesions of the pulvinar produce memory defects that correspond to the stimulation effects.

Ojemann *et al.* (1971*a*) demonstrated that direct stimulation of the left, but not the right, ventrolateral thalamus had an effect on verbal memory. The effect was very complex, being either facilitative or detrimental depending on the relation of the stimulation to the presentation. Ojemann *et al.* (1971*b*) used a distractor task, to show that left, but not right, ventrolateral thalamotomy impaired later performance on verbal recall.

We would interpret the data as indicating an impairment of either registration in or retrieval from long-term store. In a recent study, Fedio and van Buren (1974) used the same stimulation technique on the cortex to demonstrate lateralization of verbal memory effects in the left temporoparietal cortex.

The results of these stimulation studies, although suggestive, indicate complexities. The analysis of the circuit (in Fig. 5) would be simple if we could move through the circuit and find an effect of either lesion or stimulation at every part. The analysis would be even simpler if the effect of lesion and stimulation at each part were congruent. Neither of these conditions holds at present. Cingulum stimulation produces a lateralized effect. There is, however, no evidence that bilateral cingulotomy produces any permanent effect on memory. Unilateral hippocampal stimulation produces no effect. The effects of unilateral hippocampal lesions, however, are very clear.

The fornix, which is next in the circuit and which appears to be the main tract for hippocampal output, has not been subjected to direct stimulation. The reports on the effect of fornix lesions are mixed. Although a number of studies (Akelaitis,

*The appearance of perceptual errors is reasonable since the pulvinar receives visual input.

481

CEREBRAL
MECHANISMS OF
INFORMATION
STORAGE: THE
PROBLEM OF MEMORY

1943; Cairns and Mosberg, 1951; Dott, 1938; García Bengochea *et al.*, 1954) report no memory effect of bilateral section of the fornix,* there is one (Sweet *et al.*, 1959) which does demonstrate clear anterograde amnesia. The mammillary bodies have not been stimulated directly in experimental studies. Lesions of the mammillary bodies are, however, closely associated with the anterograde amnesia of the Korsakoff syndrome.

The absence of strong evidence of either a stimulation or lesion effect on the fornix is critical for any theory about the circuit as a unit. The differences between the effects of lesions and stimulation may simply indicate that some of the parts of the circuit have an excitatory function while others have an inhibitory function.

The material presented above repeatedly demonstrates lateralization effects. We should, however, note that the two halves of the brain are in close interaction. This is seen in two ways. One is, as noted earlier, in the recovery from brain damage. Recovery is relatively good when the damage is unilateral. It is relatively poor when the damage is bilateral. The other way in which the interaction is seen is in the impaired memory of commissurotomized patients (Zaidel and Sperry, 1974). Communication between the hemispheres is necessary for the efficient registration in or retrieval from long-term store. This fits well with the recent emphasis on "depth of processing" as an important aspect of registration of information in memory (Craik and Lockhart, 1972; Craik and Tulving, 1975; Glanzer and Koppenaal, 1977). Processing is "deeper" the more fully the subject considers different aspects of the meaning of a presented item or word. It is easy to see how this would require communication between the hemispheres holding special forms of information.

In conclusion, it has been shown that most of the parts of the circuit schematized in Fig. 5 have an effect on memory. The effects are, however, complex. Cingulum stimulation produces an effect; cingulum lesion does not. Bilateral but not unilateral hippocampal stimulation produces an effect; both unilateral and bilateral lesion have an effect. The rationalization of these effects has yet to be made. It is reasonable to expect complex interactions in the circuit. Stimulation at one point may be relayed to other points. Stimulation at one point may produce inhibitory effects while a lesion may eliminate these inhibitory effects. However, the complex interactions have to be specified. It is nevertheless reasonable to accept the hypothesis that the circuit functions as a unit and that the unit controls either the transfer of information to or its retrieval from long-term store.

FRONTAL LOBES

Lesions of the frontal lobes give rise to impairments of memory that differ from those found with lesions of the temporal lobes. Frontal patients show normal performance on a distractor recall task (Ghent *et al.*, 1962) but have difficulty in following instructions, difficulty in changing set, and a specific difficulty in retain-

---

*The memory testing may not have been adequate in these studies. The Akelaitis patients, for example, had undergone commissurotomy but had, with one exception, no memory defects reported. The Zaidel and Sperry (1974) study cited later shows that commissurotomy does produce a memory deficit.

ing order as opposed to item information. These types of difficulty may be basically one since, for example, following instructions ordinarily requires the ordering of a sequence of acts. Although the frontal lesions produce a different set of memory difficulties than temporal lesions, they show analogous lateralization effects.

A unilateral frontal lesion of either hemisphere makes it difficult for the patient to change strategy, to adapt to changing environmental conditions (Milner, 1971). But the specific task on which patients are hampered will vary, depending on the side of lesion. On the Wisconsin Card-Sorting Test, left frontal groups are most impaired. A small dorsolateral excision of the left frontal cortex produces impairment, while much larger lesions of the right frontal lobe may not (Milner, 1971). Conversely, right frontal patients are more impaired than left frontals on maze learning tasks (Corkin, 1965).

Milner (1973) reports data of Corsi that show the difficulty frontal patients have in ordering temporal events and also show a material-specific lateralization. In both the verbal and nonverbal forms of the test used, the subjects were shown cards bearing a pair of stimuli. In the verbal test the card had a pair of words. The subject had to decide which of the two words had been seen more recently. In some cases one of the words was new. This was designated a recognition or item memory condition. In other cases, both words had been presented before. This was designated as the recency or order condition. Right frontal lobe and right temporal lobe patients were unimpaired on both tasks. Left hemisphere groups experienced difficulty as a function of the location of cortical ablation. Left frontal patients performed well on item recognition but were impaired on recency discriminations. Left temporal lobe patients were impaired on recognition memory for items, but they performed at near-normal levels on the recency decisions. Left frontotemporal patients were impaired on both tests.

A parallel set of results is found on the nonverbal form of the test in which the items consisted of pairs of abstract art reproductions. Left hemisphere patients were unimpaired. Right frontal patients performed well on the item recognition tests but not on the recency tests. Right temporal patients were impaired on the item recognition tests but not on the recency tests. The data are clear. We find it puzzling, however, that the temporal patients are able to judge recency but are not able to recognize items. A fuller theoretical analysis of this effect is needed.

The parallel lateralization of the frontal and temporal areas is reasonable in light of the connections between the two. Hécaen and Albert (1975) discuss two neural circuits that could mediate frontotemporal interactions. The Papez circuit joins the medial frontal area to the hippocampal area through the cingulate gyrus (see Fig. 5). A second pathway joins the orbital area of the frontal lobe with the amygdala, which is interconnected with the hippocampus.

It is clear that the frontal lobes play a critical role in memory. The complete theoretical analysis of that role is, at this time, not clear. The retention of instructions and task-oriented strategies is one function that has been assigned to the frontal lobes and that has also been assigned independently to short-term store in psychological theories of memory (Atkinson and Shiffrin, 1968). Assigning the retention of instructions and task-oriented strategies to short-term store, with the frontal lobes involved in the required maintenance of information, makes sense in terms of the data we have reported above. Despite their severe memory impairment, Korsakoff and bilateral temporal patients are remarkable in their ability to carry out relatively complex cognitive tasks over a period of time. They are able to do so because the short-term store maintains these instructions; they are able to do so because the frontal lobes are intact.

483

CEREBRAL
MECHANISMS OF
INFORMATION
STORAGE: THE
PROBLEM OF MEMORY

It is more difficult to rationalize the specific impairment of the handling of order information in frontal patients. This is because there is no strong psychological theory that both differentiates and relates the processing of order and item information. The need for such a theory has been recognized and a number of proposals have been made (see Murdock, 1974, pp. 157–164). None of the proposals is, however, immediately useful for the analysis of frontal lobe functioning.

CONDUCTION APHASIA, THE REPETITION DEFICIT, AND THE MODEL OF MEMORY

A theoretical issue has recently been raised concerning the interpretation of the repetition deficit found in conduction aphasia. Warrington and Shallice (Warrington and Shallice, 1969; Shallice and Warrington, 1970) used it as the basis for revising the multiple-store model of memory. A consideration of conduction aphasia becomes, therefore, relevant to a consideration of physiolgical factors in memory.

Conduction aphasia was first distinguished as a separate form of aphasia by Wernicke (1874). Wernicke also proposed a physiological explanation of the syndrome, the breaking of the connection between Broca's area and Wernicke's area as a result of lesion of the arcuate fasciculus.

After conduction aphasia was defined by Wernicke, there was controversy over whether it existed (see Weisenberg and McBride, 1935, pp. 75–76) and, for those who accepted its existence, whether it had been appropriately named. Goldstein (1948, pp. 230–231), for example, includes its symptoms under the label "central aphasia." At present, however, both the existence of the disorder and the name "conduction aphasia" are accepted in the literature.

Benson *et al.* (1973) list the following criteria for the diagnosis of conduction aphasia, these criteria reflecting general agreement in the literature:

1. Fluent but paraphasic spontaneous speech
2. Normal (conversational) comprehension
3. Significant repetition disturbance

The three criteria above, in combination, are considered the key factors in the diagnosis of conduction aphasia. In addition to those three criteria, a number of other characteristics are associated with the disorder. These include a disturbance of naming in varying degrees of severity and a disturbance of reading. The latter, of particular interest for a point developed below, consists of relatively good comprehension in silent reading accompanied by an inability to read aloud. The inability to read aloud stems from the frequency of paraphasic output.

The present section will focus on the repetition disturbance cited above, the third criterion of conduction aphasia. Three other issues raised in connection with the repetition deficit will also be discussed subsequently—the role of item vs. order information, the role of auditory vs. visual input, and the nature of the underlying physiological damage.

The multiple-store model presented earlier has information going through the successive stores serially—sensory store, short-term store, long-term store. It is not, of course, a simple serial arrangement since the processing involves cycles of interaction between short-term and long-term store. Warrington and Shallice present data on a patient, K. F., who, they claim, has impaired short-term store but unimpaired long-term store. Therefore, they argue, short-term and long-term store must be organized in parallel rather than in series. Otherwise, if information has to go through short-term store before reaching long-term store, then impairment of short-term store should block the passage of information to long-term store. In order to support this revision two points have to be clearly established: (1) that short-term store is indeed impaired and (2) that long-term store is indeed unimpaired.

Warrington and Shallice present data on the performance of their patient, K. F., to support those two points. Supplementary data for two other patients are presented in a later study by Warrington *et al.* (1971). We do not think, however, that either of these two points is established.

The tests used to establish the two points have to meet certain requirements. The test that measures short-term store capability should not be confounded by the subject's difficulties in producing speech, i.e., by his paraphasia. The test to measure learning capability, the transfer to long-term store, should be of sufficient difficulty and complexity so that any deficit that stems from a limited short-term store has a chance to show.

We will concentrate here only on the experiments that are closely related to the evaluation of the two points and that clearly meet the requirements outlined above. Warrington and Shallice have several memory tasks that seem appropriate to test short-term store—probe recall and recognition tasks which require a simple response from the subject and should not show the effects of the subject's paraphasia. The majority of these tests indicate impairment. One, however, clearly indicates a functioning short-term store. That task is a matching task in which the patient heard a sequence of one to four items followed by another sequence of the same length. The two sequences either were identical or differed in one item. The patient was asked to indicate whether the two sequences were the same or not. Although Warrington and Shallice do not consider this a memory task, it clearly is. For sequences of four words, their patient matched correctly on 19 out of 20 trials. There are, unfortunately, no normal control data presented for comparison. The finding of good matching performance by conduction aphasics has been noted by other investigators (Strub and Gardner, 1974; Kinsbourne, 1972). Kinsbourne's two patients could match four-digit lists 0.95 and 0.80 of the time.

485

CEREBRAL
MECHANISMS OF
INFORMATION
STORAGE: THE
PROBLEM OF MEMORY

The existence of good performance on this task suggests that the repetition deficit reflects an impairment of the ability to read out information in short-term store rather than an impairment in the store itself. It also suggests that the other memory tasks showing deficit may involve a readout performance that has not been analyzed. This interpretation would make the repetition deficit have the same character as the conduction aphasics' inability to read aloud despite their ability to read silently with comprehension. Both Kinsbourne (1972) and Strub and Gardner (1974) see the repetition deficit as a readout problem. Kinsbourne sees it as arising from a processing overload, Strub and Gardner as arising from competition between processes in an impaired system.

The other point, that long-term store is indeed unimpaired, also needs further supporting evidence. At present we have some evidence of performance in the normal range for three subjects on four tasks that involve long-term store (Warrington et al., 1971)—paired associates, short story recall, free recall learning, one-trial free recall. None of these tasks, however, with the possible exception of the short story recall, pushes the limits of the subjects' capabilities, particularly capabilities sensitive to a limited short-term store. Long sequences of items do not have to be organized in these tasks. Moreover, the conduction aphasic's short-term memory problems center, as will be pointed out below, on the handling of order information. The tasks to assay the state of long-term store should focus on the registration of order information.

There are two additional characteristics of conduction aphasia that are important. One is that the performance deficits are particularly acute when the presentation is auditory (Warrington and Shallice, 1972). The other is that the deficit seems to center on the handling of order information (Dubois et al., 1964; Strub and Gardner, 1974; Tzortzis and Albert, 1974). The difficulty with sequential information may be important in the poor performance on some of the memory tasks that involve such information, e.g., probe recall tasks.

The physiological bases of conduction aphasia are clear. Most cases involve lesions of the angular and supramarginal gyri, including the arcuate fasciculus as Wernicke proposed. The lesions presumably break the communication between Broca's and Wernicke's areas. There is, however, evidence of another type of conduction aphasia which was considered by Kleist (1916). In this type the right hemisphere takes over the function of auditory comprehension of speech after a lesion of Wernicke's area in the left hemisphere. The difficulty of transferring auditory-verbal information between the two hemispheres may be the basis for the second type of conduction aphasia. Benson et al. (1973) present some evidence in support of the existence of this second type. It is, they note, distinguished behaviorally by the absence of apraxia which characterizes the other type of conduction aphasia. Kinsbourne (1972) has presented data on a patient who seems to be of the second type.

In closing, it is premature to revise the multiple-store model on the basis of the conduction aphasia data offered up to this time. The two points mentioned above have yet to be established—clear demonstration of short-term store impairment across the range of appropriate tests and clear demonstration of normal long-term store across the range of appropriate tests.

MURRAY GLANZER
AND ELISABETH O.
CLARK

Retrograde amnesia is the subject's loss of memory for information that he had presumably been able to remember at some earlier time. It is a frequent concomitant of brain damage and has, according to the literature, a number of systematic characteristics (Russell and Nathan, 1946; Williams, 1975). Two of the most striking are the following:

1. It is more pronounced for recent than remote events.
2. It tends to shrink over time, with memory for more remote events recovered first.

Retrograde amnesia can cover time periods from a few hours or less to several decades. It is likely to appear when there is anterograde amnesia.

Retrograde amnesia poses a special theoretical problem. The fact that it occurs with anterograde amnesia suggests that the two forms of amnesia involve the same type of underlying dysfunction. The usual argument is that both involve a failure of retrieval. The tendency of the retrograde amnesia to shrink identifies that amnesia particularly with retrieval failure.

Recently, data have been published that question the relation between retrograde amnesia and recency of events, characteristic 1 listed above. Sanders and Warrington (1971) used a questionnaire about news events and a recognition test of well-known faces. Both the news events and the faces could be assigned to time periods within the last 30–40 years. These tests were given to a mixed group of amnesic patients—Korsakoff, temporal lobectomy, carbon monoxide poisoning, etc.—and normal control subjects. Sanders and Warrington showed that the amnesic patients had impaired memory for all the time periods tested. There was no evidence that recent events were more likely to be lost than remote events. A study by Squire (1974) demonstrated that electroconvulsive shock treatments resulted in loss of memory for remote as well as recent events. Since his subjects were tested within an hour after treatment, the decrement in remote memory cannot be assigned to the differential effect of rehearsal over time since the trauma. This is an explanation that has been offered by Baddeley (1975) to handle the Sanders and Warrington data. In the Squire study there is, however, some evidence that memory for recent events is impaired more than for remote events.

These studies indicate, first, the need for a thorough review of the standard picture of retrograde amnesia. The data on retrograde amnesia are of critical importance for any theoretical analysis of the amnesias and therefore should be very clear. The studies also suggest the need to separate out different types of long-term memory for study, a separation that has been made in much recent work on memory. There is episodic memory, which concerns the individual's personal experiences, e.g., what he ate yesterday. There is semantic memory, which concerns certain basic information concerning the subject's language, e.g., that a bull is a male. There is also encyclopedic information about the world, e.g., that Germany was defeated in World War II. The tests used by Sanders and Warrington and by Squire are tests of encyclopedic information. It is not clear that they would have obtained the same results if they had devised tests of episodic memory, i.e., personal information. Clinical evidence of retrograde amnesia usually is centered on episodic and encyclopedic memory.

487

CEREBRAL
MECHANISMS OF
INFORMATION
STORAGE: THE
PROBLEM OF MEMORY

Theories of Amnesia

Now we are ready to consider some recent psychological theories about the basic character of the anterograde amnesias. Two opposed proposals have been made. One, referred to earlier, is that the amnesia results from faulty registration of new information in long-term store, Milner (1968a) made this proposal in terms of consolidation. Later versions of this proposal have been in terms of encoding (Baddeley and Warrington, 1973; Cermak and Butters, 1972; Cermak *et al.*, 1971, 1973, 1974; DeLuca *et al.*, 1975). Cermak and Butters further specify the encoding impairment as one of semantic encoding.

The other proposal is that the amnesia results from faulty retrieval of information from long-term store. This proposal has been presented and studied by Warrington and Weiskrantz (1970, 1973, 1974). Warrington and Weiskrantz have further specified the retrieval difficulty as stemming from an inability to cope with proactive interference. Cermak and Butters (1972) also assign a role to interference in amnesia. A recent review of these proposals and of the data in support of them is found in Baddeley (1975).

The experimental demonstrations in support of either of the two general proposals are not convincing. This is in part because the results are complicated and contradictory. More important is that the basic nature of the enterprise involved in these experimental demonstrations necessarily leads to ambiguous results. We discussed earlier the attempt to determine whether amnesia was due to registration or retrieval deficits by comparing performance on recognition and recall tasks. We noted the problems in drawing conclusions from such a comparison. More general problems are present in the work that attempts to separate registration and retrieval effects.

It is not possible to take a black box, enter an input, measure an output, and then assign a measured loss of information to either the input side of the hidden process or the output side of that process. This analysis remains indeterminate no matter how the input is varied.

If a subject is helped by partial cues, this may be because he has registered only part of the input information and with the cues can reconstruct the input, or it may be that he has registered all of the input but has a faulty retrieval procedure which is bolstered by particular cues. If a subject cannot make use of some characteristic of the item or the list, this may be because he has registered the item incompletely or because he uses those registered characteristics inefficiently in retrieval. One way out of this analytic difficulty is to attend to specific information or classes of information that the subject must have registered in long-term store before the brain damage. This type of information is isolated for study when retrograde amnesia is examined. That is why it is critical to clarify the data on retrograde amnesia and its relation to anterograde amnesia.

The recent studies of retrograde amnesia cited above have revised our view of the character of that deficit and lend some support to the hypothesis that both retrograde and anterograde amnesia reflect a common deficit. Much work, however, has to be done relating the characteristics of the retrograde to the anterograde amnesia with respect to duration, severity, specific material lost, etc., before this hypothesis can be adopted with any degree of security. Moreover, there are also certain classes of available data that will have to be accommodated before this adoption occurs. The difficulty that amnesic patients have in simple recognition has to be accounted for, however effective partial cueing is with those patients.*

The paragraph above falls into the mode of selecting either registration or retrieval as the source of impairment in amnesia. There is another alternative. The impairment may necessarily reside in both registration and retrieval. The two processes may not be separable, or both may reflect another underlying impairment. The activation view presented earlier leads easily to this formulation. In terms of a multiple-store model, amnesia is seen as a result of insufficient activation of the interchange between short-term and long-term store necessary for both registration and retrieval. Another possibility is that a basic part of the function common to storage and retrieval is lost. This may be a very simple part. The image that comes to mind is that of a librarian who has forgotten the alphabet. That librarian's performance would be impaired both in making new entries in the catalog (and placing new books appropriately) and in finding books either on the basis of call slips or through the catalog. The general activation view seems, however, most attractive at this point.

Conclusion

The effects of damage to and stimulation of the limbic system can be nicely coordinated with a multiple-store theory of memory. Some or all of the Papez circuit functions, as a unit, in the registration of new information from short-term to long-term store or in its retrieval from long-term store or in both processes. The circuit is the physiological basis for the activation of those processes. The circuit is strongly lateralized, with the left half processing verbal information and the right half processing nonverbal information. There are compensatory effects that occur in the system so that the impairment in memory performance is subtle with unilateral lesions. Severe anterograde amnesia appears only with bilateral lesions, which block compensatory functions within the circuit.

Damage to the frontal lobes produces effects, some of which fit into a multiple-store model. The maintenance of instructions, for example, may be carried out by a type of maintenance rehearsal that is usually ascribed to short-term store. The role assigned to the frontal lobes in an overall theory of memory remains, however, to be specified.

---

*Warrington and Weiskrantz have cited the fact that amnesic patients are able to learn to recognize incomplete pictures and words as evidence for defective retrieval rather than defective registration.

489

CEREBRAL
MECHANISMS OF
INFORMATION
STORAGE: THE
PROBLEM OF MEMORY

Let us return to the issue of registration vs. retrieval deficits in the amnesic symptoms of limbic damage. We have pointed out the difficulties in deciding on one of those two alternatives on the basis of current experimental approaches. A more promising way to examine the alternatives is by fuller examination of the characteristics of retrograde amnesia and their relation to the characteristics of anterograde amnesia.

In summarizing, we have again considered the issue of registration vs. retrieval. Both the registration of new information in long-term store and the setting up of retrieval routines for new information as it is registered in long-term store may, however, be jointly affected if the role of the circuit is to activate extensive communication between short-term and long-term store, the "deep processing" that permits full interpretation of new information.

Acknowledgments

We thank E. E. Coons and Samuel M. Feldman for their review and helpful comments on the chapter. We also thank the staff of the National Clearinghouse for Alcohol Information for their assistance with our literature searches.

REFERENCES*

Akelaitis, A. J. Studies on the corpus callosum. VII. Study of language functions (tactile and visual lexia and graphia) unilaterally following section of the corpus callosum. *Journal of Neuropathology and Experimental Neurology*, 1943, *2*, 226–262.

Atkinson, R. C., and Shiffrin, R. M. Human memory: A proposed system and its control processes. In K. W. Spence and J. T. Spence (eds.), *The Psychology of Learning and Motivation*, Vol. 2. New York: Academic Press, 1968.

Baddeley, A. D. Theories of amnesia. In A. Kennedy and A. Wilkes (eds.), *Studies in Long-Term Memory*. New York: Wiley, 1975.

Baddeley, A. D., and Warrington, E. K. Amnesia and the distinction between long-term and short-term memory. *Journal of Verbal Learning and Verbal Behavior*, 1970, *9*, 176–189.

Baddeley, A. D., and Warrington, E. K. Memory coding and amnesia. *Neuropsychologia*, 1973, *11*, 159–165.

Benson, D. F., Sheremata, W. A., Bouchard, R., Segarra, J. M., Price, D., and Geschwind, N. Conduction aphasia. *Archives of Neurology*, 1973, *28*, 339–346.

Blakemore, C. B., and Falconer, M. A. Long-term effects of anterior temporal lobectomy on certain cognitive functions. *Journal of Neurology, Neurosurgery and Psychiatry*, 1967, *30*, 364–367.

Brierly, J. B. The neuropathology of amnesic states. In C. W. M. Whitty and O. L. Zangwill (eds.), *Amnesia*. London: Butterworths, 1966.

Brion, S. Korsakoff's syndrome: Clinico-anatomical and physiopathological considerations. In G. A. Talland and N. C. Waugh (eds.), *The Pathology of Memory*. New York: Academic Press, 1969.

Broadbent, D. E. *Perception and Communication*. London: Pergamon Press, 1958.

Brooks, D. N., and Baddeley, A. D. What can amnesic patients learn? *Neuropsychologia*, 1976, *14*, 111–122.

Butters, N., Lewis, R., Cermak, L. S., and Goodglass, H. Material-specific memory deficits in alcoholic Korsakoff patients. *Neuropsychologia*, 1973, *11*, 291–300.

*References for this chapter were selected on the basis of relevance to the topic and clarity of the report. Some standard references have therefore been excluded.

Cairns, H., and Mosberg, W. H., Jr. Colloid cyst of the third ventricle. *Surgery, Gynecology and Obstetrics,* 1951, *92*, 545–570.

Cermak, L. S., and Butters, N. The role of interference and encoding in the short-term memory deficits of Korsakoff patients. *Neuropsychologia,* 1972, *10*, 89–95.

Cermak, L. S., and Butters, N. Information processing deficits of alcoholic Korsakoff patients. *Quarterly Journal of Studies on Alcohol,* 1973, *34*, 1110–1132.

Cermak, L. S., Butters, N., and Goodglass, H. The extent of memory loss in Korsakoff patients. *Neuropsychologia,* 1971, *9*, 307–315.

Cermak, L. S., Butters, N., and Gerrein, J. The extent of the verbal encoding ability of Korsakoff patients. *Neuropsychologia,* 1973, *11*, 85–94.

Cermak, L. S., Butters, N., and Moreines, J. Some analyses of the verbal encoding deficit of alcoholic Korsakoff patients. *Brain and Language,* 1974, *1*, 141–150.

Cermak, L. S., Naus, M. J., and Reale, L. Rehearsal strategies of alcoholic Korsakoff patients. *Brain and Language,* 1976, *3*, 375–385.

Chapman, L. F., Walter, R. D., Markham, C. H., Rand, R. W., and Crandall, P. H. Memory changes induced by stimulation of the hippocampus or amygdala in epilepsy patients with implanted electrodes. *Transactions of the American Neurological Association,* 1967, *92*, 50–56.

Corkin, S. Tactually-guided maze learning in man: Effects of unilateral cortical excisions and bilateral hippocampal lesions. *Neuropsychologia,* 1965, *3*, 339–351.

Corkin, S. Acquisition of motor skill after bilateral medial temporal-lobe excision. *Neuropsychologia,* 1968, *6*, 255–265.

Craik, F. I. M., and Lockhart, R. S. Levels of processing: A framework for memory research. *Journal of Verbal Learning and Verbal Behavior,* 1972, *11*, 671–684.

Craik, F. I. M., and Tulving, E. Depth of processing and the retention of words in episodic memory. *Journal of Experimental Psychology: General,* 1975, *104*, 268–294.

DeLuca, D., Cermak, L. S., and Butters, N. An analysis of Korsakoff patients' recall following varying types of distractor activity. *Neuropsychologia,* 1975, *13*, 271–279.

Dott, N. M. Surgical aspects of the hypothalamus. In W. E. L. G. Clark, J. Beattie, G. Riddoch, and N. M. Dott (eds.), *The Hypothalamus: Morphological, Functional, Clinical and Surgical Aspects.* Edinburgh: Oliver and Boyd, 1938.

Drachman, D. A., and Ommaya, A. K. Memory and the hippocampal complex. *Archives of Neurology,* 1964, *10*, 411–425.

Dubois, J., Hécaen, H., Maufras du Chatelier, A., and Marcie, P. Etude neurolinguistique de l'aphasie de conduction. *Neuropsychologia,* 1964, *2*, 9–44.

Fedio, P., and Ommaya, A. K. Bilateral cingulum lesions and stimulation in man with lateralized impairment in short-term memory. *Experimental Neurology,* 1970, *29*, 84–91.

Fedio, P., and van Buren, J. M. Memory deficits during electrical stimulation of the speech cortex in conscious man. *Brain and Language,* 1974, *1*, 29–42.

Fedio, P., and van Buren, J. M. Memory and perceptual deficits during electrical stimulation in the left and right thalamus and parietal subcortex. *Brain and Language,* 1975, *2*, 78–100.

Gaffan, D. Recognition memory in animals. In J. Brown (ed.), *Recall and Recognition.* New York: Wiley, 1976.

García Bengochea, F., De La Torre, O., Esquivel, O., Vieta, R., and Fernandez, C. The section of the fornix in the surgical treatment of certain epilepsies: A preliminary report. *Transactions of the American Neurological Association,* 1954, *79*, 176–178.

Gerner, P., Ommaya, A. K., and Fedio, P. A study of visual memory: Verbal and non-verbal mechanisms in patients with unilateral temporal lobectomy. *International Journal of Neuroscience,* 1972, *4*, 231–238.

Ghent, L., Mishkin, M., and Teuber, H. L. Short term memory after frontal-lobe injury in man. *Journal of Comparative and Physiological Psychology,* 1962, *55*, 705–709.

Glanzer, M. Storage mechanisms in recall. In G. H. Bower (ed.), *The Psychology of Learning and Motivation,* Vol. 5. New York: Academic Press, 1972.

Glanzer, M., and Cunitz, A. R. Two storage mechanisms in free recall. *Journal of Verbal Learning and Verbal Behavior,* 1966, *5*, 351–360.

Glanzer, M., and Koppenaal, L. The effect of encoding tasks on free recall: Stages and levels. *Journal of Verbal Learning and Verbal Behavior,* 1977, *16*, 21–28.

Glanzer, M., and Razel, M. The size of the unit in short-term storage. *Journal of Verbal Learning and Verbal Behavior,* 1974, *13*, 114–131.

Gol, A., and Faibish, G. M. Effects of human hippocampal ablation. *Journal of Neurosurgery,* 1967, *26*, 390–398.

491

CEREBRAL
MECHANISMS OF
INFORMATION
STORAGE: THE
PROBLEM OF MEMORY

Goldstein, K. *Language and Language Disturbances.* New York: Grune and Stratton, 1948.

Goodwin, D. W. Blackouts and alcohol induced memory dysfunction. In *Recent Advances in Studies of Alcoholism.* Washington, D.C.: U.S. Department of Health, Education, and Welfare, 1970, pp. 508–536.

Goodwin, D. W. Two species of alcoholic "blackout." *American Journal of Psychiatry,* 1971, *127,* 1665–1670.

Goodwin, D. W., and Hill, S. Y. Short-term memory and the alcoholic blackout. *Annals of the New York Academy of Sciences,* 1973, *215,* 195–199.

Goodwin, D. W., Crane, J. B., and Guze, S. Alcoholic "blackouts": A review and clinical study of 100 alcoholics. *American Journal of Psychiatry,* 1969, *126,* 191–198.

Goodwin, D. W., Othmer, E., Halikas, J. A., and Freemon, F. Loss of short term memory as a predictor of the alcoholic "blackout." *Nature,* 227, 1970, 201–202.

Goodwin, D. W., Hill, S. Y., Powell, B., and Viamontes, J. Effect of alcohol on short-term memory in alcoholics. *British Journal of Psychiatry,* 1973, *122,* 93–94.

Hebb, D. O. *The Organization of Behavior.* New York: Wiley, 1949.

Hécaen, N., and Albert, M. L. Disorders of mental functioning related to frontal lobe pathology. In D. F. Benson and D. Blumen (eds.), *Psychiatric Aspects of Neurological Disease.* New York: Grune and Stratton, 1975.

Horton, D. L., and Turnage, T. W. *Human Learning.* Englewood Cliffs, N.J.: Prentice Hall, 1976.

Illchysin, D., and Ryback, R. Short-term memory in non-intoxicated alcoholics as a function of blackout history. Annual Conference of the National Council on Alcoholism, Washington, D.C., 1976.

Isaacson, R. L. Memory processes and the hippocampus. In D. Deutsch and J. A. Deutsch (eds.), *Short-Term Memory.* New York: Academic Press, 1975.

Iversen, S. D. Brain lesions and memory in animals. In J. A. Deutsch (ed.), *The Physiological Basis of Memory.* New York: Academic Press, 1973.

Kinsbourne, M. Behavioral analysis of the repetition deficit in conduction aphasia. *Neurology,* 1972, *22,* 1126–1132.

Kleist, K. Über Leitungsaphasie und grammatische Störungen. *Monatsschrift für Psychiatrie und Nuerologie,* 1916, *40,* 118–199.

McLardy, T. Memory function in hippocampal gyri but not in hippocampi. *International Journal of Neuroscience,* 1970, *1,* 113–118.

Milner, B. Memory disturbance after bilateral hippocampal lesions. In P. Milner and S. Glickman (eds.), *Cognitive Processes and the Brain.* New York: Van Nostrand, 1965a.

Milner, B. Visually-guided maze learning in man: Effects of bilateral hippocampal, bilateral frontal, and unilateral cerebral lesions. *Neuropsychologia,* 1965b, *3,* 317–338.

Milner, B. Disorders of memory after brain lesions in man. Preface: Material-specific and generalized memory loss. *Neuropsychologia,* 1968a, *6,* 175–179.

Milner, B. Visual recognition and recall after right temporal excision in man. *Neuropsychologia,* 1968b, *6,* 191–209.

Milner, B. Memory and the medial temporal regions of the brain. In K. H. Pribram and D. E. Broadbent (eds.), *Biology of Memory.* New York: Academic Press, 1970.

Milner, B. Interhemispheric differences in the localization of psychological processes in man. *British Medical Bulletin,* 1971, *27,* 272–277.

Milner, B. Hemisphere specialization: Scope and limits. In F. O. Schmitt and F. G. Worden (eds.), *The Neurosciences: Third Study Program.* Cambridge, Mass.: MIT Press, 1973.

Milner, B., Corkin, S., and Teuber, H.-L. Further analysis of the hippocampal amnesic syndrome: 14-year follow-up study of H. M. *Neuropsychologia,* 1968, *6,* 215–234.

Murdock, B. B., Jr. *Human Memory: Theory and Data.* Potomac, Md.: Erlbaum, 1974.

Murdock, B. B., Jr., and Walker, K. D. Modality effects in free recall. *Journal of Verbal Learning and Verbal Behavior,* 1969, *8,* 665–676.

Neisser, U. *Cognitive Psychology.* New York: Appleton-Century-Crofts, 1967.

Newcombe, F. *Missile Wounds of the Brain: A Study of Psychological Deficits.* London: Oxford University Press, 1969.

Ojemann, G. A., and Fedio, P. Effect of stimulation of the human thalamus and parietal and temporal white matter on short-term memory. *Journal of Neurosurgery,* 1968, *29,* 51–59.

Ojemann, G. A., Blick, K., and Ward, A. A., Jr. Improvement and disturbance of short-term verbal memory with human ventrolateral thalamic stimulation. *Brain,* 1971a, *94,* 225–240.

Ojemann, G. A., Hovenga, K. B., and Ward, A. A., Jr. Prediction of short-term verbal memory disturbance after ventrolateral thalamotony. *Journal of Neurosurgery,* 1971b, *35,* 203–210.

Ojemann, R. G. Correlations between specific human brain lesions and memory changes. *Neurosciences Research Program Bulletin*, 1966, *4*, 1–65.

O'Keefe, J., Nadel, L., Keightley, S., and Kill, D. Fornix lesions selectively abolish place learning in the rat. *Experimental Neurology*, 1975, *48*, 152–166.

Ommaya, A. K., and Fedio, P. The contribution of cingulum and hippocampal structures to memory mechanisms in man. *Confinia Neurologica*, 1972, *34*, 398–411.

Papez, J. W. A proposed mechanism of emotion. *Archives of Neurology*, 1937, *38*, 725–743.

Penfield, W. Memory, autopsy finding, and comments on the role of hippocampus in experimental recall. *Archives of Neurology*, 1974, *31*, 145–154.

Peterson, L. R., and Peterson, M. Short-term retention of individual verbal items. *Journal of Experimental Psychology*, 1959, *58*, 193–198.

Postman, L. Verbal learning and memory, *Annual Review of Psychology*, 1975, *26*, 291–336.

Raisman, G., Cowan, W. M., and Powell, T. P. S. The extrinsic afferent, commissural, and association fibres of the hippocampus. *Brain*, 1965, *88*, 963–996.

Russell, W. R., and Nathan, P. W. Traumatic amnesia. *Brain*, 1946, *69*, 280–301.

Ryback, R. S. Alcohol amnesia: Observations in seven drinking inpatient alcoholics. *Quarterly Journal of Studies on Alcohol*, 1970, *31*, 616–632.

Ryback, R. S. The continuum and specificity of the effects of alcohol on memory: A review. *Quarterly Journal of Studies on Alcohol*, 1971, *32*, 995–1016.

Sanders, H. I., and Warrington, E. K. Memory for remote events in amnesic patients. *Brain*, 1971, *94*, 661–668.

Scoville, W. B., and Milner, B. Loss of recent memory after bilateral hippocampal lesions. *Journal of Neurology, Neurosurgery, and Psychiatry*, 1957, *20*, 11–21.

Shallice, T., and Warrington, E. K. Independent functioning of verbal memory stores: A neuropsychological study. *Quarterly Journal of Experimental Psychology*, 1970, *22*, 261–273.

Sidman, M., Stoddard, L. T., and Mohr, J. P. Some additional quantitative observations of immediate memory in a patient with bilateral hippocampal lesions. *Neuropsychologia*, 1968, *6*, 245–254.

Silverstein, C., and Glanzer, M. Difficulty of a concurrent task in free recall: Differential effects in STS and LTS. *Psychonomic Science*, 1971, *22*, 367–368.

Squire, L. R. Amnesia for remote events following electroconvulsive therapy. *Behavioral Biology*, 1974, *12*, 119–125.

Strub, R. L., and Gardner, H. The repetition deficit in conduction aphasia: Mnestic or linguistic? *Brain and Language*, 1974, *1*, 241–256.

Swanson, L. W., and Cowan, W. M. Hippocampo-hypothalamic connections: Origin in subicular cortex, not Ammon's horn. *Science,* 1975, *189*, 303–304.

Sweet, W. H., Talland, G. A., and Ervin, F. R. Loss of recent memory following section of fornix. *Transactions of the American Neurological Association*, 1959, *84*, 76–82.

Talland, G. A. *Deranged Memory.* New York: Academic Press, 1965.

Tzortzis, C., and Albert, M. L. Impairment of memory for sequences in conduction aphasia. *Neuropsychologia*, 1974, *12*, 355–366.

Victor, M., Adams, R. D., and Collins, G. H. *The Wernicke-Korsakoff Syndrome.* Philadelphia: F. A. Davis, 1971.

Warrington, E. K., and Shallice, T. The selective impairment of auditory verbal short-term memory. *Brain*, 1969, *92*, 885–896.

Warrington, E. K., and Shallice, T. Neuropsychological evidence of visual storage in short-term memory tasks. *Quarterly Journal of Experimental Psychology*, 1972, *24*, 30–40.

Warrington, E. K., and Weiskrantz, L. Amnesic syndrome: Consolidation or retrieval? *Nature*, 1970, *228*, 628–630.

Warrington, E. K., and Weiskrantz, L. An analysis of short-term and long-term memory defects in man. In J. A. Deutsch (ed.), *The Physiological Basis of Memory.* New York: Academic Press, 1973.

Warrington, E. K., and Weiskrantz, L. The effect of prior learning on subsequent retention in amnesic patients. *Neuropsychologia*, 1974, *12*, 419–429.

Warrington, E. K., Logue, V., and Pratt, R. T. C. The anatomical localisation of selective impairment of auditory verbal short-term memory. *Neuropsychologia*, 1971, *9*, 377–387.

Weisenberg, T., and McBride, K. E. *Aphasia,* New York: The Commonwealth Fund, 1935.

Weiskrantz, L. Experimental studies in amnesia. In C. W. M. Whitty and O. L. Zangwill (eds.), *Amnesia.* London: Butterworths, 1966.

Wernicke, C. *Der aphasische Symptomencomplex.* Breslau: Cohn and Weigert, 1874.

Whitty, C. M. W., and Lewin, W. A Korsakoff syndrome in the post-cingulectomy confusional state. *Brain,* 1960, *83,* 648–653.

Williams, M. Retrograde amnesia. In A. Kennedy and A. Wilkes (eds.), *Studies in Long-Term Memory.* New York: Wiley, 1975.

Zaidel, D., and Sperry, R. W. Memory impairment after commissurotomy in man. *Brain,* 1974, *97,* 263–272.

493

CEREBRAL
MECHANISMS OF
INFORMATION
STORAGE: THE
PROBLEM OF MEMORY

Long-Term Psychological Consequences of Cerebral Lesions

Freda Newcombe and Graham Ratcliff

Introduction

Evidence concerning the long-term consequences of brain lesions is hard to find despite the plethora of data linking disorders of cognitive function with their presumptive anatomical background. Indeed, if the modifier of the title were to be taken too literally, this chapter would be remarkable only for its brevity. But, if a case cannot yet be proven, at least some of the main issues can be raised and reasonable predictions of outcome can be based on the clinical and experimental work that has flourished in the past four decades. An early but exemplary review of some of this work by Piercy (1964) remains the best distillation of its theoretical and clinical implications.

Our knowledge of the psychological consequences of brain lesions has been both inspired and constrained by the concept of hemispheric asymmetry of functional representation. It is not within our brief to summarize work stemming from this well-entrenched concept. Rather, we must take into account modifications to this oversimplified, static, cartographic approach if useful predictions and remedial suggestions are to be made. Thus we shall have to consider such factors as the age and sex of the patient, the etiology of the lesion, the time post-onset when clinical observations and measurements are made, the pattern of recovery, and the relationship between test performance and functional efficiency in daily

Freda Newcombe and Graham Ratcliff   Neuropsychology Unit, Department of Clinical Neurology, The Churchill Hospital, Oxford, England OX3 7LJ.

life. The implicit but inevitable extrapolation from test score to "function" constitutes one of those leaps in the dark that a poet requires of his reader: the student of the neurosciences cannot always afford this willing suspension of disbelief.

With these considerations in mind, first we shall consider the sequelae of focal brain injury and the less well-studied sequelae of diffuse lesions, and then we shall discuss to what extent these clinical and experimental findings can be related to outcome and mapped onto behavior in the context of daily life. The distinction between focal and diffuse injury is difficult to justify on precise anatomical and physiological grounds. It implies relative differences in the nature and extent of brain damage and is not intended to provide more than a convenient if somewhat arbitrary way of classifying the wide variety of pathological material implied by the title of the chapter.

Focal Brain Injury

Language Disorders

There can be no doubt of the privileged role of the left hemisphere, at least for the right-handed adult, in the understanding and production of language. This conclusion, drawn from many decades of clinical and anatomical observation, was amply supported by evidence from studies of the effects of focal gunshot wounds in large populations of servicemen (Conrad, 1954; Walker and Jablon, 1961; Russell and Espir, 1961; Luria, 1970). Of 388 servicemen in the British sample (Russell and Espir, 1961) with unilateral damage to the left hemisphere, 56% were dysphasic immediately after injury and, of these, 41% still showed dysphasic symptoms on discharge from hospital. In contrast, only 2% of right-handed servicemen with right hemisphere lesions were dysphasic after the injury. In the civilian population, by far the most common cause of dysphasia is cerebrovascular accident; a recent study of a consecutive series of 850 stroke patients reported that 21% had aphasia during the acute phase (Brust *et al.*, 1976).

The question arises as to how language disorders are to be classified and whether there is a relationship between type of aphasia and pattern of recovery. The taxonomic problem is far from being solved. Groups are classified according to curious combinations of linguistic and clinical features and presumptive anatomy. Until recently, the clinician had been hard put to find a more useful operational distinction than that of an expressive or a receptive language disorder. An alternative but not very different distinction has been made between fluent and nonfluent aphasic patients that at least has the merit of using a consistent linguistic criterion: the amount and syntactic range of expressive speech (Goodglass, 1968; Geschwind, 1972). It also allows for the fact that comprehension, especially of relational words, is usually found to be imperfect in nonfluent aphasia when more than cursorily examined (Goodglass, 1968; Benson, 1977). Many patients, however, do not fit into these neat categories, and assessment procedures differ. Thus it is hazardous to compare the few studies which have addressed the question of outcome and patterns of recovery.

On the whole, more improvement can be expected in traumatic aphasia than in aphasia due to cerebrovascular disease (Butfield and Zangwill, 1946). In a sample of 53 men with focal missile wounds of the left hemisphere, examined 25 years after injury, seven still showed moderate to severe dysphasia, and 15 had slight but unambiguous symptoms of language impairment both in spontaneous speech and on formal test of vocabulary, fluency, spelling, and object naming, although these residual sequelae had not precluded a satisfactory adjustment at home and at work (Newcombe, 1969). In the civilian stroke population, the assessment of recovery is complicated by the relatively high mortality rate and the undoubted bias in selection of cases: many patients are not admitted to hospitals for examination and some with severe left hemisphere strokes cannot be tested (Oxbury, 1975).

A recent follow-up study (Brust et al., 1976) of an unselected series of stroke patients 4–12 weeks after onset reported that 25% died. Aphasic symptoms remained severe, moderate, or mild in 12%, 15%, and 29% of the group, respectively. The aphasia cleared in 19% of the cases. Regarding outcome, there are well-attested clinical findings: prognosis is related to age (Sands et al., 1969), etiology (Butfield and Zangwill, 1946), severity (Schuell et al., 1964), and, in particular, the extent of comprehension loss (Weisenburg and McBride, 1935; Wepman, 1953; Marks et al., 1957; Godfrey and Douglass, 1959; Vignolo, 1964; Kenin and Peck-Swisher, 1972). In general, a better prognosis is accorded to expressive dysphasia (e.g., Butfield and Zangwill, 1946), and, although Vignolo initially reported *relatively* more improvement in the receptive aspects of language (1964), his group has recently documented a significant improvement in oral production in a group of patients undergoing therapy (Basso et al., 1975). A recent study by Matthews and Oxbury (1975) has outlined the prognostic factors in patients with acute ischemic infarction from the neurological point of view, and data concerning the recovery of language functions in the survivors are currently under review.

Patterns of recovery are seldom taken into account (but see Bay, 1964; Brown, 1972; Kenin and Peck-Swisher, 1972; Leischner, 1976). Kertesz and McCabe (1977) have, however, completed a long-term quantitative assessment of a relatively unselected group of 93 aphasic patients, of whom 74 had infarcts or intracerebral hemorrhage. They confirmed some familiar clinical hypotheses: the prognosis for global aphasia is poor; recovery frequently occurs in patients with anomic, conduction, and transcortical aphasia; and age and initial severity of aphasia are important factors in recovery. Both these authors and Ludlow (cited by Sarno, 1976) suggest that there are characteristic and common patterns of recovery. Information about these patterns and the slope of recovery curves (Newcombe, et al., 1975) should increase predictive accuracy and perhaps also help to shape appropriate remedial techniques. The studies of Kertesz and McCabe and several others (e.g., Head, 1926; Butfield and Zangwill, 1946; Schuell et al., 1964; Vignolo, 1964; Sands et al., 1969; Sarno and Levita, 1971) confirm that most recovery takes place within 3 months of onset. But there are exceptional patients who continue to improve for much longer periods of time (Sands et al., 1969).

FREDA NEWCOMBE
AND GRAHAM
RATCLIFF

Hand preference and sex may be additional factors to consider in relation to prognosis. A more favorable prognosis for recovery of language functions has been accorded to left-handed patients (Subirana, 1958, 1969) and also to right-handed ex-servicemen with a family history of left-handedness (Luria, 1970) than for other right-handed patients, although one clinician (Roberts, 1969) has given a cautious warning that these claims may have been overemphasized. In fact, there is a dearth of critical evidence. Clinical data on the nature and extent of language deficits after unilateral lesions of either hemisphere in sinistral patients are not consistent (compare Hécaen and Sauguet, 1971; Newcombe and Ratcliff, 1973), and these inconsistencies are mirrored in studies of lateral preference in normal right- and left-handed subjects on tests of dichotic listening and recognition in the visual half-fields (compare Zurif and Bryden, 1969; Hines and Satz, 1974; Briggs and Nebes, 1976). With an emphasis on more unusual models (e.g., pathological left-handedness, bilateral speech representation), the more usual finding of speech representation in the left hemisphere for approximately two-thirds of left-handed subjects tends to be overlooked; thus the prognosis for the majority of left-handed subjects may be no better or no worse than that accorded to the right-handed patient. Normal and clinical studies treating left-handed subjects as a homogeneous group seem unlikely to produce significant results; a preliminary distinction between those presumed to have left hemisphere speech representation and the remainder could be informative (cf. Cohen and Freeman, 1977). In addition, the patent unreliability of much reported information on family histories of sinistrality must confound the attempt to evaluate this factor.

Sex may influence prognosis. Lansdell's (1962, 1964) initial observations of different patterns of deficit in men and women after unilateral temporal lobectomy were accorded little attention at the time of publication. Subsequent experimental work, critically reviewed by Fairweather (1976), has produced positive and controversial evidence; and sex-dependent behavioral effects of brain lesions have been found in physiological experiments (Goldman et al., 1974; Stein, 1974). In normal human subjects, hemispheric differences in efficiency of processing verbal and nonverbal information (inferred from dichotic and tachistoscopic experiments) have led to the suggestion that language and spatial skills are less sharply lateralized in women than in men (McGlone and Davidson, 1973; Hannay and Malone, 1976; Harris, 1976). Clinical evidence also lends support to this hypothesis: in a large group of right-handed stroke patients with unilateral cerebral lesions confirmed by computerized axial tomography, the predictable verbal-nonverbal discrepancies were statistically significant only for male patients (McGlone, 1978).

The role of speech therapy is far from clear. Two of the most recent investigations produce conflicting results: no differences between treated and untreated groups (Kertesz and McCabe, 1977) and significant gains in expressive speech for patients receiving speech therapy (Basso et al., 1975). Few studies meet the elementary requirements of control, an issue meticulously discussed in an excellent review by Sarno (1976). There is a rich store of experience in this area (Wepman, 1951, 1972; Schuell et al., 1964; Eisenson, 1973) but also a great need for systematic experiment.

Whereas disturbances of language and speech are fairly common in patients with acute left hemisphere lesions, the so-called pure or disproportionately severe disorders of reading and writing are rare. The pure alexias, interesting for the light they shed on anatomical correlates (cf. a masterly study by Déjérine, 1892; also subsequent research by Benson and Geschwind, 1969; Greenblatt, 1973), tend to persist (Ajax, 1967; Thomsen and Harmsen, 1968) and, as far as we can ascertain, there is only one report of complete recovery (Sroka *et al.*, 1973). Less pure but disproportionately severe forms of dyslexia (without dysgraphia) occur in a setting of fluent aphasia, in association with occipital lesions. Letters pose less of a problem than words, and the patient may be able to spell orally. Of particular interest in this context is a study (Hécaen *et al.*, 1952) of the long-term effects of left occipital lobectomy. It describes not only the eventual recovery of the ability to read but also a curious disinclination to do so: patients reported a feeling of discomfort after reading for more than a few minutes. The explanation of this symptom is unknown: it is yet another example of disabilities that persist and can have a profound effect on intellectual life, although they may not be detected in routine and brief "psychometric" assessment.

Disorders of reading and writing (alexia with agraphia) have usually been associated with temporoparietal lesions. However, the number of fluent aphasic patients with a disproportionately severe problem with reading and writing is small. Brown and Simonson (1957) found this pattern in 13 of the 100 dysphasic patients that they studied, while Casey and Ettlinger (1960) cite only four such cases among a group of 35 dysphasic patients drawn from an unselected sample of 700 neurological cases. In a group of over 900 men with penetrating wounds of the brain, only 11 were found to have selective difficulties with reading and writing; their lesions, as would be predicted from previous clinical and anatomical studies, clustered in the region of the angular gyrus. When alexia with agraphia occurs in a setting of fluent aphasia, the patient usually has a comparable difficulty in reading words and letters and in spelling aloud. The long-term outlook has seldom, if ever, been documented, and the few studies that are available show marked differences in the rate and extent of recovery (Mohr, *et al.*, 1973; Newcombe and Marshall, 1975; Newcombe *et al.*, 1975).

A third form of alexia, associated with frontal lobe lesions, has now been described (Benson, 1977) in some patients with Broca's aphasia who also show difficulties with writing and spelling. They are reported to find letters relatively more difficult to read than words, and they have more problems with relational words (e.g., articles, prepositions, inflections) than with content words (substantive nouns, verbs, and adjectives) at the level of both reading and comprehension.

Reading disabilities will obviously depend on the structure of the written language. Hence the different patterns of impairment that result from the use of two scripts: ideographic and phonological (Asayama, 1914; Lyman *et al.*, 1938; Sasanuma, 1975). The nature of the disorder must also depend to some extent on the former skill and training of the patient (Bastian, 1898; Elder, 1900; Poppelreuter, 1917). Nevertheless, it appears possible to distinguish linguistic categories of error, with the implication that linguistically distinct aspects of words (such as their phonological, syntactic, and semantic features) may be differentially impaired and thus associated with functionally separable performance systems

(Marshall and Newcombe, 1973, 1977; Saffran and Marin, 1975; Shallice and Warrington, 1975). The suggestion is that these different patterns of reading disorder may require different remedial programs (Morton, 1977; Patterson, 1977) and might have a different prognosis. But this is work for the future.

"Pure" agraphia (agraphia without alexia) is a very rare phenomenon. Patients have significantly more difficulty with writing than with oral spelling and spelling with alphabetic blocks (Dubois *et al.*, 1969). The disorder has sometimes been associated with the three other left parietal symptoms of the so-called Gerstman's syndrome: dyscalculia, right-left disorientation, and loss of finger order sense; and it may be associated with apraxia and left-handedness (Hécaen *et al.*, 1963). A disproportionately severe disorder of syntactic writing has been reported in confusional cases (Ferguson and Boller, 1977).

Writing disorders associated with more generalized aphasic disturbance have been studied in terms of the semantic, motor, and spatial components that may be differentially affected according to the underlying pathology (Hécaen and Kremin, 1976). These analyses, interesting in their own right, may well have a bearing on retraining programs. But, once again, their relevance has not yet been fully explored and put to the test.

Disorders of Motor Control

There seems to be a clear functional and anatomical distinction among disorders affecting (1) hand movement and the use of tools, (2) dressing, and (3) construction.

Ideomotor and Ideational Apraxia. The incidence of ideomotor and ideational apraxia is difficult to gauge, partly because there are remarkably few studies of unselected populations and also because disorders of movement have not in the past been as carefully tested as disorders of language. In one important study of over 400 unselected cases of posterior lesions (Ajuriaguerra *et al.*, 1960), only 4% of patients with either unilateral or bilateral lesions were found to have ideational apraxia whereas no patients with right hemisphere lesions developed this symptom; these data, therefore, confirm earlier work indicating the important role of the left hemisphere in praxis (Liepmann, 1900). The term "ideational apraxia" is taken to mean a disturbance in the coordinated sequencing of move-ment of the kind required, for example, to use tools. It is far from clear whether this disorder is dissociable from the disorder of gesture and the ability to make hand movements to command, which has been labeled "ideomotor apraxia." What does seem clear is that these disorders are often associated with dysphasia, and there is some evidence to suggest that this association is more than coincidental. First, let us consider the additional evidence that the left hemisphere might have a special role in motor performance (Wyke, 1971).

Semmes *et al.,* (1960) reported that unilateral wounds of the left hemisphere produce bilateral sensory deficits. Studies of normal subjects (Kinsbourne and Cook, 1971; Lomas and Kimura, 1976) have shown significant interference effects if subjects had to speak while balancing a dowel on the right hand. Then patients with left hemisphere lesions were shown to be impaired in comparison with a comparable right hemisphere group on a task requiring them to make three hand movements in succession (Kimura and Archibald, 1974). The impairment could not be ascribed solely to the sequential aspect of the task; subjects were poor at making the movements *per se*.

One interpretation of the findings has been that the left hemisphere developed a special role in skilled motor activity before it became dominant for speech (Kimura, 1976). A somewhat different interpretation (Gazzaniga, 1970) is that the factors underlying the predominance of the left hemisphere in the mediation of speech may also determine its special role in the programming of motor activity. It is equally plausible to argue that skilled motor performance and speech developed in parallel, as man's upright posture liberated his hands for the use of tools and his mouth for expression (Paillard, 1960). Whichever biological speculation is advanced, the extensive representation of hand and mouth in adjacent areas of sensory and motor cortex in man makes it likely that central lesions will often damage both motor control and speech. Indeed, if we try to envisage the functional hierarchy involved in the initiation, programming, and control of motor activity, we may postulate generators of order and sequence that command both movement and speech (recent work by Cromer, 1977, is of interest in this context). Apart from the clinical coincidence of acquired aphasia and apraxia, there is also a suggestion that children with developmental language disorders may show a disability in the control of fine distal movements of the hand and an inability to reproduce rhythmic sequences (Kracke, 1975). But how often do we assess motor skills more than cursorily either in children or in adults? We do not know whether such disorders persist or to what extent they interfere with the requirements of daily living. We know that a stroke patient may have communication problems. But is he also more clumsy and less able to use tools and manipulate the familiar objects of daily living despite intact sensorimotor function?

DRESSING APRAXIA. It is at first sight puzzling that a lesion of the left hemisphere may provoke difficulty in organizing the sequence of movements required to imitate a salute or light a cigarette whereas a lesion in the right hemisphere may make it difficult for the patient to dress himself. All these activities undoubtedly require the initiation and programming of a complicated sequence of movements. However, it might be argued that dressing apraxia, found in 22% of patients with right post-Rolandic lesions (Hécaen, 1962), involves a number of spatial transformations, e.g., the positioning of the arms with relation to the sleeves of a jacket, that are not involved to such a degree in, for example, lighting a cigarette or saluting. Different limiting factors may clearly be involved: some but not all cases of dressing apraxia can be ascribed to unilateral spatial neglect (Hécaen, 1962; Critchley, 1969). The clinical course of this symptom is unknown, but it occurs mainly in patients for whom the long-term prognosis is poor. A high percentage of patients with dressing apraxia also show constructional defects: only four of the 51 cases of dressing apraxia reported by Ajuriaguerra *et al.*, (1960) did not also involve constructional apraxia.

CONSTRUCTIONAL APRAXIA. Attempts to understand the nature of the constructional deficits that follow cerebral lesions have reflected many of the problems inherent in the study of hemispheric organization and asymmetry. There is no doubt that these deficits, usually measured in tests of drawing and block design, often follow posterior lesions of either hemisphere. In Hécaen's (1962) large sample of patients with retro-Rolandic lesions, constructional apraxia was found in 62% and 40% of patients with lesions of the right and the left hemisphere, respectively. The interesting question has been to specify whether there are quantitative or qualitative differences in the performance of these two groups of patients (Warrington, 1969) that might have a bearing on diagnosis or retraining. In the search for the different limiting factors that determine the performance of these two groups, the notion recurs that the executive capacities of the left hemisphere and the visual-perceptual capacities of the right hemisphere are involved (Hécaen *et al.*, 1951; Duensing, 1953; McFie and Zangwill, 1960; Piercy *et al.*, 1960; Warrington *et al.*, 1966). However, attempts to implicate the planning abilities of the left hemisphere (Hécaen and Assal, 1970; Collignon and Rondeaux, 1974) have not yet been substantiated (Gainotti *et al.*, 1977*b*), whereas the role of unilateral spatial agnosia in the impaired performance of groups with right hemisphere lesions seems clear-cut (Oxbury *et al.*, 1974; Gainotti *et al.*, 1977*b*). It would appear, however, that unilateral neglect (as operationally defined) may disappear after 6 months (Campbell and Oxbury, 1976) so that much would depend on *how* and *when* the groups were tested relative to the onset of their illness.

Once again, we have no evidence of the natural history of these disorders. They were certainly infrequent as a persistent consequence of missile injury. In a sample of over 200 cases seen at follow-up some 25 years later, there were only a few cases where the symptom was pronounced. These cases, however, showed conclusively that the deficit can coexist with well-preserved intelligence and verbal memory. One 60-year-old subject obtained a degree in modern languages while working full time as a civil servant but was unable to make even a mediocre copy of a geometrical figure (Rey Osterrieth, Fig. 1). Another subject, trained to be a surgeon before his right parietal injury, resumed his profession to become a successful surgical consultant. His scores on standard constructional tasks were nevertheless remarkably low (e.g., WAIS Block Design Scale score of 8) in comparison with his excellent performance on verbal intelligence and memory tasks. He was fully aware of his residual deficits and had organized his professional work accordingly.

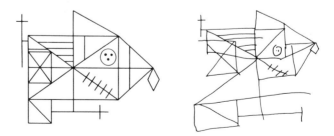

Fig. 1. Rey Osterrieth complex figure: the stimulus is on the left, the patient's copy on the right.

The perceptual deficits that follow damage to the brain are poorly understood. The visual modality has been more extensively studied than any other, but recent information indicates that even the basic question of defining the consequences of damage to the afferent visual pathway is more complex than had been supposed. The extent to which sensory disturbances affect performance on the more complex perceptual tasks is not entirely clear, and the number and generality of the terms used in the literature to describe the visuospatial disorders seen in patients with damage to the posterior part of the right hemisphere illustrate the difficulty experienced by the authors in pinpointing the nature of this deficit. Further, as with other behavioral disturbances, it is not always clear whether the perceptual deficits reported in the literature are seen only as symptoms of acute brain damage or whether they persist into the chronic phase.

DAMAGE TO THE AFFERENT VISUAL PATHWAY. Damage to the retinogeniculostriate pathway causes visual field defect, an area of elevated luminance threshold (Aulhorn and Harms, 1972), the location of which depends on the part of the visual pathway damaged. If the damage is severe enough, the threshold is raised to the point at which the patient appears to be blind in the area of the field defect. However, it now seems that "blindness" is an inadequate description of the state of vision even in dense field defects. The patient D. B. studied by Weiskrantz *et al.* (1974) and Sanders *et al.* (1974) had an almost complete left homonymous hemianopia following the surgical treatment of an angioma; this procedure presumably involved the removal of most of the striate cortex on the right side with relatively little extrastriate damage. Although D. B. had no awareness of "seeing" in his field defect, he could reach accurately for stimuli exposed in it. He could also differentiate between the letters "X" and "O" and between a grating and a homogeneous gray field such that the authors concluded that his visual acuity in the blind field was almost as good as in the symmetrical region in the good half-field. D. B. had begun to experience symptoms related to his angioma at the age of 14, some 20 years before his operation, but evidence for residual vision in scotomata, although less dramatic than that shown in D. B., has been demonstrated following lesions acquired in adulthood (Pöppel *et al.*, 1973). The neural basis of this residual capacity is not clear. The homonymous field defects have not been complete in the patients in whom it has been found, so it may depend on a spared area of striate cortex. Alternatively, sufficient information may reach the brain through a parallel pathway, or it may be that extrastriate damage, which is almost always present in occipital lesions in man, is a necessary condition for the appearance of a truly blind area of the visual field (see Weiskrantz *et al.*, 1974, for a further discussion of these possibilities). Whatever the explanation, it seems that dense visual field defects cannot always be regarded simply as areas of blindness, at least when they are caused by postgeniculate lesions (Perenin and Jeannerod, 1975).

The reverse picture, perceptual deficit in the presence of normal visual acuity and full visual fields, can be demonstrated in patients with damage to the pregeniculate part of the visual pathway. Halliday *et al.* (1972, 1973) reported that the visual evoked response was frequently delayed in patients with demyelinating disease affecting the optic nerves even when vision was apparently normal on conventional testing. Subsequent studies have revealed a perceptual correlate of this physiological phenomenon in cases with unilateral delay. A stimulus to the affected eye needs to be delivered earlier than one to the unaffected eye if the two are to appear simultaneous (Regan *et al.*, 1976). A binocularly viewed stimulus moving back and forth across the midline appears to move in an ellipse, its apparent distance decreasing when it moves toward the side of the affected eye and increasing when it moves toward the unaffected side, as in the Pulfrich phenomenon (Frisen *et al.* 1973; Rushton, 1975). The further finding that some of these patients have an impairment of color vision but not of luminance threshold (Asselman *et al.*, 1975) is not susceptible of so simple an explanation, although there appears to be an established physiological basis for such a dissociation (De Valois *et al.*, 1966; Wright and Ikeda, 1974).

Taken together, these results show that isolated aspects of visual perception may be differentially impaired by lesions quite early in the visual pathway and that alterations of perception in apparently complex tasks like the Pulfrich task may be caused by basic sensory changes. Damage to the visual pathway does not produce visual dysfunction in an all-or-none way.

The same is true for cerebral damage outside the visual pathway. We have reported the case of a patient who was unable to make use of color information following an attack of encephalitis (Newcombe and Ratcliff, 1975, Case 2; Mollon *et al.*, 1975), and Meadows's (1974) review of the literature on disturbance of color vision following cerebral lesions confirms the existence of achromatopsias which are not simply a symptom of a general reduction of visual efficiency. A further example is the defective visual localization reported by Ratcliff and Davies-Jones (1972) in patients with chronic penetrating missile wounds of the brain. The great majority of their patients with lesions involving the posterior part of either hemisphere were unable to reach accurately for a visual stimulus exposed in the half-field contralateral to the lesion. Some of these patients had field defects, usually in the lower quadrant, but the defective localization was clearly demonstrated in intact parts of the field and in patients with no field defect whatsoever. Most patients were unaware of their deficit and reported no difficulties in everyday life which seemed likely to be attributable to it. These findings, defective localization in subjectively and perimetrically normal parts of the field, are thus the reverse of those reported by Weiskrantz *et al.* (1974).

It is clear that a full visual field and normal visual acuity, even when assessed with relatively sophisticated testing methods, are no guarantee of normal visual function. Conversely, even a dense field defect does not imply complete blindness in the affected part of the field.

SENSORY DEFICITS AND COMPLEX PERCEPTUAL TASKS

There have been two main approaches to the question of whether poor performance on more complex perceptual tasks can be explained by sensory deficit. One is that exemplified by the work of Bay (1953), who argued on the basis of detailed studies of individual cases that all instances of higher-order disturbances of visual object recognition (visual agnosia) could be reduced to subtle visual field changes or to generalized intellectual deterioration. However, it seems unlikely that these changes are either a necessary or a sufficient condition for the occurrence of visual agnosia. We have seen a patient in whom no abnormality of visual sensory function could be demonstrated after exhaustive testing (Newcombe and Ratcliff, 1975, Case 1), and Ettlinger (1956) failed to demonstrate any significant relationship between the severity of sensory deficits of the kind described by Bay and the presence of visual spatial agnosia.

The other approach has been to consider whether the presence of obvious visual field defect is associated with impairment on a given perceptual or spatial test. This has been adopted by several authors, notably DeRenzi and his associates (Arrigoni and DeRenzi, 1964; DeRenzi and Spinnler, 1966a,b; DeRenzi and Faglioni, 1967; DeRenzi et al., 1968b, 1969, 1970, 1972; Faglioni et al., 1969) and the typical finding has been an interaction between presence of field defect and side of lesion, the group with right hemisphere lesion and visual field defect being most impaired. The most likely explanation for this result is that it is not the presence of a field defect *per se* which is important but that the lesions responsible for impairment in visuospatial tasks tend to be in a part of the right hemisphere, near the optic radiation, in which they are also likely to cause a field defect. There is evidence for this view: the association of field defect with impairment on some tactile tasks (DeRenzi and Scotti, 1969; DeRenzi et al., 1970) and the association of gross impairment of visual localization (Ratcliff and Davies-Jones, 1972) and visually guided maze learning (Newcombe and Russell, 1969) with upper but not lower quadrantic field defect, while the opposite pattern holds for Mooney's visual closure task (Newcombe and Russell, 1969). In fact, patients seem to adapt to homonymous hemianopia remarkably well when it is not complicated by perceptual deficits (Gassell and Williams, 1963a,b).

Nevertheless, there are some special circumstances in which visual field defect does seem to be the cause of perceptual impairment. Patients with bitemporal hemianopia following damage to the optic chiasm are blind beyond the fixation point because of overlap of the temporal field defects. This can lead to difficulty in tasks where depth perception and frequent changes of fixation between near and far objects are required. They may also experience the separation or overlapping of the two halves of the visual field, causing diplopia and the stretching or contraction of fixated objects, or the two halves may slide apart vertically (Kirkham, 1972; Ashworth, 1975). This presumably is a direct result of the field defects, because no part of the field is viewed binocularly.

One further possible cause of impairment in visuospatial tasks needs to be considered, although it is not strictly a sensory deficit. This is unilateral neglect. The argument advanced above in connection with visual field defect, that it is as common in patients with left hemisphere lesions as in those with right-sided damage, does not apply to neglect because, like visuospatial deficits, it is much commoner after right hemisphere lesions (Hécaen, 1969; Gloning et al., 1968). There is also evidence that patients with acute strokes who showed neglect in copying drawings were worse than other patients with right hemisphere damage in some other perceptual tasks (Oxbury *et al.*, 1974). However, this poor performance was still evident 6 months later when the neglect was considerably attenuated (Campbell and Oxbury, 1976). Typical perceptual and spatial deficits can also be demonstrated in patients with chronic missile wounds who show no measurable neglect (Newcombe, 1969; Newcombe and Russell, 1969; Ratcliff and Newcombe, 1973). While neglect is an obvious feature of the constructional performance of some patients with right hemisphere lesions, gross spatial distortions can be seen in parts of drawings where no elements have been omitted, in drawings which show no neglect at all, and in drawings in which the patient is working from information presumably available in memory before he acquired his cerebral lesion (e.g., see McFie *et al.*, 1950, Fig. 2).

Thus, while basic sensory disturbances and neglect may contribute to perceptual deficit and may even provide a complete explanation in individual cases, they seem to be neither a necessary nor a sufficient condition for its appearance.

CONTRIBUTION OF THE RIGHT HEMISPHERE

It is clear from a wealth of clinical and experimental evidence (recently reviewed by Oxbury, 1975) that visual perceptual deficits, when they cannot be explained by some underlying sensory change, are predominantly associated with damage to the right hemisphere. Therefore the right hemisphere presumably makes an important contribution to the analysis of complex perceptual material, but it is difficult to find a factor common to the tasks on which a right hemisphere deficit has been demonstrated that might provide a clue to the nature of this contribution.

The description "visual nonverbal tasks," besides being so general as to be of little value, would be inadequate on two grounds. First, the deficit is clearly not always limited to the visual modality. It has been demonstrated in tactile (Weinstein, 1962; Corkin, 1965; Reitan, 1964; DeRenzi *et al.*, 1968*a*) and auditory (Milner, 1962*a*) tasks, although the hemispheric asymmetry may be less marked in a tactile task than its visual equivalent (Ratcliff, 1970) and in individual cases may be present only in the visual modality (Gilliat and Pratt, 1952). Second, there have been studies investigating the discrimination of complex nonverbal shapes and patterns in which patients with left hemisphere damage were found to be as impaired as those with right hemisphere lesions (Ratcliff, 1970) or even to be significantly worse (Bisiach and Faglioni, 1974).

The label "spatial" has been applied to many tasks, and it does seem that patients with right hemisphere lesions have particular difficulty with the analysis of the spatial aspects of stimuli, but it is hard to characterize the difficulty more precisely. It is not simply an inability to locate individual points in space. Defective visual localization was neither more frequent nor more severe in the right hemisphere group in the study by Ratcliff and Davies-Jones (1972), and visual disorientation can be distinguished from the more common forms of spatial disorientation seen after damage to the right hemisphere (Benton, 1969). The deficit seems to consist more in an inability to appreciate the relative positions of stimuli or stimulus elements and to organize them into a coherent spatial framework. This is characteristic of the constructional performance of patients with right hemisphere lesions and could explain failure in some experimental tasks. Learning a stylus maze, for example, which in our laboratory is one of the tasks most sensitive to right posterior lesions (Newcombe, 1969; Newcombe and Russell, 1969; Ratcliff and Newcombe, 1973), requires that the subject learn to move in a particular direction at each choice point. To do so efficiently, he must know which choice point is which and how they are related to each other in space.

However, this description is also inadequate. The locomotor maze task—in which subjects are required to walk through a matrix of nine markers laid out on the floor of a large room along a path shown on a map that they carry with them— would also seem to require an ability to appreciate the relative positions of the markers. Yet this is a task on which a selective right hemisphere deficit has not been demonstrated. Semmes *et al.* (1955, 1963) found that patients with parietal lesions in either hemisphere were impaired, and Ratcliff and Newcombe (1973) found that only the patients with bilateral posterior lesions were significantly worse than control subjects. The nine markers used in the locomotor maze constitute a much simpler array than the 81 potential choice points in our stylus maze, and appreciation of the relative position of the markers may be sufficiently easy that it is not the factor which limits performance. In this task, unlike a stylus maze, the subject's position is constantly changing, and he must develop an absolute frame of reference instead of using his body or the maze edge (Orbach, 1959).

Just as there are studies which have used apparently spatial tasks without demonstrating a right hemisphere deficit, so there are tasks which are not obviously spatial with which such a deficit has been demonstrated. Most of these have used materials which are perceptually difficult—e.g., overlapping nonsense figures (Kimura, 1963), overlapping line drawings of objects and animals (DeRenzi and Spinnler, 1966*b*), the Mooney faces (Lansdell, 1968; Newcombe and Russell, 1969), the Gollin figures (Warrington and James, 1967*a*), the Street completion figures (DeRenzi and Spinnler, 1966*b*), letters written in unconventional script and crossed through (Faglioni *et al.*, 1969), and objects viewed from unusual angles (Warrington and Taylor, 1973). The perceptual difficulty was achieved in these studies by using particularly complex and unusual material, reducing the amount of information present, or adding irrelevant detail.

But a few studies have successfully demonstrated a right hemisphere deficit in tasks using simple material such as the matching of the slope of a line (Warrington and Rabin, 1970) or line length (Bisiach *et al.*, 1976) and the sorting of colors (DeRenzi *et al.*, 1972).

Finally, it should be mentioned that there is evidence that the right hemisphere may be involved in the processing of information about visual stimuli at a level which might be better described as cognitive than perceptual. Ratcliff (1978) showed his subjects schematic drawings of a manikin on which one of the hands was marked with a black disk (see Fig. 2). The manikin was exposed in one of four possible orientations (upright or inverted, front view or back view) which varied randomly from trial to trial. The subject's task was to say "right" or "left"

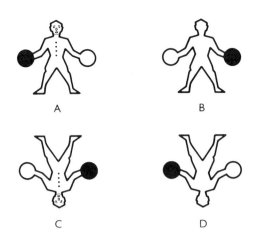

Fig. 2. Manikin task: stimuli.

depending on which hand was marked. The stimuli in the upright and inverted condition were identical apart from their orientation, yet the right posterior group was impaired relative to the left posterior group and control subjects on the inverted but not on the upright condition, where their performance was slightly better than that of men with left posterior lesions. Ratcliff interpreted these results as demonstrating a deficit, not in the perception of the stimuli, but in the performance of the mental rotation required to bring the inverted stimuli into a standard, familiar orientation prior to making the right/left judgment (Benson and Gedye, 1963).

There are thus grounds for saying that the deficits seen in patients with right hemisphere lesions are neither exclusively visual, exclusively spatial, nor perhaps even exclusively perceptual. In fact, it seems highly likely that the right hemisphere makes more than one kind of contribution in perceptual tasks, and there is evidence to suggest a different cerebral basis for at least two of these. The posterior temporal region near the parietotemporooccipital junction seems to be particularly important for the more complex perceptual tasks, while the parietal lobe is more involved in the appreciation of spatial relationships (Meier and French, 1965; Newcombe and Russell, 1969). It is also possible, of course, for patients to fail in perceptual or spatial tasks for reasons other than strictly perceptual deficit. Hence, Milner's reports of poor stylus maze learning in association with frontal and temporal lesions because of rule breaking and material-specific memory loss (Milner, 1965).

PERSISTENCE OF THE DEFICITS

Visual field defect, defective visual localization, and impairment on a spatial task (stylus maze), on a complex perceptual task (the Mooney faces), and on the manikin task described above have all been demonstrated in men with chronic missile wounds sustained 15–25 years before they were tested, and can confidently be described as long-term consequences of cerebral lesions. Unilateral neglect was not a feature of this patient group, and in Campbell and Oxbury's patients it had largely recovered 6 months after the date of the stroke. However, neglect has been reported to persist as long as 12 years (Zarit and Kahn, 1974). Delay of the visual evoked response and achromatopsia can also persist for several years. As far as we are aware, data are not available for the other deficits mentioned in this section.

MEMORY DISORDERS

The work of Milner (1958, 1966, 1968, 1970, 1973, 1975) and her colleagues at the Montreal Neurological Institute on the material-specific memory disorders associated with temporal lobe epilepsy and its surgical treatment has provided some of the most compelling evidence on hemispheric asymmetry. Briefly, these differences include the verbal memory deficits of the group with left temporal lobe lesions and the subtle impairments of visual recognition and recall of patients with right temporal lobe lesions. These differences are most striking postoperatively, but they persist. The verbal memory impairments, notable in formal testing on the delayed recall of narrative and paired associated words, are often reported by patients as difficulties in remembering fast speech, telephone messages, etc. (see also Meyer, 1959), whereas it is unlikely that the visual recognition deficits (evoked with some difficulty and often requiring a notable reduction of visual cue) have any impact on daily life except perhaps in a rare occupation demanding marked skills in pattern recognition.

Studies of the long-term consequences of temporal lobe epilepsy are not wholly consistent. One report (Blakemore and Falconer, 1967) suggested that the verbal learning deficit disappears 3–7 years postoperatively, and sooner rather than later in the case of young patients. Several factors may explain this discrepancy, including different surgical techniques and an important difference in the range of psychological testing (only the paired associate learning paradigm was used by the London group to probe for evidence of verbal memory loss).

If the deficit persists unchanged for many years, what contribution has the applied psychologist to make? What rules and strategies are available to minimize, if not bypass altogether, the practical consequences of a deficit of this kind? If Paivio (1971) is right in suggesting that there is an important alternative memory system using imagery (and there is pragmatic evidence for such a view in the place systems of the classical mnemonists), then perhaps the patient with a verbal memory deficit can exploit this strategy. There is some experimental support for this view (Jones, 1974; Richardson, 1975). As far as we know, however, this technique has not been tested in the setting of everyday life, using the plans and activities of domestic or professional life as the material to be remembered.

In contrast to these material-specific disorders are the global derangements of memory associated with bilateral brain damage. The famous case of H. M., first reported by Scoville and Milner (1957) and subsequently studied in considerable detail by Milner and her colleagues (Milner, 1962b, 1966, 1968, 1970; Milner *et al.*, 1968), dramatically illustrates the fact that global amnesia is more than the sum of the selective deficits associated with unilateral temporal lobe lesions. Few, if any, ongoing events can be recalled; and life has a dreamlike quality, according to patient H. M. and to one of the encephalitic patients described by Rose and Symonds (1960).

Such global disorders not secondary to a more generalized dementia have been found after mesial bitemporal lesions, herpes simplex encephalitis, and severe anoxic episodes (e.g., carbon monoxide poisoning, severe hemorrhage, attempted suicide by hanging). The prognosis is often grave and patients may eventually require institutional care (cf. Rose and Symonds, 1960). There has been little evidence of recovery in memory functions in published cases. Two young patients studied by Newcombe and Ratcliff (1975) showed the same severe impairment on memory tasks 5 years after the precipitating and presumptive encephalitic illness. In sheltered environments, however, they did learn a little. According to his foreman in a Remploy factory, it took M. S., then a young man in his 20s, about 18 months to learn the way from his bench to the washroom, and from his bench to the canteen; he could not take short cuts. He also acquired simple skills, e.g., using a machine to stamp press studs onto the narrow plaquet of childrens' jumpers and unpicking colored tacking threads from machine-made knitted clothing. In contrast to these skills, he was grossly impaired in formal tests of memory and construction (e.g., a WAIS Block Design raw score of 0) and was unable to select the odd man out from an array of three colored tokens. He could, however, detect differences in luminance; perhaps this explains his ability to unpick tacking threads and the surprising fact that his employers did not realize that he had color agnosia in addition to his other symptoms.

A young woman described in the same report (Newcombe and Ratcliff, 1975) was also able to make limited progress as a day patient in a hospital. Although grossly impaired on formal memory tasks and apt to forget examiners within minutes of a long interview, she did recall and recognize a social worker who spent many hours with her during her first 2 years as a hospital day patient (some 5 years after the illness). This definite albeit very limited improvement shown by two severely handicapped young patients interests us. We cannot explain it, but we note that it occurred in a sheltered, structured setting where the same therapists (professional or amateur) set the patient simple repetitive targets and supervised their performance from day to day. In this context, it is interesting that one patient learned a semiskilled motor task (a labeling machine requiring the use of a sensitive foot pedal and coordinated manual dexterity). She worked efficiently, producing over 5000 labeled swab tubes in a short working day. In contrast, she was unreliable at packing tasks, being apt to forget the position of individual items in the box, nor could she follow complicated knitting patterns, forgetting her place and forgetting to record at the end of each row. The relative preservation of motor skills and motor learning in cases of global amnesia (see also Milner, 1962b; Russell, 1966) could perhaps be fruitfully exploited in a rehabilitation setting. Patient supervision over a long period of time may nevertheless be essential.

The short-term prognosis is obviously less bleak for the transient global amnesias (Fisher and Adams, 1944; Symonds, 1966; Mumenthaler and von Roll, 1969; Benson et al., 1974) that occur mainly in elderly patients and are probably attributable to ischemic vascular lesions. In these cases, the patient may have a dense amnesia for a few hours of his life and then regain his normal competence. Reversible amnesias may also be found in conjunction with tumors of the third ventricle. We have studied one case of a middle-aged man with a colloid cyst of the third ventricle. He had a series of four operations (including the insertion of a ventricular-atrial shunt) for a recurrence of the condition and, until the last operation, recovered his memory functions and was able to resume work as an accountant. After the fourth operation, however, he remained amnesic, and became uncharacteristically lethargic and slovenly in personal appearance, an irreversible change attributed to damage to the fornix in the final operation.

The diagnosis of global amnesia is usually limited to those cases in which the disorder is not secondary to dementia. Luria (1976) now suggests that at least three different patterns of memory disorder can be observed: relatively pure memory impairments associated with cortical lesions or ventricular tumors, amnesias accompanied by disorders of orientation and seen in conjunction with thalamic lesions, and, finally, gross disturbances of memory, orientation, and personality found in patients with lesions involving the thalamus and the frontal lobes. Here the prognosis is obviously related to the etiology, but we are not aware of any studies that give relevant information in this context. Again, the need is for a precise definition of the nature and extent of disordered function, and the changes occurring with time and remedial intervention.

Deficits Associated with Frontal Lobe Lesions

It is still possible to see a patient with a large frontal lobe lesion whose impairments on standard cognitive tasks are minimal. There are, nevertheless, changes in behavior: lethargy, disinhibition, and fatuousness—a pattern more readily featured in clinical anecdote than demonstrated by quantitative test, and one often associated with orbital lesions. Neuropsychologists have tended to avoid this area of affective change. Reputable experimental paradigms are not available, and the problems of designing them require either more imagination or more interest than has been available (see Damasio, 1978, for a comprehensive review).

The few positive findings with cognitive tasks have demonstrated the perseverative trend and sluggishness in shifting from one alternative to another in a systematic fashion (Milner, 1964; Drewe, 1974) and difficulty with the well-known Stroop Task, interpreted by Perret (1974) as a problem in disregarding the familiar aspect of the stimulus when the unfamiliar one requires attention. Deficits in a certain type of verbal fluency task, in which patients have to produce words beginning with a different letter, have been found consistently (Rylander, 1948; Milner, 1964; Benton, 1968), and an ingenious, nonverbal design fluency task (Jones-Gottman and Milner, 1977) in which the subject has to create new forms rather than rely on familiar, well-practiced skills has brought out a marked right frontal deficit. Intriguing also are the data suggesting highly specific deficits in tasks requiring judgments of recency (Corsi, 1971) and estimates of size and quantity (Stevenson, 1977) whereas performance on conventional memory tasks is unimpaired. These fragments are part of a complex pattern that must one day account for the failure of the frontal lobe patient to sample the external world appropriately, to plan his performance with regard to the structure and demands of this world, to monitor his performance, and, finally, to regulate it in response to the changing environment. Clinicians have for a long time suggested that the expansion of the frontal lobe in man implies its important role in regulating and controlling social behavior (Russell, 1948). However, this hypothesis has not been systematically examined in man, and has been described in only a few patients with massive lesions (Luria, 1966) or bilateral lesions undercutting the cortex (Jarvie, 1960). Such changes can nevertheless have important consequences for long-term adjustment. Luria (1963) has commented on the poor prognosis of frontal patients compared with those with more posterior lesions; he has described patients sawing through the wood of a bench and continuing to use a sewing machine after the thread had been used up. These are gross failures observed in a handful of patients. Milder forms of such inappropriate behavior could still be a hazard in working life, although they might not be readily detectable on standard tests.

Deficits Associated with Bilateral Lesions

The interesting question about bilateral lesions is whether or not they "may entail more than a mere arithmetical doubling of the effects of a unilateral lesion" (Critchley, 1953). A positive answer to the question has been suggested on clinical grounds (Humphrey and Zangwill, 1952; Cogan, 1965) and convincingly demonstrated insofar as the global memory deficits following bilateral temporal lobe resection are concerned. But data are sparse, the problem of equating the groups for severity of damage is obvious, and on anatomical grounds alone a bilateral lesion can hardly be regarded as the sum of two discrete lesions.

One of Benton's (1968) many pioneering studies, however, does show that there is more than one answer to the question raised: on some tasks for which we may assume a strong degree of hemispheric specialization, patients with bilateral frontal lesions did no worse than those with unilateral frontal lesions, and bilateral patients were no worse than the impaired left frontal patients at fluency tasks and no worse than the impaired right frontal patients on tasks of design copy and

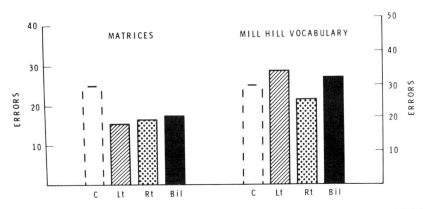

Fig. 3. Raven's Progressive Matrices and Mill Hill Vocabulary Scale: performance of men with left (Lt), right (Rt), and bilateral (Bil) gunshot wounds of the brain. The control (C) scores are derived from the standardization data.

three-dimensional construction. Benton's bilateral group was selectively impaired on tasks of time orientation and proverbs.

We addressed ourselves to this question when comparing the performance of ex-servicemen with unilateral and bilateral gunshot wounds of the brain. This population of men with stable focal lesions is particularly appropriate: they are well-matched for etiology of lesion, age when injured, interval between injury and testing, and well-preserved general intelligence (see Fig. 3).

Our comparison of the two groups showed at least three different patterns of impairment: (1) deficits that did not exceed those selectively associated with damage to either hemisphere, thus suggesting a strong degree of hemispheric specialization of function; (2) deficits exceeding those shown after unilateral injury that implied a functional contribution from both hemispheres; and (3) specific deficits that were not detected in the unilateral groups. The first pattern was clear-cut in nonsense-syllable learning and visually guided maze-learning tasks on which strong hemisphere effects would have been predicted (see Fig. 4). The tasks on which the deficits of the bilateral group exceeded those shown after unilateral injury included visual recognition tasks (see Figs. 5 and 6).

The most interesting finding from our point of view was the evidence of selective bilateral deficit demonstrated on a locomotor maze task (see Fig. 7 and Semmes *et al.*, 1955, 1963): there was virtually no overlap between the bilateral and unilateral groups, whereas on the stylus-maze task (see Fig. 8) the bilateral group had been no more impaired than the group with right posterior lesions (Fig. 9).

What are the limiting factors in the two tasks that could account for these clear-cut differences, or what additional variables in the locomotor maze task could underlie the bilateral deficit? The stylus maze requires the subject to recall and learn a sequence of movements in a fixed, two-dimensional spatial array. On the locomotor maze task, we have suggested that the subject's changing orientation

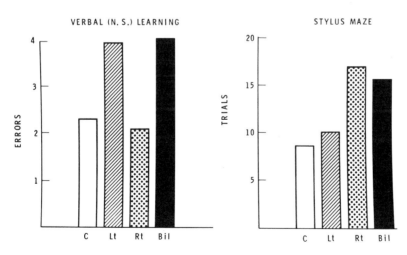

Fig. 4. Performance of men with gunshot wounds of the brain on two tasks showing a strong hemisphere effect. In neither case is the performance of the bilateral group worse than that of the more impaired unilateral group.

FREDA NEWCOMBE
AND GRAHAM
RATCLIFF

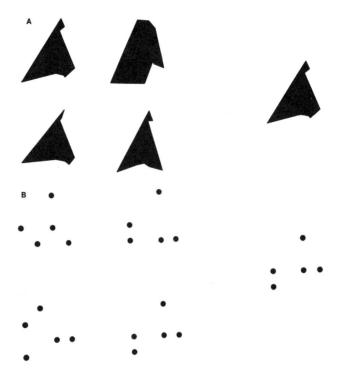

Fig. 5. Visual recognition tasks. Examples of stimuli: (A) contours and (B) dots. In each case, the target (shown on the right) was presented to the subject for approximately 2 sec. Immediately after its removal, he was required to select an identical figure from an array of four (as shown on the left of the figure).

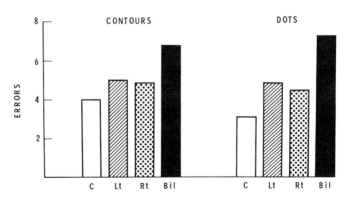

Fig. 6. Performance of men with gunshot wounds of the brain on two tasks in which patients with lesions in either hemisphere are equally impaired. The deficit in the bilateral group is significantly greater than that of either unilateral group.

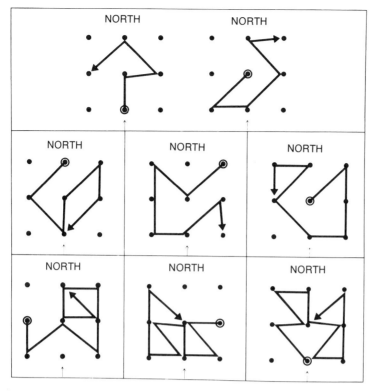

Fig. 7. Locomotor maze paths. The patient was required to walk through a matrix of nine markers laid out on the floor of a large room along the path shown on a map which he carried with him. The top two paths were used for practice.

requires an absolute frame of reference. This framework, ingeniously studied in taxi drivers learning their way in an unfamiliar town (Pailhous, 1970), may depend on a functional contribution from two hemispheres. It has in fact been suggested that their contribution may be qualitatively different (Young, 1962).

We also found that the bilateral group was significantly slower, although not necessarily less accurate, than the unilateral group on two tasks on which latencies were systematically recorded (see Figs. 10 and 11): object naming (Newcombe *et al.*, 1971) and right-left judgments on an inverted manikin (Ratcliff, 1970). Are these increased latencies characteristic of bilateral lesions? We suspect that this may be so.

DIFFUSE BRAIN DAMAGE

CLOSED HEAD INJURY

The long-term consequences of closed head injury have not been systematically studied by neuropsychologists during the past two decades, despite the relentless stream of road traffic accidents that involve mainly young people and account for 30% of admissions to hospitals for head injury (Field, 1976). It has

FREDA NEWCOMBE
AND GRAHAM
RATCLIFF

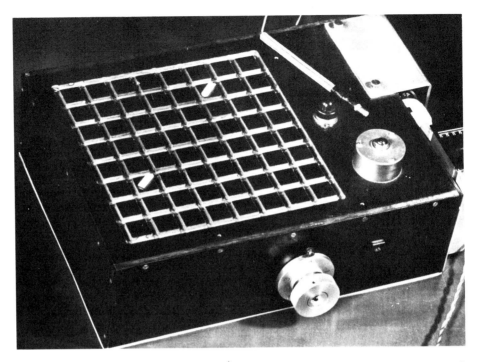

Fig. 8. Visually guided stylus-maze task. The patient was required to learn to criterion (three successive error-free trials) a ten-choice-point path that was demonstrated once by the examiner.

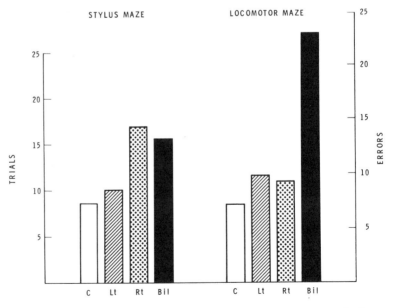

Fig. 9. Contrasting patterns of impairment of men with gunshot wounds of the brain on two maze tasks. On the locomotor maze task the bilateral group is grossly impaired, whereas neither unilateral group is significantly worse than the control group.

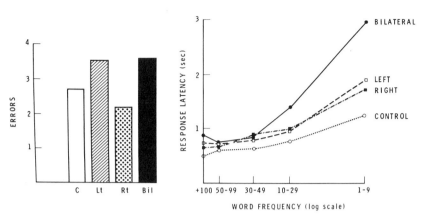

Fig. 10. Contrast between error score and latency as measures of efficiency in an object-naming task. The bilateral group differs from the left hemisphere group in speed but not in accuracy.

been estimated (London, 1967) that head injury results in approximately 1000 seriously handicapped patients in Britain each year, of whom half will never work again. Jennett (1975) has pointed out that earlier reports (MacIver *et al.*, 1958) were overoptimstic about the outcome for patients who made a good physical recovery after severe brain damage. Their optimism may have been based on recovery from dysphasia and spasticity (Miller and Stern, 1965; Najenson *et al.*, 1974; Gjone *et al.*, 1972; Westropp, 1970). Some of the physical sequelae, however, are not negligible and may have distressing consequences: slurred and monotonous speech may persist as an important social and occupational handicap.

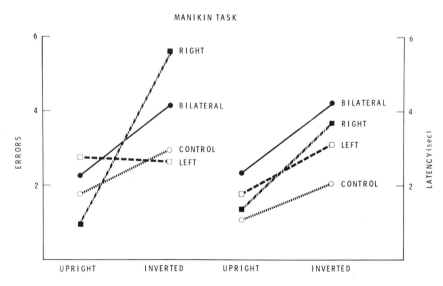

Fig. 11. Contrast between error score and latency as measures of efficiency in the manikin task. The bilateral group is slower to respond than the other groups but is not significantly less accurate.

Considerable progress has been made in developing quantitative scales to assess severity of head injury (Jennett, 1976), and the use of the Glasgow Coma Scale (Teasdale and Jennett, 1974) has produced remarkably similar patterns of severity of injury and final outcome in the large populations that have been included in a collaborative neurosurgical research program in Glasgow, Los Angeles, and Rotterdam. Those patients who have a coma of 6 hr or more achieve most of their physical recovery within 6 months; this improvement can be defined in terms of a change to the next category in a five-category outcome scale (Jennett and Bond, 1975). Clinical measures of the severity of injury encompass both diffuse (e.g., duration of coma and posttraumatic amnesia) and focal (e.g., disorders of the central nervous sytem) signs, but the so-called focal signs do not reliably indicate the presence of hematoma. Neither will a CT scan necessarily localize focal brain damage in these cases, but it may be informative regarding edema and hemorrhage.

The most widely used index of severity has been the duration of posttraumatic amnesia (PTA). This criterion, when used consistently by experienced clinicians observing patients on a day-to-day basis, shows a positive relationship with such objective measures of outcome as length of hospitalization and fitness for return to work (Russell, 1971). More recent follow-up data of 121 patients from a rehabilitation unit whose physical status and recovery in terms of capacity for independent living were carefully measured shows that a posttraumatic amnesia of more than 2 months and a duration of unconsciousness of more than 2 weeks are rarely associated with a return to fully independent living (Evans *et al.*, 1977). Nevertheless, there have been patients who achieved independent status even after 8 weeks of unconsciousness (London, 1967). Nineteen of 102 patients (studied by Lewin, 1967) who had been unconscious for more than a month returned to their former work or scholastic level, and 28 of the 92 seriously injured patients followed by Miller and Stern (1965) for over 11 years returned to work, 16 without loss of status. Clinicians concerned with the medical, counseling, and legal needs of the patient need precise criteria of severity of injury, and it is possible that further refinements can be achieved, e.g., a quantification of structural damage based on serial recordings of antigens to brain protein (Jennett, 1977) and biomathematical tools taking into account the combined effect of such predictive variables as length of unconsciousness and duration of posttraumatic amnesia.

Psychosocial changes are usually more of a subjective burden to the severely brain-damaged patient and his relatives than physical disability. An extensive study by Bond (1975) has shown that disorders of memory and personality significantly affected capacity for work and social relations and all patients with an amnesia that lasted 3–4 weeks showed some degree of mental, physical, and social handicap.

Neuropsychological work has traditionally addressed the problem of memory in closed head injury (cf. a provocative and informative review by Schacter and Crovitz, 1977). Memory deficits have consistently been found in patients with moderate and severe head injury (e.g., Richardson, 1963; Brooks, 1972; Fodor, 1972; Hannay *et al.*, 1977; Oddy, 1977), and they may persist for months and even years (Smith, 1974; Brooks, 1975). In contrast, children appear to be remarkably resilient, according to their performance on a carefully designed set of memory tasks (Chadwick, 1977). There is evidence, however, from a sample of over 100 head-injured children of impairment on an experimental word-learning task (White, 1976).

A close relationship between extent of memory deficit and severity of injury (assessed by duration of PTA) has usually been found (Russell and Smith, 1961; Norrman and Svahn, 1961; Russell, 1971; Martinius, 1977). The one study that has not replicated this finding (Smith, 1974) was carried out some three decades after injury, and the time factor may have influenced both the reconstruction of events and the outcome. Unpublished data from this laboratory show a clear-cut and persistent decrement in memory with a PTA of more than 3 weeks. In our opinion, it is unrewarding to try to unravel these discrepancies; the need is for prospective studies, using more precise and quantitative estimates of severity (including duration of unconsciousness and PTA and neurological evidence of CNS damage) and tasks that throw more light on the nature of the mnestic disturbance. In addition, recent studies carried out in laboratories in Groningen and Oxford have shown that tasks requiring serial recall of lists of unrelated words are more sensitive than conventional memory tests to the impairment found in head-injured patients (see also White, 1976). While no correlation was found between subjective complaint and performance in such tasks, there was a positive correlation between scores on such tasks and functional recovery as measured by return to work (Deelman, 1977). There was also a trend for head-injured subjects to produce intrusions from lists other than the one most recently presented, a phenomenon of interest in relation to Huppert and Piercy's (1976) studies of amnesia and location in context (Deelman, 1977). Applied research in this area will presumably develop as some of the current theoretical issues are clarified, for example, hypotheses invoking problems of decision making (Brooks, 1974a), encoding (Cermak and Butters, 1972; Cermak and Moreines, 1974), and retrieval (Warrington and Weiskrantz, 1970, 1971).

Impairment of sustained attention and speed of performance have also been well documented in cases of head injury (Conkey, 1938; Goldstein, 1942; Ruesch and Moore, 1943; Zangwill, 1976). Goldstein (1944) stressed that his patients took "much longer to react" and that the long repetitive tasks he used (reaction time tasks, continuous addition, and tests of motor power) gave "insight into . . . behavior . . . during continuous (sic) activity." Subsequent neuropsychological studies of simple and choice reaction time in patients with closed head injury show a marked deficit in choice reaction time (Norrman and Svahn, 1961; Miller, 1970; van Zomeren and Deelman, 1976) that may persist for at least 2 years (van Zomeren, 1977).

The question then arises as to whether mild cases of concussion show slight deficits, transient or permanent, of the same nature. A well-documented study (Gronwall and Sampson, 1974) suggests that this may indeed be the case. Impairment of performance in a paced serial addition task was shown in head-injured patients several weeks after they were clinically discharged as fit for work. On this basis, it has been suggested that at least some aspects of the so-called postconcussional syndrome may have a physiological basis that affects the information-processing capacity of the patient. Symptoms such as headache, dizziness, irritability, and inability to concentrate found in relatively mild cases of head injury have often been ascribed to pretraumatic personality and the pressure of compensation claims (Miller, 1966) or regarded as a posttraumatic neurosis (Lidvall *et al.*, 1974). According to Russell (1974), these symptoms have a definite physiological basis and may be averted by early and skillful rehabilitation. Financial gain is not a necessary condition for their development: they can be observed in cases where there is no compensation element (Merskey and Woodforde, 1972) and also in cases of severe disability where they are apparently unrelated to gainful employment (Dresser *et al.*, 1973). Much work requires to be done to specify what kind of cognitive and other deficits may follow relatively mild head injury. Preliminary work in this laboratory suggests that slight but significant changes may be found in tasks requiring the patient to keep track of several variables or perform relatively complicated tasks simultaneously (Saan and Thomas, 1977). Current research aims are to trace the pattern of performance in groups of patients with more severe injuries.

The disturbing behavioral changes that may follow severe head injury have been the subject of detailed clinical appraisal (Caveness and Walker, 1966; Lishman, 1973; Najenson *et al.*, 1974; Thomsen, 1974): sluggishness, irritability, emotional lability, and disturbance in patterns of feeding and sleeping have been observed, with particular reference to hypothalamic and basal brain injury (Sweet *et al.*, 1969), and depression has often been described, sometimes "emerging in a phase of partial recovery" (Merskey and Woodforde, 1972), perhaps partially attributable to increasing insight into disability. These symptoms may sometimes require psychiatric help, and it would seem appropriate to involve psychiatric outpatient clinics, especially when these clinics are attached to a general hospital or to a neurosurgical and accident service clinic.

Attempts to modify some of the behavior disturbances seen after severe head injury using operant conditioning or other techniques of behavior therapy are still in the experimental stage. A large percentage of patients, however, manage to contain what might be regarded as subclinical symptoms without psychiatric help. Oddy's (1977) study of psychosocial recovery in 54 young adults, all of whom had been unconscious for at least 24 hr immediately after the accident, included a problem checklist* with symptoms such as memory difficulties, irritability, fatigue, restlessness, and boredom. Patients and relatives independently compared pretraumatic and posttraumatic behavior. Only 20% of the patients were symptom free. Nevertheless, half of the patients had returned to full-time work for at least 2 months prior to the 6-month follow-up.

Regarding prognosis, certain general guidelines can be suggested. On the whole, the prognosis for children (for whom closed head injury accounts for about a third of general surgical admissions) is good (Jennett, 1972). One study (Flach

---

*A problem checklist of this kind is more appropriate for this population than scales designed exclusively for psychiatric and especially psychotic populations; these scales are seldom free from response bias.

and Malmros, 1972) did not detect a single case of so-called minimal brain damage, and other workers (Black, *et al.*, 1969) reported that 69% of their sample were asymptomatic, although 22% showed some behavioral disturbances such as regression, hypokinesis, and eating and sleeping problems. Behavioral rather than cognitive disturbances tend to occur after severe brain injury in children, but they are not an invariable consequence of brain damage and do not figure significantly in Chadwick's (1977) recent survey. Similarly, a better prognosis is suggested for young adults than for old patients (Brooks, 1974*b*). The prognosis tends to be less favorable when there are persistent brain stem defects (Levin *et al.*, 1976), and one detailed study of persistent anterograde amnesia in a patient with a midbrain lesion emphasizes the disabling consequences of damage to these structures (Teuber, 1969).

There is much more practical experience of rehabilitation than has ever been systematically recorded or reported (but see Walker *et al.*, 1969, and papers in the *Scandinavian Journal of Rehabilitation Medicine* that reflect special interest and skills in this area of medicine). In this context, it is interesting that one of the first studies of the potential of biofeedback techniques for neuromuscular disabilities (with a large sample of stroke patients and a well-matched control group) is in progress (Inglis, 1977). An analogous study of the power of remedial techniques for the physical and mental handicaps of the severely disabled victims of closed head injury is long overdue. Experts stress the need for early and regular contact with the patient, for whom explanation and reassurance is vital at that stage (Höök, 1969). Activity should be carefully graded and realistic targets chosen so that the patient gains confidence as he progresses. Memory problems have to be defined and remedial exercises devised accordingly. Regular, short training with a structured consistent timetable may help. Some patients with severe memory problems can be trained to use a central notice board at home (in the hall or kitchen where all members of the family write their messages). Alarm watches can be useful. In a good environment, even the most severely handicapped patient may continue to make progress years after injury, and increasing stability in work patterns have been found with increasing age (Dresser *et al.*, 1973)

DEMENTIA

The proportion of the population over 65 years of age is approximately 13% and may rise. It has been estimated that 6–10% of this population suffer from dementia (Pearce and Miller, 1973; Juel-Nielsen, 1975), of whom half are severely deteriorated; and the proportion of demented patients rises to about one in five in the group over the age of 80. A wide variety of psychological and intellectual changes are concealed by this overinclusive diagnostic label; disorientation, impaired memory, and deteriorated personal grooming are prominent features. But the course and outcome obviously depend on the etiology of the condition.

Some of these conditions are reversible. Therefore, there is a need to screen elderly confused patients. Dementia is sometimes associated with intrinsic tumors of the brain; in these cases, the prognosis will be determined and limited by the nature of the tumor and its location. More often, it is due to neuronal loss accompanied by glial proliferation and amyloid plaques. Apart from the relatively small group of patients with advanced neurosyphilis, these primary dementias are classified in two groups, Alzheimer's disease and Pick's disease, of which the former is more common. Alzheimer's disease implies generalized atrophy said to be more marked in the parietal region and in the dominant hemisphere, but this might reflect the verbal nature of tasks used to assess intellectual performance in this condition. Pick's disease is characterized by more focal cortical atrophy, involving in particular the frontal lobes. The differential diagnosis can be achieved by air encephalogram, but clinicians suggest that there is little to be gained by this invasive technique since it does not imply specific treatment or predict the rate of deterioration in an individual case (Matthews and Miller, 1972). In these diseases, therefore, neuropsychological assessment may be useful. Of more value, probably, is an attempt to modify the environment of the patient and his responses to it. The other broad group of primary dementias are attributable to multiple infarcts, usually including occlusion of the left internal carotid artery. It has been reported that the level of cognitive performance differs in the Alzheimer and vascular groups, but sampling bias is a confounding factor (Perez *et al.,* 1976).

On the face of it, the prognosis for the primary dementias must be regarded as poor. The condition has attracted little in the way of research interest, and where palliative measures have been tried in an institutional setting, there have seldom been adequate control studies. More promising remedial measures, both pharmacological and environmental, have been reviewed by Miller (1977), who selects reality orientation (Taulbee and Folsom, 1966), behavior modification (Libb and Clements, 1969), and the use of ergonomic techniques (Lindsley, 1964) to assist with the management of the demented patient. One multidisciplinary study (Brody *et al.,* 1971, 1974) of two matched groups of elderly female patients suggested that specially designed remedial programs produced a significant advantage in favor of the experimental group at the end of a year. After a further 9-month period, however, these gains had disappeared: suggestive evidence that remedial attempts to slow down the process of deterioration must be sustained.

DISCUSSION

CONCEPTUAL FRAMEWORK

Predictions regarding the outcome of brain damage require adequate models of human performance, and these are not yet available for clinical research or practice. In the meantime, hemispheric asymmetry has provided a useful if limited framework when it is flexible enough to deal with processes rather than states. One of the most intriguing of the unsolved problems concerns the true nature and extent of left hemisphere "dominance." Is the dominant hemisphere "leading even for intelligence" (Brown-Séquard, 1874; DeRenzi and Faglioni, 1965; DeRenzi *et al.,* 1966)? Does the right hemisphere play a crucial role in spatial thinking (Lhermitte *et al.,* 1928; Lange, 1936), as evidence from pathology suggests (McFie *et al.,* 1950; Ratcliff, 1978)? Despite the semantic overtones, these questions have practical relevance; the chances of a return to pretraumatic level of intellectual activity may vary accordingly for the lexicographer, the crystallographer, and the specialist in projective geometry.

In addition, there are a number of findings that do not fit so neatly into the putative dichotomy between verbal and nonverbal skills; nonverbal deficits may occur after left hemisphere lesions (Teuber and Weinstein, 1956; Russo and Vignolo, 1967; Orgass *et al.*, 1972; Masure and Tzavaras, 1976). Netley (1966) was one of the first workers to emphasize differences of strategy rather than level of performance in such patient groups. The importance of this approach has been well illustrated in subsequent experimental work: changes in task material for recognition of letters (Faglioni *et al.*, 1969), line orientation (Umiltà *et al.*, 1974), and color (DeRenzi and Spinnler, 1967) produce changes in strategy and hence in pattern of hemispheric involvement. Thus predictions as to what a patient can or cannot do may depend more on the strategies he can exploit than on the ostensible verbal or nonverbal label of the task. In turn, predictions require a more flexible model of hemispheric asymmetry that incorporates a notion of shared function and attempts to define the quantitative and qualitative contributions of the two hemispheres (Bradshaw *et al.*, 1977).

Moreover, we need to incorporate a theory of individual differences to account for the effects of injury (Marshall, 1973). There is certainly anatomical evidence of a "remarkable degree of variation from brain to brain" (Geschwind, 1974). Furthermore, the age at which the brain is damaged will be a crucial factor. Deficits must be related to myelogenetic development (Jacobson, 1975; Lecours, 1975; Yakovlev and Lecours, 1967) and stages in the acquisition of cognitive skills (Kohn and Dennis, 1974). The pattern of deficit will be a function of this inbuilt developmental program and its experience of the environment. Physiological research has yielded clear-cut evidence of the importance of these ontogenetic factors (cf. Goldman's, 1972, 1974, meticulous studies of the contrasting effects of dorsal and orbital frontal lesions in infant monkeys). Such precision is hard to achieve in mapping the consequences of pathological brain lesions in man. Consider the discrepancies in studies of language development in children with early brain lesions. Vocabulary tends to be impaired regardless of laterality of lesion (McFie, 1961), although recovery may be rapid (Basser, 1962). Alternately, language tends to be spared after early lesions of the left hemisphere (Lenneberg, 1967; Woods and Teuber, 1973). These conflicting views may be accommodated by taking into account the type of lesion (a hemispherectomy is hardly comparable with a relatively circumscribed unilateral lesion), the age at onset, the maturational status of the brain, and the aspects of language that are tested (cf. Smith, 1972, who has distinguished between the development or improvement of comprehension and expression after hemispherectomy but not of reading or writing). What does seem clear is that destruction of the traditional speech areas (Penfield and Roberts, 1959) in early childhood may result in right hemisphere or (occasionally) bilateral speech representation but that "there is always an intellectual price to pay for such plasticity" (Milner, 1973). Regarding acquired aphasia, different patterns of language disturbance follow early and late lesions: children with acquired aphasia seldom produce phonemic and semantic paraphasias, and 24 of the 32 children studied for up to a year by Alajouanine and Lhermitte (1965) reached a normal or near-normal level of performance in language tasks, although their educational achievements were limited. A similar picture was described by Byers and McLean (1962): recovery from aphasia but a decline in school performance.

The evidence for plasticity in brain organization in early childhood has its counterpart in resilience to the effects of severe deprivation during early years (Clarke and Clarke, 1976). The plasticity of the brain diminishes in time as functional specialization develops (Brown and Jaffe, 1975). Nevertheless, the young adult still has a better prognosis than the older patient in at least two different populations: wartime missile injuries (Teuber, 1975) and closed head injury (Brooks, 1976).

SEVERITY OF LESION AS A PROGNOSTIC FACTOR

The lack of precise definition or quantitative measurement must inhibit lengthy discussion of the relationship between extent of tissue destruction or damage and psychological sequelae. A strong version of Lashley's (1938) mass-action hypothesis is difficult to sustain unless very gross and selected comparisons are made. The hypothesis was not borne out by an attempt to relate size of lesion (as estimated by the neurologist on the basis of skull X-rays and surgical reports) and cognitive deficit in a population of ex-servicemen examined 25 years after unilateral missile injury (Newcombe, 1969). In a more heterogenous group of patients with cerebrovascular and space-occupying lesions, the picture could be different: a current study relating psychological sequelae and CT scan data will be informative (Vignolo, 1977). Although mass effects have not been readily demonstrated by the type of neuropsychological examination that has been fashionable, they may well affect some aspects of performance. This possibility is implied in an interesting discussion by Pillon and Lhermitte (1974) of the retardation shown by adult patients with cerebrovascular lesions or lesions due to neoplasm and trauma. Discussing the problem of fatigue, measurable only when the rate of stimulus presentation was increased, they commented: *"on a alors tendance a parler de fatigue, alors qu'il s'agit plutôt d'un abaissement des capacités fonctionnelles des réseaux physiologiquement altérés."* They regarded speed as a high-level physiological activity, a comparatively late acquisition, and one of the first changed by damage to the central nervous system.

Severity of lesion can also be translated in terms of depth of lesion. This factor was shown to be significantly related to employment status in a large group of war veterans and to be more important than site of impact in reducing the prospects of vocational rehabilitation (Dresser *et al.*, 1973). In the United Kingdom sample of ex-servicemen (Newcombe, 1969), there was a significant association between depth of injury and persistent dysphasia, a phenomenon invoked by Head (1926) to account for the persistence of dysphasia in civilian patients with cerebrovascular disease. The importance of subcortical systems and their integrative function in the use of language have been emphasized (Penfield and Roberts, 1959; Botez, 1962) if not thoroughly explored. There is evidence, however, of cognitive, linguistic, and learning deficits associated with thalamic lesions (Perret *et al.*, 1969;

Brown, 1975; Vilkki and Laitinen, 1976); and language deficits, both receptive and expressive, have been found up to 18 months after ventrolateral thalamotomy whereas no linguistic impairment was found after the larger lesion created by stereotactic pulvinotomy (Vilkki and Laitinen, 1976).

Extent of tissue destruction and depth of lesion can rarely be considered in isolation from such factors as etiology, age, IQ and cognitive habit, and neurological status. Even so, these variables may fail to account for the severity and persistence of rare disorders such as pure alexia and prosopagnosia. In some cases, we may have to take into account the possible significance of callosal lesions. In an elegant analysis of prosopagnosia, Meadows (1974) has considered a different mechanism: a particularly discrete right occipitotemporal lesion may produce negative or degraded information that results in failure to recognize faces, whereas a larger lesion (of the type occurring with right posterior cerebral artery occlusion) would put the right hemisphere mechanism out of action so that identification could be correctly made by the left hemisphere. Thus the predictive formulas that may be appropriate for trauma cases do not necessarily apply to those of vascular origin.

PSYCHOMETRIC APPROACH

Conventional psychometry is as limited and sometimes as inappropriate as that ludicrous noun—"psychometry"—suggests. The credibility gaps are all too patent. Among the victims of road traffic accident studied in this laboratory was a young woman physician whose period of unconsciousness had lasted for several weeks after the accident. A few months later, she obtained a score in the top fifth percentile on a widely used intelligence test. At that time, she was lethargic, labile, slovenly about personal grooming, and unable to run her home. Similarly, two young encephalitic patients with average intelligence quotients had disorders of memory and object recognition of such severity that they could survive only in sheltered environments. An IQ is virtually irrelevant in these cases other than to show that the disorders are not secondary to generalized intellectual deterioration. The explanation may lie in the relative imperviousness of familiar, well-practiced skills to brain injury. If, as Hebb (1942) has proposed, there are two factors involved in test performance, present intellectual power ("reasoning") and lasting changes of perceptual organization and behavior ("skill"), then we may suppose that many standard intelligence tests are tapping the latter rather than the former aspect of intellectual functioning, whereas intelligent, adaptive, behavior in the real world will require both aspects of cognition. Overlearned, well-practiced skills, such as vocabulary and the understanding and production of speech, that show a high degree of functional specialization in brain organization are presumably more vulnerable to focal lesions damaging the cortex. They are often spared in closed head injury despite the diffuse, subcortical shearing that is associated with that type of pathology (Oppenheimer, 1968; Strich, 1969).

Research on the psychological consequences of closed head injury, if not other forms of pathology, needs to be related to those brain stem arousal systems to which Penfield ascribed "primary psychological importance" and which Hebb

(1959) described as "intrinsically concerned in high mental processes and not merely an avenue of access to the cerebral cortex" (p. 267). It is known that damage to these systems may result in the arrest phenomenon described by Hunter and Jasper (1949), a paralysis rather than destruction of thought processes and a disturbance of the complicated patterns of emotion and action required in civilized adult behavior. It is plausible to suppose that residual symptoms of this disturbance could seriously handicap the prospects of an exacting professional career, a stable personal life, and perhaps the ability to drive a vehicle without undue risk.

Psychological assessment that pays attention to the source of failure and pattern of error may throw light on the nature of the disorder (cf. Saffran *et al.,* 1976; Derouesne *et al.,* 1977). This approach is reflected in work on acquired dyslexia (Marshall and Newcombe, 1973; Saffran *et al.,* 1976; Shallice and Warrington, 1975) and in studies designed to uncover the limiting factors in visuospatial disorders (e.g. Warrington and James, 1967*b,* Russo and Vignolo, 1967; Oxbury *et al.,* 1974; Gainotti *et al.,* 1977*a*).

Then, if prognosis is influenced by the degree or site of frontal lobe involvement, more sensitive techniques are required to tap those elusive disorders that recur in clinical anecdote but are seldom demonstrated with experimental rigor. We need to investigate the abilities to program, to monitor, to respond to feedback. We need to explore hypotheses emerging from physiological research, such as Teuber's (1972) concept that the prefrontal structures preset the sensory systems of the organism for future action and Deuel's (1977) version that "the frontal lobes may be working 'on line' to order motor behaviors within a time frame."

Few psychological tests tap the subject's spontaneous invention. Most require him to answer questions or respond to instructions. A possible consequence of frontal or frontothalamic damage is not that the patient fails to answer questions appropriately but that, left to himself, he will not initiate any productive activity. What test measures this tendency to "subside into silence" (Talland, 1965)? It has been demonstrated that amnesic patients who are able to code material acoustically, associatively, and semantically fail to use these strategies *spontaneously* in memory tasks (Cermak *et al.,* 1973).

Memorization is an active process. Yet many standard laboratory tasks are so structured that the patient's chances of responding normally are maximized. The external environment is less protective. There the patient has to extract the signal from relentless noise. Thus aphasic patients complain of the notorious cocktail party problem—difficulty in following and holding in mind several strands of conversation against background chatter—despite a normal performance on language tests. Patients with occipital lesions who have no difficulty in recognizing drawings of common objects have problems in detecting them against a visually noisy background (Bazhin *et al.,* 1973). Laboratory tasks probe only a narrow aspect of the business of remembering in real life. The patient is given a single-channel task (recalling words or stories), often without distraction, in a noise-attenuated environment. How different from the demands of a professional environment in which he has to keep track of several variables at once, constantly filter and select priorities, code and insert them in a temporal and spatial frame-work: intentional memory.

Furthermore, the whole area of affective change after brain damage has been neglected (but see Lishman, 1973). Yet there is no obvious reason why the psyche (apparently the target of the psychometrists) should be exclusively cognitive. As Zangwill (1976) has indicated, Fechner himself thought that "inner psychophysics would ultimately make possible a quantitative treatment not only of sensation but also of images, affects and indeed states of consciousness generally." It is, never-theless, a daunting prospect to undertake systematic enquiries where there are no clear-cut behavioral theories. But if the task of the neuropsychologist is to describe the *psychological* rather than the *cognitive* consequences of cerebral lesions, then he is hardly entitled to reject the challenge or at least should allow that it is a legitimate pursuit for his colleagues. The use of scales, designed exclusively for a psychiatric population, would hardly meet the case. There may be differences in kind between the mood changes found after damage to the central nervous system and those that occur in psychiatric illness. We do not know their etiology or natural history. They may stem directly from little-understood changes in cogni-tive efficiency. They might respond to different forms of remedial intervention.

RECOVERY AND MOTIVATION: THE INDIVIDUAL AND HIS ENVIRONMENT

Long-term quantitative studies of functional recovery are both rare and limited in scope. They are seldom mapped onto behavior in daily life or related to functional efficiency. Studies of war wound cases made this abundantly clear. Goldstein (1942) observed that "deficits found in special examinations do not always reveal conclusively the real disturbances in everyday performance." We came to the same conclusion in our study of British ex-servicemen. One ex-serviceman with a severe verbal memory deficit, measurable 25 years after a severe left temporoparietal injury, had achieved a successful career as a county archivist and had published two medieval inventories. In contrast, another man with a deep right temporal lesion, a high IQ, and no demonstrable intellectual deficits retired early after an undistinguished career as a bank clerk. Despite his superior perfor-mance in mathematical tests, he found it difficult to calculate accurately for more than short periods of time.

How then is the clinician to confront the problem of treatment and prog-nosis? And has the situation changed since Lashley (1938) suggested that "a broad clinical approach forms a better basis for prognosis than does any theoretical approach to the problem"? Past experience provides us with only the crude outlines for prediction. Prospective studies of what groups and individuals can achieve are more likely to give us insight into the possibilities and limits of recovery. Thus each patient presents a diagnostic challenge that has to be reviewed over time and related to the coordinates of daily life.

Much will depend on the individual, his constitutional makeup, and his educational status (see Dencker's important study of head injury in twins, 1958). These factors have been comprehensively reviewed by Lishman (1973), who cited Symond's cogent phrase: "it is not only the kind of injury that matters but the kind of head." Dresser *et al.* (1973) have produced behavioral evidence that employability is related to "the quality of the injured brain." The explanation, however, is obscure. Is this the resilience of overlearned skills, often cited in physiological research? Is the intelligent and stable patient more capable of discovering "coping strategies" (Goldstein, 1942; Cronholm, 1972)? Do the past experience and the resourceful environment of the gifted patient provide him with alternative possibilities of study and work?

If a patient's potential for recovery can be reliably assessed only over time, so too the time course is largely unknown. Clinical experience and traditional neuropsychological assessment show that most recovery occurs within a few months of injury. Recovery in this context refers to the results of neurological examination and performance on standard intelligence tests. There are nevertheless patients who continue to recover, albeit at a slower pace, for several years (Sands *et al.*, 1969; Newcombe and Marshall, 1975), particularly children (Black *et al.*, 1971).

The more elusive and refined aspects of intellectual activity are never measured. They may be affected by brain injury and may take time to resolve, as Brodal's (1973) illuminating autobiographical account has revealed. This distinguished scientist reported some of the symptoms that followed an embolic lesion of the posterior part of the right internal capsule. He became "much more easily tired than previously from mental work, even from ordinary conversation and reading newspapers. There was a marked reduction in the powers of concentration which made mental tasks far more demanding than before." There were also "changes in [his] powers to express himself without defects in writing and speech, in the absence of overt dysphasia." Such difficulties, perhaps overlooked in a busy outpatient clinic, could be disturbing if not disrupting to patients without insight into the nature of these disabilities. They should be taken into consideration when shaping plans for a patient's return to an exacting environment and when counseling a patient and his relatives. This is not to suggest that such symptoms are inevitable or that they persist. When present, however, they have obvious implications for the timing and grading of the remedial program.

Rehabilitation may intuitively be expected to influence prognosis, although hard evidence is signally lacking. In the case of speech therapy, there are remarkably few controlled studies of its effects (see Sarno, 1976, for an incisive review), and two of the most recent reports, both explicitly aware of the problem of selectional bias, produce conflicting data (compare the positive report of Basso *et al.*, 1975 with the negative findings of Kertesz and McCabe, 1977). Regarding unilateral spatial neglect and problems of visual scanning, often regarded as more disruptive handicaps than dysphasia, the results are again contradictory: Lawson (1962) found little evidence of transfer after systematic training, whereas Diller *et al.*, (1977) suggest that training has a favorable effect on a wide range of cognitive performance. Such fragments of information cannot be assembled into a coherent picture unless the nature of the lesion and the identity of the patient are taken into account.

The role of motivation is incalculable, and few clinicians would doubt its powerful contribution to recovery from severe brain damage (e.g., Wepman, 1953; Eisenson, 1973). We can all cite cases of phenomenal achievement that are loosely attributed to motivation, but we have no means of measuring this essential component and no knowledge of its physiological and biochemical correlates. Lashley (1938) accorded motivation an effective role in compensating for organic defect, although he was perhaps unduly pessimistic about the prospects of recovery from "the fundamental and important effects of cerebral injury . . . the defects in the capacity for organization, the lowered level of abstraction, the slowing of learning and reduced retentiveness, the loss of interest and spontaneous motivation." We wonder to what extent an inappropriate environment and lack of feedback contribute to the persistence of these symptoms. How many patients have the advantage of the regime prescribed by Schuell *et al.* (1964) and based on rehabilitation work over many years with dysphasic patients: a structured program alternating activity and rest, family counseling with an explanation of both positive and negative expectations, and a continual attempt to maintain communication. Research on feedback techniques, whether for paralyzed limbs or for disordered skills, has hardly begun. Perhaps in that area and with neuropharmacological techniques, we can hope to improve the outlook. It is as well to accept that there are limits to improvement after severe brain damage, but it is important to allow for the possibility of exceptional recovery.

References

Ajax, E. T. Dyslexia without agraphia. *Archives of Neurology,* 1967, *17.* 645–652.

Ajuriaguerra, J. de, Hécaen, H. and Angelergues, R. Les apraxies. Variétés cliniques et latéralisation lésionelle. *Revue Neurologique,* 1960, *102,* 566–594.

Alajouanine, T., and Lhermitte, F. Acquired aphasia in children. *Brain,* 1965, *88,* 653–662.

Arrigoni, G., and DeRenzi, E. Constructional apraxia and hemispheric locus of lesion. *Cortex,* 1964, *1,* 170–197.

Asayama, T. Über die Aphasie bei Japanern. *Deutsches Archiv für Clinische Medizin.* 1914, *113,* 523–529.

Ashworth, B. Neuro-ophthalmology. In W. B. Matthews (ed.), *Recent Advances in Clinical Neurology.* London: Churchill Livingstone, 1975.

Asselman, P., Chadwick, D. W., and Marsden, C. D. Visual evoked responses in the diagnosis and management of patients suspected of multiple sclerosis. *Brain,* 1975, *98,* 261–282.

Aulhorn, E., and Harms, H. Visual perimetry. In D. Jameson and L. M. Hurvich (eds.), *Handbook of Sensory Physiology,* Vol 7, Part 4. Berlin: Springer-Verlag, 1972.

Basser, L. S. Hemiplegia of early onset and the faculty of speech with special reference to the effects of hemispherectomy. *Brain,* 1962, *85,* 427–460.

Basso, A., Faglioni, P., and Vignolo, L. A. Etude contrôlée de la rééducation du langage dans l'aphasie: Comparaison entre aphasiques traités et non-traités. *Revue Neurologique,* 1975, *131,* 607– 614.

Bastian, H. C. *A Treatise on Aphasia and Other Speech Defects.* London: Lewis, 1898.

Bay, E. Disturbances of visual perception and their examination. *Brain,* 1953, *76,* 515–550.

Bay, E. Problems, possibilities and limitations of localisation of psychic symptoms in the brain. *Cortex,* 1964, *1,* 91–102.

Bazhin, E. F., Meerson, Y. A., and Tonkonogii, I. M. On distinguishing a visual signal from noise by patients with visual agnosia and visual hallucinations. *Neuropsychologia,* 1973, *11,* 319–324.

Benson, A. J., and Gedye, J. L. *Logical Processes in the Resolution of Orientation Conflict.* R.A.F. Institute of Aviation Medicine Report No. 259. London: Ministry of Defence (Air), 1963.

Benson, D. F. The third alexia. *Archives of Neurology.* 1977, *34,* 327–331.

Benson, D. F., and Geschwind, N. The alexias. In P. J. Vinken and G. W. Bruyn (eds.), *Handbook of Clinical Neurology,* Vol 4. Amsterdam: North-Holland, 1969.

Benson, D., Marsden, C., and Meadows, J. The amnesic syndrome of posterior cerebral artery occlusion. *Acta Neurologica Scandinavica,* 1974, *50,* 133–146.

Benton, A. L. Differential behavioral effects in frontal lobe disease. *Neuropsychologia,* 1968, *6,* 53–60.

Benton, A. L. Disorders of spatial orientation. In P. J. Vinken and G. W. Bruyn (eds.), *Handbook of Clinical Neurology,* Vol. 3. Amsterdam: North-Holland, 1969.

Bisiach, E., and Faglioni, P. Recognition of random shapes by patients with unilateral lesions as a function of complexity association value and delay. *Cortex*, 1974, *10*, 101–110.

Bisiach, E., Nichelli, P., and Spinnler, H. Hemispheric functional asymmetry in visual discrimination between univariate stimuli: An analysis of sensitivity and response criterion. *Neuropsychologia*, 1976, *14*, 335–343.

Black, P., Jeffries, J. J., Blumer, D., Wellner, A. M., and Walker, A. E. The post-traumatic syndrome in children: Characteristics and incidence. In A. E. Walker, W. F. Caveness, and M. Critchley (eds.), *The Late Effects of Head Injury*. Springfield, Ill.: Thomas, 1969.

Black, P., Blumer, D., Wellner, A. M., and Walker, A. E. The head-injured child: Time-course of recovery, with implications for rehabilitation. In *Head Injuries, Proceedings of an International Symposium, Edinburgh and Madrid, 1970*. London: Churchill Livingstone, 1971.

Blakemore, C. B., and Falconer, M. A. Long-term effects of anterior temporal lobectomy on certain cognitive functions. *Journal of Neurology, Neurosurgery and Psychiatry*, 1967, *30*, 364–367.

Bond, M. R. Assessment of the psychosocial outcome after severe head injury. In R. Porter and D. W. Fitzsimons (eds.), *Outcome of Severe Damage to the Central Nervous System*. Ciba Foundation Symposium 34 (new series). Amsterdam: North-Holland, Elsevier, Excerpta Medica, 1975.

Botez, M. I. The starting mechanism of speech. Paper read at the VIIIth Congress of the Hungarian Neurologists and Psychiatrists, Budapest, October 1962.

Bradshaw, J. L., Gates, A., and Nettleton, N. C. Bihemispheric involvement in lexical decisions: Handedness and a possible sex difference. *Neuropsychologia*, 1977, *15*, 277–286.

Briggs, G. G., and Nebes, R. D. The effects of handedness, family history and sex on the performance of a dichotic listening task. *Neuropsychologia*, 1976, *14*, 129–133.

Brodal, A. Self-observations and neuro-anatomical considerations after a stroke. *Brain*, 1973, *96*, 675–694.

Brody, E. M., Kleban, M. H., Lawton, M. P., and Silverman, H. A. Excess disabilities of mentally impaired aged: Impact of individualized treatment. *Gerontologist*, 1971, *11*, 124–132.

Brody, E. M., Kleban, M. H., Lawton, M. P., and Moss, M. Longitudinal look at excess disabilities in the mentally impaired aged. *Journal of Gerontology*, 1974, *29*, 79–84.

Brooks, D. N. Memory and head injury. *Journal of Nervous and Mental Disease*, 1972, *155*, 350–355.

Brooks, D. N. Recognition memory after head injury: A signal detection analysis. *Cortex*, 1974a, *10*, 224–230.

Brooks, D. N. Recognition memory, and head injury. *Journal of Neurology, Neurosurgery and Psychiatry*, 1974b, *37*, 794–801.

Brooks, D. N. Long and short term memory in head injured patients. *Cortex*, 1975, *11*, 329–340.

Brooks, D. N. Wechsler memory scale performance and its relationship to brain damage after severe closed head injury. *Journal of Neurology, Neurosurgery and Psychiatry*, 1976, *39*, 593–601.

Brown, J. W. *Aphasia, Apraxia and Agnosia*. Springfield, Ill.: Thomas, 1972.

Brown, J. W. On the neural organization of language: Thalamic and cortical relationships. *Brain and Language*, 1975, *2*, 18–30.

Brown, J. W., and Jaffe, J. Hypothesis on cerebral dominance. *Neuropsychologia*, 1975, *13*, 107–110.

Brown, J. R., and Simonson, J. A clinical study of 100 aphasic patients. *Neurology*, 1957, *7*, 777–783.

Brown-Séquard, C.-E. Dual character of the brain. No. 291 Smithsonian Miscellaneous Collections and Lecture 2 of the Toner lectures. Delivered April 22, 1874.

Brust, J. C. M., Shafer, S. Q., Richter, R. W., and Bruun, B. Aphasia in acute stroke. *Stroke*, 1976, *7*, 167–174.

Butfield, E., and Zangwill, O. L. Re-education in aphasia: A review of 70 cases. *Journal of Neurology, Neurosurgery and Psychiatry*, 1946, *9*, 75–79.

Byers, R. K., and McLean, W. T. Etiology and course of certain hemiplegias with aphasia in childhood. *Pediatrics*, 1962, *29*, 376–383.

Campbell, D. C., and Oxbury, J. M. Recovery from unilateral visuo-spatial neglect? *Cortex*, 1976, *12*, 303–312.

Casey, T., and Ettlinger, G. The occasional "independence" of dyslexia and dysgraphia from dysphasia. *Journal of Neurology, Neurosurgery and Psychiatry*, 1960, *23*, 228–236.

Caveness, W. F., and Walker, A. E. (eds.). *Head Injury*. Conference Proceedings. Philadelphia: Lippincott, 1966.

Cermak, L. S., and Butters, N. The role of interference and encoding in the short-term memory deficits of Korsakoff patients. *Neuropsychologia*, 1972, *10*, 89–95.

Cermak, L. S., and Moreines, J. Some analyses of the verbal encoding deficit in alcoholic Korsakoff patients. *Brain and Language*, 1974, *1*, 141–150.

Cermak, L. S. Butters, N., and Gerrein, J. The extent of the verbal encoding ability of Korsakoff patients. *Neuropsychologia*, 1973, *11*, 85–94.

Chadwick, O. The effect of age on initial cognitive deficits after severe head injury in children. Paper presented to the International Neuropsychological Society, Oxford, August 1–4, 1977.

Clarke, A. M., and Clarke, A. D. B. *Early Experience: Myth and Evidence.* London: Open Books, 1976.

Cogan, D. G. Ophthalmic manifestations of bilateral non-occipital cerebral lesions. *British Journal of Ophthalmology,* 1965, *49,* 281–297.

Cohen, G., and Freeman, R. Individual differences in reading strategies in relation to handedness and cerebral asymmetry. In J. Requin (ed.), *Attention and Performance, Vol. VII,* Hillside, New Jersey: Erlbaum Associates, 1978.

Collignon, R., and Rondeaux, J. Approche clinique des modalités de l'apraxie constructive secondaire aux lésions corticales hémisphériques gauches et droites. *Acta Neurologica Belgica (Bruxelles),* 1974, *74,* 137–146.

Conkey, R. C. Psychological changes associated with head injuries. In R. S. Woodworth (ed.), *Archives of Psychology,* No. 232, New York, 1938.

Conrad, K. New problems of aphasia. *Brain,* 1954, *77,* 491–509.

Corkin, S. Tactually-guided maze learning in man: Effects of unilateral cortical excisions and bilateral hippocampal lesions. *Neuropsychologia,* 1965, *3,* 339–351.

Corsi (cited by Milner, B.) Interhemispheric differences in the localization of psychological processes in man. In A. Summerfield (ed.), *Cognitive Psychology, British Medical Bulletin,* 1971, *27,* 272–277.

Critchley, M. *The Parietal Lobes.* London: Arnold, 1953.

Critchley, M. Specific developmental dyslexia. *British Journal of Hospital Medicine,* 1969, *2,* 910–911.

Cromer, R. F. Hierarchical disability in the written syntax of aphasic children. Paper presented to the International Society for the Study of Behavioural Development, Pavia, Italy, September 19–23, 1977.

Cronholm, B. Evaluation of mental disturbances after head injury. *Scandinavian Journal of Rehabilitation Medicine,* 1972, *4,* 35–38.

Damasio, A. R. Frontal lobe dysfunction. In Heilman and Valenstein (eds.), *Clinical Neuropsychology,* Oxford: Oxford University Press, 1978.

Deelman, B. Memory deficits after closed head injury. Paper presented to the International Neuropsychological Society, Oxford, August 1–4, 1977.

Déjérine, J. Contribution à l'étude anatomopathologique et clinique des différentes variétés de cécité verbale. *Comptes Rendus des Séances de la Société de Biologie et de Ses Filiales,* 1892, *4,* 61–90.

Dencker, S. J. A follow-up study of 128 closed head injuries in twins using co-twins as controls. *Acta Psychologica Neurologica Scandinavica (Suppl. 123),* 1958, *33.*

DeRenzi, E., and Faglioni, P. The comparative efficiency of intelligence and vigilance tests in detecting hemispheric cerebral damage. *Cortex,* 1965, *1,* 410–433.

DeRenzi, E., and Faglioni, P. The relationship between visuo-spatial impairment and constructional apraxia. *Cortex,* 1967, *3,* 327–342.

DeRenzi, E., and Scotti, G. The influence of spatial disorders in impairing tactual discrimination of shapes. *Cortex,* 1969, *5,* 53–62.

DeRenzi, E., and Spinnler, H. Facial recognition in brain damaged patients. *Neurology,* 1966a, *16,* 145–162.

DeRenzi, E., and Spinnler, H. Visual recognition in patients with unilateral cerebral disease. *Journal of Nervous and Mental Disease,* 1966b, *142,* 515–525.

DeRenzi, E., and Spinnler, H. Impaired performance on color tasks in patients with hemispheric damage. *Cortex,* 1967, *3,* 194–216.

DeRenzi, E., Faglioni, P., Savoiardo, M., and Vignolo, L. A. The influence of the hemispheric side of the cerebral lesion in abstract thinking. *Cortex,* 1966, *2,* 399–420.

DeRenzi, E., Faglioni, P., and Scotti, G. Tactile spatial impairment and unilateral cerebral damage. *Journal of Nervous and Mental Disease,* 1968a, *146,* 468–475.

DeRenzi, E., Faglioni, P., and Spinnler, H. The performance of patients with unilateral brain damage on face recognition tasks. *Cortex,* 1968b, *4,* 17–34.

DeRenzi, E., Scotti, G., and Spinnler, H. Perceptual and associative disorders of visual recognition. *Neurology,* 1969, *19,* 634–642.

DeRenzi, E., Faglioni, P., and Scotti, G. Hemispheric contribution to the exploration of space through the visual and tactile modality. *Cortex,* 1970, *6,* 191–203.

DeRenzi, E., Faglioni, P., Scotti, G., and Spinnler, H. Impairment of color sorting behavior after hemispheric damage: An experimental study with the Holmgren skein test. *Cortex,* 1972, *8,* 147–163.

Derouesne, J., Beauvois, M. F., and Ranty, C. Deux composantes dans l'articulation du langage oral: Preuve expérimentale de leur indépendance. *Neuropsychologia,* 1977, *15,* 143–154.

Deuel, R. K. Loss of motor habits after cortical lesions. *Neuropsychologia,* 1977, *15,* 205–216.

De Valois, R. L., Abramov, I., and Jacobs, G. H. Analysis of response patterns of L.G.N. cells. *Journal of the Optical Society of America,* 1966, *56*, 966–977.

Diller, L., Gordon, W., Weinberg, J., and Miller, J. Visual cancellation: A diagnostic and remediative tool in the rehabilitation of unilaterally brain damaged people. Paper presented at International Neuropsychological Society, Oxford, August 1–4, 1977.

Dresser, A. C., Meirowsky, A. M., Weiss, G. H., McNell, M. L., Simon, G. A., and Caveness, W. F. Gainful employment following head injury. *Archives of Neurology (Chicago),* 1973, *29*, 111–116.

Drewe, E. A. The effect of type and area of brain lesion on Wisconsin card sorting test performance. *Cortex,* 1974, *10*, 159–170.

Dubois, J., Hécaen, H., and Marcie, P. L'agraphie "pure." *Neuropsychologia,* 1969, 7, 271–286.

Duensing, F. Raumagnostische und ideatorisch-aprakitsche Störung des gestaltenden Handelns. *Deutsche Zeitschrift Nervenheilkunde,* 1953, *170*, 72–94.

Eisenson, J. *Adult Aphasia: Assessment and Treatment.* Englewood Cliffs, N. J.: Prentice-Hall, 1973.

Elder, W. The clinical varieties of visual aphasia. *Edinburgh Medical Journal,* 1900, *49*, 433–454.

Ettlinger, G. Sensory deficits in visual agnosia. *Journal of Neurology, Neurosurgery and Psychiatry,* 1956, *19*, 297–307.

Evans, C. D., Bull, C. P. I., Devonport, M. J., Hall, P. M., Jones, J., Middleton, F. R. I., Russell, G., Stichbury, J. C., and Whitehead, B. Rehabilitation of the brain-damaged survivor. *Injury: the British Journal of Accident Surgery,* 1977, *8*, 80–97.

Faglioni, P., Scotti, G., and Spinnler, H. Impaired recognition of written letters following unilateral hemisphere damage. *Cortex,* 1969, *5*, 120–133.

Fairweather, H. Sex differences in cognition. *Cognition,* 1976, *4*, 231–280.

Ferguson, J. H., and Boller, F. A different form of agraphia: Syntactic writing errors in patients with motor speech and movement disorders. *Brain and Language,* 1977, *4*, 382–389.

Field, J. H. *Epidemiology of Head Injuries in England and Wales.* H.M.S.O., 1976.

Fisher, C. M., and Adams, R. D. Transient global amnesia. *Acta Neurologica Scandinavica Supplement 9,* 1944, *40*.

Flach, J., and Malmros, R. A long-term follow-up study of children with severe head injury. *Scandinavian Journal of Rehabilitation Medicine,* 1972, *4*, 9–15.

Fodor, I. E. Impairment of memory functions after acute head injury. *Journal of Neurology, Neurosurgery and Psychiatry,* 1972, *35*, 818–824.

Frisen, L., Hoyt, W. F., Bird, A. C., and Weale, R. A. Diagnostic uses of the Pulfrich phenomenon. *Lancet,* 1973, *2*, 385–386.

Gainotti, G., Caltagirone, C., and Miceli, G. Poor performance of right brain-damaged patients on Raven's coloured matrices: Derangement of general intelligence or of specific abilities? *Neuropsychologia,* 1977a, *15*, 675–680.

Gainotti, G., Miceli, G., and Caltagirone, C. Constructional apraxia in left brain-damaged patients: A planning disorder? *Cortex,* 1977b, *13*, 109–118.

Gassell, M. M., and Williams, D. Visual function in patients with homonymous hemianopia Part II. Oculomotor Mechanics. *Brain,* 1963a, *86*, 1–36.

Gassell, M. M., and Williams, D. Visual function in patients with homonymous hemianopia. Part III. The completion phenomenon; insight and attitude to the defect; and visual functional efficiency. *Brain,* 1963b, *86*, 229–260.

Gazzaniga, M. A. *The Bisected Brain.* New York: Appleton-Century-Crofts, 1970.

Geschwind, N. Language and the brain. *Scientific American,* 1972, *226*, 76–83.

Geschwind, N. Late changes in the nervous system: An overview. In D. G. Stein, J. J. Rose, and N. Butters (eds.), *Plasticity and Recovery of Function in the Central Nervous System.* New York: Academic Press, 1974.

Gilliatt, R. W., and Pratt, R. T. C. Disorders of perception and performance in a case of right-sided cerebral thrombosis. *Journal of Neurology, Neurosurgery and Psychiatry,* 1952, *15*, 264–271.

Gjone, R., Kristiansen, K., and Sponheim, N. Rehabilitation in severe head injuries. *Scandinavian Journal of Rehabilitation Medicine,* 1972, *4*, 2–4.

Gloning, I., Gloning, K., and Hoff, H. *Neuropsychological Symptoms and Syndromes in Lesions of the Occipital Lobe and the Adjacent Areas.* Paris: Gauthier-Villars, 1968.

Godfrey, C. M., and Douglass, E. The recovery process in aphasia. *Canadian Medical Association Journal,* 1959, *80*, 618–624.

Goldman, P. S. Developmental determinants of cortical plasticity. *Acta Neurobiologiae Experimentalis,* 1972, *32*, 495–511.

Goldman, P. S. An alternative to developmental plasticity: Heterology of CNS structures in infants and adults. In D. G. Stein, J. J. Rosen, and N. Butters (eds.), *Plasticity and Recovery of Function in the Central Nervous System.* New York: Academic Press, 1974.

Goldman, P. S., Crawford, H. T., Stokes, L. P., Galkin, T. W., and Rosvold, H. E. Sex-dependent behavioral effects of cerebral cortical lesions in the developing rhesus monkey. *Science,* 1974, *186,* 540–542.

Goldstein, K. The two ways of adjustment of the organism to cerebral defects. *Journal of Mount Sinai Hospital,* 1942, *9,* 504–513.

Goldstein, K. Physiological aspects of convalescence and rehabilitation following central nervous system injuries. Symposium on Physiological Aspects of Convalescence and Rehabilitation (A Keys, ed.), 1944.

Goodglass, H. Studies on the grammar of aphasics. In S. Rosenberg and J. Koplin (eds.), *Developments in Applied Psycholinguistics Research.* New York: Macmillan, 1968.

Greenblatt, S. H. Alexia without agraphia or hemianopsia. *Brain,* 1973, *96,* 307–316.

Gronwall, S., and Sampson, H. *The Psychological Effects of Concussion.* Auckland: Auckland University/ Oxford University Press, 1974.

Halliday, A. M., McDonald, W. I., and Mushin, J. Delayed visual evoked response in optic neuritis. *Lancet,* 1972, *1,* 982–985.

Halliday, A. M., McDonald, W. I., and Mushin, J. Visual evoked response in diagnosis of multiple sclerosis. *British Medical Journal,* 1973, *4,* 661–664.

Hannay, H. J., and Malone, D. R. Visual field effects and short-term memory for verbal material. *Neuropsychologia,* 1976, *14,* 203–209.

Hannay, H. J., Levin, H. S., and Grossman, R. G. Closed head injury and recognition memory. Paper presented at the International Neuropsychological Society, Oxford, August 1–4, 1977.

Harris, L. J. Sex differences in spatial ability: Possible environmental, genetic, and neurological factors. In M. Kinsbourne (ed.), *Hemispheric Asymmetries of Function.* Cambridge: Cambridge University Press, 1976.

Head, H. *Aphasia and Kindred Disorders of Speech.* Cambridge: Cambridge University Press, 1926.

Hebb, D. O. The effect of early and late brain injury upon test scores, and the nature of normal adult intelligence. *Proceedings of the American Philosophical Society,* 1942, *85,* 275–292.

Hebb, D. O. Intelligence, brain function and the theory of mind. *Brain,* 1959, *82,* 260–275.

Hécaen, H. Clinical symptomatology in right and left hemispheric lesions. In V. B. Mountcastle (ed.), *Interhemispheric Relations and Cerebral Dominance.* Baltimore: Johns Hopkins Press, 1962.

Hécaen, H. Aphasic, apraxic and agnosic syndromes in right and left hemispheric lesions. In P. J. Vinken and G. W. Bruyn (eds.), *Handbook of Clinical Neurology,* Vol. 4. Amsterdam: North-Holland, 1969.

Hécaen, H., and Assal, G. A comparison of constructive deficits following right and left hemispheric lesions. *Neuropsychologia,* 1970, *8,* 289–304.

Hécaen, H., and Kremin, H. Neurolinguistic research on reading disorders resulting from left hemisphere lesions: Aphasic and "pure" alexias. In H. A. Whitaker and H. Whitaker (eds.), *Studies in Neurolinguistics,* Vol. 2, Chapter 8. New York: Academic Press, 1976.

Hécaen, H., and Sauguet, J. Cerebral dominance in left-handed subjects. *Cortex,* 1971, *7,* 19–48.

Hécaen, H., Ajuriaguerra, J. de, and Massonet, J. Les troubles visuoconstructifs par lésions pariétooc-cipitales droites. Rôle des perturbations. *Encéphale,* 1951, *1,* 122–179.

Hécaen, H., Ajuriaguerra, J. de, and David, M. Les déficits fonctionnels après lobectomie occipitale. *Monatsschrift für Neurologie und Psychiatrie,* 1952, *123,* 239–291.

Hécaen, H., Angelergues, R., and Douzenis, J. A. Les agraphies. *Neuropsychologia,* 1963, *1,* 179–208.

Hines, D., and Satz, P. Cross-modal asymmetries in perception related to asymmetry in cerebral function. *Neuropsychologia,* 1974, *12,* 239–247.

Höök, O. Comments on rehabilitation of the brain-injured. In A. E. Walker, W. F. Caveness, and M. Critchley, (eds.), *The Late Effects of Head Injury.* Springfield, Ill.: Thomas, 1969.

Humphrey, M. E., and Zangwill, O. L. Effects of a right-sided occipito-parietal brain injury in a left-handed man. *Brain,* 1952, *75,* 312–324.

Hunter, J., and Jasper, H. H. Effects of thalamic stimulation in unanaesthetised animals. *Electroencephalography and Clinical Neurophysiology,* 1949, *1,* 305–324.

Huppert, F. A., and Piercy, M. Recognition memory in amnesic patients: Effect of temporal context and familiarity of material. *Cortex,* 1976, *12,* 3–20.

Inglis, J. Biofeedback and the re-education of neuromuscular disabilities after stroke. Paper presented to the International Neuropsychological Society, Oxford, August 1–4, 1977.

Jacobson, M. Brain development in relation to language. In E. H. Lenneberg and E. Lenneberg (eds.),

Foundations of Language Development: A Multidisciplinary Approach. New York: Academic Press, 1975.

Jarvie, H. Problem-solving deficits following wounds of the brain. *Journal of Mental Science,* 1960, *106*, 1377–1382.

Jennett, B. Head injuries in children. *Developmental Medicine and Child Neurology,* 1972, *14*, 137–147.

Jennett, B. Scale, scope and philosophy of the clinical problem. In R. Porter and D. W. Fitzsimons (eds.), *Outcome of Severe Damage to the Central Nervous System,* Ciba Foundation Symposium 34 (new series). Amsterdam: Elsevier, Excerpta Medica, 1975.

Jennett, B. Assessment of the severity of head injury. *Journal of Neurology, Neurosurgery and Psychiatry,* 1976, *39*, 647–655.

Jennett, B., and Bond, M. Assessment of outcome after severe brain damage. *Lancet,* March 1, p. 480, 1975.

Jones, M. K. Imagery as a mnemonic aid after left temporal lobectomy: Contrast between material-specific and generalized memory disorders. *Neuropsychologia,* 1974, *12*, 21–30.

Jones-Gotman, M., and Milner, B. Design fluency: The invention of nonsense drawings after focal cortical lesions. *Neuropsychologia,* 1977, *15*, 653–673.

Juel-Nielsen, N. Epidemiology. In J. G. Howells (ed.), *Modern Perspectives in the Psychiatry of Old Age.* New York, Brunner-Mazel, 1975.

Kenin, M., and Peck-Swisher, L. A study of pattern of recovery in aphasia. *Cortex,* 1972, *8*, 56–68.

Kertesz, A., and McCabe, P. Recovery patterns and prognosis in aphasia. *Brain,* 1977, *100*, 1–18.

Kimura, D. Right temporal lobe damage. *Archives of Neurology (Chicago),* 1963, *8*, 264–271.

Kimura, D. The neural basis of language qua gesture. In H. Whitaker and H. A. Whitaker (eds.), *Studies in Neurolinguistics,* Vol. 2. New York: Academic Press, 1976.

Kimura, D., and Archibald, Y. Motor functions of the left hemisphere. *Brain,* 1974, *97*, 337–350.

Kinsbourne, M., and Cook, J. Generalized and lateralised effects of concurrent verbalization on a unimanual skill. *Quarterly Journal of Experimental Psychology,* 1971, *23*, 341–345.

Kirkham, T. E. The ocular symptomatology of pituitary tumours. *Proceedings of the Royal Society of Medicine,* 1972, *65*, 517–518.

Kohn, B., and Dennis, M. Somatosensory functions after cerebral hemidecortication for infantile hemiplegia. *Neuropsychologia,* 1974, *12*, 119–130.

Kracke, I. Perception of rhythmic sequences by receptive aphasic and deaf children. *British Journal of Disorders of Communication,* 1975, *10*, 43–51.

Lange, J. Agnosien und Apraxien. In O. Bumke and O. Foerster (eds.), *Handbuch der Neurologie,* Vol. VI. Berlin: Springer, 1936.

Lansdell, H. A sex difference in effect of temporal-lobe neurosurgery on design preference. *Nature (London),* 1962, *194*, 852–854.

Lansdell, H. Sex differences in hemispheric asymmetries of the human brain. *Nature (London)* 1964, *203*, p. 550.

Lansdell, H. Effect of extent of temporal lobe ablations on two lateralized deficits. *Physiology and Behavior,* 1968, *3*, 271–273.

Lashley, K. S. Factors limiting recovery after central nervous lesions. *Journal of Nervous and Mental Disease,* 1938, *88*, 733–755.

Lawson, I. R. Visual-spatial neglect in lesions of the right cerebral hemisphere. *Neurology,* 1962, *12*, 23–33.

Lecours, A. R. Myelogenetic correlates of the development of speech and language. In E. H. Lenneberg and E. Lenneberg (eds.), *Foundations of Language Development,* Vol. 1. New York: Academic Press, 1975.

Leischner, A. Aptitude of aphasics for language treatment. In Y. Lebrun and R. Hoops (eds.), *Recovery in Aphasics.* Amsterdam: Swets and Zeitlinger BV, 1976.

Lenneberg, E. H. *Biological Foundations of Language.* New York: Wiley, 1967.

Levin, H. S., Grossman, R. G., and Kelly, P. J. Aphasic disorder in patients with closed head injury. *Journal of Neurology, Neurosurgery and Psychiatry,* 1976, *39*, 1062–1070.

Lewin, W. Severe head injuries. *Proceedings of the Royal Society of Medicine,* 1967, *60*, 1208–1212.

Lhermitte, J., de Massary, J., and Kyriaco, N. Le rôle de la pensée spatiale dans l'apraxie. *Revue Neurologique,* 1928, *50*, 895–903.

Libb, J. W., and Clements, C. B. Token reinforcement in an exercise program for hospitalized geriatric patients. *Perceptual Motor Skills,* 1969, *28*, 957–968.

Lidvall, H. F., Linderoth, B., and Norlin, B. Causes of the post-concussional syndrome. *Acta Neurologica Scandinavica Supplement 50*, 1974.

Liepmann, H. Das Krankheitsbild der Apraxie ("motorischen Asymbolie") auf Grund eines Falles von einseitiger Apraxie. *Monatsschrift für Psychiatrie und Neurologie*, 1900, *8*, 15–44, 102–132, 182–197.

Lindsley, O. R. Geriatric behavioral prosthetics. In R. Kastenbaum (ed.), *New Thoughts on Old Age*. New York: Springer, 1964.

Lishman, W. A. The psychiatric sequelae of head injury: A review. *Psychological Medicine*, 1973, *3*, 304–318.

Lomas, J., and Kimura, D. Intrahemispheric interaction between speaking and sequential manual activity. *Neuropsychologia*, 1976, *14*, 23–33.

London, P. S. Some observations on the course of events after severe injury of the head. *Annals of the Royal College of Surgeons of England*, 1967, *41*, 460–479.

Ludlow, cited by Sarno, M. T. The status of research in recovery from aphasia. In Y. Lebrun and R. Hoops (eds.), *Recovery in Aphasics*. Amsterdam: Swets and Zeitlinger BV, 1976.

Luria, A. R. *Restoration of Function after Brain Injury*. Oxford: Pergamon Press, 1963.

Luria, A. R. *Human Brain and Psychological Processes*. New York: Harper and Row, 1966.

Luria, A. R. *Traumatic Aphasia*. The Hague: Mouton, 1970.

Luria, A. R. *The Neuropsychology of Memory*. New York: Wiley, 1976.

Lyman, R. S., Kwan, S. T., and Chao, W. H. Left occipitoparietal brain tumour with observations on alexia and agraphia in Chinese and English. *Chinese Medical Journal*, 1938, *54*, 491–516.

MacIver, I. N., Lassman, L. P., Thompson, C. W., and McLeod, I. Treatment of severe head injuries. *Lancet*, 1958, *2*, 544–550.

Marks, M., Taylor, M., and Rusk, H. A. Rehabilitation of the aphasic patient: A survey of three years' experience in a rehabilitation setting. *Neurology*, 1957, *7*, 837–843.

Marshall, J. Some problems and paradoxes associated with recent accounts of hemispheric specialization. *Neuropsychologia*, 1973, *11*, 463–470.

Marshall, J. C., and Newcombe, F. Patterns of paralexia: A psycholinguistic approach. *Journal of Psycholinguistic Research*, 1973, *2*, 175–199.

Marshall, J. C., and Newcombe, F. Variability and constraint in acquired dyslexia. In H. A. Whitaker and H. Whitaker (eds.), *Studies in Neurolinguistics*, Vol 3. New York: Academic Press, 1977.

Martinius, J. Performance and activation in children following brain trauma. Paper presented to the International Neuropsychological Society, Oxford, August 1–4, 1977.

Masure, M. C., and Tzavaras, A. Perception de figures entrecroisées par des sujets atteints de lésions corticales unilatérales. *Neuropsychologia*, 1976, *14*, 371–374.

Matthews, W. B., and Miller, H. *Diseases of the Nervous System*. Oxford: Blackwell, 1972.

Matthews, W. B., and Oxbury, J. M. Prognostic factors in stroke. In R. Porter and D. W. Fitzsimons (eds.), *Outcome of Severe Damage to the Central Nervous System*. Ciba Foundation Symposium 34 (new series). Amsterdam: North-Holland, Elsevier, Excerpta Medica, 1975.

McFie, J. Intellectual impairment in children. *Journal of Neurology, Neurosurgery and Psychiatry*, 1961, *24*, 361–365.

McFie, J., and Zangwill, O. L. Visual-constructive disabilities associated with lesions of the left cerebral hemisphere. *Brain*, 1960, *83*, 243–260.

McFie, J., Piercy, M. F. and Zangwill, O. L. Visual-spatial agnosia associated with lesions of the right cerebral hemisphere. *Brain*, 1950, *73*, 167–190.

McGlone, J. Sex differences in functional brain asymmetry. *Cortex*, 1978, *14*, 122–128.

McGlone, J., and Davidson, W. The relation between cerebral speech laterality and spatial ability with special reference to sex and hand preference. *Neuropsychologia*, 1973, *11*, 105–113.

Meadows, J. C. Disturbed perception of colours associated with localized cerebral lesions. *Brain*, 1974, *97*, 615–632.

Meier, M. J., and French, L. A. Lateralized deficits in complex visual discrimination and bilateral transfer of reminiscence following unilateral temporal lobectomy. *Neuropsychologia*, 1965, *3*, 261–272.

Merskey, H., and Woodforde, J. M. Psychiatric sequelae of minor head injury. *Brain*, 1972, *95*, 521–528.

Meyer, V. Cognitive changes following temporal lobectomy for relief of temporal lobe epilepsy. *Archives of Neurology and Psychiatry*, 1959, *81*, 299–309.

Miller, E. Simple and choice reaction time following severe head injury. *Cortex,* 1970, *6*, 121–127.

Miller, E. The management of dementia: A review of some possibilities. *British Journal of Social and Clinical Psychology,* 1977, *16*, 77–83.

Miller, H. Mental sequelae of head injury. *Proceedings of the Royal Society of Medicine,* 1966, *59*, 257–266.

Miller, H., and Stern, G. The long-term prognosis of severe head injury. *Lancet,* 1965, 30 January, 225–229.

Milner, B. Psychological defects produced by temporal lobe excision. *Research Publications of the Association for Research in Nervous and Mental Disease,* 1958, *36*, 244–257.

Milner, B. Laterality effects in audition. In V. B. Mountcastle (ed.), *Interhemispheric Relations and Cerebral Dominance.* Baltimore: Johns Hopkins Press, 1962*a.*

Milner, B. Les troubles de la mémoire accompagnant des lésions hippocampiques bilatérales. In *Physiologie de l'Hippocampe.* Colloques Internationaux No. 107. Paris: C.N.R.S., 1962*b.*

Milner, B. Some effects of frontal lobectomy in man. In J. M. Warren and J. Akert (eds.), *The Frontal Granular Cortex and Behavior.* New York: McGraw-Hill, 1964.

Milner, B. Visually-guided maze learning in man: Effects of bilateral hippocampal, bilateral frontal and unilateral cerebral lesions. *Neuropsychologia,* 1965, *3*, 317–338.

Milner, B. Amnesia following operation on the temporal lobes. In C. W. M. Whitty and O. L. Zangwill (eds.), *Amnesia.* London: Butterworths, 1966.

Milner, B. Visual recognition and recall after right temporal-lobe excision in man. *Neuropsychologia,* 1968, *6*, 191–209.

Milner, B. Memory and the medial temporal regions of the brain. In K. H. Pribram and D. E. Broadbent (eds.), *Biology of Memory.* New York: Academic Press, 1970.

Milner, B. Hemispheric specialization: Scope and limits. In F. O. Schmitt and F. G. Worden (eds.), *The Neurosciences: Third Study Program.* Cambridge, Mass.: MIT Press, 1973.

Milner, B. Psychological aspects of focal epilepsy and its neurosurgical management. In D. P. Purpura, J. K. Penny, and R. D. Walter (eds.), *Advances in Neurology.* New York: Raven Press, 1975.

Milner, B., Corkin, S., and Teuber, H.-L. Further analysis of the hippocampal amnesic syndrome: 14-year follow-up study of H. M. *Neuropsychologia,* 1968, *6*, 215–234.

Mohr, J. P., Sidman, M., Stoddard, L. T., Leicester, J., and Rosenberger, P. B. Evolution of the deficit in total aphasia. *Neurology,* 1973, *23*, 1302–1312.

Mollon, J., Polder, P., Newcombe, F., and Ratcliff, G. The Maid from Banbury re-visited. Paper presented to the Experimental Psychology Society, Oxford, April 8–9, 1975.

Morton, J. In-depth study of a phonemic dyslexic. Paper presented to the Experimental Psychology Society, Oxford, July 7–9, 1977.

Mumenthaler, M., and von Roll, L. Amnestische Episoden: Analyse von 16 eigenen Beobachtungen. *Schweizer Medizinische Wochenschrift,* 1969, *99*, 133–139.

Najenson, T., Mendelson, L., Schechter, I., David, C., Mintz, N., and Groswasser, Z. Rehabilitation after severe head injury. *Scandinavian Journal of Rehabilitation Medicine,* 1974, *6*, 5–14.

Netley, C. Processing of visual information by patients with localised cerebral lesions. Ph.D. thesis, University of London, 1966.

Newcombe, F. *Missile Wounds of the Brain: A Study of Psychological Deficits.* London: Oxford University Press, 1969.

Newcombe, F., and Marshall, J. C. Traumatic dyslexia: Localization and linguistics. In K. J. Zülch, O. Creutzfeldt, and G. C. Galbraith (eds.), *Cerebral Localization.* New York: Springer-Verlag, 1975.

Newcombe, F., and Ratcliff, G. G. Handedness, speech lateralization and ability. *Neuropsychologia,* 1973, *11*, 399–407.

Newcombe, F., and Ratcliff, G. G. Agnosia: A disorder of object recognition. In F. Michel and B. Schott (eds.), *Les Syndromes de Disconnexion Calleuse chez L'Homme.* Lyon: Colloque International de Lyon, 1975.

Newcombe, F., and Russell, W. R. Dissociated visual perceptual and spatial deficits in focal lesions of the right hemisphere. *Journal of Neurology, Neurosurgery and Psychiatry,* 1969, *32*, 73–81.

Newcombe, F., Oldfield, R. C., Ratcliff, G. G., and Wingfield, A. Recognition and naming of object drawings by men with focal brain wounds. *Journal of Neurology, Neurosurgery and Psychiatry,* 1971, *34*, 329–340.

Newcombe, F., Hiorns, R. W., Marshall, J. C., and Adams, C. B. T. Acquired dyslexia: Patterns of deficit and recovery. In R. Porter and D. W. Fitzsimons (eds.), *Outcome of Severe Damage to the Central Nervous System.* Ciba Foundation Symposium 34 (new series). Amsterdam: Elsevier, Excerpta Medica, North-Holland, 1975.

Norrman, B., and Svahn, K. A follow-up study of severe brain injuries. *Acta Psychiatrica Scandinavica,* 1961, *37*, 236–264.

Oddy, M. Social recovery from severe head injury in young adults. Paper presented to the International Neuropsychological Society, Oxford, August 1–4, 1977.

Oppenheimer, D. Microscopic lesions in the brain following head injury. *Journal of Neurology, Neurosurgery and Psychiatry,* 1968, *31*, 299–306.

Orbach, J. Disturbances of the maze habit following occipital cortex removals in blind monkeys. *Archives of Neurology and Psychiatry,* 1959, *81*, 49–54.

Orgass, B., Poeck, K. Kerschensteiner, M., and Hartje, W. Visuo-cognitive performance in patients with unilateral hemispheric lesions. *Zeitschrift für Neurologie,* 1972, *202*, 177–195.

Oxbury, J. M. The right hemisphere and hemispheric disconnection. In W. B. Matthews (ed.), *Recent Advances in Neurology.* Edinburgh: Livingstone, 1975.

Oxbury, J. M., Campbell, D. B., and Oxbury, S. M. Unilateral spatial neglect and impairments of spatial analysis and visual perception. *Brain,* 1974, *97*, 551–564.

Pailhous, J. *La Représentation de l'Espace Urbain.* Paris: Presses Universitaires de France, 1970.

Paillard, J. The patterning of skilled movements. *Handbook of Physiology,* 1960, *67*, 1679–1708.

Paivio, A. *Imagery and Verbal Processes.* New York: Holt, Rinehart and Winston, 1971.

Patterson, K. Reading impairment of some aphasic patients. Paper presented to the Experimental Psychology Society, Oxford, July 7–9, 1977.

Pearce, J., and Miller, E. *Clinical Aspects of Dementia.* London: Baillière Tindall, 1973.

Penfield, W., and Roberts, L. *Speech and Brain-Mechanisms.* Princeton, N.J.: Princeton University Press, 1959.

Perenin, M. T., and Jeannerod, M. Residual vision in cortically blind hemiphields. *Neuropsychologia,* 1975, *13*, 1–7.

Perez, F. I., Stump, D. A., Gay, J. R. A., and Hart, V. R. Intellectual performance in multi-infarct dementia and Alzheimer's disease: A replication study. *Journal Canadien des Sciences Neurologiques,* 1976, *3*, 181–187.

Perret, E. The left frontal lobe of man and the suppression of habitual responses in verbal categorical behaviour. *Neuropsychologia,* 1974, *12*, 323–330.

Perret, E., Kohenof, M., and Siegfried, J. Influences de lésions thalamiques unilatérales sur les fonctions intellectuelles, mnésiques et d'apprentissage de malades Parkinsoniens. *Neuropsychologia,* 1969, *7*, 79–88.

Piercy, M. The effects of cerebral lesions on intellectual function: A review of current research trends. *British Journal of Psychiatry,* 1964, *110*, 310–352.

Piercy, M., Hécaen, H., and Ajuriaguerra, J. de. Constructional apraxia associated with unilateral cerebral lesions—left and right sided cases compared. *Brain,* 1960, *83*, 225–242.

Pillon, B. and Lhermitte, F. Désignation et dénomination à différents rhythmes chez des patients atteints de lésions cérébrales. *Neuropsychologia,* 1974, *12*, 55–63.

Pöppel, E., Held, R., and Frost, D. Residual visual function after brain wounds involving the central visual pathways in man. *Nature (London)* 1973, *243*, 295–296.

Poppelreuter, W. *Die psychischen Schädigungen durch Kopfschuss im Kriege 1914-1916: Die Störungen der niederen und hoheren Sehleistungen durch Verletzungen des Okzipitalhirns.* Leipzig: Voss, 1917.

Ratcliff, G. G. Aspects of disordered space perception. D.Phil. thesis, University of Oxford, 1970.

Ratcliff, G. G. Spatial thought, mental rotation and the right cerebral hemisphere. *Neuropsychologia,* 1978, in press.

Ratcliff, G. G., and Davies-Jones, G. A. B. Defective visual localisation in focal brain wounds. *Brain,* 1972, *95*, 49–60.

Ratcliff, G. G. and Newcombe, F. Spatial orientation in man: Effects of left, right, and bilateral posterior cerebral lesions. *Journal of Neurology, Neurosurgery and Psychiatry,* 1973, *36*, 448–454.

Regan, D., Milner, B. A., and Heron, J. R. Delayed visual perception and delayed visual evoked potentials in the spinal form of multiple sclerosis and in retrobulbar neuritis. *Brain,* 1976, *99*, 43–66.

Reitan, R. M. Psychological deficits resulting from cerebral lesions in man. In J. M. Warren and M. Akert (eds.), *The Frontal Granular Cortex and Behaviour.* New York: McGraw-Hill, 1964.

Richardson, F. Some effects of severe head injury: A follow-up study of children and adolescents after protracted coma. *Developmental Medicine and Child Neurology,* 1963, *5*, 471–482.

Richardson, J. T. E. The effect of word imageability in acquired dyslexia. *Neuropsychologia,* 1975, *13*, 281–288.

Roberts, L. Aphasia, apraxia and agnosia in abnormal states of cerebral dominance. In P. J. Vinken and G. W. Bruyn (eds.), *Handbook of Clinical Neurology*, Vol. 4. Amsterdam: North-Holland, 1969.

Rose, F. C., and Symonds, C. A. Persistent memory defect following encephalitis. *Brain*, 1960, *83*, 195–212.

Ruesch, J., and Moore, B. E. Measurement of intellectual functions in the acute stage of head injury. *Archives of Neurology and Psychiatry*, 1943, *50*, 165–170.

Rushton, D. Use of the Pulfrich pendulum for detecting abnormal delay in the visual pathway in multiple sclerosis. *Brain*, 1975, *98*, 283–297.

Russell, I. S. Animal learning and memory. In D. Richter (ed.), *Aspects of Learning and Memory*. London: Heinemann, 1966.

Russell, W. R. Functions of the frontal lobes. *Lancet*, March 6, 1948, p. 356.

Russell, W. R. *The Traumatic Amnesias*. London: Oxford University Press, 1971.

Russell, W. R. Recovery after minor head injury. *Lancet*, November 30, p. 1315, 1974.

Russell, W. R., and Espir, M. L. E. *Traumatic Aphasia*. London: Oxford University Press, 1961.

Russell, W. R., and Smith, A. Post traumatic amnesia in closed head injury. *Archives of Neurology*, 1961, *5*, 4–17.

Russo, M., and Vignolo, L. A. Visual figure-ground discrimination in patients with unilateral cerebral disease. *Cortex*, 1967, *3*, 113–127.

Rylander, G. Personality analysis before and after frontal lobotomy. *Research Publications of the Association for Research in Nervous and Mental Disease*, 1948, *27*, 691–705.

Saan, R., and Thomas C. Early changes in memory. Paper presented to the International Neuropsychological Society, Oxford, August 1–4, 1977.

Saffran, E. M., and Marin, O. S. M. Semantic errors in paralexia. Paper given at the 3rd annual meeting of the International Neuropsychological Society, Florida, February 5–7, 1975.

Saffran, E. M., Marin, O. S. M., and Yeni-Komshian, G. H. An analysis of speech perception in word deafness. *Brain and Language*, 1976, *3*, 209–228.

Sanders, M. D., Warrington, E. K., Marshall, J., and Weiskrantz, L. "Blindsight": Vision in a field defect. *Lancet*, April 20, 707–708, 1974.

Sands, E., Sarno, M. T., and Shankweiler, D. Long-term assessment of language function in aphasia due to stroke. *Archives of Physical Medicine and Rehabilitation*, 1969, *50*, 202–207.

Sarno, M. T. The status of research in recovery from aphasia. In Y. Lebrun and R. Hoops (eds.), *Recovery in Aphasics*. Amsterdam: Swets and Zeitlinger BV, 1976.

Sarno, M. T., and Levita, E. Natural course of recovery in severe aphasia. *Archives of Physical and Medical Rehabilitation*, 1971, *52*, 175–186.

Sasanuma, S. Kana and Kanji processing in Japanese aphasics. *Brain and Language*, 1975, *2*, 369–383.

Schacter, D. L., and Crovitz, H. F. Memory function after closed head injury: A review of the quantitative research. *Cortex*, 1977, *13*, 150–176.

Schuell, H., Jenkins, J. J., and Jiménez-Pabón, E. *Aphasia in Adults*. New York: Harper and Row, 1964.

Scoville, W. B., and Milner, B. Loss of recent memory after bilateral hippocampal lesions. *Journal of Neurology, Neurosurgery and Psychiatry*, 1957, *20*, 11–21.

Semmes, J., Weinstein, S., Ghent, L., and Teuber, H.-L. Spatial orientation in man after cerebral injury. 1. Analyses by locus of lesion. *Journal of Psychology*, 1955, *39*, 227–244.

Semmes, J., Weinstein, S., Ghent, L., and Teuber, H.-L. *Somatosensory Changes after Penetrating Brain Wounds in Man*. Cambridge, Mass.: Harvard University Press, 1960.

Semmes, J., Weinstein, S., Ghent, L., and Teuber, H.-L. Correlates of impaired orientation in personal and extrapersonal space. *Brain*, 1963, *86*, 747–772.

Shallice, T., and Warrington, E. K. Word recognition in a phonemic dyslexic patient. *Quarterly Journal of Experimental Psychology*, 1975, *27*, 187–200.

Smith, A. Dominant and nondominant hemispherectomy. In W. Lynn Smith (ed.), *Drugs, Development, and Cerebral Function*. Springfield, Ill.: Thomas, 1972.

Smith, E. Influence of site of impact on cognitive impairment persisting long after severe closed head injury. *Journal of Neurology, Neurosurgery and Psychiatry*, 1974, *37*, 719–726.

Sroka, H., Solsi, P., and Bornstein, B. Alexia without agraphia: With complete recovery. *Confinia Neurologica*, 1973, *35*, 167–176.

Stein, D. G. Some variables influencing recovery of function after central nervous system lesions in the rat. In D. G. Stein, J. J. Rosen, and N. Butters, (eds.), *Plasticity and Recovery of Function in the Central Nervous System*. New York: Academic Press, 1974.

Stevenson, J. Cited by T. Shallice in Dyslexia or Frontal Lobe Functions. Paper presented to the Experimental Psychology Society, Oxford, July 7–9, 1977.

Strich, S. J. The pathology of brain damage due to blunt head injuries. In A. E. Walker, W. F. Caveness, and M. Critchley (eds.), *The Late Effects of Head Injury*. Springfield, Ill.: Thomas, 1969.

Subirana, A. The prognosis in aphasia in relation to cerebral dominance and handedness. *Brain*, 1958, *81*, 415–425.

Subirana, A. Handedness and cerebral dominance. In P. J. Vinken and G. W. Bruyn (eds.), *Handbook of Clinical Neurology*, Vol. 4. Amsterdam: North-Holland, 1969.

Sweet, W. H., Ervin, F., and Mark, V. H. The relationship of violent behaviour to focal cerebral disease. In S. Garattini and E. B. Sigg (eds.), *Aggressive Behaviour*. Proceedings of the International Symposium on the Biology of Aggressive Behaviour. Amsterdam: Excerpta Medica, 1969.

Symonds, C. Disorders of memory. *Brain*, 1966, *89*, 625–644.

Talland, G. A. *Deranged Memory: A Psychonomic Study of the Amnesic Syndrome*. New York: Academic Press, 1965.

Taulbee, L. R., and Folsom, J. C. Reality orientation for geriatric patients. *Hospital and Community Psychiatry*, 1966, *17*, 133–135.

Teasdale, G., and Jennett, B. Assessment of coma and impaired consciousness. A practical scale. *Lancet*, 1974, *2*, 81–84.

Teuber, H.-L. Neglected aspects of the posttraumatic syndrome. In A. E. Walker, W. F. Caveness, and M. Critchley (eds.), *The Late Effects of Head Injury*. Springfield, Ill.: Thomas, 1969.

Teuber, H.-L. Unity and diversity of frontal lobe functions. *Acta Neurobiologiae Experimentalis*, 1972, *32*, 615–656.

Teuber, H.-L. Effects of focal brain injury on human behavior. In D. B. Tower (ed.), *The Nervous System*, Vol. 2:. *The Clinical Neurosciences*. New York: Raven Press, 1975.

Teuber, H.-L., and Weinstein, S. Ability to discover hidden figures after cerebral lesions. *Archives of Neurology and Psychiatry*, 1956, *76*, 369–379.

Thomsen, I. V. The patient with severe head injury and his family. *Scandinavian Journal of Rehabilitation Medicine*, 1974, *6*, 180–183.

Thomsen, I. V., and Harmsen, I. V. Retraining in a case of agnosic alexia. *Folia Phoniatrica*, 1968, *20*, 342–347.

Umiltà, C., Rizzolatti, G., Marzi, C. A., Zamboni, G., Franzini, C., Camarda, R., and Berlucchi, G. Hemispheric differences in the discrimination of line orientation. *Neuropsychologia*, 1974, *12*, 165–174.

van Zomeren, A. H. Long term recovery of reaction time after closed head injury. Paper presented to the International Neuropsychological Society, Oxford, August 1–4, 1977.

van Zomeren, A. H., and Deelman, B. G. Differential effects of simple and choice reaction after closed head injury. *Clinical Neurology and Neurosurgery*, 1976, *79*, 81–90.

Vignolo, L. A. Evolution of aphasia and language rehabilitation: A retrospective exploratory study. *Cortex*, 1964, *1*, 344–367.

Vignolo, L. A. Personal communication, 1977.

Vilkki, J., and Laitinen, L. V. Effects of pulvinotomy and ventrolateral thalamotomy on some cognitive functions. *Neuropsychologia*, 1976, *14,* 67–78.

Walker, A. E., and Jablon, S. *A Follow-up Study of Head Wounds in World War II*. V. A. Medical Monograph. Washington, D.C.: U.S. Government Printing Office, 1961.

Walker, A. E., Caveness, W. F., and Critchley, M. (eds.). *The Late Effects of Head Injury*. Springfield, Ill.: Thomas, 1969.

Warrington, E. K. Constructional apraxia. In P. J. Vinken and G. W. Bruyn (eds.), *Handbook of Clinical Neurology*, Vol 4. Amsterdam: North-Holland, 1969.

Warrington, E. K., and James, M. Disorders of visual perception in patients with unilateral cerebral lesions. *Neuropsychologia*, 1967*a*, *5*, 253–266.

Warrington, E. K., and James, M. Tachistoscopic number estimation in patients with unilateral cerebral lesions. *Journal of Neurology, Neurosurgery and Psychiatry*, 1967*b*, *30*, 468–474.

Warrington, E. K., and Rabin, P. Perceptual matching in patients with cerebral lesions. *Neuropsychologia*, 1970, *8*, 475–487.

Warrington, E. K., and Taylor, A. M. The contribution of the right parietal lobe to object recognition. *Cortex*, 1973, *9*, 152–164.

Warrington, E. K., and Weiskrantz, L. Amnesic syndrome: Consolidation or retrieval? *Nature (London)*. 1970, *228*, 628–630.

Warrington, E. K., and Weiskrantz, L. Organisational aspects of memory in amnesic patients. *Neuropsychologia*, 1971, *9*, 67–73.

Warrington, E. K., James, M., and Kinsbourne, M. Drawing disability in relation to laterality of cerebral lesion. *Brain,* 1966, *89,* 53–82.

Weinstein, S. Differences in effects of brain wounds implicating right or left hemispheres: Differential effects on certain intellectual and complex perceptual functions. In V. B. Mountcastle (ed.), *Interhemispheric Relations and Cerebral Dominance.* Baltimore: Johns Hopkins Press, 1962.

Weisenburg, T. H., and McBride, K. E. *Aphasia: A Clinical and Psychological Study.* New York: Commonwealth Fund, 1935.

Weiskrantz, L., Warrington, E. K., Sanders, M. D., and Marshall, J. Visual capacity in the hemianopic field following a restricted occipital ablation. *Brain,* 1974, *97,* 709–728.

Wepman, J. M. *Recovery from Aphasia.* New York: Ronald, 1951.

Wepman, J. M. A conceptual model for the processes involved in recovery from aphasia. *Journal of Speech and Hearing Disorders,* 1953, *18,* 4–13.

Wepman, J. M. Aphasia therapy: A new look. *Journal of Speech and Hearing Disorders,* 1972, *37,* 203–214.

Westropp, C. Long term care in cases of severe head injury. *Rehabilitation,* 1970, No. 72, 51–53.

White, S. R. Mnemonic strategies in normal and head-injured children. D.Phil thesis, Oxford University, 1976.

Woods, B. T., and Teuber, H.-L. Early onset of complementary specialization of cerebral hemispheres in man. *Transactions of the American Neurological Association,* 1973, *98,* 113–117.

Wright, M. J., and Ikeda, H. Processing of spatial and temporal information in the visual system. In F. O. Schmitt and F. G. Worden (eds.), *The Neurosciences: Third Study Program.* Cambridge, Mass.: MIT Press, 1974.

Wyke, M. The effects of brain lesions on the performance of bilateral arm movements. *Neuropsychologia,* 1971, *9,* 33–42.

Yakovev, P., and Lecours, A.-R. The myelogenetic cycles of regional maturation of the brain. In A. Minkowski (ed.), *Regional Development of the Brain in Early Life.* Oxford: Blackwell, 1967.

Young, J. Z. Why do we have two brains? In V. B. Mountcastle (ed.), *Interhemispheric Relations and Cerebral Dominance.* Baltimore: Johns Hopkins Press, 1962.

Zangwill, O. L. Thought and the brain. *British Journal of Psychology,* 1976, *67,* 301–314.

Zarit, S. H., and Kahn, R. L. Impairment and adaptation in chronic disabilities: Spatial inattention. *Journal of Nervous and Mental Disease,* 1974, *159,* 63–72.

Zurif, E. B., and Bryden, M. P. Familial handedness and left-right differences in auditory and visual perception. *Neuropsychologia,* 1969, *7,* 179–187.

PART VII

Toward Understanding the Mechanisms of Consciousness

Beyond Commissurotomy: Clues to Consciousness

Joseph E. LeDoux, Donald H. Wilson, and Michael S. Gazzaniga

Introduction

When the inevitable topic of nature of consciousness is approached in the light of modern brain research, the experienced student has come to brace himself for the mellifluous intonations of someone's personal experience and ideas on the matter, as opposed to data. Yet we all listen dutifully, because ultimately the business of the serious neuroscientist is to figure out the mechanisms of brain and mind.

One of the most thoughtful and experienced neuroscientists in the world on this issue is Roger W. Sperry. His offerings on the subject reflect what can be called the "it" analysis. Consciousness or "it" is this or that, present or not present, and the like. In his words, it is an "emergent property or cerebral activity . . . and is an integral component of the brain process that functions as an essential constituent action and exerts a directive holistic form of control over the flow pattern of cerebral excitation" (Sperry, 1969). Thus Sperry, after years of thought, feels it necessary to instruct a beleaguered yet lackadaisical field of professional brain and behavior scientists that mental properties of the brain are real, and they are on top, and they can exert control over the individual elements that upon interaction give rise to mental phenomena. It is testimony to thinking at the time that this needed saying, and Sperry's papers as usual are extremely important in focusing future work on important questions. Yet in no way should such overviews be

Joseph E. LeDoux   Department of Neurology, Cornell University Medical College, New York, New York 10021   Donald H. Wilson   Department of Neurosurgery, Dartmouth Medical School, Hanover, New Hampshire 03755   Michael S. Gazzaniga   Department of Neurology, Cornell University Medical College, New York, New York 10021.

constructed as insights into the mechanism of consciousness per se. These types of analyses deal with consciousness as a single impenetrable entity.

The operational properties and mechanism of conscious experience thus remain largely unidentified. Yet it is in this area that we personally find our own research program directed, and it is our experiemental studies on the "how" of consciousness that occupy this chapter.

In the following, we will describe our observations on one truly unique individual, case P. S. P. S.'s uniqueness among split-brain patients centers around the psychological robustness of his right hemisphere. Although only his left hemisphere can talk, other linguistic skills are extensively represented in both half-brains (Gazzaniga and LeDoux, 1978; Gazzaniga et al., 1977), and most of what follows deals with observations made possible by this special neurological circumstance.

SPLIT CONSCIOUSNESS

Much of the intrigue surrounding the split-brain studies of the early 1960s (Gazzaniga et al., 1962, 1963, 1965) was related to the possibility that the mechanisms of human conscious experience were doubly represented following brain bisection. While the conscious properties of the left hemisphere were apparent through the patient's verbal behavior, the view that the right hemisphere was also worthy of conscious status was widely criticized. Sir John Eccles, for example, asserted that the psychological capacities of the right hemisphere were best described as "automatisms" (Eccles, 1965). Others, such as Donald MacKay (1972), argued that unless it could be shown that each separated half-brain has its own independent system for subjectively assigning values to events and settings and response priorities, the split brain could not be viewed as a split mind.

In a series of tests aimed at specifying the nature and extent of linquistic representation in P. S.'s right hemisphere, we lateralized pictures of objects to his mute half-brain and asked him to spell the name of the object by selecting letters from a group and arranging them in proper sequence (Gazzaniga and LeDoux, 1978; Gazzaniga et al., 1977). His capacity to respond in this situation raised the question of whether he might also be able to spell his answer to subjective and personal questions directed to his mute right hemisphere. This seemed to be the opportunity to assess whether the right hemisphere, along with the left, could possess conscious properties following brain bisection.

We generated a series of questions that could be visually presented exclusively to the right hemisphere (LeDoux et al., 1977). This was accomplished by verbally stating the question, except that key words in the question were replaced by the word "blank," and then the missing information was exposed in the left visual field, which effectively lateralized visual input to the right half-brain. Subsequently, P. S. was asked to spell his answer by selecting and arranging letters from two complete alphabets (made up of "Scrabble" letters).

The first question asked was "Who 'blank'?" The key words lateralized to the right hemisphere on this trial were "are you?" Our expectations were met! As his eyes scanned the 52 letters available, his left hand reached out and selected the "P," set it down, and then proceeded to collect the remaining letters needed to spell "Paul" (Fig. 1). Overflowing with excitement, having just communicated on a personal level with a right hemisphere, we collected ourselves, and then initiated the next trial by saying, "Would you spell the name of your favorite 'blank'?" Then "girl" appeared in the left visual field. Out came the left hand again, and this time it spelled "Liz," the name of his girlfriend at the time. On the next two trials, the question was the same, but the key words were "person" and then "hobby." "Car" was the reply to hobby, and "Henry Wi Fozi" was the response to his favorite person (Henry Winkler is the real-life name of the television character, Fonzie, that P. S., a 15-year-old boy, idolizes). Another question was "What is tomorrow?" He correctly spelled "Sunday." He spelled "automobile race" as the job he would pick. This is interesting, because the left hemisphere frequently asserts that "he"

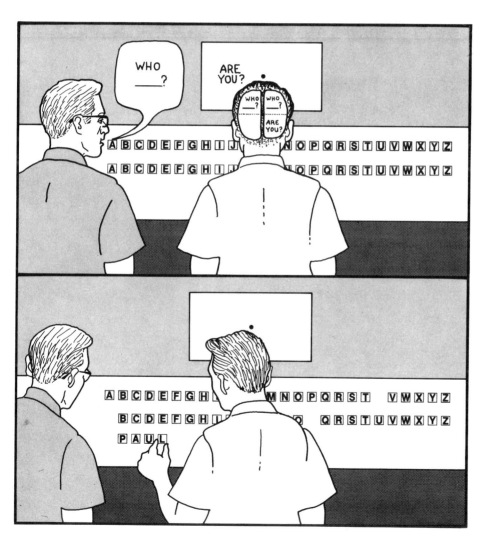

Fig. 1. Volitional expression by the mute hemisphere (see text).

JOSEPH E. LEDOUX,
DONALD H. WILSON,
AND MICHAEL S.
GAZZANIGA

wants to be a draftsman. In fact, shortly after the test session we asked P. S. what sort of job he would like to have, and he said, "Oh, be a draftsman." Finally, we asked the right hemisphere to spell its "mood." It spelled "good."

These observations suggested to us that the right hemisphere in P. S. possesses qualities that are deserving of conscious status. His right hemisphere has a sense of self, for it knows the name it collectively shares with the left. It has feelings, for it can be describe its mood. It has a sense of whom it likes, and what it likes, for it can name its favorite people and its favorite hobby. The right hemisphere in P. S. also has a sense of the future, for it knows what day tomorrow is. Furthermore, it has goals and aspirations for the future, for it can name its occupational choice.

It is important to emphasize that these responses were self-generated by P. S.'s right hemisphere from a set of infinite possibilities. The only aid provided was the two alphabets from which he could select letters at will. The fact that this mute half-brain could generate personal answers to ambiguous and subjective questions demonstrated that in P. S. the right hemisphere has its own independent response priority determining mechanisms, which is to say its own volitional control system.

Thus it would appear that the right hemisphere, along with but independent of the left, *can* possess conscious properties following brain bisection. In other words, the mechanisms of human consciousness *can* be split and doubled by split-brain surgery.

Since P. S. is the first split-brain patient to clearly possess double consciousness, it seems that if we could identify the factor that distinguishes his right hemisphere from the right hemisphere of the other split-brain patients, we would have a major clue to the underlying nature of conscious processes. That factor is undoubtedly the extensive linguistic representation in P. S.'s right hemisphere. As we have seen, his right hemisphere can spell, and, in addition, it can comprehend verbal commands as well as process other parts of speech and make conceptual judgments involving verbal information (Gazzaniga and LeDoux, 1978; Gazzaniga *et al.*, 1977). While it is possible that the conscious properties observed in his right hemisphere are spuriously associated with these linguistic skills, the fact remains that in all other patients where linguistic sophistication is lacking in the right hemisphere so too is the evidence for consciousness.

Observations such as these immediately raise the question of whether nonhuman organisms are conscious. However, the clear distinction between the conscious status of the left and right hemispheres of most split-brain patients (P. S. excluded) adds an important qualification to this question. Unless it could be shown that nonhumans possess conscious powers that surpass those of the right hemisphere of most split-brain patients, then the criticisms levied against the conscious status of these right hemispheres also apply to nonhumans. Still it is not our intent to deny the possibility of some form of conscious awareness in nonhumans. Instead, our point is that while nonhumans may be found to be aware and even self-aware, they are nevertheless not aware in the unique ways and to the extent made possible by the human verbal system. Consequently, our aim in the following is to identify and examine some of the mechanisms through which the verbal system contributes to the creation of consciousness, as we as humans experience it.

The person is usually engaged in much more activity than can possibly enter consciousness at once, and, in our opinion, much of what does enter is what is registered by the verbal system. It is the one system that is capable of continuously monitoring our overt behavioral activities, as well as our perceptions, thoughts, and moods. In taking note of, integrating, and interpreting these events, we believe that the verbal system provides for a personal sense of conscious reality.

In the following, we will examine how further observation on P. S. shed light on these mechanisms. Again, it is only through the novel experimental situation involved in testing such a patient that these mechanisms, which we feel are basic to man, are exposed.

As a result of having bilateral representation of language comprehension, P. S. is able to act in response to verbal commands exclusively presented to either hemisphere but can only describe verbally the left hemisphere stimuli (Gazzaniga and LeDoux, 1978; Gazzaninga *et al.*, 1977). The observations of relevance here involve the manner in which his left hemisphere dealt with our queries as to why he was responding in a certain way to commands known directly by the right half-brain alone. In brief, when P. S. was asked "Why are you doing that?" his talking left hemisphere was faced with the cognitive problem of explaining a discrete overt movement of great clarity carried out for reasons truly unknown to it.

In trial after trial, the left hemipshere proved extremely adept at immediately attributing cause to the action. When "laugh," for example, was presented to the right hemisphere, P. S. commenced laughing, and when asked why, said, "Oh, you guys are really something" (Fig. 2). When the command "rub" was flashed, the subject, with the left hand, rubbed the back of his head. When asked what the command was, he said "itch." Here again, the response was observed by the left hemisphere, and the subject immediately characterized it. Yet that he said "itch" instead of "rub" shows that he was guessing. In the same way, he could be quite accurate when the command had less leeway for multiple description, as in the case of the word "boxer." The test instruction was to "assume the position of . . ." P. S. correctly assumed the pugilistic position, and when asked what the word was, he said "boxer." But on subsequent trials, when he was restrained, and the word "boxer" was flashed, the left hemisphere said it saw nothing. Moments later, when released, however, he assumed the position, and said, "OK, it was 'boxer.'"

Similar responses were observed in other tests. Pictures of objects were lateralized to his right hemisphere and P. S. was required to spell out the name of the object by selecting and arranging "Scrabble" letters, as described earlier. If while spelling the word he was asked to name the object he had seen, the left hemisphere's verbal response was consistent with the information available externally, but inconsistent with the true state of affairs known only by the right hemisphere. For example, after the picture of a playing card was flashed to his right hemisphere, and he began to select letters, we asked P. S. what the object was. Looking down at the letters "c," "a," and "r," he said "car." However, as this response was being emitted by the left hemisphere, the left hand and the right hemisphere completed the word by adding the final letter "d." The left hemisphere then said, "Oh, it was a card," and P. S. smiled.

JOSEPH E. LEDOUX,
DONALD H. WILSON,
AND MICHAEL S.
GAZZANIGA

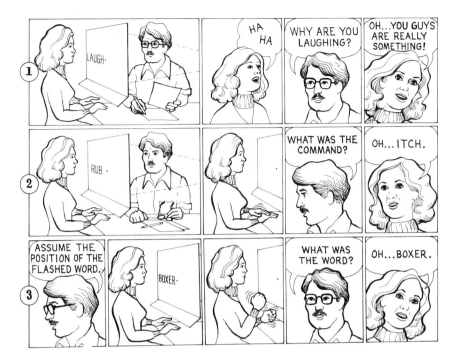

Fig. 2. When a series of commands were presented to the right hemisphere, each evoked a response. Although the left hemisphere did not know what the command was, it attempted to account for the response. When the command was *laugh* or *rub,* the left hemisphere instantly "filled in." When the response was less equivocal, the reason generated for the action was quite accurate, as with the word *boxer.*

In another series of observations, we simultaneously presented each hemisphere with a different object-picutre, and the P. S. was required to select the picture choice cards that best related to the flashed stimuli (Gazzaniga and LeDoux, 1978). Thus if "cherry" was one of the stimuli flashed, the correct answer might have been "apple" as opposed to "toaster," "chicken," or "glass," with the superordinate concept being, of course, "fruit." Using this procedure (which was developed by Marjorie Pinsley for testing aphasic patients) it was possible to escalate the subtlety of the cognitive requirement without changing the test design or response demands on the subject.

It was clear that each hemisphere under the simultaneous presentation could perform. Only rarely did the response of one side block a response from the other. In general, each hemisphere pointed to the correct answer on each trial.

What is of particular interest, however, is the way the subject verbally interpreted these double-field responses. When a snow scene was presented to the right hemisphere and a chicken claw was presented to the left, P. S. quickly and dutifully responded correctly by choosing a picture of a chicken from a series of four cars with his right hand and a picture of a shovel from a series of four card with his left hand. The subject was then asked "What did you see?" "I saw a claw and I picked chicken, and you have to clean out the chicken shed with a shovel" (Fig. 3).

In trial after trial, we saw this kind of response. The left hemisphere could easily and accurately identify why it had picked its answer, and then subsequently, and without batting an eye, it would incorporate the right hemisphere's response into the framework. While we knew exactly why the right hemisphere had made its choice, the left hemisphere could merely guess. Yet, the left did not offer its suggestion in a guessing vein, but rather as a statement of fact as to why that card had been picked.

These varied observations on P. S. offer us the opportunity to consider whether we were not observing a basic mental mechanism common to us all. We feel that the conscious verbal self is not always privy to the origin of our actions, and when it observes the person behaving for unknown reasons, it attributes cause to the action as it if knows, but in fact it does not. It is as if the verbal self looks out and sees what the person is doing, and from that knowledge it interprets a reality. This notion is reminiscent of the well-known theory of cognitive dissonance, which suggests how one's sense of reality, one's system of beliefs about the world, arises as a consequence of considering what one does (Festinger, 1957).

Implicit in the idea that self-consciousness involves, at least in part, verbal consideration of sensory-motor activities is the assumption that the person or self

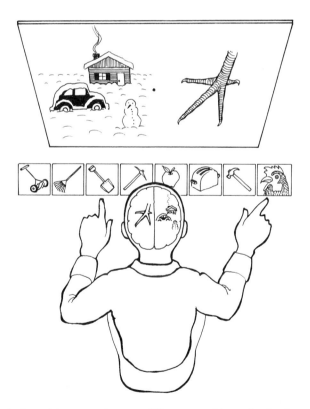

Fig. 3. The method used in presenting two different cognitive tasks simultaneously, one to each hemisphere. The left hemisphere was required to process the answer to the chicken claw, while the right dealt with the implications of being presented with a snow scene. After each hemisphere responded, the left hemisphere was asked to explain its choices. See text for implications.

is not a unified psychological entity, such that the conscious self comes to know the other selves through overt behavior. In other words, what we are suggesting is that there are multiple mental systems in the brain, each with the capacity to produce behavior, and each with its own impulses for action, that are not necessarily conversant internally. This point is well illustrated by the results of an experiment conducted by Dr. Gail Risse on patients who, for medical reasons, had one hemisphere anesthetized (Risse and Gazzaniga, 1978). When this left hemisphere was put to sleep, these patients completely lost the capacity to produce and understand speech. During this time, an object was placed in the patient's left hand, which projects mainly to the awake and linguistically void right hemisphere. When the left hemisphere had recovered, the patients were totally unable to name the object that had been in the left hand, but could nevertheless pick it out from a group of several objects by pointing to it. These data suggest that information encoded in the absence of the verbal system is uninterpretable by the verbal system when it returns to normal functioning. In other words, the verbal system encodes information in its special way, and the other systems do the same. Moreover, it would seem that when information is encoded by other than the verbal system, the person is not consciously aware of the information, as the patients showed no indication that they knew how they responded correctly, or, for that matter, that they had responded correctly.

These data allow for a rather radical hypothesis. Could it be that in the developing organism a constellation of mental systems exists, each with its own values and response probabilities? Then, as maturation continues, the behaviors that these separate systems emit are monitored by the one system we come to use more and more, namely, the verbal, natural language system. Gradually, a concept of self-control develops such that the verbal self comes to know some (though surely not all) of the impulses for action that arises from the other selves, and it tries either to inhibit these impulses or free them, as the case may be. Indeed, it could be argued that the process of psychological maturation in our culture is largely the process through which the verbal system learns to regulate, in accord with social standards, the behavioral impulses of the many selves that dwell inside of us.

The model being proposed here, then, is clear. We believe that the split-brain observations, combined with the sodium amytal data, paint a unique view of the mental properties of the brain. The mind is not a psychological entity, but a sociological entity, being composed of many submental systems. What can be done surgically and through hemisphere anesthetization may only be exaggerated instances of a more general phenomenon. The uniqueness of man, in this regard, is his ability to verbalize and in so doing create a personal sense of reality and conscious unity out of the multiple mental systems present.

EMOTION AND CONSCIOUSNESS

The last set of observations to be described here provides new insights into the nature of cognitive-emotional interactions and at the same time points out how the verbal system is capable of monitoring internal psychological states, in addition to overt behavioral activities.

On the verbal commands test described earlier, where a word was lateralized to the right hemisphere and P. S. was instructed to perform the action described by the word, his reaction to the word "kiss" proved revealing (Gazzaniga and LeDoux, 1978; Gazzaniga *et al.*, 1977). Although the left hemisphere of this adolescent boy did not see the word, immediately after "kiss" was exposed to the mute right hemisphere, the left blurted out, "Hey, no way, no way. You've got to be kidding." When asked what it was that he was not going to do, he was unable to tell us. Later, we presented "kiss" to the left hemisphere and a similar response occurred: "No way. I'm not going to kiss you guys." This time, however, the speaking half-brain knew what the word was. In both instances, the command "kiss" elicited an emotional reaction that was detected by the verbal system of the left hemisphere, and the overt verbal response of the left hemisphere was basically the same, regardless of whether the command was presented to the right or left half-brain. In other words, the verbal system of the left hemisphere seemed to be able to accurately read the emotional tone of the word seen by the right hemisphere alone.

This observation, which suggests that emotion is encoded in a directionally specific manner, is inconsistent with the currently accepted cognitive theory of emotion (Schachter, 1975). According to the cognitive theory, emotional arousal is nonspecific. The affective tone of emotion is viewed as being determined by the cognitive apprehension of the external situation in which the arousal occurs. However, in P. S., the left hemisphere appeared to have experienced emotion in the absence of cognition. The following experiment was thus aimed at evaluating the reality of this phenomenon (LeDoux and Gazzaniga, 1978).

We selected a number of words that repeatedly appear in P. S.'s verbal behavior. It was assumed that personal words would be more likely to elicit measurable emotional responses than neutral words. Following the lateralized visual exposure of a word, P. S. was encouraged to verbally rate the word on a preference scale. The scale values included "like very much," "like," "undecided," "dislike," and "dislike very much." When the word was presented to the left hemisphere, the verbal judgment was made by the hemisphere that saw the word. However, when the word was lateralized to the right hemisphere, the left hemisphere had to verbally respond to a word it did not see.

We obtained 21 left hemisphere ratings of words lateralized to the right hemisphere. Twelve right hemisphere words were rated, some as many as three times, others only once.

Figure 4 compares the left hemisphere rating of each word on the first left hemisphere trial with the first successful right hemisphere trial (an unsuccessful right hemisphere trial was one on which the word could be named; such ratings were counted as left hemisphere trials). In only one instance ("Nixon") did the left hemisphere rating of right hemisphere words differ by more than one scale value from the left hemisphere rating of the same words after left hemisphere exposure.

It thus appears that the emotional value of a stimulus is encoded in a

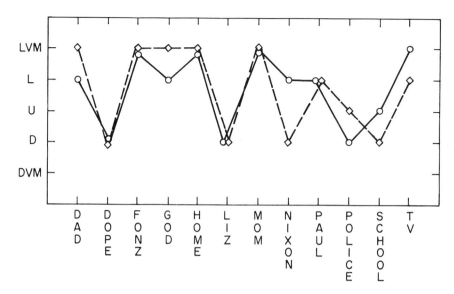

Fig. 4. Left hemisphere verbal rating of stimuli exposed to the left and right hemispheres. Data points represented by open squares connected by dotted lines indicate right hemisphere exposure, and open circles connected by solid lines indicate left hemisphere exposure. In only one instance ("Nixon") did the ratings differ by more than one scale value.

directionally specific manner. Although the perceptual nature of a stimulus exposed to the right hemisphere was unavailable to the conscious process of the left hemisphere, the emotional tone of the stimulus was nevertheless represented in the conscious awareness of the left hemisphere. Consequently, while cognitions surely initiate emotional reactions, and while visceral arousal is nonspecific, on the neural level, emotion appears to be specifically encoded. Although our data speak only to directional (positive-negative) encoding, it seems likely that qualitative emotional distinctions (as between joy and love) might be similarly encoded.

What possible mechanisms could be invovled in the type of emotional encoding suggested here? As noted, P. S. is a callosum-sectioned patient, which means that his anterior commissure was surgically spared (Wilson, et al., 1977). Anatomical studies have shown that the human anterior commissure derives its fibers from the temporal lobe and from subcortical "limbic" structures, in particular the amygdala, and projects to the same regions in the other hemisphere (Klinger and Gloor, 1960). Evidence that the interhemispheric limbic connections are intact and functioning in P. S. is provided by our observation that like other anterior commissure-intact patients (Risse *et al.*, 1977) and unlike split-brain patients with anterior commissure sections (Gordon and Sperry, 1969) P. S. shows interhemispheric transfer of olfactory information. Given the role of the amygdala in emotion in addition to olfaction (Papez, 1937; MacLean, 1949; Kluver and Bucy, 1937; Mark and Ervin, 1970), the interlimbic connections of the anterior commissure could well be responsible for the interhemispheric emotional judgments observed in P. S.

Recent elucidation of the pharmacological properties of opiate receptor sites in the brain suggests a concentration of these sites in the amygdala (Kuhar *et al.*,

1973). Also concentrated in the amygdala are nerve terminals utilizing morphine-like peptides (enkephalins) as the neurotransmitter (Snyder, 1977). These peptides bind to the opiate receptor sites, and this action has been linked with emotional mechanisms. Thus it is possible that the neural mechanisms of emotional encoding seen in P. S. involve the opiate receptor sites in the amygdala and the interamygdala connections of the anterior commissure.

At the psychological level, the observation that the verbal system can accurately read the emotional tone precipitated by an external stimulus without knowing the nature of the stimulus allows speculation concerning the nature and variability of our mood states. The idea that we are intrigued with is that the person is not always aware of the origin of his moods, just as he is not always aware of the origin of his actions. In other words, the conscious self appears to be capable of noticing that the person is in a particular mood without knowing why. It is as if we become subtly conditioned to particular visual, somatosensory, auditory, olfactory, and gustatory stimuli, and while such conditioning can be, it is not necessarily within the realm of awareness of the conscious self. When in Florence, for example, one can be focused on David and feel so aroused, awed, and inspired that unbeknownst to the verbal system the brain is also recording the scents, noises, and the total gestalt of that remarkable city. The emotional tone conditioned to these subtle aspects of the experience might later be triggered in other settings because of the presence of similar or related stimuli. The person, puzzled by his affective state, might ask himself, "Why do I feel so good today?" At this point, if the Florentine experience is not recalled (registered by the verbal system), the process of verbal attribution may take over and concoct a substitute, although perhaps very plausible, explanation. In short, the environment has ways of planting hooks in our minds, and while the verbal system may not know the why or what of it all, part of its job is to make sense out of the emotional and other mental systems and in so doing allow man, with his mental complexity, the illusion of a unified self.

We thus feel that the verbal system's role in creating our sense of conscious reality is crucial and enormous. It is the system that is continually observing our actual behavior, as well as our cognitions and internal moods. In attributing cause to behavioral and psychological states, an attitudinal view of the world, involving beliefs and values, is constructed, and this becomes a dominant theme in our own self-image.

REFERENCES

Eccles, J. *The Brain and The Unity of Conscious Experience.* The 19th Arthur Stanley Eddington Lecture. Cambridge: Cambridge University Press, 1965.

Festinger, L. *A Theory of Cognitive Dissonance.* Evanstown, Ill.: Row, Peterson, 1957.

Gazzaniga, M. S. and LeDoux, J. E. *The Integrated Mind.* New York: Plenum, 1978.

Gazzaniga, M. S., Bogen, J. E., and Sperry, R. W. Some functional effects of sectioning the cerebral commissures in man. *Proceedings of the National Academy of Sciences,* 1962, *48*, 1765.

Gazzaniga, M. S., Bogen, J. E., and Sperry, R. W. Laterality effects in somesthesis following cerebral commissurotomy in man. *Neuropsychologia,* 1963, *1*, 209–221.

Gazzaniga, M. S., Bogen, J. E., and Sperry, R. W. Observations in visual perception after disconnection of the cerebral hemispheres in man. *Brain,* 1965, *88*, 221–236.

Gazzaniga, M. S., LeDoux, J. E., and Wilson, D. H. Language, praxis, and the right hemisphere: Clues to some mechanisms of consciousness. *Neurology,* 1977, *24*, 1144–1147.

Gordon, H., and Sperry, R. W. Lateralization of olfactory perception in surgically separated hemispheres of man. *Neuropsychologia, 7,* 111–120.

Klinger, J., and Gloor, P. The connections of the amygdala and of the anterior temporal cortex in the human brain. *Journal of Comparative Neurology,* 1960, *115*, 333–369.

Kluver, H., and Bucy, P. C. Psychic blindness and other symptoms following bilateral temporal lobectomy in monkeys. *American Journal of Physiology,* 1937, *119*, 352–353.

Kuhar, M. J., Pert, C. B., and Snyder, S. H. Regional distribution of opiate receptor binding in monkey and human brain. *Nature,* 1973, *245, 447–450.*

LeDoux, J. E., and Gazzaniga, M. S. On the nature and mechanisms of human conscious experience. *Scientific American,* 1978, in press.

LeDoux, J. E., Wilson, D. H., and Gazzaniga, M. S. A divided mind: Observations on the conscious properties of the separated hemispheres. *Annals of Neurology,* 1977, *2*, 417–421.

MacKay, D. Personal communication cited in M. S. Gazzaniga. One brain—two minds? *American Scientist,* 1972, *60*, 311–317.

MacLean, P. O. Psychosomatic disease and the visceral brain. *Psychosomatic Medicine,* 1949, *11*, 338–353.

Mark, V. H., and Ervin, F. R. *Violence and the Brain.* New York: Harper and Row, 1970.

Papez, J. W. A proposed mechanism of emotion. *Archives of Neurology and Psychiatry,* 1937, *3*, 230–251.

Risse, G. L., and Gazzaniga, M. S. Well-kept secrets of the right hemisphere: A sodium amytal study. *Neurology,* 1978, in press.

Risse, G. L., LeDoux, J. E., Springer, S. P., Wilson, D. H., and Gazzaniga, M. S. The anterior commissure in man: Functional variation in a multisensory system. *Neuropsychologia,* 1977, *16,·* 23–31.

Schachter, S. Cognition and contralist—Peripheralist controversies in motivation and emotion. In M. S. Gazzaniga and C. W. Blakemore (eds.), *Handbook of Psychobiology.* New York: Plenum, 1975.

Snyder, S. H. Opiate receptors and internal opiates. *Scientific American,* 1977, *236,* 44–56.

Sperry, R. W. A modified concept of consciousness. *Psychological Reviews,* 1969, *76*, 532–536.

Wilson, D. H., Reeves, A., Culver, C., and Gazzaniga, M. S. Cerebral commissurotomy for control of intractable seizures. *Neurology,* 1977, *27*, 708–715.

Index